OXFORD MEDICAL PUBLICATIONS

Women's Health

OXFORD GENERAL PRACTICE SERIES

Editorial Board

Godfrey Fowler, John Hasler, Jacky Hayden, Iona Heath, and Clare Wilkinson

Women's Health
Fourth Edition

Oxford General Practice Series • 39

Edited by

Ann McPherson

General Practitioner, Oxford

and

Deborah Waller

General Practitioner, Oxford

Oxford : New York : Tokyo

OXFORD UNIVERSITY PRESS

Oxford University Press, Great Clarendon Street, Oxford OX2 6DP

Oxford New York
Athens Auckland Bangkok Bogata Bombay Buenos Aires Calcutta
Cape Town Chennai Dar es Salaam Delhi Florence Hong Kong Istanbul
Karachi Kuala Lumpur Madrid Melbourne Mexico City Mumbai
Nairobi Paris São Paolo Singapore Taipei Tokyo Toronto Warsaw

Oxford is a trade mark of Oxford University Press

Published in the United States
by Oxford University Press Inc., New York

A catalogue record for this book is available from the British Library

Library of Congress Cataloging in Publication Data
(Data available)

ISBN 0 19 262 750 3

Printed in Great Britain by
Biddles Ltd,
Guildford & King's Lynn

PREFACE TO
FOURTH EDITION

Exit the title 'Women's Problems' and enter 'Women's Health' along with a second editor. Why? Because the breadth of the book (and it is just a little bit more paunchy as well!) has greatly increased. All the old chestnuts are still there – but fully revised and containing all the most recent 'evidence-based' material from clinical trials. Menstrual problems, pre-menstrual syndrome, menopause, contraception, cystitis, incontinence, eating disorders (with a practical step-by-step guide for treatment in primary care), unwanted pregnancy, sexual and emotional problems, cervical screening, and breast cancer have all had the treatment.

In addition there are new and original chapters on hospital referrals – 'Referral to specialist clinics', on how and why they vary; 'Variations in hospital treatment rates for common conditions' with an emphasis on female conditions; 'The role of primary health care in promoting the health of women' written by a practice nurse; 'Chronic pelvic pain and its management' to replace the previous chapter which only dealt with endometriosis; 'Infertility' with details of how to investigate couples in general practice and a section on miscarriage; and finally a chapter on 'Complementary medicine and women's health' which reviews evidence concerning widely-used Complementary therapies.

Authors have been chosen with great care, for their expertise in the field. Many are women, and most have first hand experience of general practice. Following the success of the 'Controversies section' in the Cervical cytology chapter in the 3rd edition, most chapters now also include this.

Deborah Waller is the new editorial addition. Two minds are better than one when trying to undertake a critical appraisal of such an extensive field, and it certainly makes the work more fun.

Oxford   A. M.
March 1997   D. W.

Dose schedules are being continually revised and new side-effects recognized. Oxford University Press makes no representation, express or implied, that the drug dosages in this book are correct. For these reasons the reader is strongly urged to consult the pharmaceutical company's printed instructions before administering any of the drugs recommended in this book.

CONTENTS

Contents

CONTRIBUTORS

Christine A'Court is a GP in Oxfordshire. Trained in Oxford and at St Thomas's Hospital, London, she worked mainly in internal medicine, then clinical research in the Intensive Therapy Unit. Her interests include the evaluation of medical practice, orthodox and complementary, and she represents GPs on the Blackie Scientific and Ethical Research Committee, London, which evaluates proposals and allocates funds for research into homeopathy.

Joan Austoker is Director of the CRC Primary Care Education Group, University of Oxford Department of Public Health and Primary Care and Reader in Public Health and Primary Care. She conducts research on breast and cervical screening, particularly relating to the role of primary care teams and the acceptability of screening programmes. She has published books for primary care on both breast and cervical screening.

Jane Clarke is a Consultant Surgeon at the Oxford Radcliffe Trust in Oxford. She was appointed in 1992 as a General Surgeon with a special interest in breast disease and breast screening. Her main area of clinical research relates to the use of hormone replacement therapy in patients who are at high risk of developing breast malignancy.

Jean Coope has worked in general practice for over 30 years and has specialized in the care of menopausal women and treatment with hormone replacement therapy. She has carried out original research on the clinical effects of oestrogen and blood-clotting and is a member of the World Health Organization's Scientific Research Committee on the Menopause which met in Geneva in June 1994. She is also the Editor of the *Journal of the British Menopause Society*.

Angela Coulter has been Director of the King's Fund Development Centre since 1993. Prior to joining the King's Fund, Angela had 10 years' experience in health services research at the University of Oxford, where she directed the Health Services Research Unit. She has published widely on primary care and women's health and has a particular research interest in treatment options for menorrhagia.

Lis Davidson is a GP and has worked in inner-city Liverpool for the past 10 years. She also works at the Brook Advisory Centre on a regular basis as well as being on the management committee. She is a trainer in general practice and an instructor in family planning. When doing none of the above she enjoys playing on her allotment, learning to dance the salsa, and the company of women.

Fiona Duxbury was a GP in London from 1986 to 1992, and helped to establish 'health advocacy' interpreting services in primary care for the Bangladeshi and Turkish communities in Hackney. On first coming to Oxfordshire in 1992, she worked in a semi-rural practice in Bicester, and became interested in the clinical consequences of child sexual abuse, violence, and rape. She is currently a job-sharing GP principal in Blackbird Leys, Oxford.

Adriane Fugh-Berman is chair of the US National Women's Health Network, a science-based advocacy organization, and author of *Alternative medicine: what works* (Odonian Press, 1996), a review of clinical trials. Formerly coordinator of field investigations for the Office of Alternative Medicine at the US National Institute of Health, she is currently medical officer for the Contraceptive Development Branch of the National Institute of Child Health and Human Development. A GP in Washington, D.C., she practises herbal and nutritional medicine.

Katy Gardner is a GP in inner-city Liverpool. She has been involved in women's health and well woman clinics since the early seventies, with a special interest in premenstrual syndrome. She has counselled women with PMS over many years both in her own practice, at Liverpool Brook Advisory Clinic, and via informal women's health networks. She has experienced severe PMS herself.

Susanna Graham-Jones qualified from St Mary's, London and then trained in psychiatry and general practice in Oxford. She was a lecturer and principal in general practice in Liverpool from 1985 until 1993, when she returned to Oxford as a lecturer in the Department of Public Health and Primary Care. She is a member of Women in Medicine.

John Guillebaud is Medical Director of the Margaret Pyke Family Planning Centre. In 1992 he was appointed by University College, London as Professor of Family Planning and Reproductive Health, the first practising gynaecologist in the world to be given a personal chair in this field. Believing with UNICEF that, globally, 'Family planning could bring more benefits to more people at less cost than any other technology now available to the human race', he is frequently called on in an advisory or consultancy capacity by Government and official national and international bodies. He is author or co-author of six books and more than 250 other publications for the medical profession and the general public, on population and the environment, birth control, and women's health issues. He considers it opportune for this book that during his training he worked as a locum in a variety of general practices in the north and south of England.

Susan Harrison is a Psychosexual Therapist and Counsellor working in general practice. She has been involved in the training and supervision of psychosexual therapists since 1976. She has a special interest in enabling GPs and other members of the primary health care team to deal with psychosexual problems, particularly among older people.

Keith Hawton is a Professor of Psychiatry at Oxford University and Consultant Psychiatrist at the Warneford Hospital in Oxford. In addition to working as a general psychiatrist he has extensive research and clinical experience in the fields of sexual medicine, suicidal behaviour, and general hospital psychiatry. He has taken a particular interest in women's sexual disorders and their treatment, and is also involved in research into the outcome of depression in women. He has extensive research publications and is the author, co-author, or editor of nine books including the two Oxford University Press publications, *Sex therapy: a practical guide* and *Cognitive behaviour therapy for psychiatric problems: a practical guide.*

Sally Hope is a GP in Woodstock with a special interest in women's health. She is a founder member of the 'Primary Care Group in Gynaecology'.

Kim Jobst. Until taking up a post in the University Department of Integrative Medicine at the Royal Homoeopathic Hospital, Glasgow, Dr Jobst was Clinical Director of the Oxford Project To Investigate Memory and Ageing (OPTIMA), Oxford University. Trained in acupuncture as a medical student, his interest in the work of Jung has led him to train as an analytical psychologist. He is Chairman of the Blackie Homoeopathic Foundation Scientific and Ethical Research Committee and is on the Scientific Advisory Board of the Center for Complementary Medicine at Columbia University, New York.

Jacqueline Jolleys. Having retired from a career in academic general practice on health grounds, Dr Jolleys has gained experience in health services management and is now an independent health care consultant. For the past 10 years she has researched and continues to study patients with incontinence and/or benign prostatic hypertrophy. She has published widely in this field through which she has gained international recognition.

Rosemary Kay is a Lecturer/Practitioner at Oxford Brookes University. She works as a Practice Nurse in central Oxford and her main interest is in family planning and women's health. In collaboration with others, she has published a paper on free condom distribution in general practice and is currently engaged in research into provision of primary health care for teenagers. She is a module leader on the family planning course (ENB 901) and women's health screening module.

Stephen Kennedy is a Senior Fellow in Reproductive Medicine/Honorary Consultant in the Nuffield Department of Obstetrics and Gynaecology, Oxford. His research interests include pelvic pain and the genetics and epidemiology of endometriosis.

Gill Lockwood is a Clinical Research Fellow at the Oxford Fertility Unit at the John Radcliffe Hospital, Oxford. Her first degree was in Philosophy, Politics, and Economics at Oxford and following a Masters course in Applied Statistics at Oxford she worked for the Cabinet Office as a Statistician. A career change, inspired by a medical documentary, took her back to Oxford to read medicine. As well as clinical IVF, teaching reproductive endocrinology and working for a research doctorate on the polycystic ovarian syndrome, she lectures and broadcasts regularly on ethical aspects of fertility treatment.

Anneke Lucassen is a Clinical Lecturer in the Nuffield Department of Medicine, Oxford and an Honorary Senior Registrar in Clinical Genetics. She is interested in the genetics of common diseases, including common cancers. Particular areas of interest include the integration of research findings in this area, such as new molecular genetic information, into evidence-based clinical practice.

Ann McPherson works as a GP in Oxford with 5 other partners, including Deborah Waller, the co-editor of this fourth edition. She has, for many years, had a special interest in the health of women and adolescents. Her previous publications on women's health include *Cervical screening: a practical guide, Miscarriage*, and the first three editions of *Women's problems in general practice*. Her books for teenagers, which include *Diary of a teenage health freak, I'm a health freak too*, and *Fresher Pressure*, introduce medical information for teenagers in a new fiction form. She has recently developed a training pack for GP registrars on adolescent health and is presently writing the *Woman's Hour book of women's health*. She lectures and broadcasts on women's health problems.

Klim McPherson has been Professor of Public Health Epidemiology at the London School of Hygiene and Tropical Medicine since 1991. Prior to this, he was University Lecturer in Medical Statistics in the Department of Public Health and Primary Care, University of Oxford. He has special interests in medical uncertainties, the long-term effects of the use of hormones by women both for contraception and hormone replacement therapy, and involving patients in decision-making. He has been the principal investigator in many research studies, including the investigation of the long-term effects of various gynaecological treatments for women, and has over 270 publications in scientific journals. He was Head of the Unit of Health Promotion Sciences in the Department of Public Health and Policy at the LSHTM between 1991–95. He is married to a well-known GP in Oxford.

Pippa Oakeshott qualified from Cambridge in 1975 and is a Lecturer in General Practice at St George's Hospital Medical School, London. She is also a part-time GP in an inner-London practice, and mother of three children. Her main research interest is in improving management of cervical chlamydia infection in general practice.

Julie Parkes has been a GP for 10 years and GP Vocational Training Scheme Course Organizer for 8 years, initially in London and now in Oxford. She is at present doing an MSc in evidence-based health care at Oxford University and is a member of the Centre for Evidence-Based Medicine at the John Radcliffe Hospital.

Margaret Rees is an Honorary Senior Clinical Lecturer in Obstetrics and Gynaecology at the John Radcliffe Hospital in Oxford. She is a medical gynaecologist. She has been undertaking research into the process of menstruation, its psychological implications, and the control of the endometrium since the late 1970s. Currently her research is focusing on endometrial angiogenesis using *in vitro* systems.

Diana Sanders is a Chartered Counselling Psychologist working in Oxfordshire Mental Health NHS Trust. She specializes in cognitive therapy in the Oxford city community mental health team, working in primary care settings. She has researched psychological therapies for somatic problems, and has a long-standing interest in women's health, including research on the premenstrual syndrome.

Deborah Waller is a GP working with Ann McPherson in a group practice in central Oxford. She has particular interests in student and women's health and has spent the last few years developing a practical approach to help young women with eating problems in primary care.

Jacqueline Wootton is managing Editor of the *Journal of Alternative and Complementary Medicine*, published in New York, and directs the Informatics Project at the Rosenthal Center for Complementary and Alternative Medicine, Columbia University. She is on the Advisory Board of GIFTS (Global Initiative For Traditional Systems) of Health, Oxford, UK, and is also on the Advisory Board for the international Cochrane Collaboration Complementary Field.

CHAPTER ONE

Women's health and its controversies – an overview

Ann McPherson and Deborah Waller

Although this book is about women's health, it would be a mistake to regard it as offering a competitive attitude between the sexes as to who dies earlier, who has more illnesses, who consults most, and who has the most mental illness. What we are interested in are those specific illnesses which are unique to women and those diseases of women which make a significant contribution to the burden of general practice. Indeed, it is worth noting that nature appears to view men as the 'weaker' or more vulnerable sex. More males are born than females and this is almost universal in the animal kingdom. Presumably this is to compensate for the increased death rate that occurs amongst men at almost all stages of life.

So why has women's health moved on over the last three decades from simply concentrating on childbirth? The rise of feminism, the increasing number of women doctors, the more international nature of medicine, and the increasing political power of women have all played their part. These four areas have contributed to the establishment of the cervical and breast cancer screening programmes, now well-established in the UK and starting to yield benefits.

Although, as general practitioners (GPs), the bulk of our work is dealing with non-life-threatening illness, included in this chapter are tables and figures which look at women's and men's mortality and serious morbidity in the UK and Europe to help put women's health into a more general perspective:

Fig 1.1 looks at causes of death by age and sex;

Table 1.1 looks at the approximate number of women in England and Wales who die from various causes at different ages;

Figs 1.2a and 1.2b look at the incidence of the 10 commonest cancers for men and women in the UK;

Table 1.2 gives the lifetime risk of developing common cancers for men and women;

Fig 1.3 gives the 5-year relative survival rates for different cancers for men and women. These survival rates are for people with cancer in all stages of its development;

Fig 1.1 *Causes of death by age and sex, England and Wales, 1992*
(Source: OPCS Mortality Statistics, 1992. Copyright 1992. Reproduced by permission of the Controller of HMSO and of the Office for National Statistics)

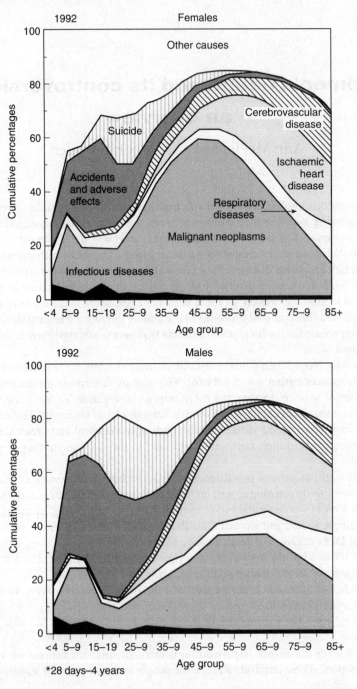

Table 1.1 *Approximate number of women in England and Wales who will die from the various causes listed (Beral, V., personal communication)*

	Before age 25	Before age 50	Before age 75
Breast cancer	1 in 200 000	1 in 200	1 in 30
Lung cancer	1 in 500 000	1 in 800	1 in 40
Heart attack	1 in 100 000	1 in 700	1 in 14
Stroke	1 in 40 000	1 in 500	1 in 35
Accidental death	1 in 400	1 in 200	1 in 100

Fig 1.4 looks at common causes of death over the last three decades in people under 65;

Table 1.3 looks at the deaths from cancer, cerebrovascular disease, and diseases of the circulatory system in countries in Europe.

Women tend to live longer than men. They outnumber men from the age of 50, with 63% of the population over 75 being female, and by age 85, 75%. But with the extra years available comes the question of how worthwhile these years are. Neither men nor women want extra years of suffering or a twilight existence. Although expectation of life is going up for men and women, when active life between the sexes is analysed in greater detail, the 'gain' for women disappears. The expectation of life without disability for both men and women is increasing far more slowly than is life expectancy, with 60% of women over the age of 80 living alone (Silman 1987). Because of this, some of the new agendas concern euthanasia and 'care of the elderly'.

The 1990s has seen what could have been a welcome shift to community care, supporting people in their own homes, if at all possible, rather than institutionalizing them. The lack of resources, however, has often meant that this is non-care in a non-community with women bearing the brunt of this, both as carers and those being cared for.

The historical perspective

The development of contemporary medical attitudes to women's health can be best understood within an historical and social context.

There have always been differences between the health problems of men and women, and even in primitive hunter–gatherer societies it is not difficult to imagine that the major causes of death would have been different for the sexes. In more recent history much of the emphasis on women's health has concentrated on childbearing, but, with the advent of more effective contraception and the conquest of infection, the broader and subtler aspects of women's, as against men's, health have become apparent.

The general health of both women and men has improved dramatically since the 1800s. In 1840 the expectation of life at birth for men was 40, and in 1993 it was 74; while for women in 1840 it was 42, and 79 in 1993. The

Fig 1.2a *Ten commonest cancers for women, UK, 1988*
(Source: Cancer Research Campaign, 1994)

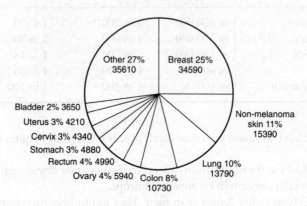

(a)

Fig 1.2b *Ten commonest cancers for men, UK, 1988*
(Source: Cancer Research Campaign, 1994)

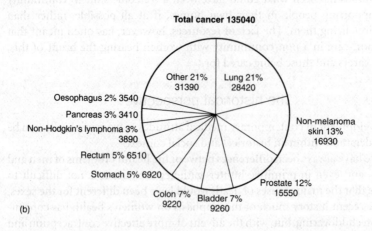

(b)

Table 1.2 *Estimates of the percentage cohort who develop cancer over a lifetime and the lifetime risk*

Site (Females)	%	risk
Breast	8.6	1 in 12
Skin (non-melanoma)	5.0	1 in 20
Lung	3.8	1 in 26
Colon	3.1	1 in 33
Ovary	1.8	1 in 55
Rectum	1.5	1 in 67
Cervix	1.4	1 in 72
Stomach	1.4	1 in 72
Uterus	1.3	1 in 75
Bladder	1.1	1 in 93
Site (Males)	**%**	**risk**
Lung	9.1	1 in 11
Skin (non-melanoma)	5.7	1 in 18
Prostate	4.4	1 in 23
Bladder	2.8	1 in 35
Colon	2.6	1 in 38
Stomach	2.4	1 in 42
Rectum	2.0	1 in 50
NHL	1.1	1 in 93
Pancreas	1.1	1 in 95
Oesophagus	1.0	1 in 96

Source: Cancer Research Campaign 1994

main cause of death in the 1800s, and even in the early part of this century, in both sexes, was infectious diseases. The heroines of novels and opera wasted away with consumption or died tragically in childbirth. Even as late as between 1921 and 1930, records show that tuberculosis accounted for 26% of deaths in women under the age of 45 and that maternal mortality (mainly puerperal fever) in the same age group accounted for 17% of deaths. Many factors, both specific to women and general to both sexes, played a part in the eradication of these causes of death, particularly improvements in the general standards of living including better nutrition, improved housing and sanitation, public health measures, more effective contraception, safer childbirth, the introduction of antibiotics, the treatment of anaemia, and other medical advances.

From 1911, the Health Insurance Act entitled specific groups of working men and working women, depending on income, to the services of a panel doctor and free medicine. This, however, did not cover hospital treatment or give help to a dependant – other than a maternity grant to the working man's wife. For example, according to the 1911 census only 10% of married women were working outside the home, so that health care facilities were not

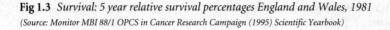

Fig 1.3 *Survival: 5 year relative survival percentages England and Wales, 1981*
(Source: Monitor MBI 88/1 OPCS in Cancer Research Campaign (1995) Scientific Yearbook)

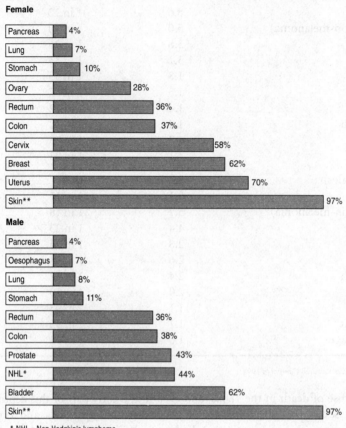

Female

Pancreas	4%
Lung	7%
Stomach	10%
Ovary	28%
Rectum	36%
Colon	37%
Cervix	58%
Breast	62%
Uterus	70%
Skin**	97%

Male

Pancreas	4%
Oesophagus	7%
Lung	8%
Stomach	11%
Rectum	36%
Colon	38%
Prostate	43%
NHL*	44%
Bladder	62%
Skin**	97%

* NHL = Non-Hodgkin's lymphoma
** Excluding malignant melanoma

available to 90% of married women unless they were paid for. It would be untrue to say that there were no free health care facilities for women working at home, as provision was made for advice to be given in the local authority or voluntary infant welfare clinics and municipal antenatal clinics which were being developed at this time. These were available to those who were pregnant or who had just had a baby. Women used these clinics – many not until later on in the pregnancy – for antenatal advice, but very few were seen for postnatal check-ups.

Further evidence concerning women's illnesses was provided by the Women's Health Enquiry Committee, which, in 1939, received over a thousand

Fig 1.4 *UK death rates for people aged under 65: by gender and selected cause of death*
(*Source: Office of Population Censuses and Surveys; General Register Office (Scotland); General Register Office (Northern Ireland) in Social Trends, 1996*)

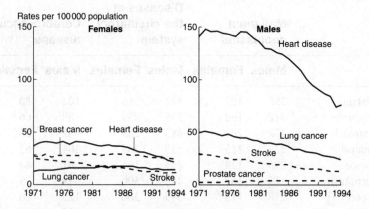

replies from working-class, married women to a questionnaire sent out via health visitors. It was found that the ailments most mentioned were anaemia, headaches, constipation, rheumatism, gynaecological trouble, dental problems, varicose veins, and ulcerated legs. From the results, the Committee felt that only a third were actually in poor health. Although many women who replied had consulted a doctor, only a very small number (5%) felt that they had received any 'health' teaching.

A study looking at illness, incapacity, and medical attention among adults in 1947–49 (Logan 1950) reflected the official figures of the changing morbidity patterns immediately before and after the introduction of the National Health Service (NHS). The main difference between the years 1947–48 and 1948–49 was that medical consultation rates increased over the whole country. The increase was 6% for men under the age of 65 and 9% for those over that age. For women the increases were much greater, 18% for the younger age group and 22% for the older women. Therefore there can be little doubt that before the start of the NHS many women failed to seek medical advice for economic reasons, but once the final disincentive was removed they consulted their doctors more for the same relative amount of sickness. The NHS theoretically provides free health care for all, and although women are no longer discriminated against in the same direct economic way as prior to 1948, the continuing differences in the use of the health service facilities by different social classes give some indication of the complexities involved.

The influences of fashion and finances on health

The classification of ailments raises the question of how society, and the individual within society, define disease. Changing patterns of what has classically

Table 1.3 *Death rates[1] for selected diseases EC comparison, 1992*

	Malignant neoplasms		Diseases of the circulatory system		Cerebrovascular disease	
	Males	Females	Males	Females	Males	Females
Austria	257	157	473	316	102	80
Belgium[2]	312	160	379	239	80	66
Denmark	272	204	443	263	81	65
Finland	232	135	535	289	104	83
France	295	129	255	151	61	44
Germany	273	162	473	300	99	79
Greece	218	113	395	300	125	126
Irish Republic	271	187	504	302	85	78
Italy[3]	284	146	376	248	105	81
Luxembourg	303	160	413	272	112	102
Netherlands	295	160	370	214	74	63
Portugal	222	126	447	317	231	176
Spain[3]	255	119	335	242	97	82
Sweden	197	143	421	244	74	61
United Kingdom	275	182	450	266	91	80
EC average	273	151	395	251	94	77

Rates per 100 000 population

[1] Age standardized
[2] Data are for 1989
[3] Data are for 1991
Source: World Health Organization in Social Trends (1996)

been considered pathological disease and the increasing medicalization of areas such as childbirth, sex, disease prevention, relationship problems, etc., are, in part, responsible for the relatively high rate that women attend GP surgeries. These changes have led to an increasing awareness of 'health fashions' which are based to a variable degree on new scientific evidence. Changes in fashion are particularly abundant in the area of women's health; examples are the changing attitudes towards the menopause, premenstrual tension, eating disorders, and 'faddish' diets. Other examples, perhaps less specific to women but still very female dominated, are demands for counselling, alternative therapies, and more recently, Prozac.

Although there is naturally little direct reference to such risqué areas in Victorian literature, it is possible that some characters, Mrs Nickleby for instance, were, in fact, menopausal. However, the lack of references to the menopause in literature may not only have been due to prudery but also to the fact that far fewer women succeeded in surviving long enough to experience it! Doctors were slow to accept menopausal symptoms as a problem to which they could offer any contribution until patients and the media forced them to take notice. In this atmosphere of increased awareness, the drug companies devoted themselves to producing and marketing suitable hormone replacement therapy. Thus the interdependency of medical, pharmaceutical, and lay interests has encouraged the view that symptoms of the menopause are pathological. Nevertheless, permanent cessation of menstruation is something that happens to all women and cannot therefore in itself be classified as disease, though it is likely that some women will have symptoms which do need treatment. The symptoms themselves are not the only determining factor of therapy. As always in medicine, they have to be balanced against the side-effects of the therapy used. Prevention of osteoporosis and heart disease and prolongation of an active sexual life by the use of hormone replacement therapy (HRT) is being presented by the drug companies as the only way forward for women in their middle years; an attitude challenged by others who have anxieties about increased risks of breast cancer, and cannot believe that it is the norm for all women to need hormone replacement. Unfortunately, the arguments are becoming polarized, with the ever-printworthy Germaine Greer almost labelling some women as HRT wimps, and some doctors comparing the use of HRT with 'needing to wear glasses' for age-onset presbyopia or describing the menopause as 'nature's mistake'. Some women will undoubtedly benefit from hormone replacement, while others will suffer more than they gain. What is certain is the uncertainty that still remains.

However, uncertainty in health is something that women of all ages have to face. Pill scares occur with monotonous frequency. The uncertainty associated with so-called 'user-friendly', third-generation, oral contraceptive pills versus the 'thrombo-friendly', second-generation, old-fashioned standbys has been complicated by the cost-cutting agenda of the government and the profit motives of the drug companies. Scientific truth, information for GPs, and choices for women are often obscured by the media angst.

Environment, social class and disease

Fashion and market values are only two of many influences. Social factors are also important in the way they affect women's health. It is women who are often represented as being depressed in advertisements in medical magazines and journals. They may be represented in this way for good reason, and sociological studies have helped to give GPs insight into some of the environmental influences on the health of women. As long ago as 1978 Brown and Harris looked at depression in a random sample of women in South London (there was no similar study for men), and their findings confirmed what had been for many GPs a clinical impression. They found that the incidence of depression was significantly greater in the lower social classes and identified certain vulnerability factors that preceded the depression. These included loss of mother in childhood, three or more children aged less than 14 living at home, lack of a confiding or intimate relationship with a husband or boyfriend, and lack of full- or part-time work. The effect of employment was especially interesting, as even when all the other factors were present, many more women developed depression if they did not have paid employment. This is a finding that is in line with more recent research and with the rising levels of unemployment and has important implications for medical practice. Other important findings were that less than half the women with clinical symptoms of depression had seen their GP, and only a small minority of those who had were then referred to a psychiatrist.

The differing standard mortality ratios in men, by occupation and social class, are well-documented (for example, the Black Report 1980), but the implications of the differences for women have received less attention. For instance, why is the incidence of cervical cancer in coalminers' wives so much higher than in doctors' wives? And not only do women appear to suffer from the effects of their husband's occupation, but also more directly from their own occupations and their own social class.

Data are now available to look directly at the effects of women's occupations on various disease processes. Social class differences in mortality, however, are best seen when married women are tabulated according to their husband's occupation rather than their own, so it is important that social class differences are looked at in both ways – by the husband's occupation and the woman's. The observations that women working in the textile industry appear to have a higher incidence of vascular disease as well as the apparent increase of spontaneous abortion rates in female anaesthetists suggest that women's occupations themselves also affect morbidity. In the US such findings have led to claims that certain occupations should be closed to women, unless they agree to be sterilized, because of risks to a potential fetus. Almost all ill health and mortality is increased in social classes IV and V, a fact present from birth with the doubling of perinatal mortality and the tripling of infant mortality rates in babies born to women of these classes. Of course, classifications of social class are traditionally likened to a temperature taken with a thermometer – they tell you something is wrong without being able to define what it is; but the effects of social class on health permeate almost every aspect of health care. It is too early to assess the health implications of short-term contracts, job insecurity, and the isolation of working from home.

General environmental influences, such as the effects of exercise, diet, and weight on coronary artery disease and of smoking on the incidence of lung cancer, have also been examined more thoroughly in men than in women. Nevertheless, coronary artery disease is the main cause of death in women (albeit less so than in men) and the cessation rate among female smokers is less than that in male smokers. In 1950, women in Britain smoked half as many cigarettes as their male contemporaries, while in 1980 they smoked nearly as many, and by the 1990s, in younger age groups, women smoked more than men. Not surprisingly, therefore, the rates of lung cancer in women are soaring. The anti-smoking health education programme has made attempts to aim messages specifically at women (usually only during pregnancy) with notable lack of success. Little attention has been paid to why there are differences in the changing smoking patterns in men and women, but recent information on smoking habits emphasizes the need for the GP to use different tactics when counselling women and to tailor advice to different groups of women.

Diet and exercise are two further areas in which men and women behave in different ways. The HMSO *Social trends* figures for 1996 show that 16% of women are obese compared to 13% of men and that there was little difference between the consumption of red meat and butter between men and women, but that in the 18–39 age group, twice as many men as women ate fried foods. Women generally attributed more importance to diet as an influence on health than men, but alas, many of us still remain fat!

There are signs from the General Household Survey that more women are taking part in sports and other physical activities than in previous years, but this still remains less than for men. In 1993–94, 72% of men and 57% of women in the UK took part in at least one physical activity in the 4 weeks prior to interview for the General Household Survey.

What do women worry about?

Little is known about women's anxieties and attitudes to health, and yet this information is highly relevant in the planning of services if we are to meet women's needs appropriately. The popular Radio 4 programme, *Woman's Hour*, in 1994 commissioned a survey of 533 women over 16, with interviews at home, to determine their anxieties and attitudes to health. The sample was representative of women throughout Britain in age, social class, and working status. Only one in 10 women described their health as excellent, but nearly 50% said their health was very good. 10% of the women felt they were not in control of their lives and 73% of these suffered from stress or nerves, compared with 46% of the whole sample. Fig 1.5 and Table 1.4 show what women worry about and the top 10 worries within each age group. A third of all the women worried about being overweight. Other common concerns were breast cancer, reduced mobility, effects of stress on health, appearance, and becoming senile.

Self-help

Women are becoming ever better informed and increasingly want to take more responsibility for their own treatment choices. Self-help for women has always been an alternative to professional care but has recently become something of a growth industry. It is by no means new, and in the past it may have come from a similar impetus to the contemporary movement. There is a manuscript dating from 1500 that was re-issued in 1981 under the title *Medieval woman's guide to health*. This was produced, as the editor comments, 'because women were dissatisfied with their treatment at the hands of male physicians and were endeavouring to instruct one another as to how to help themselves with their gynaecological problems'.

Fig 1.5 *What do women worry about?*

(Source: BBC Broadcasting Research survey on women's health, Aug, 1994)

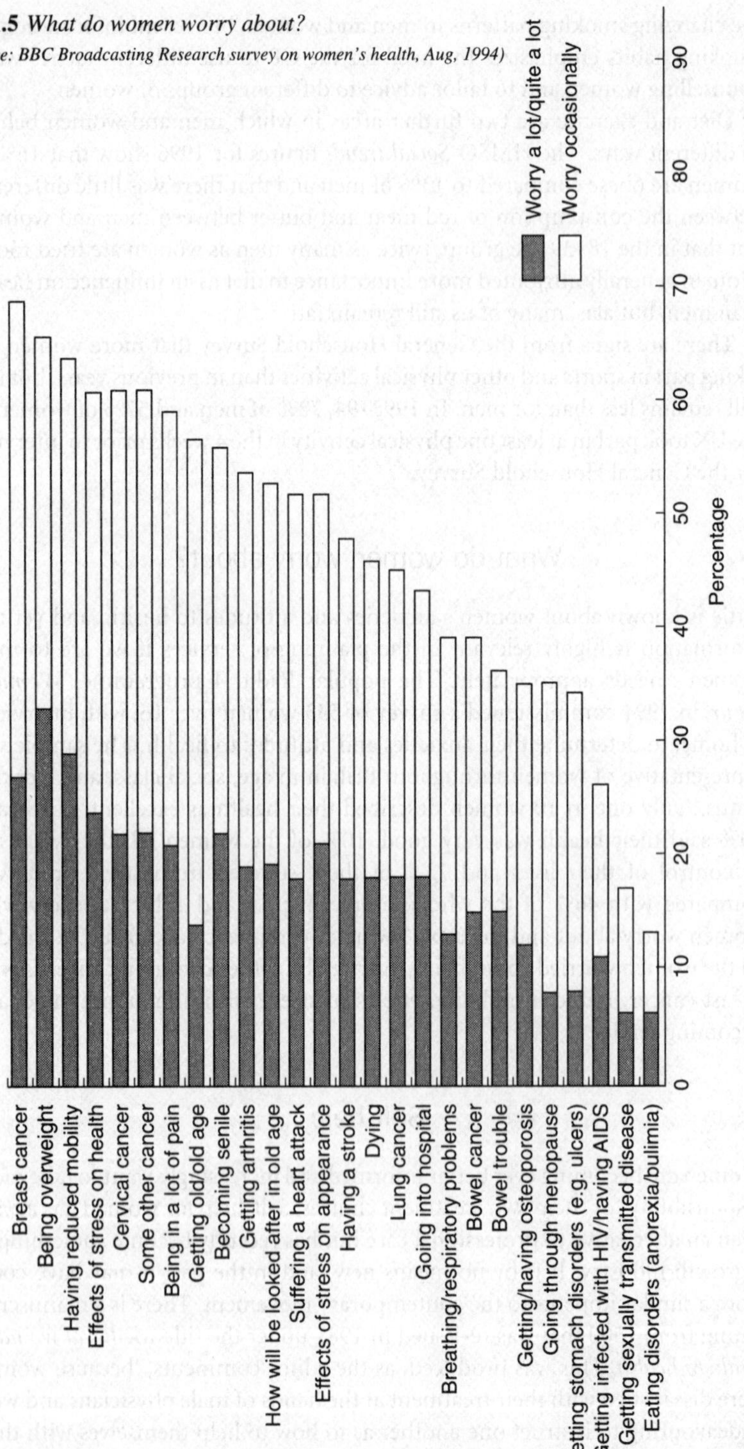
Worry a lot/quite a lot
Worry occasionally
Percentage
0
10
20
30
40
50
60
70
80
90
Breast cancer
Being overweight
Having reduced mobility
Effects of stress on health
Cervical cancer
Some other cancer
Being in a lot of pain
Getting old/old age
Becoming senile
Getting arthritis
How will be looked after in old age
Suffering a heart attack
Effects of stress on appearance
Having a stroke
Dying
Lung cancer
Going into hospital
Breathing/respiratory problems
Bowel cancer
Bowel trouble
Getting/having osteoporosis
Going through menopause
Getting stomach disorders (e.g. ulcers)
Getting infected with HIV/having AIDS
Getting sexually transmitted disease
Eating disorders (anorexia/bulimia)

Table 1.4 *How do worries vary by age?*

16–24	%	25–44	%	45–64	%	65+	%
Breast cancer	82	Breast cancer	78	Reduced mobility	76	Reduced mobility	72
Cervical cancer	77	Stress on health	75	Senility	68	Arthritis	65
Stress on appearance	73	Cervical cancer	74	Breast cancer	67	Senility	64
Overweight	69	Overweight	72	Overweight	65	Looked after in old age	62
Being in a lot of pain	69	Other cancer	68	Other cancer	61	Being in a lot of pain	56
Dying	68	Getting old	63	Stroke	60	Stroke	51
Other cancer	67	Reduced mobility	62	Stress on health	60	Getting old	49
HIV/AIDS	64	Being in a lot of pain	59	Looked after in old age	58	Overweight	47
Stress on health	61	Stress on appearance	57	Heart attack	58	Other cancer	40
Lung cancer	59	Arthritis	55	Cervical cancer	54	Heart attack	39
				Arthritis	54	Going into hospital	39
						Bowel trouble	39

Source: BBC Broadcasting Research Survey on Women's Health, (1994)

The publication of *Our bodies, ourselves*, as a modern counterpart, by a group of non-medical women in Boston in 1971, produced a focus for women on the possibilities and increased self-respect that self-help in health might offer them. The book challenged the idea that help was only the medical profession's prerogative – the authors all having experienced 'frustration and anger towards specific doctors and the medical maze in general'; and the basic aim was 'learning to understand, accept, and be responsible for our physical selves'. In the US the book rapidly became a bestseller but when the first UK edition was published in the late 1970s it went unheralded. The difference in the reactions to the text and its philosophy in the two countries may, in part, have been because in the early 1970s American medicine, including family planning and child health, was almost entirely male-dominated (only 7% of doctors were female), whereas in the UK there were relatively more women doctors (though they were still in the minority) and certainly in the areas of family planning and child health it was very likely that women patients would come into contact with women doctors.

The Bristol Cancer Centre is one example where women have rejected the conventional 'high-tech, toxic-perceived' option as the answer to breast cancer, and have turned instead to the alternative holistic approach offered by such centres. Unfortunately, research to compare outcomes of conventional treatment versus the Bristol Centre approach was foreshortened when the Bristol Centre was falsely accused of higher death rates, resulting in polarization of the two approaches. There is room for many different approaches and they need to be evaluated with an open mind.

Polarization of positions on natural, self-help, and conventional medicine has led to some curious outcomes. Women, rightly, are wary of medicines which are known to have side-effects. However, in a perverse kind of way, the knowledge of the side-effects of drugs used, for example in the treatment of the menopause, has led to the use of untried natural remedies for many disorders. There is a general misconception that the word 'natural', as in natural remedies, automatically means safe. However, this is clearly not so; for example it is possible to take an overdose of vitamins, and some so-called natural diets are, in fact, deficient in some basic elements. Ginseng, vitamins, diets, herbs, homeopathy, and so on, though fashionable as natural remedies at the moment, have mostly never been properly assessed either for their efficacy or for their side-effects (see Chapter 20). Nevertheless, it is likely that there are far more benefits than disadvantages in the movement towards self-help.

This apparent interest by women in self-help is perhaps because in their role as carers, women have to be more sensitive to the emotional side of well-being – something that they obviously felt was sadly lacking in many of the medical services provided. The health areas in which women are able to support each other are many – as represented by such organizations as Breast Cancer Care, Rape Crisis Centres, The National Childbirth Trust, The Postnatal Support Group, etc. For a complex variety of reasons women predominate, both as users and as providers, whichever way health in the community is considered. With the continuing shortfall in NHS financing, self-help has become an integral part of the health service.

Consultation rates

GPs see more women patients than men and give them more medicine. Why is this? Who are these women? What illnesses do they have, and what medicines do they take?

There are, of course, more women than men in the community as a whole – the slightly larger number of males than females in the community up to the age of 45 being more than offset by the longevity of women. In England and Wales in 1990, of the 3.6 million individuals aged 75 or more, 63% were women. Thus the diseases of ageing, for example dementia and cancer, will tend to be diseases affecting women.

Information on consultation rates comes from the General Household Survey (a continuous monitor of a random sample of the population) and the fourth national morbidity survey conducted by a non-random set of GPs in 1991–92 (McCormick *et al.* 1995). Thus the consultation rates are collected in different ways and at different times and sometimes with different results.

Although it may appear that women do consult their doctors more often than men from the crude figures – and crude they are – it does also seem that women actually suffer more from disease and do not simply consult more often for each episode of illness. Much of the disease is 'gender related'. There is still a difference, but the differences between men and women are much smaller once consultations which are not for illness are removed; and virtually disappear after consultations for pregnancy and childbirth and diseases of the male and female genitourinary systems are excluded.

The reasons for which women and men consult their doctors also show differences. For instance, women consult more for endocrine/nutritional/metabolic diseases, diseases of the blood and reproductive organs, mental disorders, diseases of the circulatory system, genitourinary disorders, and muscular and connective tissue disorders. A further category of complaints entitled 'symptoms and ill-defined conditions' is twice as common in women. The category for which consultation rates are commoner in males is accidents, poisoning, and violence. Consultation rates are roughly the same in both sexes for infectious and parasitic diseases, diseases of the nervous system (excluding mental disorders), diseases of the respiratory system, and disorders of the digestive system and of the skin, though in nearly all these the female/male ratio slightly favours the females.

A further difficulty lies in interpretation of the consultation statistics because of the question of who deals with what problems where. For instance, the figures for consultation rates with GPs show that for genitourinary problems in the 25–44 age group there were approximately 10 times as many patient consultations for women as for men (26% compared with 2.5%). These consultations in women cover a wide range of problems such as menstrual irregularities, abortion, menopausal problems, vaginal discharge, etc. The equivalent problems in men, such as urethral discharge, are most likely to be dealt with in hospital venereal disease or genitourinary clinics. Likewise, men may consult their GP for injuries, but are also likely to go directly to hospital for treatment.

Parents (usually women) have other sources of medical advice, such as child health clinics, which will not be documented as their own consultation. Those who run child health clinics well-recognize that the problems they most frequently encounter, such as feeding problems, sleep problems, etc., have as much to do with the stresses and strains on women as parents in our present society as any actual illness in the child.

Consultation rates are, therefore, hardly an accurate reflection of illness. The GP is consulted for only one in 18 illness episodes, the rest being 'coped with' without formal medical consultation; while there is an average of 11 lay consultations for every medical consultation (Morrell 1976). This rate is a reflection of what patients and doctors consider as appropriate to be dealt with by the GP, and goes some way towards demonstrating the actual workload he or she has to deal with.

Medications

If women appear to like their doctors' company then it is also clear that they consume a diet rich in pills, both prescribed and non-prescribed. The General Household Survey (1995), for instance, showed that in a fortnight previous to the survey, half the women and a third of the men reported that they had taken prescribed medicine, and another study showed that twice as many women as men had treated themselves (17% versus 8%). This pattern did not apply to girls under the age of 15, where the reverse was true, so that one cannot conclude that early experience plays a significant role, although girls may see their mothers taking tablets as being a part of female adult life. However, a study in Oxfordshire in 1985 of 14-year-olds showed that 77% of girls had taken medicines in the previous 4 weeks compared to 63% of boys.

The prescribing practices of GPs can provide valuable information. A GP-based study over 3 years (Jones *et al.* 1984) showed that twice as many women as men received psychotropic drug prescriptions, and women were three times more likely than men to have had a psychotropic drug in the past, and other studies have shown similar patterns. Women were not only prescribed drugs more often, the drugs were also prescribed for longer periods of time.

Whether consultation rates and prescribing rates are linked or not, it does seem that women take more pills and it is difficult to find the reason, though obviously both patients and doctors are involved. Regular contact with services such as family planning, antenatal care, and child health clinics might encourage women to think of drug-taking as acceptable. Further, women as shopper-consumers – at whom most advertisements are directed – have, in shops and elsewhere, more easy access to medicines; and women's magazines, with their widespread circulation, give further credence to the idea of taking medicines to cure certain ills. These ideas must remain speculative and do not give the full explanation. If they did, one would expect to see a more significant difference between the sexes in the self-medication rates compared with the prescribed rates, and the studies done in this are conflicting. It may be that, historically, women have tended to take medicines and pills whereas men have taken alcohol. Laudanum and various other tonics containing psychotropic components might have been the mother's little helper of Victorian times, replaced now by diazepam, Prozac, and other such drugs; throughout this time beer drinking and the group psychotherapy camaraderie in the pubs and other leisure centres have probably been the equivalent medication available to men!

Perhaps doctors have a preconceived idea that the male patient should be able to cope without help and that the female 'being the weaker sex' needs the support of drugs. A quick glance through the drug advertising in medical journals still reinforces the picture of the downtrodden woman patient as a headachy, premenstrual, depressed person with chronic backache and lines of worldly care across her face, in obvious need of immediate help from her GP, probably in the form of a prescription.

Further information about prescribed medicines and perceived general health was gathered from over 6000 adults (3429 women) by interview (Breeze *et al.* 1994). 42% of women and 32% of men were taking prescribed drugs. As would be expected, the number of medicines taken was related to age (e.g. only 1% of 16–44 year-old women were taking four or more medicines, compared to 21% of women aged 75 years and over). When age groups were compared by sex, a higher proportion of women than men were taking medicines in every age group.

Looking at the types of medicine taken, 21% of women aged 45–64 were taking endocrine drugs (largely hormone replacement therapy). 1% or less of women were taking medicines for genitourinary conditions. 17% of all women were taking medicines affecting the central nervous system, 15% the cardiovascular system, and 6% the gastrointestinal system, and the proportion taking medicines in these three categories increased markedly with age. The contraceptive pill was excluded from the analysis. When men and women were compared, of those who reported longstanding problems of the musculo-skeletal, digestive, endocrine, or metabolic systems, women were more likely than men to be taking medication. There were no sex differences for other chronic illnesses. For all age groups, the number of medicines taken was higher for those who reported poorer health. Those who said they had a longstanding illness were more likely to be taking medicines affecting the cardiovascular or central nervous systems. However, 35% of those with a longstanding illness or disability were taking no medicines.

Women doctors

Women are not only the main users of the health service but are also, as nurses, midwives, health visitors, hospital ancillary staff, radiographers, physiothera-pists, etc., to a large extent the providers. On the other hand, the majority of doctors are still men, but in 1991, for the first time, over 50% of the medical student intake throughout the country were women.

The Department of Health, in its recent report on opportunities for women doctors, showed that at consultant level, in all hospital medical specialties, only 15% were women, which is much lower than might be expected given the previous percentage of female medical graduates. Even in general practice, in 1995 only 28% of partners were women, though this is an improvement on the 19% in 1985.

Women are more likely to be part-time at some stage in their career, with one in three women working part-time compared with one in 20 men. The future of general practice looks as if it will be increasingly female and therefore will need to be more flexible. The number of GPs rose by 10% over the last 10 years: this is largely accounted for by the rise in the number of female GPs many of whom are working part-time, with a decrease in the number of full-time equivalents. Over the same period the overall number of GP registrars has fallen by 20%, but the number of female registrars has risen by 11%.

Recent results from cohort studies (Allen 1996) of British medical graduates comparing career preferences in 1983 and 1993, found an overall decline in those wanting to enter general practice. This was found to be true for both sexes but the decline was greatest amongst the men; 40% to 17% as against 52% to 34% for women. In other words, twice as many women as men are now attracted by general practice. Recruitment to general practice is now an acute problem, yet there is continuing talk of a primary care-led NHS, which still assumes a medical workforce mainly made up of men working full-time in general practice for 40 years. Few regional health authorities have addressed the problem of part-time training, and many have not yet faced up to the fact that a large part of their potential workforce will not continue training, or be available in specialties where they are needed, unless part-time working facilities and crèches/nurseries are provided. Having more women GPs can be seen as an asset or problematical. A study in one group practice looked at consultation patterns of male and female partners (two male and two female). There was no truth in the myth that the women doctors did not pull their weight with regard to the number of consultations carried out. They saw more women patients than their male counterparts; the women partners had a slightly higher, or at least an equal, consultation rate than their male colleagues; and doctor-initiated appointments were higher for women patients of women doctors than for their male patients.

Apart from problems of recruitment there are also worries about job satisfaction. The Institute of Manpower Studies in 1990 found that only 59% of married women with certified vocational training had principal posts, compared to 85% of married male GPs. More women GPs than men were dissatisfied with their current employment status. However, women doctors are more likely than other professional women to continue working once they have children. It is children that interfere with career achievement. Even in the age of the 'new man', full-time working women have an average of 17 hours a week less leisure time than men. The data on the outcomes of different types of child-care arrangements are conflicting. There is a tension. The medical profession is producing evidence to suggest that it may affect a child adversely to be in some types of child care for more than 20 hours a week in the first year of life. But at the same time so little is still being done to enable women doctors (or any other women in the health service) to fulfil their potential by appropriate part-time training schemes and career posts.

What do women want from their doctor?

During the last two decades there have been various studies to look at women's preference of sex of doctor. They all show that some women want to see a woman doctor, especially younger women and for certain conditions, e.g. gynaecological and maternity. However, the surveys show variation, probably dependent on the way the data were collected. In 1984 the Women's National Commission surveyed 5840 women and whereas 72% felt women should be offered the choice of a female or male doctor for hospital treatment, preference for a female GP was 18%, though higher (35%) in the younger age group. The main reasons given for wanting a female were that: (a) as a woman she would have a better understanding of women's problems (82%); and (b) a female doctor would be easier and less embarrassing to talk to (70.5%).

The more recent Woman's Hour study (1994) found 66% had a male GP, 23% a female, and 11% saw both. 19% wanted a woman, 10% a man, and 28% said it depended on the problem. 43% said it made no difference. What people wanted was a good doctor, though in this study 45% found female doctors were more understanding. 45% wanted more time with their doctor, 90% felt doctors were overworked, nearly 50% felt doctors were too ready to prescribe drugs, and 35% felt that doctors had little patience with women stress sufferers. There were also some areas that women had particular difficulty with. They found discussion about sexual difficulties, having an internal examination, undressing in front of the GP, breast problems, and talking about sexually transmitted diseases problematical. There may be similar problems in men, but we have no figures. The young women found these areas more difficult than the older women.

Conclusion

We have, in this introduction, presented some ideas influencing women's health in general, but also, more specifically, in relation to general practice. It is obvious, when reviewing the facts available, that they are open to many inter-pretations. Nevertheless, we hope that the issues raised provide a background for the chapters of this book which deal largely with the more specific problems for which women consult their GPs. Just as it has been traditionally necessary for a surgeon to be aware of the female/male differences in the anatomy, it is be-coming increasingly important to consider the subtler female/male differences in behaviour and attitudes to disease during GP training.

The rapidly developing field of molecular biology promises to have a huge impact on medicine in the future. Our understanding of the molecular pathol-ogy of many diseases, such as cancer, arteriosclerosis, neuropsychiatric illness, and congenital malformations, is increasing. It is too early to say whether the application of DNA technology to these problems will revolutionize their management or even prevent them. If we take this a step further, as we gain more control over the human genome we may be in a position to modify the human phenotype more or less as we please. This raises complex ethical questions and is likely to be a major issue facing society in the future.

Many changes are taking place in the health service. It is an ideal opportunity to monitor the provision of care. In all aspects of medicine, including women's health, there is a realization that interventions must become more evidence based. Women are not asking for a separate health system, but within a comprehensive system there needs to be proper evaluation of alternative ways of providing health care to women in order to find the most effective way forward.

References and further reading

Allen, I. (1996). Career preferences of doctors. *British Medical Journal*, 313, 3.

BBC Broadcasting Research Survey on Women's Health (1994) for *Women's Hour*. Personal communication.

Black, D. (1980). *Inequalities in health*. Report of a Research Working Group. Department of Health and Social Security, London.

Breeze, E. *et al.* (1994). *Health survey for England*. HMSO, London.

Brown, G. and Harris, T. (1978). *Social origins of depression*. Tavistock Publications, London.

Cancer Research Campaign (1994). *Factsheet* 1.1.

Cancer Research Campaign (1995). *The challenge we face – the latest cancer statistics*. Scientific Yearbook 1995–6.

Cartwright, A. and Anderson, R. (1981). *General practice revisited*. Tavistock Publications, London.

Central Statistical Office (1996). *Social trends* 26. HMSO, London.

Department of Health (1991). *Your health: a guide to services for women*. O/N 13916 (HSSH) J1299NJ. DoH, London.

Dunnell, K. (1995). Population review: (2) Are we healthier? *Population Trends*, **82**, HMSO.

General Household Survey Annual Reports (1995). HMSO.

Jones, L., Simpson, D., Brown, A.C., *et al.* (1984). Prescribing psychotropic drugs in general practice: three year study. *British Medical Journal*, **289**, 1045–8.

Lambert, T., Goldacre, M., Edwards, C., and Parkhouse, J. (1996). Career preferences of doctors who qualified in the United Kingdom in 1993 compared with those qualifying in 1974, 1977, 1980, and 1983. *British Medical Journal*, **313**, 19–24.

Logan, W.P.D. (1950). Illness, incapacity and medical attention among adults, 1947–1949. *Lancet*, **i**, 773–6.

Macfarlane, A. (1990). Official statistics and women's health and illness. In *Women's health counts* (ed. H. Roberts). Routledge, London.

McCormick, A., Fleming, D., and Charlton, J. (1995). *Morbidity statistics from General Practice: Fourth National Study 1991–92*. OPCS, Series MB5 no.3. HMSO, London.

Morrell, D.C. and Wale, C.J. (1976). Symptoms perceived and recorded by patients. *Journal of the Royal College of General Practitioners*, **26**, 398–403.

OPCS. (1994). *Mortality statistics – general, 1992*. Series DHI no.27. HMSO, London.

Newman, L. (1992). Second among equals. *British Journal of General Practice*, **42**, 71–4.

Preston-Whyte, M.E., Fraser, R.C., and Beckett, J.L. (1983). Effect of a principal's gender on consultation patterns. *Journal of the Royal College of General Practitioners*, **255**, 654–8.

Report of a Women's National Commission Ad Hoc Working Group (1984). *Women and the health service*.

Rowland, B. (ed.) (1981). *Medieval women's guide to health*. Croom Helm, London.

Silman, A.J. (1987). Why do women live longer and is it worth it? *British Medical Journal*, May, 1311.

The Boston Women's Collective (1971). *Our bodies ourselves*. Simon and Schuster, New York.

CHAPTER TWO

The role of primary health care in promoting the health of women

Rosemary Kay, Ann McPherson, and Deborah Waller

Introduction

This chapter aims to provide a framework of ideas for the primary health care team to look at women's special needs, and to develop an overall health promotion strategy. It will look particularly at the needs of women at different ages, the *Health of the Nation* targets and how they relate to women's health, and the methods of delivery of health information and health promotion. Smoking, alcohol, nutrition and exercise will be explored in detail, and evidence as to whether a primary health care team has a role in these areas will be addressed.

Many issues relevant to women's health promotion are looked at elsewhere in this book. These include family planning, breast and cervical screening, and emotional problems.

Definitions of health promotion

Health promotion is generally agreed to include three main kinds of activity, which often overlap (Tannahill 1985), and the primary health care team clearly has a role in all three:

1. *Health education.* The provision of readily available information on healthier lifestyles for patients, and how to make the best use of health services, with the intention of enabling people to make rational health choices and of ensuring awareness of the factors determining the health of the community.

2. *Prevention of ill health.* Measures to reduce the risk of disease and disability, for example, screening for breast and cervical problems.

3. *Health and protection.* Derived from the tradition of public health and includes legal, fiscal, and political measures and regulations to prevent ill health, for example, seat belt laws, tax on cigarettes and alcohol, and fluoridation of water. Doctors have an important role in influencing the development of healthy public policy because they hold positions of influence at local, regional, and national levels.

The seven ages of health promotion for women

At first, the female infant muling and puking in the health visitor's arms at the child health clinic.

Then the whining, smoking schoolgirl with her menarche and acne, truanting like snail, away from school to pub.

Then the sighing lover's early morning creep for emergency contraception with woeful ballad of tale made to her mate's burst condom.

Then the working woman cum harassed mother, full of strange myths, Evening Oil of Primrose, Prozac, and health-ladened oaths.

Then the fully-screened, round-bellied, hot-flushed matriarch, full of HRT.

The sixth age shifts into the deserted, shrinking osteoporotic, all wise figure of fun, with spectacles on nose.

The last scene of all that ends this strange, eventful history is second childishness and Alzheimer's, sans teeth, sans eye, sans taste, sans man, sans everything.
(With acknowledgement and apologies to W. Shakespeare)

To facilitate assessment of their varying health promotion needs, women can be looked at in different age groups. The seven ages of women for this purpose are: childhood, teenage, pre-child bearing years, reproductive years, pre-menopausal, menopausal, and elderly.

Childhood

Health promotion for this age group in general practice is principally the responsibility of the health visitors, ensuring immunizations are given and by supporting parents, giving information on breast-feeding, diet, and accident prevention. There is really no differentiation between males and females.

Teenage years

The teenage years are a time of experimentation and risk-taking behaviour. Teenagers are able to assimilate health information for themselves. Although teenagers in general are a healthy group, 30% will visit their general practitioner (GP) in any 3-month period, mainly with minor illnesses (Macfarlane 1987). Information can be given opportunistically during these consultations. Teaching teenagers how to use the surgery and telling them what is available, together with the assurance of confidentiality, are probably the most important areas in the way of health promotion in this age group. A recent survey in London found that 25% of teenage girls 'felt that the discussion with their GP could be relayed to their parents against their wishes' (Donovan 1996, personal communication). Sexual health is an important area for health promotion in this group, though only one in five 15-year-old girls are sexually active. Information about emergency contraception and sexually transmitted diseases, with the provision of free condoms, require the practice to be open, realistic and supportive if things go wrong (Williams *et al.* 1994). As regards smoking, most young people already know about the risks of smoking, but for girls, linking risks with contraception and use of the contraceptive pill is a useful way to broach the subject. Teenagers rarely come to talk about alcohol and drugs problems, although parents will seek advice and information in this area. The teenage years are a time when young women may give up healthy pursuits such as organized sport, although many of them will take part in aerobics and it is encouraging to see that the gap in activity between men and women in their late teens and twenties is narrower than in previous decades. There are two extremes – excessive exercisers and the non-exercisers. Both can cause problems later; the former may have an adverse effect on bone density, the latter on obesity and heart disease. Lastly, dieting is extremely common amongst teenage girls and may lead to the development of eating disorders in susceptible individuals. Healthy eating and avoidance of fad diets are important with regards to health promotion, as well as the detection and appropriate help for young women with eating disorders.

Receptionists, nurses, and doctors need to be non-judgemental. Issues relating to sexuality and contraception should be raised appropriately. One study showed that teenagers did want information about contraception but did not want advice on relationships. Waiting rooms can be made less awesome with music (if not Radio One for the sake of other patients!), appealing notice boards, and a good selection of teenage magazines (these are read by 40% of teenage girls and are an important source of health information). Confidentiality is a major worry of young people and needs to be emphasized. Notices assuring all patients of confidentiality along with information about emergency contraception should be displayed in waiting rooms. If teenagers feel comfortable coming to the practice they are more likely to use it as a health resource.

Pre-childbearing years

Areas of health promotion to be addressed are: contraceptive advice, cervical smears (see Chapter 12), and pre-conceptual counselling. Evidence shows that 25% of women feel they do not get enough information from their GPs about contraception. They would like more choices about the different methods and more information about side-effects, including written information (FPA 1996). Pre-conception is the time to check rubella status and arrange for immunization if necessary, and to tell women about folic acid supplements. Information advising women to start taking folic acid 3 months before conception can be displayed on posters in the waiting rooms. One audit, in a general practice in Oxford, showed that 51% of women were not taking folic acid when they became pregnant (McIntyre 1996, personal communication). Women on anti-convulsants are at a higher risk of having a child with spina bifida and it is particularly important to target this group of women before conception to give advice on the potential teratogenicity of their medication, as well as the need to be on folic acid. They are easily identifiable as they are likely to be getting repeat prescriptions. Leaflets giving preconception advice are also available in various languages.

Reproductive years

Women are likely to attend the practice in their own right for contraception during these years, or otherwise while accompanying their children with their various ills. If not already done, the risk factors for heart disease should be recorded and appropriate advice given. This can be done opportunistically or at a well woman clinic. Blood pressure should be checked 3-yearly and weight, height, and BMI recorded. If there is a family history of premature heart disease a cholesterol test should be offered. Advice on diet and exercise should also be given. There is evidence that patients have reported changing their eating habits when they receive dietary recommendations from their practice (Baron *et al.* 1990). Cervical smear status should be checked opportunistically. Breast awareness can be discussed, although it is uncertain how effective this is in reducing breast cancer in later years. If there is a family history of breast cancer or ovarian cancer these need to be addressed and screening considered (see p. 118).

Antenatal

This is another time when folic acid supplements should be discussed. Antenatal clinics are an ideal place for health information, as there is evidence that it is a time when women are receptive to health messages, including the importance of smoking cessation.

Postnatal

Midwives and health visitors are key contacts with women postnatally. They have the opportunity to visit the home and offer advice on such areas as accident prevention for children, immunizations, breast-feeding, a healthy diet, infant growth and development, and sleep problems. Detection of the early signs of postnatal depression is important at this stage, with the provision of increased support and referral if necessary.

Pre-menopausal

Periods

Periods often change in character from the late thirties onwards. Cycles may become shorter with heavier periods. Women are often surprised and worried by this and may consult for advice. Information on what is normal and abnormal will help them to cope with the changes that happen at this time.

Premenstrual syndrome (PMS)

Some women are aware of premenstrual symptoms throughout their lives. PMS becomes a problem for others in their late thirties and early forties. Diary cards are invaluable in helping to diagnose true premenstrual symptoms (see Chapter 9).

Breast awareness

Many women will already be 'breast aware', checking their breasts regularly. This should be encouraged as it is a time when women generally begin to worry more about breast cancer.

Menopausal

Breast and cervical screening

From the age of 50, all women in Britain are called for a mammogram under the national screening programme. Not all women take up this offer, some because they just never get around to going, some because they are too frightened, and some because they do not want to have a mammogram. They should be fully informed about the benefits of screening and encouraged to attend. There is some evidence that mammography uptake is increased if GPs discuss it opportunistically. One way of enabling this is to flag the notes of women who have not attended for screening. Routine cervical smears are offered up to the age of 65 (Chapter 12).

Menopausal symptoms

Information on the menopause and its management should be available. There are pros and cons of hormone replacement therapy. The relative benefits of osteoporosis and heart disease prevention should be weighed up with each individual woman, against the possible side-effects of treatment (e.g. weight gain, bloating, nausea) and the small increase in breast cancer risk with long-term use. Only when fully informed is she in a position to make a decision about whether or not to take it.

Hypertension

Regular blood pressure checks should be offered as blood pressure often rises after the menopause in women. Heart disease is still the main cause of death in women, and the risk factors can be identified and appropriate treatment and advice given.

Elderly

All practices are now involved in providing health checks to the over-75s as part of their terms of service under the 1990 GP contract. A study on elderly health checks found that 43% of those patients who had been assessed had some unmet need (Brown *et al.* 1992). Health checks have proved more popular with patients than with health professionals. Home visits do enable some problems to be picked up which could be missed at the surgery, for example, the smell of urine because of incontinence, social isolation, poor diet, poor compliance with medication. Seven out of 10 of the population over the age of 80 are female. Dementia and arthritis are mainly women's diseases. Carers are also likely to be women and may be in deteriorating health themselves. They often carry the burden of caring for older relatives and may be suffering from stress-related disorders. Caring for carers should be part of the community care programme to help provide, in collaboration with social services, more effective support for the elderly population. In reality, funds are insufficient and help is seldom available. However, ensuring that the appropriate allowances are applied for, can be one positive way of helping older women.

Urinary incontinence

Incontinence is common among women (see Chapter 16), particularly in those who have had children. Many sufferers never consult their doctor about it, because they find the subject embarrassing and think that doctors regard it as only a minor inconvenience. However, it can be successfully diagnosed and managed in general practice. Asking about it routinely at well women clinics may enable women who find it a disabling problem to be motivated to try a treatment programme.

Health of the Nation targets relating to women

What are they? In 1992, the Department of Health (DoH) set national health targets, most of them to be achieved by the years 2000–2005. These cover coronary heart disease and stroke, mental illness, cancers, HIV/AIDS and sexual health, and accidents.

The targets relating to women are:

1. Coronary heart disease (CHD) and stroke
    Objectives:
    - To reduce death rates for both CHD and stroke in people under 65 by at least 40%.
    - To reduce the death rate for CHD in people aged 65–74 by at least 30% by the year 2000.
    - To reduce the death rate for stroke in people aged 65–74 by at least 40% by the year 2000.

    Health promotion:
    These to be achieved by stopping smoking, taking more exercise, treating hypertension, and improving diet.

2. Mental illness
    Objectives:
    - To improve significantly the health and social functioning of mentally ill people.
    - To reduce the suicide rate by at least 15% by the year 2000 and in those with severe mental illness by at least 33%.

    There were 1500 female suicides in 1992. Asian women are three times more likely than other groups to commit suicide.

    Health promotion:
    These to be achieved by being alert to the causes of suicide, recognizing depression in patients, treating patients with adequate doses of antidepressant, asking about suicidal thoughts.

3. Cancers
    Objectives:
    - To reduce ill health and death caused by lung cancer, breast and cervical cancer, and skin cancer.

Lung cancer
- To reduce the death rate by 15% in women under 75 by the year 2010, from 24.1 per 100 000 to no more than 20.5 per 100 000.
- In addition to the overall reduction in prevalence, at least a third of women smokers to stop smoking at the start of their pregnancy by the year 2000.
- To reduce smoking prevalence among 11–15 year-olds by at least 33% by 1994 from about 8% in 1988 to less than 6%.

Breast cancer
- To reduce the death rate for breast cancer in the population invited for screening by at least 25% by the year 2000 from 95.1 per 100 000 to no more than 71.3 per 100 000

Cervical cancer
- To reduce the incidence of invasive cervical cancer by at least 20% by the year 2000 from 15 per 100 000 in 1986 to no more than 12 per 100 000.

Skin cancer
- To halt the year on year increase in the incidence of skin cancer by 2005.

Health promotion:
These to be done by helping women to stop or reduce smoking, encouraging and offering cervical and breast cancer screening, and discouraging sunbathing and sunburn.

4. HIV/AIDS and sexual health
   Objectives:
   - To reduce the number of unwanted pregnancies.
   - To reduce the incidence of sexually transmitted diseases and HIV infection.
   - To reduce the rate of conceptions among girls under 16 by at least 50% from 9.5 per 1000 to no more than 4.8 per 1000.

Overall, women resident in England have 150 000 abortions each year, most of the unwanted pregnancies resulting from failure to use, or failure of, contraception.

Health promotion:
These to be done by encouraging use of family planning and contraceptive services (including advertising availability of emergency contraception) and use of precautions against sexually transmitted diseases.

5. Accidents
   Objectives:
   - To reduce ill health, disability, and death caused by accidents.

Health promotion:
These to be done by taking care with prescribed drugs when driving, not

drinking and driving, and keeping medicines under lock and key. For over-65s to encourage regular eye checks and checking of safety and lighting in people who have fallen at home.

Priorities for health promotion

Healthy eating

The facts

Diet. Most women in the UK eat too much fat and not enough fruit and vegetables. They have a higher intake of saturated fat as a percentage of energy than men, and a lower average polyunsaturated: saturated fat ratio. Women's dietary fibre intake is also lower than men's. Fruit and vegetables are rich sources of antioxidants (vitamins C, E, and B carotene) and there is increasing evidence that antioxidants may protect against coronary heart disease (CHD). Fruit and vegetable intake is low in Britain and there is a marked social class difference, with lower income families eating fewer green vegetables and fresh fruit, along with more fat, than those with higher incomes. Among women in the UK, there is a strong inverse relationship between obesity and social class which is not found in men. Women with a high waist: hip ratio are at particularly high risk of CHD.

Obesity. Long-term prospective studies amongst women show that as Body Mass Index (BMI) increases the risk of CHD increases. Even mild to moderately overweight women (BMI 25–30) have significantly increased risk of CHD. The influence of obesity on CHD is mainly due to effects on blood pressure, cholesterol, and diabetes. Moreover, there is a synergistic effect between obesity and other CHD risk factors, particularly smoking and diabetes. There has been a large increase in the proportion of obese women in Britain (BMI over 30) from 8% in 1980 to 16% in 1992. 45% of women now have a BMI over 25, i.e. are overweight or obese (OPCS 1992). The increased prevalence of obesity is due partly to increased intake of dietary fat and partly to increasingly inactive lifestyles.

Cholesterol. Below the age of 50, cholesterol levels in women are lower than in men, but in older age groups the majority of people with high cholesterol levels are women. By the age of 55, the majority of women have cholesterol levels over 6.5 mmol/1, and as many as a third have levels over 7.8 mmol/1. Much of the high total cholesterol levels in women is accounted for by higher high density lipoprotein (HDL) levels – the protective cholesterol fraction – and this may be why CHD is less common in women than men. The sex difference in HDL levels reduces after middle age; post-menopausal women have an increase in total and low density lipoprotein (LDL) cholesterol and a relative fall in HDL levels.

Research shows that lowering blood cholesterol levels in men reduces their risk of CHD. However, there are no primary prevention trials involving women, so there is no actual evidence on which to base advice on what is a

---

Box 2.1 *Managing moderate/severe obesity (Freeman and Newman 1994)*

1. Take a long-term view
2. Try and stop further weight gain and discourage 'yo-yo' dieting
3. Set realistic goals for weight loss (e.g. a woman weighing 20 stone needs to lose 1 lb a week for 84 continuous weeks if she is to get down to 14 stone). It is easier to set short-term goals with small steps
4. Treat medical complications
5. Concentrate on establishing different patterns of eating rather than new patterns of dieting

---

safe level of cholesterol in older women and when to intervene to reduce levels for CHD protection. For women with established CHD there is now evidence that reducing cholesterol levels reduces the risk of major coronary events from the Scandinavian Simavastatin Survival Trial (1994). In this study the number of women involved was too small to show a significant reduction in mortality though this was found to be so in the whole sample.

What do we want women to do?

Healthy diet. We want women to eat a healthy diet, whatever that is. A cynic, with some justification, might claim that the experts' opinions on what is a healthy diet have changed over the years. Currently we want women to eat:

(1) less overall fat and especially less saturated fat, e.g. substituting olive oil for other oils in cooking;
(2) regular meals rather than snacking and grazing as these snacks are likely to be highly processed with a high fat content;
(3) more fresh fruit and vegetables;
(4) less red meat and more fish and white meat;
(5) an increased intake of fibre.

Controlling obesity. Dieting *per se*, though practised at some time by up to 70% of the female population, does not seem to work, with 98% of women having regained the weight they lost and often gaining more within 2 years of the weight loss. In recent years, commercial and self-help weight loss programmes (e.g. Weight Watchers) have become very popular. These groups have the potential to offer a comprehensive approach to weight loss with personal involvement and ongoing support. However, they often encourage unrealistic expectations, sometimes through misleading advertising. Moreover, there is very little published research data evaluating popular diets and weight loss programmes, especially their long-term effects.

There is also substantial evidence suggesting that weight fluctuation ('yo-yo dieting') is associated with increased morbidity and mortality. In the Framingham cohort, weight variability in women was associated with a 38% increase in CHD morbidity and 55% increase in CHD mortality. The effects of unintentional weight loss were not separated from intentional weight loss in this analysis, so it is not possible to conclude that dieting is positively harmful to obese individuals, though it may not carry any health benefits.

Very low calorie diets (VLCDs) provide less than 800 calories a day as a liquid diet, and contain sufficient protein, vitamins, and minerals for health. They are usually reserved for people who are at least 30% overweight and can be dangerous in mildly obese people due to excessive protein losses. They should always be administered under medical supervision. In women they produce weight losses of up to 20 kg in 3–4 months (two to three times more than more conventional diets). Unfortunately, women who lose weight on VLCDs tend to regain as much as 50% of their lost weight in the year following treatment, even if they successfully modify their lifestyle.

Exercise is an integral part of standard weight reduction programmes, though even prolonged strenuous activity will only 'burn off' a relatively modest number of calories. Psychological factors may be more important here: every time a person is active this reinforces a change in lifestyle. People should be encouraged to chose activities they enjoy, even if these are not particularly strenuous, and to be as active as possible to encourage cognitive change. Epidemiological data now suggests that even modest activity may have considerable health benefits.

As well as increasing the level of physical activity, weight reduction programmes focus on the modification of eating habits. The emphasis is on changing eating behaviour to restrict calorie absorption as well as increasing energy expenditure through exercise. **Behaviour treatment** has been extensively researched and several 'user friendly' treatment manuals have been produced (e.g. the LEARN programme, Brownell 1994). The data suggest that while behaviour treatment is effective in the short term, the relapse rate is disappointingly high.

Drug treatments for obesity should only be considered for patients who fail to lose weight or maintain their weight loss following conventional therapy and should always be used as part of a programme of calorie restriction and exercise. It is generally recommended that medication is only prescribed under specialist supervision. A number of drugs are licensed for the treatment of obesity; dexfenfluramine and fluoxetine are both serotonin re-uptake inhibitors and are the least likely to cause problems of abuse and dependence. Both these drugs lead to good short-term weight loss, but weight gain recurs on cessation of the drug unless there are permanent changes in lifestyle and eating behaviour.

For severe obesity, in addition to the above, **surgery** may need to be considered. Jaw wiring has the advantage of being temporary, but weight loss during jaw wiring tends to be regained in the months following removal of the wire. Gastric restriction (stomach stapling or banding) or gastric bypass operations are both possibilities. Both are major operations with long-term side-effects, but the weight loss achieved is maintained. Operative mortality is less than 0.5%, whereas mortality due to severe obesity is between three to 12 times greater than normal, so there may be an argument in favour of surgery, especially when the psychological benefits are considered.

What role for primary health care and does intervention work?

Most influence on diet comes from national food policy, price of food, advertising, general education, and cultural influences. Giving information about a healthy diet is probably poorly done in primary care except in very general terms. Women at high risk of CHD, with known raised lipoproteins and cholesterol, can be especially targeted with appropriate low-fat diets, and where indicated, lipid-lowering medication.

There has been little evidence to show that encouragement by GPs and practice nurses to eat more healthily is effective, although the most recent results from the OXCHECK study were more encouraging, with evidence of dietary advice being heeded (ICRF 1995). Rather than simply advising women to reduce the fat content of their diet from 40% to 35%, time should be taken to explain how to reduce fat in terms of actual meals. Very little is known about what goes on within households (Dowler 1994). Food provision is still mostly a woman's task but her partner and children may also have strong opinions on what they want to eat. Women may simply not be able to buy healthy foods because the money is not available. For many women on low incomes, income supplements are too low to allow them to purchase a regular, healthy diet.

Exercise

The facts

Exercise is good, but why, and are there any disadvantages? Prevention of obesity, protection from osteoporosis, reduction of stress as well as reduced risk of developing cardiovascular disease, non-insulin-dependent diabetes mellitus, colon cancer, and possibly breast cancer are some of the benefits cited (Fentem 1994). Most of the studies on physical exercise compare physically active men with their sedentary counterparts and few provide information about women. Despite their inadequate representation in the research literature it is thought that non-white men and women of all racial and ethnic groups seem to accrue the same relative benefits from activity as white men (Powell 1996).

Skeletal muscle, tendon, and connective tissue functions are enhanced by exercise, resulting in increased stamina with increased capacity for work and reduction in the risk of injury. Exercise also helps joint function with improved range of movement, lubrication of joints, and maintenance of flexibility. At any age, including the elderly, some exercise results in people being able to work harder, longer, and with less effort. This is also true of the physically disabled where involvement in some exercise enables them to remain independent for longer, continue working, and avoid institutional care.

The best evidence for benefit of exercise concerns reduction of CHD, with men who exercise having half the risk of the sedentary. In contrast, in the few studies at present there is insufficient evidence to conclude that physical inactivity is an independent risk factor for women. But some of the known risk factors for CHD in women such as hypertension, obesity, non-insulin-dependent diabetes, and lipoprotein levels are modified favourably by physical activity. Total cholesterol is unaffected by exercise from cross-sectional and longitudinal studies but it does have an effect on HDL cholesterol among both endurance-trained women and those taking more moderate amounts of exercise such as walking. Accompanied weight loss produces more marked changes in the lipoproteins. The mechanism of effect is still under debate but may include increased activity of the enzyme lipoprotein lipase. The exercise needed to affect CHD has to use the body's large muscle groups. Unfortunately, the activity sustained during a normal day's work appears to be insufficient to confer CHD benefit, though getting women who do little activity during their everyday lives to increase it can confer other benefits in, for example, mobility. Insulin sensitivity and glucose tolerance have both been shown to improve with exercise in laboratory studies which may be the mechanism of benefit on non-insulin-dependent diabetes and in obesity.

Regular weight-bearing exercise, by maintaining and increasing mineral content of bone, prevents osteoporosis and the potential for fractures of the vertebrae, hip, and wrist. Women of all ages, from 20–80, who exercise at least three times a week, have a higher bone density than those who are sedentary. Exercise in women starts to have a negative effect on bone density only when it is of such quantity and frequency to produce amenorrhoea and low oestrogen levels.

How much do women exercise? In Britain and other developed nations less than 50% of adults are regularly active. The Allied Dunbar National Fitness Survey showed that one-third of men and two-thirds of women would find it difficult to sustain walking at a moderate pace (3 mph up a 5° slope). Less women than men participate in sports and other physical activities, but the gap has narrowed over time. In 1993–94, 57% of women and 72% of men in the UK took part in at least one activity in the 4 weeks before being interviewed for the General Household Survey. Walking was the most popular physical activity for women with keep fit/yoga and swimming being the next most popular. In 1993, 20% of women had not taken part in any activity of a moderate or vigorous level in the preceding 4 weeks (OPCS 1993).

What role for primary health care and does intervention work?

We should be careful in using the word 'sport' when promoting exercise to women. It may remind them of negative experiences at school which have a strong influence on the way they approach physical activity as they get older. Women's own leisure time is rarely a priority within their daily schedule. Emphasis on weight loss and looking and feeling good may help in promoting exercise. The younger the woman starts to take regular exercise the more likely she is to continue into later life (Rhodes 1994). Some local authorities allow GPs to prescribe use of exercise facilities free for patients who would benefit from them. Advertising exercise facilities in the waiting room and running exercise classes at the surgery have all been tried, but with minimal evaluation.

As with dietary changes, promoting exercise involves multi agency support if it is to have an impact. The media gives very little attention to women's sport so it is perhaps not surprising that women see sport primarily as a male activity. Any campaign to encourage women to take part in exercise programmes should use women to promote it. 'Friends for fitness' was a successful campaign run by Thames Television which promoted the social aspect of exercise and did not depend on facilities. The message was to find a friend and get fit. Seven thousand women took part, and 8 months after the promotion 50% of the women were still doing some sort of exercise,

What do we want women to do?

We would like to encourage women to increase their levels of physical activity in any way they choose. No one knows the 'right' level of exercise. The latest recommendations from the NIH Consensus Development Panel on Physical Activity and Cardiovascular Health (1996) suggest at least 30 minutes of activity of moderate intensity on most, preferably all, days of the week. The phrase 'physical activity' rather than 'exercise' was used so that most people could incorporate this into their daily lives. But even getting women to walk rather than take the car, walk upstairs rather than take the lift, and walk fast rather than slowly are all improvements on no exercise or activity. Unless exercise is enjoyable and can be included in a woman's normal daily routine it is unlikely to be sustained regularly.

Alcohol

The facts

It is now thought that light to moderate alcohol intake confers a protective effect against CHD, ischaemic stroke, and cholesterol gallstones. These benefits become clear in post-menopausal women. High levels of alcohol intake are associated with serious health and social problems. Hypertension, liver cirrhosis, cardiovascular disease, cancers of the mouth, pharynx, and oesophagus are all dose-related diseases. Heavy, long-term consumption is also associated with mental illness, neurological disease, and liver cancer. Some studies have shown a link between breast cancer and alcohol consumption, but no causal relationship has yet emerged. Drinking in pregnancy, other than at very low levels, is also associated with particular risks to fetal and early infant development and there may be an increased risk of miscarriage.

Women who are heavy drinkers are more likely to become victims of alcohol-related aggression such as rape. Attempts to quantify the effects of heavy drinking in women on marital breakdown have been made, and there is some evidence that, not surprisingly, the divorce rate is very high (nine out of ten marriages end in divorce compared to one in three when the man is alcoholic) (Bigby 1995).

Women of all ages drink less than men in general. The GHS survey (1993) showed that 14% had not had a drink during the past 12 months compared with 7% of men. 58% drank less than 8 units per week and one in eight women drank more than 14 units per week. Only 2% of women drank over 35 units per week.

Although alcohol affects women and men in similar ways there are some important differences. However, research data in this area is very limited. The prevalence of most alcohol-related diseases is much lower in women than men in Britain because women drink less. Women weigh less than men on average, and when the gender differences in tissue concentrate of water and rates of alcohol metabolism are considered, as well as possible increased vulnerability to tissue damage at equivalent alcohol levels, women should be advised to drink less than men.

What role for primary health care and does intervention work?

Most doctors are pessimistic about being able to influence and help excessive drinkers, yet there is evidence that as many as two-thirds respond well to treatment. Drinking habits are often hard to break and the patient needs to be highly motivated to change her drinking pattern. Ambivalence can be addressed by asking her to draw up a balance sheet of the pros and cons of continued drinking. She should then set realistic goals for changing her lifestyle. The best way to do this is probably to aim for achievable short-term goals at first (e.g. 3 weeks abstinence) and then to report back to the doctor.

The first approach for help is often made by the spouse and it may be a good idea to involve the spouse in consultations, partly to give the true picture and also to help the family find a way of life that does not involve drinking. Laboratory tests (GGT, MCV, and blood alcohol levels) are useful, objective means of monitoring progress. Regular appointments to review progress and set agreed goals are essential. It is often useful to ask the patient to keep a drinking diary as this helps her to identify circumstances in which she is likely to drink, to make changes, and to check progress. Patients and their families may find self-help guides, as well as self-help groups, useful. The first 6 months of progress will usually give a good indication of longer-term prognosis. Relapses are very common: learning from relapses and developing strategies to prevent further recurrences are all part of recovery.

What do we want women to do?

The latest guidelines on sensible drinking were compiled by a Department of Health Inter-Departmental Working Group (1995). The advice is based on daily rather than weekly alcohol consumption. This was thought to give a better indication as to how much an individual should drink on a single occasion to avoid excessive drinking bouts and their attendant health and social risks. For women, the health benefit in terms of mortality and morbidity from all causes relates to post-menopausal women and the major part of this can be obtained by drinking 1 unit of alcohol per day, with the maximum health advantage lying between 1–2 units per day. Regular consumption of 2–3 units per day does not accrue any significant health risk. However, consistently drinking 3 or more units per day is not advised because of the progressive health risk it carries. For men, the maximum health advantage lies between 1–2 units per day; regular intake of 3–4 units per day does not accrue any significant health risk.

The health benefits are more evident from daily drinking, and may be lost with binge drinking. After an episode of heavy drinking, it is advisable to refrain from drinking for 48 hours to allow tissues to recover.

Pregnant women and those trying to conceive should not drink more than 1–2 units of alcohol once or twice week, and should avoid episodes of intoxication.

Smoking

The facts

Smoking kills over 30 000 women a year in the UK. It is now the most preventable cause of illness in women. Smoking has declined in adults but this decline has been slower in women, particularly women who are at social disadvantage. Women in manual socio-economic groups are one and a half times more likely to be smokers than those in non-manual groups and those in unskilled manual work are three times more likely to be smokers than those in professional work. With the stresses of poverty, unemployment, and child care, smoking can be seen by women as the one luxury in their lives and each cigarette 'helps women to cope with the demands made upon her' (Amos 1994).

Both female and male smoking has continued to decline over the last two decades. The prevalence for women was 42% in 1972 (for men, 52%) and 28% in 1992 (for men, 29%). In the younger age groups things are not so encouraging. Cigarette smoking is now more common amongst girls than boys. In 1996, by the age of 16, 30% of girls and 26% of boys were regular smokers (McCMiller and Plant 1996). The prevalence is the same in the 16–19 age group and although there are various theories put forward to explain this we do not really know why. Once women start smoking they are less likely to give up. Teenage magazines still have photographs of popular role models, like Madonna, smoking. Girls are concerned about their body image and think that smoking will help keep them thin. Much cigarette advertising is targeting women, even using 'slim' in the brand name. Girls whose family and friends smoke are more likely to take up smoking. Women smokers, like men, have increased mortality rates from CHD, lung cancer, chronic obstructive lung disease, and peripheral vascular disease. There are also some problems caused by women smoking that are specific to women (Batten 1996).

Menstruation. There appears to be an association between smoking and abnormal menstrual patterns though PMT is not affected.

Menopause. The menopause occurs 2–3 years earlier in smokers. Smoking is also a risk factor for loss of bone density and osteoporosis.

Cervical cancer. Female smokers have up to a four times higher risk of developing this cancer and duration of smoking is also important.

Oral contraception (combined pill). There is a tenfold increased risk of heart attack, stroke, or other cardiovascular disease in women who take the pill and smoke and this is even more marked in women over 45.

Pregnancy. Smoking can reduce fertility; there is an increased risk of miscarriage, complications during pregnancy, stillbirth, and perinatal mortality as well as low birth weight. Babies of mothers who smoke are lighter than those of non-smokers. Pregnancy provides a strong incentive to give up smoking (Batten 1996). Recent evidence shows that women are more likely to quit at this time if they are older (over 30), have a partner who does not smoke, are of higher social class, and have higher educational levels. One in four women will stop smoking during pregnancy and 40% will cut down consumption prior to or during a pregnancy, but there is a high relapse rate in the quitters with 40% having resumed smoking 3 months postpartum.

What role for primary health care and does intervention work?

There is good evidence that women know that smoking is dangerous even if they cannot exactly quantify the risk. Most but not all women want to give up smoking. There is little value in just telling women to stop smoking without taking their personal views and circumstances into consideration. They need practical help and support. There is a balance of risk and benefits – more money in the pocket, reduced risk of disease, smelling fresher, improved taste, against the perceived benefits of weight control, pleasure, and relaxation. There is evidence that simple cessation advice from GPs during routine consultations is more effective than no advice for some smokers; in a trial in general practice, cessation rates at 1 year were 5% for the brief advice group compared with 1% in the non-intervention control group (Russell *et al.* 1979). Meta-analyses have shown that nicotine replacement as patches, gum, or spray doubles the cessation rate to 10% at 1 year when compared with placebo as long as there is continued support from doctors and/or nurses (Silagy *et al.* 1994). Nicotine replacement is especially effective in heavy smokers. Relapses are common but there is evidence that the relapse should not be seen as a failure but rather a stage on the road to success. None of these studies have looked at women specifically. The results from smoking cessation groups are not very encouraging. However, women may be attracted by groups linked to their workplace, particularly if the cessation message is directed at their level. Smoke-free environments at work encourage women to stop smoking and support them in their efforts (Jacobson 1994).

Banning tobacco advertising would probably be the most effective measure to reduce smoking nationally. In Norway, tobacco advertising was banned in 1975 and it is now one of the few developed countries where significant falls in smoking rates have occurred and girls smoke less than boys.

When asked, most doctors and nurses say they need more training to help people give up smoking. When trying to help women stop smoking it is worth remembering that not all smokers will be receptive to help at all times. A useful model is to see giving up smoking in terms of a series of stages:

Stage 1: precontemplation – the woman is not thinking of quitting and could be called the 'happy smoker';
Stage 2: contemplation – the woman is thinking of quitting, the 'unhappy smoker';
Stage 3: preparation – she is thinking of quitting within the next month;
Stage 4: ready for action;

Stage 5: action;
Stage 6: learning how to stay stopped;
Stage 7: maintenance – staying stopped in the longer term.

Possible interventions that can be instigated in general practice are: brief advice including setting a quit date, written information, nicotine replacement, follow-up appointments to discuss smoking, and the use of carbon monoxide monitors. None of these interventions have been evaluated in a gender specific way.

The Health Education Authority (HEA) looked at smoking in pregnancy and issued guidance for all health professionals supporting pregnant women who want to stop smoking (1993). They identified the approaches most likely to succeed and these included: one-to-one contact; recognizing and addressing personal and social circumstances; assessing motivation; tailoring intervention to individual need; offering support and follow-up; offering alternative approaches e.g. community based projects; trying again after a failed first attempt, and use of carbon monoxide monitors.

What do we want women to do?
Not to start smoking;
To give up or reduce if they are smokers;
To give up during pregnancy.

CHD prevention – are women getting a fair deal?

Health professionals, the public, and the media tend to label CHD as a male problem. There is evidence that women with CHD are referred later for medical treatment and diagnostic tests. Health professionals may also be less likely to offer women advice on CHD prevention and women themselves may not see health messages about CHD as being relevant to them (Sharp 1994). The major risk factors for CHD – smoking, high cholesterol, and raised blood pressure – are the same for women as for men although women seem to tolerate the risks better as their risk of CHD is less than men. The potential for prevention is great. Women need to know about CHD and be aware of the risks. Health professionals need to be more aware of CHD among women and training for medical and nursing staff should include the possibilities for prevention and the modification of risk factors for women. Smoking is the most preventable cause of CHD. It is becoming much more common amongst low-income women who find it hardest to give up. Girls are much more likely to smoke than boys. Strategies need to be developed to tackle these areas. Tobacco advertising should be banned. Women's magazines could promote anti-smoking in their fashion, editorial, and advertising space (Sharp 1994). Promotion of exercise from an early age and as a part of long-term education is needed to produce positive attitudes among girls and women to physical activity. Diets need to be improved as, on average, women eat less fruit and vegetables and too much fat. This is particularly the case for poorer women who feel they cannot afford a healthier diet.

More research needs to be done on CHD in women generally, as most of the data comes from men. We need to know how to motivate changes in behaviour amongst girls and women. Research is needed on the benefits and risks of lowering cholesterol levels in healthy women and on how to manage high cholesterol levels in women. Also, more research is needed into the effects of HRT on CHD risks. The present consensus is that HRT, both oestrogen and combined preparations, is cardioprotective with claims of up to 50% reduction in risk of CHD. Other risks and benefits need assessing when an individual woman decides on whether to take long-term HRT as preventive treatment. Women with known CHD, or a strong family history of CHD, should be amongst those targeted to consider HRT for prevention rather than just as a treatment of menopausal symptoms.

Organization of services

Money for health promotion within practices now has to be applied for locally and applications are assessed by a local health promotion committee. Details will therefore vary around the country but a bid for monies can be based on this chapter. Organization of health promotion in each practice should be based on an assessment of the needs of the individual practice population. A practice profile of woman patients, including age, socio-economic status, and ethnicity is the first step and should take account of the practice turnover. For example, if there is a large, ethnic minority population of young women who do not speak English, resources need to be diverted into areas such as contraception and antenatal care, and this might include leaflets in the relevant language and interpreters/liaison officers. In East London, it was found that, contrary to the beliefs of GPs in the area, such women were enthusiastic about cervical screening once they understood the purpose of the test, and these kinds of consultations could provide a forum for wider aspects of health promotion (Naish et al. 1994). There is a subtle way in which people weigh up the desirability of behaviour change and 'trade off' positive and negative aspects of health-related behaviours. Local knowledge of the population and the opportunities for one-to-one interaction which exist in the general practice setting are extremely important resources in providing health promotion and advice (Backett et al. 1994).

Who should provide the service?

A national study looking at CHD prevention reported that individual members of the primary health care team had their own distinct areas of health promotion activity, but the division was not a result of coherent planning. It seemed to be more a product of the contract which devolved the work to the practice nurse and hindered the broader, team-based approach to planning and delivery of health promotion in relation to the needs of the practice population (Calnan et al. 1994). Time is an important factor. More health promotion is achieved when appointments are extended from 7.5 minutes to 10 minutes, and shortage of time was cited as a major factor by GPs in their failure to realize their potential in health promotion (Wilson *et al.* 1992). This may account for health checks being seen as the remit of the practice nurse, who is perceived to have more time to offer patients. However, this may not always be true, as often the nurse has shorter consultations than the GP. It may be a question of feeling someone else should be doing it, not oneself. Health promotion is seen as an integral part of the health visitor's role, although traditionally she has focused on the under 5's. With the latest changes in health promotion reimbursement, local practice priorities can now be based on local needs. However, very little has really been done to explore these avenues in proper scientific ways.

Methods of delivering the services

Opportunistic consultations

Seventy per cent of patients are seen every 3 years and 90% every 5 years. For women this figure may be even higher. These consultations provide an opportunity for health promotion and, in particular, a chance to target high-risk groups. When people are invited to attend special clinics or health checks, Hart's 'inverse care law' comes into play; it tends to be the frequent consulters who turn up, whilst those most at risk and likely to benefit more fail to attend.

Clinics

The well woman clinic. This is an appropriate place to promote women's health in general practice. Consultations can be spaced more widely, either at 10 or 15 minute intervals and, by the very name of the clinic, women understand that they do not need to be ill to attend and so will not be accused of 'wasting the doctor's time'. Women have been interviewed on their views as to the desirability of GP intervention in their lifestyle habits (Stott and Pill 1990). Most respondents expected issues to be relevant to their presenting problem. The well woman clinic may meet this expectation. Having more time for each consultation may improve the quality of care (Howie *et al.* 1991). Howie found that there was more patient satisfaction and more health promotion being done when longer consultations were offered. Well woman clinics are usually staffed by women; another factor that may encourage patients to attend. Patients can be given the choice to see either a doctor or nurse. Issues such as contraception, period problems, menopausal symptoms, problems with fertility, etc. can be addressed. In a well woman clinic set-up in general practice, whatever women consult for, time is available to look at wider health needs – for example, a young woman requiring contraception can be advised about safer sex and risks of HIV, follow-up can be offered to the woman who is trying to give up smoking, and women can be called up who may have experienced an early menopause following hysterectomy.

Teenage clinics. These have had limited success in general practice probably due to the perception the teenagers have of their doctor's surgery. How do we make our practice attractive and available as a provider of health care to teenagers? The clinics that have been successful often have a specific area set aside for the young people which provides loud music and facilities for making drinks, such as are found at the Brook Advisory Centres. A separate entrance is an advantage, with the clinic staffed with welcoming people providing an informal atmosphere. The 'Hint' project in Nottingham (Daniel 1992) provides a model of holistic health care reflecting the needs of young people. The centre which the teenagers have helped to design is a large area providing a wide range of facilities, including counselling rooms, treatment rooms, nursery, kitchen, arts and craft area, cafe, gym, etc. These facilities are obviously not possible in general practice but some aspects can be incorporated. A number of the targets set by the *Health of the Nation* document (DoH 1996) are particularly applicable to young people. A GP in London invited all the 16-year-olds in the practice to attend a birthday consultation to try and give them access to the health services that were on offer (Donovan 1988). There was only a 50% take-up of the offer and others have had an even poorer response. Other studies are currently in progress to evaluate teenage clinics. Clinics may not be appropriate for all practices but we still need to avoid frightening off young people when they do come to the practice. Once they attend, the opportunities to offer health promotion do exist.

Contraception/family planning clinics. If a practice advertises family planning clinics, women may consider that there are doctors and nurses who are specifically interested and trained in this area. Eighty per cent of all women attend their general practice for family planning advice rather than the community family planning clinic, and with cuts in resources, more women may go to their doctor as the choice in family planning services no longer exists. The advantages of a clinic can be that staff are switched on to the subject and so can offer a comprehensive service looking at wider issues of health relevant to contraception.

Menopause clinics. These clinics are described in detail elsewhere in the book (p. 366) but it is worth mentioning them as an opportunity to give health promotion advice.

Groups

Groups have been tried in primary care for weight reduction, smoking cessation, and even exercise with varying and limited success. Participants need to be highly motivated and group leaders experienced.

Information

Leaflets

The HEA produce leaflets on a limited number of conditions and the Family Planning Association produce quality leaflets on all aspects of contraception. These can be displayed in the waiting areas but it is also probably worth having some leaflets of a personal nature, such as incontinence or sexually transmitted

Fig 2.1

Dietary quiz

Circle the answer you choose – all answers are listed on the board in the waiting room. You are welcome to discuss any queries with the doctor or nurse.

1. Cholesterol in the diet is the most important factor to consider when wanting to lower blood cholesterol levels   True/False/Don't know

2. Polyunsaturated fats and monosaturated fats are both advised
   True/False/Don't know

3. Foods labelled 'low fat' are advised   True/False/Don't know

4. Foods which include vegetable oils in place of animal fats are advised
   True/False/Don't know

5. A vegetable oil containing over 50% coconut oil is recommended
   True/False/Don't know

6. Foods containing 'hydrogenated oil' are recommended
   True/False/Don't know

7. A cheese containing 25% fat is recommended   True/False/Don't know

8. Any margarine is advised in preference to butter as it is lower in fat
   True/False/Don't know

9. Oily fish should be eaten three times a week   True/False/Don't know

10. People with moderately raised cholesterol levels can eat up to six eggs a
    week providing dietary fat is low   True/False/Don't know

11. Dietary fibre is only good for the bowels and specific types of fibre do not
    reduce blood cholesterol levels   True/False/Don't know

12. Greek yoghurt contains as much fat as double cream
    True/False/Don't know

13. Brie and Camembert–full fat cheeses–can be recommended to people with
    raised blood cholesterol   True/False/Don't know

14. Lower fat dairy products, such as skimmed milk, contain as much calcium as
    the full fat alternative   True/False/Don't know

15. Vegetarian diets are recommended for all because they are always low in fat
    and high in fibre   True/False/Don't know

16. Dietary fat restriction is of benefit to the whole population because calories will
    fall and it is desirable for everyone to lose weight   True/False/Don't know

(Oxfordshire Community Dietitians)

Fig 2.1 *continued*

Answers

1. This is FALSE. The most important factor to consider when wanting to lower blood cholesterol levels is reducing saturated fats in the diet.

2. TRUE. Olive oil is a monounsaturated fat. Polyunsaturated fats and monounsaturated fats both help reduce cholesterol levels in the blood.

3. FALSE. Foods which are labelled 'low fat' will contain 50% less fat than the original product but they might be the 'wrong' sort of fat, i.e. saturated fats.

4. FALSE. There are some vegetable oils, notably coconut oil, which are saturated fat and often used in blended vegetable oils. Sunflower and rapeseed oil are unsaturated fats and recommended.

5. FALSE. As in No. 4–coconut oil is a saturated fat.

6. FALSE. Hydrogenated oils are saturated fats. Remember that if you keep reheating polyunsaturated oil in a chip pan it will become hydrogenated.

7. TRUE. Hard cheeses like Cheddar and Double Gloucester contain 30–50% fat. Edam contains 25% and is therefore lower in fat although it is saturated fat.

8. FALSE. Margarines can be just as high in fat as butter–particularly hard margarines, you have to check the labels to see if the fats contained in the product are unsaturated.

9. NOT KNOWN. It is believed that oily fish is useful in lowering cholesterol levels but it is not known how often it should be eaten. Fish oils contribute to healthy eating.

10. TRUE. Eggs contain cholesterol but reducing cholesterol in the diet will have little effect on blood cholesterol levels–lowering your saturated fat intake will help reduce blood cholesterol levels.

11. FALSE. Dietary fibre, particularly oats, pulses, beans and peas, and fruit containing pectin (like blackcurrants, plums, apricots, etc.) probably help reduce blood cholesterol levels.

12. FALSE. Greek yoghurt contains 10% fat, while double cream contains 40% fat.

13. TRUE. They are both fairly low in fat, 20–25%, so can be included in a low fat diet.

14. TRUE. If anything, lower fat dairy products contain more calcium than full fat alternatives.

15. FALSE. Although the message is increase your fibre and lower your fat intake, not all vegetarian food is recommended.

16. FALSE. If you are normal weight you need to replace the lost fat with carbohydrates or you will lose weight.

diseases, in the toilets where they can be accessed privately. However, the distribution and availability can be a problem. Many are produced by drug companies and may not cover the subject matter in the way that the practice would like. Many have not been evaluated so we are uncertain of their efficacy. With computer technology, leaflets can be written 'in-house' and printed to a reasonable standard.

A recent survey organized by the Family Planning Association Contraceptive Education Service stated that 89% of women wanted to receive both spoken and written information but that only 38% received any information in writing (Contraceptive Education Service 1996). If this finding is true for health promotion generally, then we should be providing leaflets more often when giving health advice. It has been estimated that only about 30% of the content of any consultation with a health worker is remembered and the backup of leaflets is likely to reinforce any health promotion message.

Posters

Time can be spent in producing health messages on moveable boards which can be changed between waiting-rooms. These can be regularly updated. Patients say they read and remember the subject of waiting-room posters. They can increase awareness of health promotion issues (Ward and Hawthorne 1994). Some examples are shown in Figs 2.1–2.3. Practices can make seasonal changes to these boards and respond to topical events such as pill scares. Posters can advertise the recommended use of folic acid prior to pregnancy, emergency contraception availability, and the pros and cons of HRT. When specific clinics are in progress there is the opportunity of relating the health education boards to the clinic, such as 'What do you know about taking your pill? A quiz' at a contraception clinic.

Patient health records

The parent-held record for child health has proved very popular and effective. Some practices have issued cards for women telling them about cervical screening results. An extension of this idea would be the provision of patient-held records in the area of women's health but this is yet to be developed and evaluated.

Educational videos

One of the problems of many of the videos that are currently available is that they are funded by drug companies and are either overtly or covertly promotional. There is a need for well-produced, well-researched, independent videos for women to watch in the surgery or to borrow. Interactive videos for women on issues relating to the menopause, breast cancer choices, and uterine problems have been developed and evaluated in the USA, and studies are underway to evaluate them here, though it is likely that CD Rom will be the medium for future information.

Fig 2.2. *Example of health education board on the menopause*

Menopause
HRT – to take or not to take

- Many women have no problem during this time but others get a variety of symptoms which can vary from **MINOR** to **VERY UNPLEASANT**.

- Some women notice *cycle changes* in their late 30's or early 40's *(pre-menopausal)*.

- This is likely to be due to *hormone changes*. Around the time of the menopause *(peri-menopause)* a number of symptoms can be distressing; **VAGINAL DRYNESS, HOT FLUSHES, NIGHT SWEATS, INSOMNIA, LACK OF CONFIDENCE, MOOD SWINGS, LOSS OF SEX DRIVE –**

  these symptoms, if they occur, can continue for a number of years.

- The Menopause is the moment periods stop. A year after this is often referred to as the *post-menopause*.

- **HRT** *(hormone replacement therapy)* is very useful in controlling symptoms in the *peri-menopausal* years, although some women do get side-effects.

- There are few risks associated with taking **HRT** for up to 5 years.

- **PREVENTION OF HEART DISEASE AND OSTEOPOROSIS** (brittle bones): Taking **HRT** for 5–10 years probably reduces the risk of these problems which do increase as you get older. However if you take **HRT** for more than 10 years there is likely to be increased risk of breast cancer. The **BENEFITS** of **HRT** need to be weighed against the **RISKS**. We are happy to discuss these with you at any time or at the Well Woman Clinic on Tuesdays.

- **BOOKS** which may be helpful:

  The change: women, ageing and the menopause by Germaine Greer

  Menopause without medicine by L. Ojeda

  Dr Miriam Stoppard's practical guide to the menopause

Telephone helpline

Practices could advertise their telephone number as being a helpline to patients. This would be of particular benefit to women using or needing contraception as such queries can usually be dealt with quickly and clearly.

Fig 2.3 *Example of practice leaflet or health education board*

What do you know about taking your pill?

A quiz on the combined pill

1. What would you do if you missed a second-to-last pill in your packet?

2. When will you start your first packet of pills?

3. What would you do if you vomited 6 hours after taking your pill?

4. If you get some bleeding while taking your pills, are you contraceptively safe?

5. How many hours are you allowed to forget your pill before taking extra contraceptive precautions?

6. If you forget your pill, how many days do you need to take extra contraceptive precautions?

7. If you want to delay a 'period', what would you do?

8. If you start your packet on a Sunday, which day of the week will you start your next packet?

9. If you had to choose the most unsafe pills to forget in the packet, would it be Day 1, Day 8, or Day 20?

10. Does the pill protect you from HIV infection?

Answers attached

Please feel free to discuss any queries with the doctor or nurse

By advertising the number on the notice boards or on practice leaflets it gives women permission to use the services in this way. The nurses, if trained appropriately, can often manage these calls without causing overload for the doctors.

Library

A few practices do have libraries open to patients but they are an underdeveloped resource. Libraries can provide information for patients as well as for staff but are only of use if they are regularly updated and easy to access.

Training

In-house training within the primary health care team has been a very neglected area. Training is by no means specific to women's health, but by focusing on this area, protocols can be written and agreed with all members to help ensure consensus on preventive health care.

It is important that training is available to receptionists so that they can be aware of health issues that they themselves can promote. For example, the receptionist who is trained to pick up the emergency contraception request when it may be only alluded to by the patient can be pivotal in preventing an unwanted pregnancy. The nurse who is trained to listen actively to women when they present for routine appointments may pick up on other important issues relevant to health promotion.

Community nurse courses designed for health visitors, district nurses, and practice nurses are available in most areas and these offer training in health promotion. Other modular courses cover smear-taking, women's health screening, family planning, and focus on the wider issues of holistic health care. 'Nurse specialist' courses are being developed, for example, in the field of family planning, the ENB A08, to train nurses to become independent practitioners in their specialty. The training undertakes to ensure that the students act appropriately within their role following frameworks of care and protocols, and to acknowledge the limits of their expertize.

GPs perceive a lack of expertize amongst themselves in practising preventive medicine although it is known that the therapeutic power of the doctor is greater than appreciated and promoting health can be achieved with the skills they already possess (Davies 1991). Many opportunities exist for exposure to health promotion ideas both during vocational training and subsequent PGEA courses, but practical training in effective interventions is very limited.

References and further reading

ABC of Alcohol, 3rd edn. *British Medical Journal.*

Amos, A. (1994). Smoking patterns among girls and women. Why do they smoke? In *Coronary heart disease: are women special?* (ed. I. Sharp). 71–80. National Forum for Coronary Heart Disease Prevention, London.

Backett, K., Davison, C., and Mullen, K. (1994). Lay evaluation of health and healthy lifestyles: evidence from three studies. *British Journal of General Practice*, **44**, 277–80.

Baron, J.A., Gleason, R., Crowe, B., and Mann, J.I. (1990). Preliminary trial of the effect of general practice based nutritional advice. *British Journal of General Practice*, **40**, 137–41.

Batten, L. (1996). Smoking and women. *Maternal and Child Health*, **21**, No. 6, 147–9.

Bigby, J. and Cyr, M. (1995). Alcohol and drug abuse. *Primary care of women* (ed. K.J. Carlson and S.A. Eisenstat). Mosby, St. Louis.

Brown, K., Williams, E.I., and Groom, L. (1992). Health checks on patients 75 years and over in Nottinghamshire after the new GP contract. *British Medical Journal.* **305**, 619–21.

Brownell, K.D. (1994). The LEARN programme for weight control (6th edn) (ed. Edmonds). American Health Press, W.A.

Calnan, M., Cant, S., Williams, S., and Killoran, A. (1994). Involvement of the primary health care team in coronary heart disease prevention. *British Journal of General Practice*, **44**, 224–8.

Contraceptive Education Service (1996). *Contraceptive choices.* Family Planning Association.

Daniel, S. (1992). Teenage Health Centre Development Project. Publicity material.

Davies, P. (1991). Health promotion in general practice. *Australian Family Physician*, **20**, 28–9.

Department of Health (1995). Sensible drinking: the report of an inter-departmental working group. HMSO, London.

Department of Health (1996). The health of the nation: what you can do about it. HMSO, London.

Donovan, C.F. (1988), *Health Trends* Is there a place for adolescent screening in general practice? **20**, 64.

Dowler, E. (1994). Diet: what are the policy implications for women? In *Coronary heart disease: are women special?* (ed. I. Sharp) National Forum for Coronary Heart Disease Prevention, London. 119–32.

Fentem, P.H. (1994). Benefits of exercise in health and disease. *British Medical Journal.* **308**, 1291–5.

Freeman, C. and Newton, R. (1994). Eating disorders. In *Women's problems in general practice* (3rd edn). (ed. A McPherson), 424–7. Oxford University Press, Oxford.

Hart, J.T. (1971). The inverse care law. *Lancet*, **1**, 405–12.

Health Education Authority (1993). Smoking and pregnancy: guidance for all health professionals supporting pregnant women who want to stop smoking. HEA, London.

Howie, J.G.R., Porter, A.M.D., Heaney, D.J., *et al.* (1991). Long to short consultation ratio: a proxy measure of quality of care for general practice. *British Journal of General Practice*, **41**, 48–54.

Imperial Cancer Research Fund OXCHECK Study Group (1995). Effectiveness of health checks conducted by nurses in primary care: final results of the OXCHECK Study. *British Medical Journal* **310**, 1099–1104.

Jacobson, B. (1994). Policy implications for women and smoking. Is there a special case for action? In *Coronary heart disease: Are women special?* (ed. I. Sharp) National Forum for Coronary Heart Disease Prevention, London. 81–8.

MacMiller, P. and Plant, M. (1996). Drinking, smoking and illicit drug use among 16 and 17 year olds in the United Kingdom. *British Medical Journal*, **313**, 394–7.

Macfarlane, A., McPherson, A., McPherson, K. *et al.* (1987). Teenagers and their health. *Archives of Disease in Childhood*, **62**, 1125–9.

NIH Consensus Conference (1996). Physical activity and health: NIH Consensus Development Panel on Physical Activity and Cardiovascular Health. *Journal of the American Medical Association*, **267**, 241–6.

Naish, J., Brown, J., and Denton, B. (1994). Intercultural consultations: investigations of factors that deter non-English speaking women from attending their GPs for cervical screening. *British Medical Journal*, **309**, 1126–8.

Office of Population Censuses and Surveys (1993). Health Survey for England. HMSO, London.

Powell, K. and Pratt, M. (1996). Physical activity and health. *British Medical Journal*, **313**, 126–117.

Rhodes, D. (1994). Patterns of physical activity among women: what are the policy implications? In *Coronary heart disease: are women special?* (ed. I. Sharp) National Forum for Coronary Heart Disease Prevention, London. 163–72.

Russell, M., Wilson, C., Taylor, C., *et al.* (1979). Effect of GPs' advice against smoking. *British Medical Journal*, **2**, 231–5.

Scandinavian Simvastatin Survival Study Group (1994). Randomised trial of cholesterol lowering in 4444 patients with coronary heart disease: 45. *Lancet*, **344**, 1383–9.

Sharp, I. (1994). *Attitudes to women and coronary heart disease: are women special?* National Forum for CHD Prevention.

Silagy, C., Mant, D., Fowler, G., and Lodge, M. (1994). Meta-analyses of efficacy of nicotine replacement therapies in smoking cessation. *Lancet*, **343**, 139–42.

Stott, N.C. and Pill, R.M. (1990). 'Advise yes, dictate no'. Patients' views on health promotion in the consultation. *Family Practice*, **7**, 125–31.

Tannahill, A. (1985). What is health promotion? *Health Education Journal.* **44,** 167–8.

Ward, K. and Hawthorne, K. (1994). Do patients read health promotion posters in the waiting-rooms? A study in one general practice. *British Journal of General Practice,* **44,** 583–5.

Williams, E.C., Kirkman, R.J., and Elstein, M. (1994). Profile of young people's advice clinic in reproductive health, 1988–93. *British Medical Journal,* **309,** 786–8.

Wilson, A., McDonald, P., Hayes, L., and Cooney, J. (1992). Health promotion in the general practice consultation: a minute makes a difference. *British Medical Journal,* **304,** 227–30.

CHAPTER THREE

Referrals to specialist clinics

Angela Coulter

Introduction

Women are more frequent users of health services than men. They are more likely to report both acute and chronic illnesses and they live longer than men on average, so it is not surprising to find that they consult general practitioners (GPs), dentists, and opticians more often (OPCS 1995a). They are also more likely to be referred to hospital outpatient clinics and to be admitted for hospital treatment (Department of Health 1995). As gatekeepers to specialist services, GPs' referral decisions are key determinants of hospital use.

The rates at which GPs refer to specialist outpatient clinics are known to vary widely. On average, GPs make about five referrals per 100 consultations, or about 12 referrals per 100 registered patients per year, but many studies have shown that referral thresholds differ, both between individual GPs and between practices. The extent of variation between individual GPs is hard to estimate because they have different working hours and see different types of patients, but rates are known to vary between practices by at least threefold or fourfold (Wilkin and Smith 1987; Noone et al. 1989).

Sex differences in outpatient referrals

In one of the largest studies of outpatient referrals, the Oxford Region Referral Study, GPs in 36 practices in Berkshire, Buckinghamshire, Northamptonshire, and Oxfordshire (combined study population 480 000) kept records of all their referrals to specialist clinics over a 10-month period in 1990–91 (Bradlow et al. 1992). Fig 3.1 shows the distribution of referrals by age and sex.

The referral rate for women was 146 per 1000 female population per annum, as compared to 104 per 1000 males. Women were more likely to be referred than men in all but the youngest and oldest age groups, with particularly high rates of referral in the middle years. Referrals to obstetrics were excluded from these data, so pregnancy does not account for the higher rate of referral among women between the ages of 25–54, but we know that women in these age

Fig 3.1 *Age and sex-specific referral rates*

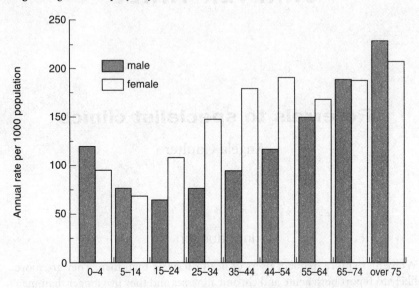

groups consult their GPs more often than men and the referral patterns mirror consultation rates quite closely (OPCS 1995*b*).

Just 15 conditions accounted for more than a quarter of the referrals in the study (Fig 3.2). The high incidence of conditions such as breast lumps (which topped the list of conditions referred to general surgeons), menorrhagia, and requests for sterilization and termination of pregnancy go some way to explaining the higher referral rate among women, but gender-specific conditions do not explain all of the difference. Women predominated in referrals to each of the specialties with the exception of general surgery and ENT (Table 3.1).

Referrals to gynaecology account for much of the excess rate of referral among women. Fig 3.3 shows the 10 problems most commonly referred to gynaecology clinics. These 10 problems accounted for nearly two-thirds of the referrals to gynaecologists in the study. In most cases the referral represents a request for a temporary transfer of responsibility for the care of the patient. In the case of gynaecology, GP participants in the study indicated that in 69% of cases the patient was being referred because the GP wanted the specialist to take over the management of the problem, 27% were referred for diagnosis or investigation with the expectation that management of the condition would continue to be the GP's responsibility, while the reason for referral in the remaining cases was to seek the specialist's advice or to reassure the patient.

Quality of primary care and referrals

Menorrhagia (excessive regular menstrual blood loss), which tops the list of referrals to gynaecology clinics, provides an interesting case study of the links between practice patterns in primary care and use of secondary care. Since

Fig 3.2 *Top fifteen problems referred to specialist outpatient clinics (for both sexes)*

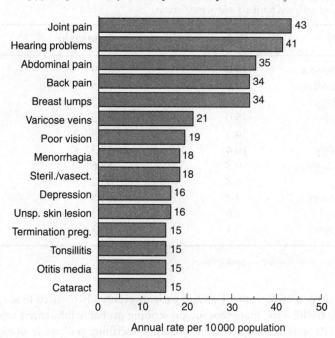

this condition can either be managed wholly in general practice or referred to gynaecology clinics for specialist treatment, it illustrates the important connection between the effectiveness of general practice treatment and the demand for specialist intervention.

Menorrhagia is a very common reason for consultation in general practice. On average, a GP can expect 5% of female patients in the 30–49 age group to consult for excessive menstrual blood loss in a year (Peto *et al.* 1993). In most cases, a course of drug therapy is the first-line treatment for this problem and specialist investigation is not necessary, yet a high proportion of women who consult with this problem end up being referred to hospital. In a cohort study of 348 women consulting GPs with a complaint of heavy menstrual bleeding, 89% tried a course of drug therapy, but 60% were eventually referred to a gynaecologist, and most of these eventually underwent surgical treatment (hysterectomy or endometrial ablation) (Coulter *et al.* 1994*a*).

The high rate of referral was unexpected since there are a number of drugs available which can reduce menstrual blood loss by around 50% (Effective Health Care 1995). However, a systematic review of the randomized controlled trials of the different drug treatments showed that the most commonly prescribed drugs were the least efficacious (Coulter *et al.* 1995*a*). For example, norethisterone, the drug which was most often prescribed to reduce menstrual blood loss, has not performed at all well in clinical trials when used at the recommended doses. Drugs, such as tranexamic acid, which are better supported by evidence of efficacy, were hardly ever prescribed. It was

Table 3.1 *Outpatient referral rates (per 000 population per annum) by specialty an percentage of referred patients who were female*

Specialty	Rate	% female
General surgery	24.8	48.9
General medicine	19.6	53.5
Gynaecology	15.7	99.3*
Orthopaedics	15.0	51.5
ENT	14.3	49.7
Dermatology	10.4	57.3
Opthalmology	9.8	58.6
Psychiatry	5.8	60.2
Rheumatology	4.2	60.8
Paediatrics	3.6	51.1
Plastic surgery	3.1	64.3

* Includes male patients referred to infertility clinics

not surprising, therefore, that GPs and patients eventually resorted to surgical treatment. In this case, inappropriate prescribing probably influenced referral rates. If GPs were to adopt evidence-based prescribing policies it would be interesting to see what would happen to referral rates for menstrual disorders.

Patients' preferences have also been shown to influence referral decisions. In the above-mentioned cohort study, patients who had a preference for surgical treatment were more likely to be referred than those who had no such preference, showing that GPs' decisions are often sensitive to patients' wishes (Coulter *et al.* 1994*b*). GPs' views and preferences can also influence the outcome. For example, there is some evidence that male and female doctors have different practice styles. In the menorrhagia cohort study, patients of women GPs were slightly less likely to be referred than patients who consulted men GPs, and fewer of the women doctors' patients received surgical treatment, although the differences were quite small (Coulter *et al.* 1995*b*). It is possible that women GPs are more reluctant to refer and spend more time trying alternatives to surgery. This may be because they are more confident about managing menorrhagia in general practice, perhaps because they tend to see more patients with gynaecological problems than their male colleagues. What-ever the reasons for differences in referral rates, it is clear that GPs' decisions play an important part in determining the likelihood that their patients will be admitted to hospital.

Explaining variations in referral rates

Many studies have looked for associations between referral rates and variables related to different characteristics of patients, doctors, or practices in an attempt to discern systematic patterns which might explain the variations in

Fig 3.3 *Top ten problems referred to gynaecology*

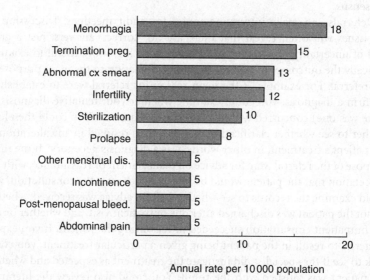

rates. No clear patterns have emerged (Wilkin 1992). The differences in rates do not appear to be related to differences in patterns of disease or case mix, to the social class composition of practice populations, to the age or experience of the doctors, to structural features of practices, or to the relative accessibility of hospital services. All these factors probably play some part in determining the differences but they cannot explain much of the variation.

We do know, however, that individual GPs and practices exhibit distinctive referral patterns which tend to remain consistent over time. We are left with the conclusion, therefore, that decisions about whether and when a referral is appropriate are complex and involve consideration of social, organizational, and personal factors as well as clinical signs and prognostic indicators. In the absence of clear, scientifically-based guidelines, doctors are likely to make different decisions according to the circumstances as they perceive them. These differences are probably influenced by doctors' attitudes to risk and uncertainty and the constellation of habits and experience that distinguish personal practice styles.

Auditing referrals

It is important to remember that referral rates in themselves do not reveal anything very useful about the quality of care. There is nothing intrinsically 'good' about an average referral rate. We know very little about the consequences of high and low referral rates and therefore should not leap to the conclusion that high referrers are wasting resources or that low referrers are depriving their patients of beneficial treatment. The existence of variations merely highlights the fact that doctors disagree about appropriate treatment and points to the need to seek evidence on which to build a scientifically-based consensus.

Referrals can make interesting topics for audit meetings. Discussion of the issues will often reveal that there are no 'correct' answers, just a great deal of uncertainty. Instead of comparing rates, it is more useful to examine critically the outcomes of referral decisions in relation to the main purpose of the referral. For example, if the main reason for referral were to establish or confirm a diagnosis, you could examine whether your tentative diagnosis (if there was one) concurred with the specialist's diagnosis. You could then look further to see whether clarification of a diagnosis resulted in any alteration of the patient's treatment, in other words, was a diagnosis necessary? If the main purpose of the referral were for advice on management or reassurance, with the expectation that the patient would be referred back after the consultation, you could examine the records to see whether helpful advice was received, whether or not the patient was discharged after one outpatient visit, and whether or not the outpatient consultation succeeded in reassuring the patient. If you expect a referral to result in the patient being given a particular treatment, you could look to see if the specialist did instigate the treatment as expected and whether the patient was satisfied with the result. You could also review the literature to see if the treatment was likely to have been effective and appropriate for the patient. Critical examination of referrals will help to ensure that specialist services are used efficiently.

Sharing decision-making

The menorrhagia example showed that patients' preferences can influence the decision to refer. It is usually important to take account of patients' views when deciding on appropriate management of their problem and referral decisions are no exception. The high non-attendance rate in outpatient clinics may in part be due to a failure to explore patients' beliefs about the necessity or desirability of referral. Grace and Armstrong (1986, 1987) gave questionnaires to 306 patients referred to hospital outpatient clinics, asking for their views on the reason for the referral, whether they thought the GP could have done more before referring them, whether they considered the referral was necessary, and whether they felt they had been referred to the most suitable consultant. The same questions were asked of the GP and the consultant involved. Patients, GPs, and consultants disagreed on the reason for the referral in two-thirds of the cases and there was also disagreement about the necessity and suitability of many of the referrals. These findings illustrate the need for clear communication of the reasons for referral to both specialists and patients. Poor communication can result in considerable wasted effort and resources.

Patients are sometimes dissatisfied by their GP's failure to refer them for specialist attention, although they do not always make their views known. A survey by the College of Health of a representative sample of 2338 adults in the UK found that one in five people would have liked to have been referred for a second opinion, but two-thirds of them failed to convey this desire to their GP

(College of Health 1991). Again, time spent discussing why a referral is not felt to be necessary may help to reduce misunderstandings. If the patient is anxious, a referral for a second opinion may be justified, but it is important that the consultant knows that this is the reason for referral.

Sometimes referrals are initiated by patients. For example, in making referrals for termination of pregnancy, sterilization, or infertility treatment, GPs are usually responding to requests by the patient. Others are triggered by screening tests routinely carried out in primary care, for example, referrals for abnormal cervical smears or breast lumps. But usually the decision is much less clear-cut and the way in which the patient describes her symptoms, the effect on her quality of life, her concerns about her health, and her treatment preferences are all factors which the GP has to take into account.

Eliciting and imparting all relevant information in a consultation so that the patient is fully informed stretches the skills of the most experienced GP. There is growing interest in developing better methods for informing patients about their medical conditions and the risks and benefits of treatment options, in order to encourage them to participate in decisions about their care. Experiments are under way to develop and evaluate leaflets, videos, audiotapes, and decision boards which give patients access to reliable overviews of the research evidence. These are intended as aids to clinical decision-making, recognizing that an average consultation time of 10 minutes does not leave GPs much time to promote true, shared decision-making.

Interactive videos have been developed in the US to inform patients about treatment choices for a number of common diseases, including breast cancer, benign uterine conditions (menorrhagia, fibroids, dysmenorrhea, endometriosis), and hormone replacement therapy (Kasper et al. 1992). Initial results from studies evaluating the use of interactive videos have been encouraging (Shepperd et al. 1995) but we need to know more about the effect of this form of information-giving on the doctor–patient relationship, on subsequent treatment decisions, and on health outcomes and patients' well-being. There are grounds for optimism. We know that most patients want more information than they often receive – lack of information about their illness and treatment is the commonest complaint in surveys of patient satisfaction – and there is already some evidence that involving patients in treatment decisions leads to more satisfactory doctor–patient relationships and better health outcomes (Greenfield et al. 1985; Kaplan et al. 1989). What we need now is the means to ensure that the ideal of shared decision-making can become a reality.

Conclusions

Referral decisions are both important and difficult. Many of the common conditions affecting women's health lack clear evidence-based guidelines on when a referral is appropriate. In these situations it is important to ensure that patients are informed about the choices and encouraged to participate in decisions. Good communication is vital in ensuring appropriate use of specialist services.

References and further reading

Bradlow, J., Coulter, A., and Brooks, P. (1992). *Patterns of referral*. Health Services Research Unit, Oxford.

College of Health (1991). Which way to health. February, 32–5.

Coulter, A., Peto, V., and Jenkinson, C. (1994a). Quality of life and patient satisfaction following treatment for menorrhagia. *Family Practice*, **11**, 394–401.

Coulter, A., Peto, V., and Doll, H. (1994b). Patients' preferences and general practitioners' decisions in the treatment of menstrual disorders. *Family Practice*, **11**, 67–4.

Coulter, A., Kelland, J., Peto, V., and Rees, M. (1995a). Treating menorrhagia in primary care: an overview of drug trials and a survey of prescribing practice. *International Journal of Health Technology Assessment*, **11**, 456–471.

Coulter, A., Peto, V., and Doll, H. (1995b). Influence of sex of general practitioner on management of menorrhagia. *British Journal of General Practice*, **45**, 471–5.

Department of Health (1995). *Health and personal social services statistics for England 1995*. HMSO, London.

Effective Health Care (1995). *The management of menorrhagia*. Nuffield Institute for Health, Leeds; NHS Centre for Reviews and Dissemination, York; and Royal College of Physicians, London.

Grace, J.F. and Armstrong, D. (1986). Reasons for referral to hospital: extent of agreement between the perceptions of patients, general practitioners and consultants. *Family Practice*, **3**, 143–7.

Grace, J.F. and Armstrong, D. (1987). Referral to hospital: perceptions of patients, general practitioners and consultants about necessity and suitability of referral. *Family Practice*, **4**, 170–5.

Greenfield, S., Kaplan, S., and Ware, J. (1985). Expanding patient involvement in care. *Annals of Internal Medicine*, **102**, 520–8.

Kaplan, S., Greenfield, S., and Ware, J. (1989). Assessing the effects of physician–patient interactions on the outcomes of chronic disease. *Medical Care*, **27**, S110–26.

Kasper, J., Mulley, A.G., and Wennberg, J.E. (1992). Developing shared decision-making programs to improve the quality of health care. *Quality Review Bulletin*, **18**, 182–90.

Noone, A., Goldacre, M., Coulter, A., and Seagroatt, V. (1989). Do referral rates vary widely between practices and does supply of services affect demand? *Journal of the Royal College of General Practitioners*, **39**, 404–7.

Office of Population Censuses and Surveys (1995a). *General Household Survey 1993*. HMSO, London.

Office of Population Censuses and Surveys (1995b). *Morbidity statistics from general practice. Fourth national study 1991–1992*. HMSO, London.

Peto, V., Coulter, A., and Bond, A. (1993). Factors affecting general practitioners' recruitment of patients into a prospective study. *Family Practice*, **10**, 207–11.

Shepperd, S., Coulter, A., and Farmer, A. (1995). Using interactive videos in general practice to inform patients about treatment choices: a pilot study. *Family Practice*, **12**, 443–7.

Wilkin, D. (1992). Patterns of referral: explaining variation. In *Hospital referrals* (ed. M. Roland and A. Coulter). Oxford University Press, Oxford.

Wilkin D, and Smith, A. (1987). Varations in general practitioners' referral rates to consultants. *Journal of the Royal College of General Practitioners*, **37**, 350–3.

CHAPTER FOUR

Variations in hospital treatment rates for common conditions

Klim McPherson

In the overall provision of health care various proportions of gross national product (GNP) are expended in different countries. These vary between nearly zero to upwards of 15% in the US. This expenditure goes predominantly on hospital care, as opposed to primary care or prevention. The total proportion spent on health care is usually higher the more the GNP per capita; rich countries spend proportionally more on health care than poorer countries. Also, generally, the higher the proportion spent on primary care the lower the expenditure per capita, which may be why the UK spends a low proportion (7%) for its wealth.

Clearly these expenditures can be affected by health policy, but with difficulty because acute hospital medicine has enormous prestige and is usually perceived as being essential. In the US 1% of a large GNP is spent on intensive care alone, where the admission rates are five times higher than in England. Many poorer countries (like Albania, for example) on the other hand spend less than 3% of a tiny GNP on all health care. These differences epitomize the kind of issues to be discussed in this chapter.

Of the eight most common surgical procedures in this country, five are predominantly for women, three being concerned with female reproductive organs (dilatation and curettage, hysterectomy, and ovarian surgery). It is thus interesting to examine which are really appropriate and which are not. There is, however, apparently no upper limit to what could be provided in the name of (expensive) curative medicine. This is because some admissions are *de facto* much more discretionary than is commonly imagined. Hence the essence of any coherent admission policy must rely on establishing what is cost-effective, given many other sensible ways of using scarce resources. Evidence about which admissions are highly discretionary is useful, so the role of clinical discretion itself can be better understood.

It is clear that, with or without budgets, general practitioners (GPs) are the major gatekeepers of the NHS, responsible for rationing expensive hospital care. They would clearly prefer to do this on the basis of clinical need, but often the health gain associated with hospital admission is not as well-established as might have been thought, even by the specialists. We know this must be true from the evidence on medical practice variations which provide some insight into the uncertainties concerning effectiveness and appropriateness of much of medical care. This, simply stated, demonstrates that, in all countries and in communities within countries (e.g. district health authorities), much that is provided is not properly assessed under any coherent, scientific or public policy on priorities for better health. If they had been, the variations observed in the population-based rates of admission would not be as great as they are, given what we know about natural differences in illness rates.

Variation in population-based rates of hospital admission

Studying variations in admission rates

Hospital admission rates might naively be expected to be related closely to disease incidence (McPherson 1994). However, the process of admission is a complex amalgamation of the effects of supply of hospitals, operating theatres, waiting lists, doctors, nurses, GPs, and other medical facilities as well as prevailing health beliefs, expectations of patients and their cultural setting, and so on. That these are important complexities in the determination of hospital admission in many cases can be supported by the diverse and extensive litera-ture which reports the phenomenon in many different settings. For example, the best estimates of the crude admission rates for selected surgical operations in developed countries is shown in Table 4.1.

Clearly, a chapter could be devoted to each of these operations and the pos-sible reasons for the quite marked and systematic differences in their utilization rates between countries analysed (McPherson 1989). Obviously the US, which spends 15% of its GNP on a fee-for-service system, has all sorts of incentives to intervene rather than not (among those who can afford to pay for the care), when in doubt. But for something like acute appendicitis the opportunities for real clinical discretion are more limited than for treating menorrhagia, for example. Nonetheless, some cultures seem to assume different thresholds for intervention even for the symptoms of acute appendicitis, on the quite robust assumption of broadly similar true incidence rates. Coronary bypass grafting is determined not only be medical need but also by some strong medical and cultural preferences, for example, the preference for all hospitals to have cardiac surgical facilities to attain some sort of overall credibility threshold. Expensive supply of facilities tends to induce a demand of its own (Wennberg 1982).

It is possible that people in these different countries are demanding these various levels of intervention from their respective health care systems, but this is most unlikely. It is worth noting that to propose a randomized trial to determine the appropriate level of intervention for painful gallstones, in which one group was offered intervention rates prevalent in the UK and the other the high rates of the US or Canada (see Fig 4.1), would be regarded as ethically unjustifiable in both communities for opposing reasons. This is one reason

Table 4.1 *Reported annual admission rates for selected surgical procedures in the early 1980's per 100 000 population*

	Tonsil-lectomy	CBPG	Cholecys-tectomy	Ing. hernia	Prosta-tectomy	Hyste-rectomy	Cataract	Appendi-ctomy
Australia	115	32	145	202	183	405	101	340
Canada	89	26	219	224	229	479	139	143
Denmark	229	?	21	?	?	234	255	188
Ireland	256	4	91	100	52	124	123	245
Japan	61	1	2	67	?	90	35	149
Netherlands	421	5	131	175	116	381	68	149
New Zealand	102	2	99	211	191	431	95	169
Norway	45	13	30	78	238	120	71	64
Sweden	65	?	140	206	111	48	145	168
Switzerland	51	?	49	116	?	?	22	74
UK	26	6	78	154	144	250	98	131
US	205	61	203	238	308	557	294	130

Fig 4.1 *Cholecystectomy rates by age, sex and country (from McPherson, 1988)*
(Source: Chris Ham (Editor). Health Care Variations. London: King's Fund Institute, 1988. Reproduced by permission)

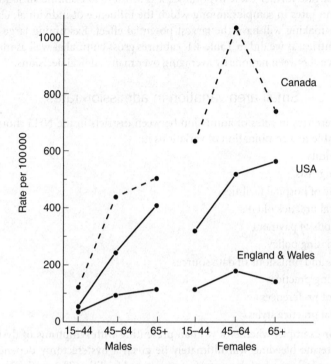

why, as we shall discover, so little is apparently known about the outcomes of these common procedures used at different symptomatic thresholds.

Glover, in 1938, first noted large differences in tonsillectomy rates which related, in his view, most strongly to 'variations of medical opinion on the indications for operation'. In the US, variations were recorded and analysed in 1969 (Lewis 1969) and internationally in 1968 (Pearson 1968), leading to the conclusion that the incidence of common procedures seemed hardly to relate to disease rates at all, and was often more closely determined by supply of beds and preferences of doctors. Even operations like appendicectomy, as we have seen, for acute appendicitis seemed to vary systematically by geography as well as by illness rates. Hysterectomy for benign indications has been frequently cited as being highly discretionary and determined by demand from women, but there is little evidence to support this (Coulter 1985). What is clear is that systematic attempts to relate admission rates to underlying disease rates have mostly failed (Weinberg 1977).

Thus an important hypothesis, strongly suggested by this work, is the extent to which differences in clinical opinion do determine admission rates, since such differences could also be attributable to variations in the quality of care as well as to genuine, patient or doctor, uncertainties about the appropriateness of care at different levels of intervention. Often variations in hospitalization rates are a manifestation of a tendency to treat at different thresholds of disease in an apparently progressive (but usually essentially benign) disease process. To investigate further these hypotheses it is sensible to examine variations in admission rates in samples among which the influence of individual, clinical decision-making will have the largest potential effect. Examining large areas like countries, as we did in Table 4.1, captures gross cultural as well as medical differences between nations by averaging over many clinical decisions.

Small area variation in admission rates

The differences in rates of admission between districts in the NHS should be attributable to a combination of variations in:
- morbidity
- waiting-lists
- supply of hospital facilities
- referral practice of GPs
- methods of payment
- purchasing policy
- errors and omissions in data sources
- labelling practices
- patient preferences
- clinical practice styles.

Thus, for example, whether a woman presenting with symptoms of dysfunctional uterine bleeding will ultimately be given a hysterectomy depends on exogenous influences of the supply of people and facilities. The availability and preferences for private practice, the budgets available for this kind of surgery, and the clinical preferences of the gynaecological team are all determined entirely ignorant of her individual needs. But most of the overall supply factors are determined by characteristics of the population in which she lives, which on average would be similar to neighbouring districts.

The assumption that the extent of clinical uncertainty about appropriateness can be measured by the amount of small area variations in admission rates, depends on important endogenous factors, such as illness rates being similar between neighbouring districts (McPherson 1982). It is difficult to know what the main causes for the variation between small areas in any one country are, but the 'small area variation' argument (Knickman 1994) assumes that they are due to different medical opinion, uncertainties, and clinical practice style. There may be other plausible explanations, such as supply factors, but the most likely cause of otherwise unexplained variations between districts would be differences in clinical opinion.

Some admissions rates do have variations which look like the variation we see between districts for the incidence of cancer and cause-specific mortality rates but others are much more variable. Variations in genuine illness rates tend not to have more than a twofold range, while admissions can have tenfold ranges in their rates.

A formal examination of small area variations in rates (McPherson 1988) gives rise to a different set of figures to those seen when comparisons are made between countries. For example, while hysterectomy rates vary enormously between countries they vary little between small areas in a single country, suggesting some strong national consensus for quite different thresholds of intervention in each country. It is also observed that the amount of variation is approximately constant in different countries for particular kinds of admission, whether or not the prevailing rates are similar (McPherson 1982). Thus some kinds of admission appear to be variable and others not.

Of the admissions which are not variable, appendicectomy and hysterectomy stand out. Of the highly variable procedures the most variable is carotid endarterectomy for stroke prevention (McPherson 1996) but also excision of the vas deferens. Clearly, the first depends on expertize and clinical opinion on appropriate indications and the second is, probably almost uniquely, led by individual 'patient' demand.

Table 4.2 shows admissions to hospital, categorized by the amount of variation between districts, observed in four regional health authorities. Admissions for both sexes are included for comparison purposes but it is clear which admissions exhibit the most discretion.

Clearly, many of the admission designations in Table 4.2 will represent alternative treatments for which admission is necessary, and sometimes may reflect multiple admission of a single person in the study period (1991–93). The more variable conditions represent interventions for which there may be many indications. However, as a crude categorization of the variability of hospitalization for surgical or medical indications, as they are provided for populations in England and Wales, this is a first step in understanding an important dimension of the process. Those admissions for which variation between neighbouring districts already exhibits around sixfold differences in admission rates, cannot be regarded as always necessary. More detailed information on appropriate indications and good prior evidence for benefit would be required.

The eight most common surgical procedures consist of four procedures predominantly for women; namely dilatation and curettage, which is four times as common as hysterectomy, which in turn is about as common as varicose vein surgery and operations on the ovary. Moreover, cataract surgery (which is half as common as dilatation and cutterage and because of the age structure largely performed for women) and cholecystectomy are much more common among women.

Around 50% of both surgical and medical admissions are of a kind for which the variation exhibited is between three and fourfold. Only around 13% of surgical admissions and less than 1% of medical admissions have characteristic variation which is less than threefold between small neighbouring areas. Allowing for all the problems of artefact, designation, and definition this is not how hospital admission is commonly viewed. Most would believe that the majority of admissions would be associated with indications for which there was little doubt. Exactly the opposite is shown to be true; most have a measured variation which is higher than fourfold.

Table 4.2 *Tabulation of common hospital admissions by the observed small area variation in age and sex standardized rates. England and Wales 1991–93*

Range of rates between districts	Surgical admissions	Medical admissions
Less than twofold	Hernia repair Colectomy	
Two to threefold	Hysterectomy Appendectomy Proctectomy	
Three to fourfold	Prostatectomy Hip replacement Tonsillectomy Cholecystectomy Knee replacement Coronary bypass Varicose veins D&C Cataract Haemorrhoidectomy Pacemaker insertion	Stroke Rheumatism Pneumonia and influenza ABRI
Four to eightfold	Adenoidectomy Aorta-iliac-femoral bypass	Diabetes Ischaemic heart disease TIA Chronic obstructive pulmonary disorder
More than eightfold	Excision of vas deferens Carotid endarterectomy	Hypertensive disease

Conclusions

These medical practice variations can often be justified by reference to individual experiences and differing interpretations of the research literature. In circumstances of genuine uncertainty too, decisions have to be made and practice styles inevitably emerge from uncontrolled, observational clinical experience. Clearly, much that is done in hospital is influenced to some degree by essentially irrelevant exogenous factors such as waiting-lists, local variations in staff, peer pressures, etc., which may inadvertently lead to practice styles which cannot be justified or are only poorly justified (Irvine, 1995). More clearly still, the research literature itself is generally so extensive that to be completely cognizant of it, and all its implications, is not compatible with any significant commitment to patient care. Thus when variations are largely determined by medical practice, this does not itself imply any information about which rates are appropriate (Sackett 1995).

This leads to a simplifying distinction between causes of measured district variation of 'uncertainty' and 'ignorance'. The distinction between them is that the former is not informed by scientific evidence, because the research has not been completed or is inadequate. The second is simply that the scientific evidence that there is, is ignored, forgotten, never understood or read, to varying degrees and is justified, if at all, by citing biased or misleading information. The bulk of the relevant research literature points overwhelmingly towards uncertainty as being most important, but the kind of uncertainty being held responsible is not necessarily acknowledged explicitly. Indeed, often it is vehemently denied, which is one reason why this work is important. Practice styles develop and evolve in different milieux on the basis of experience and understanding and consolidate as firmly justified. That these styles are often different is a measure of the state of the hard evidence or its comprehension.

The recent research and development (R&D) emphasis in the NHS on evidence-based medicine and on research is directed at the former, while the R&D dissemination agenda is directed at the latter. Presumably a widespread acceptance and practice of evidence-based medicine would reduce that observed variation which was attributable to the latter. An indirect method of monitoring the acceptance of evidence-based medicine, in particular circumstances, is therefore to monitor changes in variation which might follow the widespread availability of reliable information from the systematic reviews and dissemination strategy.

It is, however, quite remarkable that hysterectomy, once a highly discretionary operation (Leape 1990) is now one of the least variable of common operations. It is possibly even more remarkable that the differences between countries in hysterectomy rates is now also narrowing; the rates in the US are coming down and those in this country have stabilized at around 60% of the US rate. This is, in part, due to publicity about rates of discretionary operations (Coulter 1988) and possibly, in part, due to a growing international consensus. Dilatation and curettage, on the other hand, is lacking in justification among women under 40 (Dyck 1977) and is still practised, and overall remains a highly discretionary procedure.

Clearly though there is a lot of research to be done, not only on the likely consequences of discretionary hospitalizations but also on understanding the individual woman's preferences for the various treatment options. Mostly women believe that hospital admission is a matter for their advisors, because they do not appreciate the true levels of manifest uncertainty.

References and further reading

Coulter, A. and McPherson, K. (1985) Socioeconomic variations in the use of common surgical operations. *British Medical Journal*, **291**, 183–7.

Coulter, A. McPherson, K., and Vessey, M.P. (1988) Do British women undergo too few or too many hysterectomies? *Social Science and Medicine*, **27** (9), 987–94.

Coulter, A., Klassen, A., MacKenzie, I., and McPherson, K. (1993) Dilatation and curettage: is it used appropriately? *British Medical Journal*, **306**, 236–9.

Dyck, F., Murphy, F., Murphy, J., *et al.* (1977) Effect of surveillance on the number of hysterectomies in the province of Saskatchewan. *New England Journal of Medicine*, **296**, 1326.

Glover, J.A. (1938) On the incidence of tonsillectomy in school children. *Proc. Royal Society of Medicine*, **31**, 1219–36.

Irvine, C. Baird, R., Lamont, P., and Davies, A. (1995) Endarterectomy for asymptomatic carotid artery stenosis. *British Medical Journal*, **311**, 1113–4.

Knickman, J.R. and Foltz A-M. (1994) Regional differences in hospital utilization. How much can be traded to population differences? *Medical Care*, **22**, 971–86.

Leape, L., Park, R., Solomon, D., *et al.* (1990) Does inappropriate use explain small area variations in the use of health services? *Journal of the Medical Association*, **263**, 669.

Lewis, C.E. (1969) Variations in the incidence of surgery. *New England Journal of Medicine*, **281**, 880–4.

McPherson, K. (1988) Variations in hospitalisation rates: Why and how to study them. In *Research report 2–health care variations. Assessing the evidence* (ed. Chris Ham), pp. 15–20. King's Find Institute, London.

McPherson, K. (1989) International differences in medical care practices. In *International comparison of health care financing and delivery: data and perspectives*. Health Care Financing Administration, annual supplement.

McPherson, K. (1994). Chapter 8. In *The epidemiological imagination: A reader*, (ed. J. Ashton). Open University Press, Buckingham.

McPherson, K., Wennberg, J., Hovind, O. *et al.* (1982) Small area variations in the use of common surgical procedures: an international comparison. *New England Journal of Medicine*, **307**, 1310.

McPherson, K., Downing, A., and Buirski, D. (1996). *Systematic variation in surgical procedures and hospital admission rates.* Research Report, PHP Publication, 23 London School of Hygiene and Tropical Medicine.

Pearson, R.J.C., Smedby, B., Berfenstam, R., *et al.* (1968) Hospital case loads in Liverpool, New England and Uppsala: an international comparison. *Lancet*, **2**, 559–66.

Sackett, D. and Rosenberg, W. (1995) The need for evidence-based medicine. *Journal of the Royal Society of Medicine*, **88**, 620–4.

Wennberg, J. and Gittleson, A. (1975) Small area variations in health care delivery. *Science*, **18**, 1102–8.

Wennberg, J. and Fowler, F. (1997). A test of consumer contribution to small area variations in health care. *Journal of the Maine Medical Association*, **68**, 8, 275–9.

Wennberg, J.E., Barnes, B.A., and Zubkopf, M. (1982) Professional uncertainty and the problem of supplier-induced demand. *Social Science and Medicine*, **16**, 811–20.

CHAPTER FIVE

Breast problems

Joan Austoker, Ann McPherson, Jane Clarke,
and Anneke Lucassen

Introduction

Breast cancer is the commonest cancer in women, accounting for 20% of all new female cases. Overall in the UK it is estimated that about one in 12 women will develop the disease at some stage in their life. A diagnosis of breast cancer is likely to herald the onset of significant physical and psychological difficulties for the patient, as well as gloom and despair in her family and carers. Although our understanding of breast cancer has increased enormously over the last two decades and treatment has become more rational, progress is slow, but there has been improvement in case survival in the last few years.

Breast diseases of all sorts account for a substantial number of consultations each year in general practice. General practitioners (GPs) can expect to see around 30 new presentations per 1000 women a year relating to breast disease, with problems ranging from mild breast pain to actual breast cancer. Only 5.8% of women (of all ages) presenting to their GP with a breast disorder, and an even smaller proportion of younger women, are found to have breast cancer (RCGP, OPCS: Fourth National GP Morbidity Survey 1991–92 (1995)). It can be difficult to differentiate the conditions and therefore there has been an increase in the number of referrals to specialists from general practice of up to 80% in some age groups mainly for what is eventually diagnosed as benign breast disease. In 1981, 26% of referrals were found to be malignant whereas now the level is 10%.

This chapter focuses on both breast cancer and the management of benign breast disease since the latter forms the majority of the consultations for breast symptoms in general practice and as such constitutes a large cost to the NHS in terms of medical, nursing, and administrative time. It is also a cause of a great deal of anxiety in the women who have these symptoms. We begin by considering the epidemiology of breast cancer and the strategies available to promote its early diagnosis. We then discuss the management of a woman who presents with symptoms of breast disease, including information on examining the breasts. The general management of benign breast disease is considered in some detail. This is followed by sections dealing with the diagnosis and treatment of both early and advanced breast cancer. We conclude with a consideration of the adverse effects of treatment and the psychological aspects of breast cancer.

Epidemiology

The size of the problem

In 1991 in the UK, 34 500 women were newly diagnosed with breast cancer, and in 1995 14 080 died from it (Cancer Research Campaign 1996). Four thousand new cases occur in women under the age of 45 per year. Of every 1000 women aged 50, two will recently have had breast cancer diagnosed and about 15 will have had a diagnosis made before the age of 50, giving a prevalence of approximately 2%. The incidence is increasing slowly, particularly among elderly women, by about 1–2% per year. There has also been a short-term increase in incidence in women aged 50–64 related to the onset of the screening programme.

Breast cancer is the leading cause of female cancer death in the UK, accounting for 20% of these deaths. However, in Scotland lung cancer deaths have exceeded those from breast cancer since 1984. There are 900 deaths from breast cancer per year in women under 45 and it is the commonest single cause of death from all causes in women aged 35–54. The UK is in the unenviable position of having the highest breast cancer mortality rate worldwide. Between the late 1950s and early 1970s in England and Wales mortality in women aged 15–44 increased by 16% but since the late 1980s the breast cancer death rate has started to fall. The decline has been greatest in younger women: since 1985–89 breast cancer mortality rates decreased by 14% in women aged 20–49; by 11% in women aged 50–69; and by 5% in women aged 70–79 (Fig 5.1). Various theories have been put forward to explain this decline. Although changes in childbearing patterns in previous decades and changes in assigning cause of death play a part, it is thought that better treatment for early breast cancer is mainly responsible. It is too soon and across too wide an age span to be due to the National Health Service Breast Screening Programme which was only phased in gradually from 1988 (Beral *et al.* 1995; Quinn *et al.* 1995).

The aetiology of breast cancer

Many studies of the aetiology of breast cancer have been reported and there is a vast literature. Only a very brief review will be given here. More comprehensive information can be found in Hulka and Stark (1995) and McPherson *et al.* (1995).

Family history

Between 5–10% of breast cancer in western countries is now thought to be due to inherited susceptibility. The genetic susceptibility is inherited as an autosomal dominant with limited penetrance. This means that it can be transmitted through either sex and that some family members may transmit the gene

Fig 5.1 *Breast cancer mortality in England and Wales, 1950–93*
(Source: Beral et al., 1995)

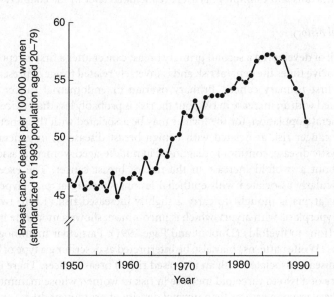

without developing the cancer themselves. Several breast cancer genes have so far been isolated.

BRCA1 (Breast Cancer 1), the first breast cancer gene to be isolated, is on the long arm of chromosome 17. It is carried by approximately one in 883 women and responsible for 2% of breast cancers in women under 70 years and 8% of all breast cancers in women under 30 years of age (Ford *et al.* 1995). It is associated with 3% of ovarian cancers and implicated in 80% of families with a predisposition to both breast and ovarian cancer. Over 100 different mutations of BRCA1 have already been identified. BRCA2 is on the long arm of chromosome 13. A few cases of breast cancer arise from mutations in the p53 tumour suppressor gene on the short arm of chromosome 17. Other breast cancer genes are likely to be identified. Some families affected by breast cancer also show an excess of other cancers, i.e. ovarian, colon, and prostate cancer which can be attributed to the same inherited gene. A woman is more likely to carry a genetic mutation if the breast cancer occurs at a young age, she develops bilateral breast cancer, or another epithelial cancer. Women in high risk families have only a 50:50 chance of inheriting the defective gene. A woman with a strong family history is unlikely to have inherited a gene if she is unaffected by age 65. Certain ethnic groups may be more susceptible. A recent population survey of Ashkenazi Jews revealed that approximately 1% carry the BRCA1 mutation, making familial breast and ovarian cancer attributable to this mutation potentially the most common serious single gene disease yet identified in any population group (Struewing 1995; Collins 1996). Thirty-eight per cent of Jewish women with breast cancer under the age of 30 have germ-line BRCA1 mutations.

A woman's risk of developing breast cancer is two or more times greater if she has a first degree relative with the disease diagnosed before the age of 50. Further details and examples of cases are included later in the chapter.

Medical history

The risk of developing a second primary breast cancer after a first is reported to be up to five times the general risk and is inversely related to age at presentation of the first primary cancer. Primary ovarian or endometrial cancer is also associated with an increase in risk, but the risk is probably less than twice that of the general population, for the former may be associated with the genetic role.

The cancer risk associated with benign breast disease is, in general, low. Fibrocystic disease, commonly diagnosed in middle-aged women, is associated with about a twofold increase in the risk of breast cancer. The excess risk is particularly associated with epithelial lesions showing atypia. Hyperplasia without atypia is thought to carry a slightly increased risk (1.5 to twofold), while hyperplasia with atypia, which is uncommon, shows a moderate increase in risk (four to fivefold) (Dupont and Page 1991). Particular mammographic patterns (Wolfe patterns) may also be interpreted as describing a type of benign breast disease associated with an increased risk of breast cancer. There is some evidence of a two to threefold increase in risk in women whose mammograms show dysplasia or a greater than normal density of prominent ducts.

Menstrual factors

An early onset of menarche is associated with a two to threefold increase in breast cancer risk. This effect is reduced after the menopause. One study has found that breast cancer cases established regular menstrual cycles more rapidly than controls, and that the combination of early menarche (age 12 years) and early establishment of regular cycles (within 1 year of menarche) was associated with a more than threefold increase in risk (Henderson *et al.* 1984).

For individual women, menopause before the age of 45 leads to a twofold reduction in risk compared with menopause occurring after age 55. Artificial menopause induced by surgical treatment has a protective effect similar to that of natural menopause.

These findings all indicate a positive association between the number of menstrual cycles and the risk of breast cancer. The possible carcinogenic role of oestrogen has been widely explored. Other hormones have also been invest-igated but the precise relationship between endogenous hormones and breast cancer risk remains unclear.

Reproductive factors

An early full-term pregnancy has an important protective effect. Women who deliver their first child before age 20 have approximately half the risk of breast cancer of nulliparous women, or of women whose first child is born when they are aged 30–35 years. The risk is highest in women whose first full-term pregnancy occurs after the age of 35 years, although other factors also contribute to the high risk in this group. High parity is associated with early age at first birth, but there is some evidence that high parity may itself provide some additional protection.

The protection gained from an early first pregnancy is operative only if the pregnancy continues to term. Some recent studies have suggested that first tri-mester abortion before first full-term pregnancy is associated with a substantial increased risk of breast cancer, but this finding has not been replicated in all studies. Abortions after the first full-term pregnancy probably do not carry any increased risk.

The independent effect of lactation on risk remains a subject of continuing debate. A protective effect of lactation has been reported in several studies (e.g. Byers *et al.* 1985; McTiernan and Thomas 1986).

Exogenous hormones

Breast cancer is a hormonal cancer. The effects of hormonal supplementation, whether taken as oral contraception and/or HRT, on breast cancer is of enor-mous concern. Even if there is only a small increased risk from exposure to these hormones the effect on breast cancer rates could be substantial as breast cancer itself is common and both oral contraceptives and HRT are widely used.

Oral contraceptives. In recent years various case control studies have reported an association between oral contraceptive use and breast cancer at a young age (e.g. UK National Case Control Study Group 1991). Other studies have failed to find such an association. A systematic review (Collaborative Group on Hor-monal Factors in Breast Cancer 1996) pooled the results from 54 case control studies involving 53 297 women with breast cancer and 100 239 without it, to compare the past exposure to oral contraceptives and breast cancer. If one looks at all women who have been exposed to the pill regardless of age, length of use, family history, parity, etc. then the women who have used the pill do not appear to have an increased risk of breast cancer. However, these studies indicated that there is a 24% increased risk in those women who are currently using the pill or have recently stopped the pill. This risk disappears over the next 10 years after stopping the pill. Of course, pill users tend to be young women for whom the risk of breast cancer is relatively small (16 per 10 000 cumulative cases in women under the age of 35) and therefore a 24% increased risk for them will not be very dramatic (17.5 per 10 000). However, for women aged 40 or more who are on the pill an increase of 24% will be more important (see Chapter 6). This risk appears to be independent of how long women have been on the pill. One important question relating to length of use of the pill before first-term pregnancy remains inadequately addressed, even by these data, as only a very small proportion of women in these studies had used the pill for a long time (more than 5 years) before their first full-term pregnancy. The problem is that long-term use before first term pregnancy is something that has only fairly recently become common with changing contraceptive and social practice. Unfortunately this meta-analysis cannot address the long-term consequences for women when they reach the age of high breast cancer risk if they took the pill for a long time when they were young. For short-term use before first pregnancy and long-term use in parous women it appears that we can now be reassuring.

The meta-analysis also found that breast cancers diagnosed in those women on the pill were clinically less advanced than among non-users, though this may be because of increased surveillance and therefore earlier diagnosis. The increased risk of breast cancer among current users and decline in risk after stopping the pill supports the theory that oral contraceptives might be working as tumour promoters; i.e. making them grow faster, rather than as carcinogenic factors, i.e. initiating the cancer.

Another unanswered question is what happens to the breast cancer risk in women who have been on the pill for most of their fertile years and then take HRT for many years, as once again this is a recent phenomenon.

HRT. The relationship between HRT and breast cancer also remains controversial (McPherson 1995). Most of the long-term, follow-up data available are based on the effect of oestrogen alone, which was used before combined supplements were introduced in the 1980s because of the risk of inducing endometrial cancers with unopposed oestrogens. Meta-analyses of oestrogen alone have shown that long-term use (more than 10 years) may increase the risk of breast cancer by 50%. A more recent study (Colditz *et al.* 1995) showed the risk increased after only 5 years of use and that combined preparations did not appear to reduce risk as some people had hoped. The new estimates of risk for breast cancer in women using HRT prophylactically will probably still give a net gain in years of life so long as the effects on risk revert to normal after the supplements are stopped and the protective effects on heart disease last long after they are stopped, but we do not know the answer to these two questions yet.

It is difficult to assess risk for an individual woman and to quantify the balance between benefits and risk. For a 50-year-old woman the baseline lifetime risk of coronary heart disease is around 45%, of hip fracture is 15%, and of breast cancer is 8%. How women view these risks as well as the effect that HRT has on quality of life in the short term in relieving menopausal symptoms together with possible side-effects, her own family history, her fears and prejudices, will vary (McPherson 1995).

Weight, diet, and alcohol

Most studies indicate that breast cancer risk is directly proportional to relative weight, with obese women experiencing an increased risk of 1.5 to twofold. This increased risk is restricted to post-menopausal women.

The issue of diet as a cause of breast cancer has been dominated by work on fat intake. The association between dietary fat intake and breast cancer is contentious and, at the present time, remains unresolved. Some have judged the evidence convincing enough to warrant dietary recommendations, others find the evidence very weak (Boyd *et al.* 1993). Population correlation studies have suggested that animal fat or meat consumption may be of primary importance in determining breast cancer risk. However, individual case control studies have provided only very weak evidence confirming this finding and a large prospective study of nurses has failed to show any relationship between fat intake and subsequent breast cancer during the first 4 years of follow-up.

The relationship between alcohol consumption and breast cancer is also still the subject of debate.

Ionizing radiation

There is direct evidence of the carcinogenic effect of radiation on breast cancer risk, both from Japanese atomic bomb survivors and from women exposed to high doses of ionizing radiation in the management of mastitis and pulmonary TB. The extent of risk is directly proportional to the radiation dose and inversely proportional to the age of the woman at the time of exposure.

This relationship has raised anxieties about the use of mammographic screening. However, the probability of a middle-aged woman developing breast cancer as a result of a single, modern mammographic examination is very low – perhaps one in 2 million. This risk is far outweighed by the potential benefits of screening (see below).

Non-risk factors

A number of factors have been considered as possible indicators of breast cancer risk but should now be considered as 'non-risk factors'. These include exposure to diazepam and hair dyes, and the occurrence of cholecystectomy and thyroid disease. Importantly, cigarette smoking is a non-risk factor, but this does *not* imply that it is a protective factor.

Breast cancer screening

The latest national survival figures for England show that an average of 64% of women diagnosed with breast cancer in 1983–85 were alive 5 years later (Cancer Research Campaign 1996). The stage at which a woman has her breast cancer diagnosed greatly influences her survival chances. Generally speaking, the earlier the breast cancer is diagnosed, the better are the survival rates (see Table 5.1). By identifying tumours earlier in their evolution, effective treatment is expected to be curative in a greater proportion of women. This is the basis of population-based screening discussed below.

While not all small cancers can be cured, there is now evidence that smaller tumours of less than 15 mm are often found to be less aggressive and are less likely to spread than bigger ones. There is thus considerable potential for reducing population mortality from breast cancer by a systematic approach to improving the stage at presentation by early detection. About 70–80% of screen-detected cancers may have a good prognosis. At the initial screen approximately 20% of cancers may be *in situ* and 50% of invasive cancers detected by the screening programme are 15 mm or less across (this is smaller than a new 5p piece). Up to 70% of important abnormalities detected by screening are impalpable but it detects only 95% of breast cancers.

Breast screening by mammography has been demonstrated to be of value by rigorous randomized controlled trials (Day 1991). There have, in addition,

Table 5.1 *Breast cancer stage and 5–year relative survival*

Stage	Description	% 5–year relative survival
I	Small mobile tumour less than 2 cm and confined to the breast. No lymph node involvement	84
II	As I, but with some nodal involvement, or larger tumours (2–5 cm) with or without nodal involvement. No known distant metastases	71
III	Locally advanced tumour possible attached to the chest wall. Nodal involvement. No known distant metastases	48
IV	Distant metastases present	18
All stages		63

Source: CRC Factsheet 6 (1996)

been a number of non-randomized, population-based breast screening trials. For women aged 50 years and over at entry into the trials, all trials show a reduction in breast cancer mortality although the results are not statistically significant in all cases. The randomized trials show a reduction in breast cancer mortality ranging from 20–40% and the design of these trials has been such as to avoid the problems of bias. A recent meta-analysis shows that mammographic screening significantly reduces breast cancer mortality in women aged 50–74 years after 7–9 years of follow-up, regardless of screening interval or number of mammographic views (overall summary relative risk 0.74–95%, CI 0.66–0.83). (Kerlikowske *et al.* 1995).

Benefits versus adverse effects

With any screening programme there are benefits and adverse effects. The benefits include:
- improved prognosis because of earlier diagnosis
- less radical treatment as earlier diagnosis
- reassurance for those with negative test results.

The adverse problems include:
- discomfort and pain of mammography
- reassurance to those who have a false negative result
- anxiety and psychological morbidity for those with false positive results
- over-diagnosis of minor abnormalities
- unnecessary tests and interventions for those with false positive results
- knowledge and stigmatization with a disease with no difference in outcome
- risks of radiation.

The list of disadvantages may appear long but the disadvantages have to be

---

Box 5.1 *Breast screening: ways to decrease anxiety*

- Women should be prepared in advance for the possibility of receiving an invitation – use posters and leaflets in the practice in the 6 months before the practice is screened
- Breast screening should be presented in the context of other preventive checks and health-related behaviours
- The routine nature of the programme should be emphasized
- Women should be sent comprehensive information about the service from the screening programme with their invitation letter
- Waiting times should be short at the screening unit
- Effective communication with women at each stage should be a priority
- Women should know when to expect their results and how they will receive them
- Women should be aware of the meaning of a positive result
- Women should be prepared in advance about a possible recall
- Letters of recall should be comprehensive, giving a reason for the recall, and offering as much reassurance as possible
- Time between notification and results and the recall appointment should be minimal
- Communication and support both by the GP and breast care nurse at the centre will be required at this time for women who are recalled
- Non-attenders are a special group – GPs can send them further advice about breast screening and offer to discuss it with them
- Care should be taken to reduce false reassurance and ensure women understand the objective of breast screening – that is, detection not prevention

Source: Austoker (1995a)

---

seen within the context of the main advantage: improved prognosis for many women with screen-detected cancer. The adverse problems have to be taken seriously, evaluated, and attempts made to reduce them wherever possible. There are various times at which anxiety can be increased or decreased during the different stages of the screening programme. Box 5.1 lists ways to try and minimize anxiety.

Compression of the breast against the X-ray plate during screening is uncomfortable for the majority of women. Three large studies involving over 7000 women showed that 81% experienced discomfort, classified as actual pain by 46% of women, and severe by 7% (McIlwaine 1993). In the majority this pain was fortunately short-lived. Over 60% women saw a cervical smear test and venepuncture as more uncomfortable.

There is no evidence that there is increased anxiety found in women invited to attend for breast cancer screening (Walker *et al.* 1994). Nine out of 10 women who are recalled for further investigation do not have cancer. There is increased anxiety in women who need recall. While for most women shown to have false positives this increased anxiety is not sustained in the long term (Cockburn *et al.* 1994), a substantial number of women continue to suffer intense anxiety for many months and even years (Lerman 1991).

There is over-diagnosis of some small, well-differentiated and *in situ* cancers which are unlikely to have caused any trouble during the patient's lifetime. However, Swedish and Finnish studies have shown this problem to be small and limited to the first mammographic examination (Tabar *et al.* 1992; Hakama *et al.* 1995). The problem of advancing the number of years of knowing one is a breast cancer patient (lead time bias) remains unsolved. For a percentage of women there is no benefit to having their cancer diagnosed earlier as the prognosis remains unaltered, either because it is metastatic and the treatment for them makes no difference to outcome, or because delay in diagnosis would not affect outcome.

Calculations have been made to assess the likelihood of mammography actually causing cancer. This depends on the radiation dose and age at screening. For every 2 million women aged over 50 who have been screened by means of a single mammogram, radiation may cause one extra cancer after 10 years. If one is increasing the number of mammograms by increased frequency and increased number of views this figure will obviously be greater, but compared with an incidence of breast cancer that approaches 2000 in every million women aged 60 this risk is very small.

The UK screening programme

Since March 1988, health authorities in the UK have been phasing in the national breast screening programme. By the end of 1994 all eligible women had been invited to be screened.

Guidelines

- Age
  –all women aged 50–64
  –women aged 65 and over may be screened on request not more than once every 3 years
  –women under 50 are not offered routine screening
- Frequency
  –3-yearly
- Views
  –Initial screening by two views
  –Subsequently single oblique view

Guidelines for special groups

Women with a family history. Women with a strong family history under the age of 50 may be offered mammograms outside the screening programme, but at present this varies in different parts of the country. Women aged 50 and over with a strong family history are offered 3-yearly screening within the programme unless there are mammographic or clinical indications to be screened more frequently.

Women with symptoms between routine mammography. Women need to know that if they develop symptoms between routine screens, these should be reported to the GP and, after examination, referral made if necessary.

Women with breast cancer – Women aged 50 and over with breast cancer should remain on the call/recall system and continue to have mammography at least every 3 years on the other breast, and in the case of breast conservation, on the treated breast. In practice, many of these women will have more frequent mammograms.

Non-attenders. If a woman does not attend for mammography her GP will be informed. This should then be recorded in the notes or computer record in a way that will alert the next person to see the woman. Several studies have looked at the effect of GP on the uptake of breast screening. A study in the US showed that the most important factor predicting whether a woman attended for mammography was whether her GP discussed it with her or not. Women were 4–12 times more likely, depending on their age, to attend for screening after such a discussion even if it was only very brief and/or simple. Such opportunities are often missed as shown by a study in south east London when it was noted that only 7% of women attending for breast screening had discussed it with their GP although 63% had actually seen their doctor in the previous month.

Organization of the screening programme

All eligible women from a whole general practice are invited for screening every 3 years after the addresses and status of the women have been checked for accuracy by the primary health care team. Screening by whole practice rather than screening a third of the women from a practice each year allowed for better concentrated information and publicity initially. However, the disadvantage of this approach is that women who reach 50 just after the practice has been called for screening will not actually get screened until they are almost 53.

Results

The coverage by the screening programme in England was 64% of women aged 50–64 at 31 March 1995 (DoH 1996). Coverage varies with regional health authorities with the Thames regions being the lowest, mainly because of a more mobile population giving problems with accurate address registers.

In the UK, 1 507 607 women in the target group were invited for screening in 1994–95 (NHSBSP 1996). Sixty-five per cent of the women invited for screening had been screened at least once before. The overall acceptance rate among women aged 50–64, invited for the first time, is improving: almost 75% in 1994/1995 compared with 71% who accepted at the beginning of the programme. Only a third of women who had previously refused screening attended at the second time of asking. Ninety per cent of women who have attended before come back again. The acceptance rate in all categories falls with age.

Overall, of the women screened, 5% were referred for assessment. The rate varied depending on whether it was the first screen or not. At a woman's first attendance there is a higher chance of finding disease which has been there for some time than at her subsequent attendance. Various benign conditions which can give rise to an initial abnormal result will need investigation at the first visit but not thereafter. The first screen is called the prevalent screen and the second and subsequent screens the incident screen. For 1994–95, about 7.2% of women who were in the first (prevalent) round were referred compared to 3.4% in the second or subsequent (incident) rounds. Cytological tests were carried out in one in five of those referred and diagnostic histology on one in 10. For the prevalent screen for women aged 50–64, the number of cancers detected was 5.9 per 1000 women screened: the detection rate was lowest at 4.7 per 1000 for women aged 50–54 and was 9.5 per 1000 for women aged 60–64 (NHSBSP 1996). For the incident screen, the cancer detection rate was 4.3 per 1000 women screened. For the prevalent screen, the *in situ* rate was 19% and 52.8% of invasive cancers were less than 15 mm. For the incident screen the figures were 19% and 55% respectively.

Controversies in breast screening

Interval of screening

Interval cancers are a major determinant of the success or otherwise of a screening programme. An interval cancer is defined as one in which there is histological confirmation of a primary breast cancer within 3 years of a negative screen. Interval cancers in the UK programme have been observed to be almost twice the rate of those observed in the Swedish study on which the UK screening programme was modelled. For example, in East Anglia they were 24%, 59%, and 79% of the expected underlying incidence in the absence of screening in the 1st, 2nd, and 3rd years after a negative screen whereas the corresponding figures in the Swedish study were 17%, 30%, and 56% (Day *et al.* 1995). Subsequent rereading of the original negative mammograms (in a blind situation) resulted in a recommendation of recall in 70% of them, suggesting that sensitivity of the test related to training of radiologists may, in part, account for the high interval cancer rate. A study from the north western region also found a higher proportion of interval cancers than expected (31%, 52%, and 82%) (Woodman *et al.* 1995). The incidence of interval cancers in the third year after screening approached that which would have occurred in the absence of screening and suggests that the 3-year interval between screens is too long and should be reduced to 2 years. If these figures for interval cancers continue then the estimated mortality reduction will be nearer 18% than the 25% specified in the *Health of the Nation* target for breast cancer.

Two mammographic views or one

The standard screening technique used in the NHS breast screening programme from its inception in 1988 was a single view of each breast: the mediolateral oblique view. A randomized controlled trial, completed in 1994, showed that two-view mammography detected 24% more women with breast cancer than one view mammography (Wald *et al.* 1995). The proportion of women recalled for assessment was 15% lower with two views (6.9%) than with one view (8.1%). The odds of a recalled woman having breast cancer was one in 10 with two-view mammography and one in 14 with one-view mammography. Therefore, from January 1995, a change in policy was introduced: a second (cranio-caudal) view should also be taken at a women's first screening appointment, to enable radiologists to decide with greater certainty whether or not recall for further investigation is required. Independently 50% of screening programmes had been operating this policy for sometime. Introduction of two views at the prevalent screen, together with other measures, is expected to contribute to a decrease in the number of interval cancers. If all other factors (such as the interval) are optimal this could reduce breast cancer mortality by 34% in screened women compared with a reduction of 27% with one view. At present, subsequent screening mammography will usually involve only one view, although a reduction in false positive rate is likely to be seen at subsequent examinations if two views were carried out, but this has not yet been quantified (Wald *et al.* 1995).

Screening under 50

Breast cancer in women under 50 is less common than in women over 50, therefore the number of cancers identified in any screening programme will be less. There is evidence to suggest that the sensitivity of mammography appears to be lower in women in this age group. There is uncertainty about the effectiveness of mammographic screening in women under 50 and the results to date indicate that mortality is not significantly reduced in this age group, although evidence is now accruing that there may be a greater benefit than was originally thought. There still remains differences of opinion as to the effectiveness as well as cost-effectiveness of such a policy and consensus guidelines vary in different countries. A meta-analysis of eight RCTs (Smart *et al.* 1995) looked at outcomes with follow-up over 7–18 years. These results suggested that there could be a 23% benefit to women aged 40–49 invited for screening, but they excluded the Canadian National Breast Screening Study which showed an excess mortality from breast cancer of 36% in women aged 40–49 years. Two other meta-analyses (both also excluding the Canadian results) showed no overall benefit in screening women under 50 (Elwood *et al.* 1993; Kerlikowske *et al.* 1995). This issue is currently the subject of a large study in the UK.

Should women be screened before going on HRT?

Current guidance from the DoH Advisory Committee on Breast Cancer Screening states that women do not require a baseline mammogram prior to starting HRT and being on HRT does not mean that a woman should start screening at a younger age or be screened more frequently than is currently available with the NHS breast screening programme. Several studies have demonstrated that a considerable number of women on HRT (25–30%) show a pronounced increase in fibroglandular tissue, especially those on combined oestrogen/progestagen therapy (Kaufman *et al.* 1991; Vd Mooren *et al* 1993). This increase in mammographic glandular density has implications for the detection of malignant lesions, and can cause concern for radiologists, especially in populations being screened for breast cancer. It is also an issue for women under 50 who commence HRT prior to being eligible for the screening programme, whose mammograms may be difficult to interpret when they do enter the programme. Many people believe that because of this problem a baseline mammogram should be taken prior to commencing HRT, irrespective of age.

Should young women with a strong family history of breast cancer be screened?

The appropriate management of those women with a strong family history of breast cancer (who may carry BRCA1 or BRCA2 mutations) is a matter of profound uncertainty (Hoskins *et al.* 1995). In the absence of absolute evidence of benefit for mammographic screening in women under 50, it is not possible to formulate a management policy with any degree of certainty (Collins 1996). Current recommendations vary from centre to centre. In general, mammographic screening is recommended from age 35 years either annually, or biennially together with annual clinical examination (which is also of unproven benefit). In the absence of evidence of benefit, the slight risk from radiation becomes a concern. It is also important to ensure that women understand the limitations of screening. At present, women are unaware of the uncertainties and believe that screening offers them a real chance of reducing their susceptibility. A national strategy for management of women with a strong family history of breast or ovarian cancer is currently being prepared. This should enable data from throughout the country to be pooled in order to assess the efficacy of the strategy. A randomized controlled trial is not deemed feasible as high risk women are unlikely to accept being randomized to the 'no screening' arm.

Should women conduct breast self-examination (BSE)?

The role of routine breast self-examination following a set technique is controversial (Mant 1992). In the past, BSE has been advocated as a means of promoting the early diagnosis of breast cancer, both as an adjunct to screening and as a technique in its own right. None of the studies of BSE have shown a reduction in breast cancer mortality in women carrying out BSE compared with controls, though some studies showed somewhat more favourable tumour characteristics in BSE performers than controls. As the studies were not randomized the results are subject to a number of biases. This means that any differences in stage observed in BSE performers does not guarantee a survival benefit. The BSE studies showed a low, positive predictive value for presented breast lumps. This means that only a small proportion of women with a 'positive' test result will, on further investigation, be shown to have breast cancer. All studies to date have experienced difficulty in achieving good acceptance rates.

Evidence about the effectiveness of different approaches to BSE instruction is inadequate and conflicting. There is also considerable variation and inconsistency in suggested techniques, both between studies and, on occasion, within studies.

BSE is therefore a procedure for which there is only fragmentary evidence of benefit and, furthermore, which only a small minority of women practice despite a high awareness of its existence. There is currently no evidence to support the view that BSE should be regarded as a primary screening technique, nor that it should be conducted on a routine basis following a set technique which requires formal instruction. However, most breast cancers (over 90%) are found by women themselves, and we need to optimize the chances of them doing so. Accordingly, in the UK a more general breast awareness is being encouraged, based on knowing what is normal, knowing what changes to look out for, and, above all, encouraging the prompt reporting of any such changes. A leaflet, *Be breast aware*, has been produced. GPs and practice nurses will play an important role in facilitating the raising of breast awareness.

Women need to know what is normal for them, how to look and feel their breasts, what changes to look out for, and to report changes without delay. Breast self-examination is a regular, ritualistic exercise following a strict set of guidelines whilst breast self-awareness involves the woman being aware of her breasts and using convenient opportunities to feel them and see how they alter during the cycle if pre-menopausal The difference between being breast aware and BSE is difficult to appreciate fully both for women and health professionals!

Consultation with a woman with breast symptoms

The most important aspect of management for any patient presenting with a problem related to the breast is to exclude malignancy and in so doing provide effective reassurance to the patient. The level of anxiety induced by breast symptoms may in some women be of such magnitude as to impede their ability to seek medical help, and these women may present to their GP with a hidden agenda offering some totally unrelated reasons for consultation. Alternatively, denial may take over and some women with symptoms of malignancy delay so long that their prognosis is adversely affected (Phelan *et al.* 1991). While some women are genuinely ignorant of the sinister implications of their symptoms, the majority understand their symptoms but are characterized by a diversity of beliefs and behaviour including an overwhelming fear of doctors, hospitals, illness in general, and cancer in particular (Fallowfield 1991). Several studies report that delayers are generally older women of lower socio-economic class, less well-educated than non-delayers, more depressed or anxious, and more pessimistic about the treatment or fearful of the consequences of surgery (Williams *et al.* 1976). Thus all patients who present to their GP with a lump or other symptom related to their breasts should be seen without delay in order to exclude cancer where possible and thus alleviate anxiety. If there is any doubt in the GP's mind as to the cause of the problem, prompt diagnostic procedures or referral can then be instituted.

Table 5.2 *History-taking in a patient with a breast problem*

Symptom	Relevant questions
Lump	When did you notice the lump?
	Does it change with the menstrual cycle?
	Did it appear gradually or suddenly?
	Does it hurt?
Breast pain	How long has the pain been present?
	Is it associated with a lump?
	Is it bilateral or unilateral?
	Is it generalized or focal
	What is its relation to the menstrual cycle?
	How does it interfere with your lifestyle?
Nipple discharge	Is it bilateral or unilateral?
	Does it come from a single or multiple point(s)/duct(s)
	Is it milky (galactorrhoea)? Watery (serous)? Bloody? Green?
	Does it occur spontaneously?
	How much discharge is there, and how frequently does it occur?
	Have you noticed any associated changes in the nipple?

The consultation process for a women with breast symptoms

As with all presenting complaints, the first essential is for the doctor to take an appropriate history. The age and menstrual status of the patient should be noted together with an accurate account of the symptoms. The history is divided into two parts. The first is that of the presenting complaint, and the second is to ascertain whether the patient has any risk factors which make her more likely to develop breast cancer compared with the baseline population. Table 5.2 outlines the appropriate questions depending on whether the presenting complaint is a lump, pain, or a nipple-related problem.

To establish the risk factors, the following questions should be asked:

1. Is there a history of breast cancer in the family? If so, how many family members are involved, are they first or second degree relatives, and at what age did they develop the disease? (The relative risk being greatest with a history of pre-menopausal, first degree relatives, especially if the disease is bilateral.)

2. What is the parous state of the patient and, if relevant, how old was she at her first pregnancy? (Nulliparity and delay in first pregnancy to over the age of 35 being associated with an increased risk.)

3. Is there a past history of those 'benign' breast conditions which are known to predispose to the development of breast cancer? (i.e. multiple papillomatosis, atypical ductal hyperplasia, phyllodes tumour, and lobular carcinoma *in situ.*)

4. Is she currently taking any hormonal preparations? If so, what, and for how long?

Finally, the history should enquire as to her general health and whether she is taking any other drugs such as antidepressants, antihypertensives, H2 receptor antagonists, or opiates. A carefully-taken history will begin to shape one's index of suspicion. Age plays an important part in this as breast lumps are increasingly likely to be malignant as the age of the patient increases. Women under the age of 30 rarely develop breast cancer but even in this group the diagnosis should be considered. Other presenting symptoms and signs may be those of metastatic disease, such as anaemia, unexplained backache, ascites, or abdominal pain.

Examination of the breasts

The breasts should always be examined systematically. Inspection of the breasts, with the woman sitting facing the doctor, may reveal a change in outline, size, or shape of the breast and puckering or dimpling of the skin or nipple. These changes may be accentuated if the patient presses her hands on her hips or elevates the arms. Any pain or discomfort associated with a lump should be ascertained. Palpation of the breasts should be carried out with the flat of the fingers in a systematic fashion so that each part of the breast is examined. The patient should be positioned so that the nipple/areolar complex is central in the breast. For most women this is achieved by having the head of the couch at 45 degrees with her arms above her head, but the larger the breast the more horizontal she will need to be. If a lump is present the doctor needs to assess its position and size, whether it is discrete or diffuse, whether it is smooth or irregular, tender or painless, mobile or fixed. Any discharge should be inspected, its colour noted and, if facilities are available, tested for occult blood. Finally, the axillae and supraclavicular fossae should be examined and the neck palpated for cervical nodes.

Benign breast disease

About 50% of women in the UK will experience symptoms of benign breast disease during their reproductive years (Hughes *et al.* 1989). Compared with breast cancer there has been relatively little work on the epidemiology of benign breast disease, despite the fact that now only about 10% of patients attending breast clinics will turn out to have breast malignancy, whereas in 1981 26% were malignant.

Classification of benign breast disease

The management of benign breast conditions is critically dependent on an

Table 5.3 *A broad classification of benign breast disorders*

1. ANDI (Aberration of Normal Development and Involution)
    - (a) Development
Lobular	Fibroadenoma
Stromal	Adolescent hypertrophy
    - (b) Cyclical change
Hormonal activity	Mastalgia
	Nodularity– focal/diffuse
    - (c) Involution
Lobular	Cyst formation
	Sclerosing adenosis
2. Duct ectasia/periductal mastisis
3. Epithelial hyperplasias
4. Conditions with well-defined aetiology, for example,
    Lactational abscess
    Traumatic fat necrosis

Reproduced with kind permission of Professor L. Hughes

understanding of the normal and histological processes within the breast and the aberrations which lead to symptoms and physical signs. Terminology in benign breast conditions has been confused by a multiplicity of terms which do not relate accurately to clinical or histological patterns and which are not based on sound concepts of pathogenesis. The ANDI classification (Aberrations of Normal Development and Involution) (Hughes *et al.* 1987) has been put forward as a nomenclature based on pathogenesis to replace the division of benign breast disorders into normal and disease (see Table 5.3). It recognizes that a spectrum exists for most conditions which extends from normal through mild abnormality to aberrations and finally disease. An important point in the classification is the replacement of the term 'disease' by 'disorder'. It recognizes that most breast complaints are due to disorders based on the normal processes of development, cyclical changes, and involution. Such disorders occasionally become frankly abnormal and then can be considered as disease. The main benign breast disorders which will be considered in this section are fibroadenomas, cysts, breast pain, nodularity, and nipple discharge and infection of the breast.

The four major symptoms

The four major symptoms which women present with are lumps, nipple discharge, nipple retraction, and pain. Faced with a lump, the GP needs answers to the following questions: who found the lump (patient, partner, or physician, or nurse), was its onset sudden or gradual, is it single or multiple, is it diffuse, is it smooth or are the margins irregular, and is it mobile or tethered? If nipple discharge is being complained of the GP should note whether it is spontaneous or present only on expression, if it is scanty or profuse, unilateral or bilateral, from single or multiple ducts, and what colour, i.e. milky (galactorrhoea), green, watery (serous), or bloody. With regard to nipple retraction, there are several features which will help in diagnosis – the length of the history, whether it is unilateral or bilateral, transient or permanent, partial or complete, linear or ferential, and real or apparent (e.g. eroded nipple). Similarly, there are specific features of breast pain which will aid diagnosis – its cyclicity, whether it is diffuse or well-localized, whether it is unilateral or bilateral, if it is confined to the breast, and whether it originates in the breast or elsewhere.

General principles of management and referral

Having taken a history and examined the patient, the GP has to ask whether a true breast lump is present. Sometimes lumps are within the skin, such as sebaceous cysts, or are deep to the breast, such as a costochondral junction. Some women may experience a lump or lumpiness as part of the menstrual cycle or in association with pregnancy.

If there is definitely no lump, and no other significant abnormality has been found in the history and examination, or the symptoms can be satisfactorily explained as being due to trauma or hormonal fluctuations, reassurance should suffice even if a specific diagnosis cannot be made. Care should be taken to ensure that the patient is not harbouring a particular fear of breast cancer (cancer phobia) which might necessitate further reassurance, or even investigation and/ or referral. The woman should always be advised about breast awareness and invited to re-consult should there be any further problems.

In a substantial percentage of women complaining of breast symptoms, especially those in their thirties or forties with lumpy breasts, it may be more difficult for the GP to make a definite diagnosis. Sometimes it can be helpful to ask the woman to return at a different time in the menstrual cycle, especially after a period, for another examination. If at the second examination there is some abnormality, nodularity, or thickening, referral to a specialist is probably the safest course of action.

The finding of a persistent, discrete lump requires that a specific diagnosis is reached and this may require referral to hospital, preferably to a specialist breast clinic (Yelland *et al.* 1991). Box 5.2 shows the conditions that should be referred to a specialist and Box 5.3 shows those conditions that can be managed, at least initially, by the GP. There is now good evidence that outcomes for breast cancer are better if women with breast cancer are treated in specialist centres. A study in Scotland showed that the 5-year survival rate was 9% higher and the 10 year survival rate 8% higher for patients cared for by specialist surgeons (Gillis and Hole 1996). A reduction in risk of dying of 16% (95% CI 6–25%) was found after adjustment for age, tumour size, socio-economic status, and nodal involvement. The benefit of specialist care was apparent for all age groups, for small and large tumours, and for tumours that did and did not affect the nodes and was consistent across all socio-economic categories. Therefore if a woman presents to the GP with a breast problem that needs referral she should be referred to a surgeon with a specialist interest in breast disease in a specialist centre. Unfortunately, this is not happening uniformly across the country

Box 5.2 *Conditions that require referral to a surgeon with a special interest in breast disease: summary*

Lump
- Any new discrete lump
- New lump in pre-existing nodularity
- Asymmetrical nodularity that persists at review after menstruation
- Abscess
- Cyst persistently refilling or recurrent*

Pain
- If associated with a lump
- Intractable pain not responding to reassurance, simple measures such as wearing a well-supporting bra, and common drugs
- Unilateral persistent pain in post-menopausal women

Nipple discharge
- All women aged 50 and over
- Women under 50 with:
  - bilateral discharge sufficient to stain clothes
  - bloodstained
  - persistent single duct

Nipple retraction or distortion, nipple eczema

Change in skin contour

Family history

Request for assessment by a woman with a strong family history of breast cancer (referral to a family cancer genetics clinic where possible)

*If the patient has recurrent multiple cysts, and the GP has the necessary skills, then aspiration is acceptable

Source: Austoker et al. (1995b)

Box 5.3 *Women who can be managed, at least initially, by their GP*

- Young women with tender, lumpy breasts and older women with symmetrical nodularity, provided that they have no localized abnormality
- Women with minor and moderate degrees of breast pain who do not have a discrete palpable lesion
- Women aged under 50 who have nipple discharge that is from more than one duct or is intermittent and is neither bloodstained nor troublesome

Source: Austoker et al. (1995b)

Fig 5.2 *Relative frequency of breast disorders*
(Source: Austoker et al., 1995b)

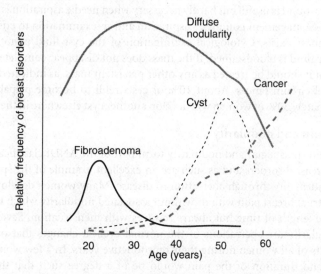

(Sainsbury *et al.* 1995). The very act of referral will undoubtedly induce anxiety and so the GP should advise the woman as to what is likely to happen to her in the way of investigations when she attends the hospital – such as aspiration cytology, core biopsy, ultrasound, and mammography.

Breast lumps – fibroadenomas and cysts

Benign, discrete breast masses are most commonly fibroadenomas or breast cysts. These two conditions have different age distributions. The relative frequency of breast conditions against age is shown in Fig 5.2. Fibroadenomas account for about 12% of all palpable, symptomatic breast lumps (Dent and Cant 1989). They are particularly common in the 15–30 age group. They tend to be spherical, have a rubbery consistency, a smooth surface, and are extraordinarily mobile (hence the alternative name of 'breast mouse'). About 5% of fibroadenomas will grow progressively, 20% will regress, but the majority will remain the same size, becoming less distinct after the menopause. The diagnosis is made by a combination of clinical examination, ultrasound, and aspiration cytology. Since they are benign and without a malignant potential they can be safely left *in situ*, but some women request excision.

Breast cysts are most common in the 40–50 years age group. In more than 50% of patients they are multiple and are most often in the upper outer quadrant. They are the commonest abnormality in patients presenting to a breast clinic (Haagensen 1986). They are frequently asymptomatic and noted accidentally by the patient when touching the breast but can be accompanied by pain, especially if they are tense or have developed rapidly. The clinical findings of cysts vary with the degree of intracystic tension. A cyst can be completely missed if it is soft, but misdiagnosed as cancer if it is hard. The single passage of a fine (21 g) needle into every discrete lump to exclude a cyst may save the patient much distress. Mammography alone is of limited use as it is difficult to differentiate cysts from fibroadenomas, or indeed from well-defined carcinomas. Ultrasound is useful but hardly necessary when needle aspiration is readily available. Management comprises aspiration and re-examination to ensure no residual mass exists. Cytological examination of the cyst fluid is not useful unless the fluid is bloodstained. If the mass does not disappear completely after aspiration it should be treated as any other persistent mass, as indicated by the individual circumstances. About 10% of cysts refill to become palpable and approximately 50% of women will develop another cyst elsewhere in the breast.

Breast pain and nodularity

Breast pain (mastalgia) and nodularity form part of the ANDI classification of benign breast disorders and as such are an excellent example of the spectrum from abnormality through aberration to disease. Many women develop mild, premenstrual breast pain with or without associated nodularity which lasts for a variable length of time but always resolves with menstruation. Severe pain and nodularity are aberrations of the normal cyclical changes that occur in the breasts of all women during their reproductive years. In a few women the severity and duration of the pain would be of a degree such that the term disorder could be applied. Pain alone or a painful lump is the presenting symptom in about 50% of women attending a breast clinic and a lump alone or painful lump is the presenting symptom in approximately 70% of cases (Dixon and Sainsbury 1993).

During an ongoing evaluation of the NHS breast screening programme breast referral guidelines, preliminary results show that although 90% of the referrals for breast pain are due to benign lesions, most women believe referral to a specialist is indicated for breast pain.

There are three main clinical syndromes of mastalgia. The commonest (75% of total) is cyclical mastalgia which shows a definite relationship to the menstrual cycle and is often associated with nodularity of varying degree, maximal in the outer upper quadrant and which shows a similar cyclical variation. It presents most commonly during the third decade of life and tends to be of a chronic, relapsing nature with resolution of the symptoms around the time of the menopause. The second-largest group, non-cyclical mastalgia, has no relationship to the menstrual cycle and tends to present a decade later with a shorter duration of symptoms that resolve spontaneously in about 50% of cases. The pain tends to be well-localized in the breast and nodularity is less prominent than in the cyclical group. Some of these patients have a tender area in the chest wall, palpation of which may 'trigger' their pain. In this subgroup, injection of this spot with a mixture of methyl prednisolone and lignocaine may be of benefit. The third group is Tietze's syndrome which is not true breast pain, but pain occurring in the costochondral junction. The pain is felt in the region of the breast that overlies the costal cartilage, and so typically is felt within the medial quadrants of the breast and worsens when pressure is applied to the affected cartilage.

The aetiology of mastalgia is unclear. The long-held views about water retention have not been substantiated in well-controlled clinical trials and it is more likely that there are abnormalities in the control mechanisms of the pulsatile secretion of gonadotrophins and/or prolactin. The relationship of the Pill to mastalgia is unclear. There does not appear to be any constant correlation between the brand of pill, its hormonal content, and the occurrence of breast pain. The use of HRT in peri- and post-menopausal women is a well-known cause of mastalgia and is treated by withdrawing the exogenous oestrogen completely or using a low-dose, combined preparation for a short time only. If clear pathological causes of pain can be excluded, such as abscess, periductal mastitis, and malignant disease, most patients can be managed by explanation of the likely physiological nature of the symptoms and reassurance that they do not have cancer. However, in about 15% of women the pain is so severe that it affects their lifestyle and requires treatment. Bromocriptine, danazol, gamolenic acid (GLA), and tamoxifen have all been shown in placebo controlled trials to be useful in the treatment of breast pain. Diuretics, the most popular treatment in general practice, progestogens, and B 6 have not been shown to be any more efficacious than placebo. Danazol, a synthetic steroid with anti-gonadotrophic properties, is the most effective treatment for women with severe cyclical mastalgia. At a dose of 200 mg daily it can relieve symptoms in 70% of women, and the dose can be lowered to 100 mg either daily or on alternative days after the first 2 months of treatments. Side-effects include hirsutism and weight gain. Evening primrose oil, a natural source of GLA, has been shown to reduce pain, tenderness, and nodularity in 60% of patients at a dose of 300 mg of GLA daily. Its low incidence of side-effects makes it especially useful, and so is recommended as first-line treatment.

Bromocriptine reduces the secretion of prolactin. At a dose of 2.5 mg twice daily it is helpful in women with cyclical mastalgia but not in those with non-cyclical mastalgia. However, 20% of women experience side-effects such as nausea, vomiting, and dizziness, sufficient for them to terminate treatment. Tamoxifen has been found to improve mastalgia at a dose of 10–20 mg daily, but it does not have a product licence for use in mastalgia and so is best restricted to use in a specialized clinic. LHRH analogues have been investigated, and although they are an effective treatment for breast pain the side-effect profiles are unacceptable.

Nipple discharge

Nipple discharge is a relatively uncommon presenting complaint but women may present because they fear the diagnostic implications, because it is socially embarrassing, or because it is in association with another breast symptom such as a lump. If it is the latter, then the lump will take precedence as far as investigation is concerned (see Fig 5.3). Nipple discharge is potentially most significant when it occurs spontaneously and as the dominant symptom. Three main groups of discharge are described: bloody, coloured opalescent, and milky. A serous, serosanguinous, or frankly bloodstained discharge all carry the same significance. They are usually due either to a hyperplastic epithelial lesion or duct ectasia (see below). The epithelial hyperplasia is usually benign, due to

Fig 5.3 *Nipple discharge*
(Source: Austoker et al., 1995b)

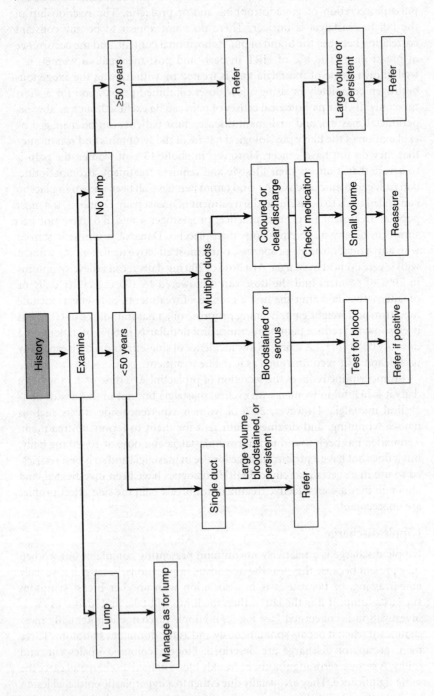

one or more duct papillomas, but the risk of malignancy increases with age, being much greater after the menopause. The discharge from a duct papilloma usually arises from a single duct and a nodule may be felt below the skin which, upon pressure, results in a small jet of discharge from the duct. Galactorrhoea is the term used to describe secretion of human milk from the breast unrelated to breast-feeding. Its cause is usually physiological but may be due to medication such as phenothiazines, butyrophenones, or metoclopramide. Only rarely is it due to a pituitary tumour.

Discharges other than sanguinous or milky can, for most purposes, be considered together and are not associated with an increased risk of cancer. They occur more commonly in the later years and can be very profuse. Multiple ducts of one or both breasts are involved and the underlying pathology is usually duct ectasia. (Not everyone may find it easy to distinguish single from multiple ducts.) The discharge can be nearly any colour and in about 50% of cases contains blood. This disorder may also present with nipple inversion, inflammatory masses, abscess formation, and mammillary fistulae.

The management of nipple discharge depends on its nature and the age of the patient. The management of galactorrhoea is that of the underlying cause and bromocriptine may be of use if the discharge is profuse. In a young patient with a bloodstained discharge, the risk of malignancy is so low as to require simple observation after a full assessment has been made. However, in women over 45, the risk of malignancy is such that excision of the affected duct(s) is appropriate. The use of appropriate antibiotics, especially those effective against anaerobic organisms, can help resolve the inflammatory element of duct ectasia but are not appropriate for the treatment of discharge alone (in the absence of an inflammatory mass). A coloured, opalescent discharge only requires treatment by duct excision if it is so copious as to require the use of pads. The laying open of a single mammary duct fistula is usually effective in allaying chronic recurrent abscesses.

Infection of the breast

The most common cause of breast abscess in general practice is in lactating women although its incidence appears to be decreasing (Benson 1982). The vast majority of puerperal infections are caused by *Staphylococcus aureus* but there are a substantial number of cases of non-infective mastitis, where the early symptoms are identical. These symptoms of a painful, red, and swollen breast often with some constitutional upset. Emptying the breast, either by suckling or expression, is of vital importance and these days it is *not* advised to stop feeding from the affected side. An anti-pyretic/anti-inflammatory drug is recommended and in the case of non-infective mastitis this should resolve the symptoms within 24 hours. Flucloxacillin, 500 mg four times a day, is the antibiotic of choice in the presence of infection and in most cases will arrest the process at the cellulitic phase. However 5–10% of women will go on to develop an abscess requiring surgical drainage. In young, non-lactating women, periareolar sepsis is frequently associated with cigarette smoking, whilst in the older woman, periductal mastitis/duct ectasia, sometimes associated with inverted nipples and a chronic nipple discharge, is the commonest cause. In these cases, the causative organ is more likely to include an anaerobe. Recurrent infections may result in a mamillary fistula which will need surgical treatment.

Malignant breast disease

Diagnosis of palpable lesions

The confident diagnosis of breast cancer involves the 'triple assessment' – clinical examination, radiology, and pathological confirmation. Surgery remains the commonest primary treatment for breast cancer and in recent years there has been an increasing tendency to obtain a pre-operative diagnosis so that patients can be counselled before surgery and the various treatment options discussed. The two main methods of obtaining a pre-operative tissue diagnosis are fine needle aspiration cytology (FNAC) and core biopsy (Sloane 1991). The advantage of a core biopsy is that structural as well as cytological information can be obtained, which is especially important in distinguishing *in situ* from infiltrative carcinomas. However, FNAC offers distinct advantages in that it is a quick, simple technique and the slide can be processed and reported immediately, hence reducing the length of time the patient has to wait for a diagnosis and thereby reducing anxiety. Furthermore, it enables future management to be planned at the first visit, reducing clinical visits. If either FNAC or core biopsy fails to make the diagnosis, an 'open' surgical biopsy is sometimes required, and can be carried out under general or local anaesthetic.

Diagnosis of impalpable mammographic lesions

The use of mammography in the investigation of symptomatic patients or as a screening test presents the problem of diagnosing mammographic abnormalities which are impalpable. Special radiological and surgical localization techniques and highly-skilled pathology are required for these patients and sterotactic FNAC +/– core biopsy are both important means of reaching a diagnosis in a patient with an impalpable lesion. MRI is also an investigative tool which is starting to be used in these cases.

Treatment of breast cancer: early stage disease

The management of breast cancer has changed significantly over the past two decades and continues to do so. The aims of clinicians involved are twofold – the first is to eradicate local disease and prevent local and regional recurrence (achieved mainly by a combination of surgery and radiotherapy) and the second is to prolong survival by the use of adjuvant systemic agents (as micrometastatic disease may be present at the time of diagnosis despite negative staging investigations (Sacks and Baum 1993)). The choice of treatment combinations for any individual patient will depend on the characteristics of the

Table 5.4 *Survival at 10 years of patients with breast cancer according to the involvement of axillary lymph nodes*

All patients	45.9%
Negative axillary lymph nodes	64.9%
Positive axillary lymph nodes	24.9%
1–3	37.5%
>4	13.4%

Source: Miller et al. (1995)

tumour, the size of the breast, whether nodal metastases are present, and patient preference.

Prognostic factors

There are many factors involved in the staging of breast cancer and the important prognostic factors should be determined when trying to decide on treatment and predict survival (Miller *et al.* 1995).

Tumour size correlates directly with survival; the smaller the tumour the better the prognosis. Patients with tumours less than 2 cm have 5-year survival rates between 84–90% compared to 60% for patients with tumours >5 cm.

Axillary node involvement is the single most important prognostic factor. There is direct correlation between survival and the level and number of axillary nodes involved (Table 5.4). Axillary nodes are routinely biopsied or removed to assess the stage of the cancer (Bundred *et al.* 1995). Whether the nodes are sampled or cleared is controversial and varies from centre to centre.

Metastases and where they occur affect survival. Although there may be micro invasion at time of diagnosis, demonstrable metastases carry a worse prognosis. If the metastases are only in the supraclavicular site the prognosis is better than other sites.

Histological type and grade. Invasive tumours are now classified as those of special type (tubular, cribriform, medullary, mucoid, papillary, and lobular) or of no special type. The former have a better prognosis than the latter. Tumours are also classified according to histological grade dependent on the differentiation and mitotic activity of the cells.

Vascular and lymphatic invasion by tumour cells is found in 25% of patients with breast cancer. There is a doubling of the rate of local recurrence after wide excision or mastectomy and short-term systemic relapse is more common.

Hormone and growth factor receptors are found in some breast cancers. Oestrogen receptors (know as ER status) help predict the response to hormonal manipulation. ER status can be measured and graded. Generally, women who are post-menopausal are more likely to have tumours that are ER positive, whilst in pre-menopausal women the ER status is more likely to be negative or weakly positive. More and more, decisions as to whether to have hormonal treatment or not are being guided by ER status. A false- negative or not measuring ER status can be a mistake. ER-positive tumours are more likely to respond to hormonal treatment such as tamoxifen than ER-negative ones, but it is not always so. The presence of epidermal growth factor receptors within the membrane of breast cancer cells is inversely correlated with the presence of oestrogen receptors and is associated with a diminished period free of relapse and reduced overall survival. Patients whose tumours are positive for epidermal growth factor receptors are unlikely to respond to hormonal treatment.

DNA content measures the amount and type of DNA in the cells to help assess how rapidly the cancer cells are dividing. If the cancer cells have the correct amount of DNA in a cell they are called diploid, whilst if the amount of DNA is abnormal they are know as aneuploid. Thirty per cent of breast cancer tumours are diploid and have a better prognosis. There are also many other markers of proliferation that have been developed to help in assessment.

The presence of certain oncogenes, tumour suppressor genes, proteases, and second messenger systems are all used to try and assess prognosis.

Survival curves

When women are diagnosed with breast cancer many want to know how likely they are to live or die. The available survival curves at 5 and 10 years have to be treated with caution as treatments have changed and there is now evidence of better prognosis for some women because they are treated with adjuvant therapy/or oophorectomy.

Surgery

Almost all women with early breast cancer will be offered some form of surgery. Although the risk of local recurrence is reduced, there is no evidence that survival is prolonged by radical surgery compared with local removal of the tumour. Hence there has been a recent trend towards more conservative surgery, either alone or, more commonly, in conjunction with radiotherapy. Where the disease is confined to the breast alone, surgery might be sufficient to achieve cure (Baum *et al*, 1994). In all other cases the surgical procedure has two aims – firstly to remove the tumour and reduce the chances of local recurrence, and secondly to provide important information with regards to prognosis and tumour stage by performing a regional lymph node dissection. The surgical options to the breast itself include either wide local excision of the tumour (partial mastectomy) or removal of the whole breast (simple mastectomy). In certain cases patient preference will influence the decision-making process, but in general terms large tumours, tumours in a central position, and tumours in small breasts make conservative surgery less feasible as in these circumstances the cosmetic result will be poor. Hence, tumours which are larger than 4 cm, retroareolar, or multifocal are most commonly treated by mastectomy in order to obtain adequate control of the disease, and vascular invasion, nodal involvement, and extensive preinvasive disease are additional indications, as these factors are associated with an increased risk of local recurrence after wide local excision. The surgical dissection in the axilla is either limited to 'sampling' of representative nodes (which, although providing staging information, does not adequately treat the involved axilla) or a 'clearance' of all nodal tissue (which gives excellent staging information and treats involved nodes but will overtreat the 'negative' axilla).

For those patients who are not suitable for breast conservation, some form of breast reconstruction may be requested. This may either be performed at the time of the mastectomy or delayed until a later date. In general terms, reconstruction of the breast can be performed either by replacing the breast with an implant (containing either silicone or saline) or using a myocutaneous flap (Watson *et al.* 1995). The simplest type of reconstruction involves placing a prosthesis behind the pectoral muscle. If the nipple has been preserved and minimal skin removed (a subcutaneous mastectomy), the correct-sized implant can be placed at the time of operation. If, as happens more commonly, a simple mastectomy has been necessary, an inflatable prosthesis is used which is inserted in a deflated state and then inflated gradually over a period of time by injection of saline through a subcutaneous injection 'port'. This stretches the chest wall skin over the prosthesis until the desired size is achieved. Although this procedure is simple it has the disadvantage that it is difficult to achieve the natural shape of the breast, and so it is most suitable for reconstructing small breasts which are not particularly ptotic. A long-term problem with this operation is the formation of a 'capsule' of scar tissue around the prosthesis which can distort the breast and cause pain. In addition, this operation is not suitable as a delayed technique if the chest wall has been irradiated as the skin loses its elasticity.

Reconstruction using tissue flaps involves the use of the skin and subcutaneous tissue from either the back (latissimus dorsi flap) or lower abdomen (TRAM flap). The advantage of the former is that it is a simpler operation with good flap survival, but most women need a prosthesis in addition to the flap in order to achieve sufficient bulk of tissue. The TRAM is probably the 'gold standard' operation for breast reconstruction, but it is a lengthy procedure with a higher complication rate and a longer recovery period.

Radiotherapy

Radiotherapy is given daily or three times a week over several weeks. Very small, good-prognosis tumours and pre-invasive ductal disease (DCIS) are sometimes treated by wide excision alone without the need for radiotherapy, but with these exceptions adjuvant radiotherapy is usually given to the residual breast tissue following conservative surgery in order to reduce the risk of local recurrence to a level comparable to that following more radical surgery.

The likelihood of local recurrence after breast-conserving surgery and radiotherapy has varied widely in different studies with reported rates of between 0–22%. Factors involved in this variation include: the completeness of the excision, presence of an extensive *in situ* component, presence of lymphatic vascular invasion, and high tumour grade (Dixon 1995). The 12-

year follow-up of the randomized trial from the United States National Cancer Institute, comparing the outcome in women with early breast cancer after total mastectomy alone or after lumpectomy with or without radiotherapy, showed no difference in survival between the three groups. The incidence of ipsilateral tumour recurrence was 35% in the lumpectomy alone group as against 10% in the lumpectomy and radiotherapy group (Fisher *et al.* 1995). Other studies have shown that radiotherapy after lumpectomy reduces local recurrence from about 20% to 5%. A recent overview of nine trials found that radiotherapy produced substantial reduction in local recurrence, with three times fewer recurrences when radiotherapy was added to surgery (Early Breast Cancer Trialists' Collaborative Group 1995). An overview of data from early radiotherapy trials suggested that radiotherapy had a detrimental effect on long-term survival. More recent trials including patients treated with more modern techniques do not show this. There is even some evidence from the meta-analysis of nine trials that radiotherapy seems to reduce the risk of death from breast cancer but this is still counterbalanced by an increased risk of death from other causes leading to no difference in overall survival.

Following mastectomy, radiotherapy is given to those patients who are thought to have the greatest risk of local recurrence following surgery alone, such as patients with large primary tumours, especially those with a poor grade with positive nodes. In addition, those patients having less than a full surgical clearance of the axilla, and those who demonstrate pathological involvement of lymph node samples, benefit from post operative radiotherapy to prevent uncontrollable axillary recurrence. Radiotherapy to the axilla following a radical dissection is not recommended because of the severe lymphoedema of the arm that can result from this combined approach.

Systemic therapy

Systemic treatment may either be given pre-operatively (primary medical treatment or neoadjuvant therapy), or post-operatively (adjuvant therapy), and it may be in the form of either cytotoxic chemotherapy or hormonal manipulation.

Neoadjuvant treatment

As a rule, patients are chosen for neoadjuvant treatment if they present with large tumours, especially if they are of poor grade. The rationale behind this approach is that tumour response to any regime can be assessed by clinical and radiological measurement, and in the case of non-response, the treatment can be changed. Using adriamycin containing chemotherapy, response rates of up to 70% have been described. A further advantage of this approach is that in patients who respond, the surgical procedure need be less radical than that possible before the chemotherapy, hence a wide local excision may become feasible rather than a mastectomy. It is hoped that tumours treated in this way may have a better outcome than when treated in a more conventional fashion, but this is yet unproven and the morbidity of the treatment is such that only poor prognosis tumours are appropriate. If it is known that the tumour is likely

Table 5.5 *Numbers of extra 10-year survivors from treatment of 100 middle-aged women with stage II breast cancer (NB absolute benefit might be about half as great in stage I) (R. Peto, personal communication)*

Allocated treatment	Numbers of extra 10-year survivors per 100 treated (best estimate)
Age over 50	
Tamoxifen alone for 5 years	8
Multiple-agent cytotoxic chemotherapy alone (e.g. 6 months or more of CMF	5
Tamoxifen + chemotherapy	12
Age under 50	
Ovarian ablation alone	11
Multiple agent chemotherapy alone	10
Ovarian ablation + chemotherapy	at least 12
Tamoxifen for 5 years	8

to be sensitive to hormonal treatment (if, for example, a biopsy had shown the tumour to be ER positive), or if the patient is elderly and not suitable for aggressive chemotherapy then tamoxifen may be given as a neoadjuvant treatment.

Adjuvant systemic therapy

Clinical trials of adjuvant therapy have established that both cytotoxic chemotherapy, the anti-oestrogen tamoxifen, and ovarian ablation can reduce 10-year mortality from breast cancer and increase the period of disease-free survival. A recent overview showed that there was a 12% increase in 10-year survival in women with stage II disease and 6% for stage 1 (Table 5.5). This meta-analysis of almost all known adjuvant trials of either tamoxifen or chemotherapy concluded as follows (Early Breast Cancer Trialists' Collaborative Group 1992):

1. Tamoxifen given daily for 5 years as immediate treatment reduces recurrence both for pre and post-menopausal women.
2. Tamoxifen at a dose of 20 mg per day taken for 2 years or more following local therapy produces a reduction in 10-year mortality from breast cancer, especially in women aged 50 and over (post-menopausal women).
3. Combination chemotherapy, particularly CMF-based regimens (cyclo-phosphamide, methotrexate, 5-fluorouracil), produces a 10-year mortality reduction, especially in women under 50 (pre-menopausal women).
4. There is no evidence that continuing CMF treatment for longer than 6 months is more effective.
5. Both chemotherapy and tamoxifen significantly reduce recurrence rates

among both younger and older women. The combination is more effective than either treatment alone for women over 50.

6. Ovarian ablation, either by surgery or radiotherapy, reduces 10-year mortality in pre-menopausal women.

7. Tamoxifen reduces the risk of getting cancer in the opposite breast by 40%.

In general, the data suggest that the smaller the risk of relapse for the individual patient then the smaller would be the absolute benefit of adjuvant therapy and so the greater would be the relative importance of any toxic side-effects of that therapy.

With this principle in mind, some simple guidelines emerge. In post-menopausal, node-positive and node-negative patients, 5 years of tamoxifen has little toxicity and definite benefits. In younger women there is also some benefit but the anti-oestrogenic side-effects are more likely to cause problems with hot flushes and night sweats, and so the benefit has to be weighed against quality of life, especially if the tumour is known to be ER poor. Pre-menopausal, node-positive women will benefit most from cytotoxic chemotherapy, which can then be followed by 5 years of tamoxifen. For patients who relapse on hormonal treatment it is worthwhile trying a second line treatment such as a progesterone, an LHRH agonist, or an aromatase inhibitor.

Screen-detected lesions

Before the advent of the national breast screening programme, ductal carcinoma *in situ* (DCIS) constituted less than 5% of all breast cancers, but now the figure is approximately 20%. If untreated it is estimated that about 40% of patients with this condition will develop invasive disease, hence the treatment of (DCIS) is an important issue as an increasing number of patients are diagnosed by screening. Unfortunately, there is not yet a consensus as to how small, localized lesions should be best treated nor how to distinguish who are the 40% of women with DCIS that will progress, but trials in the UK and US are ongoing to compare conservative surgery alone, surgery and radiotherapy, surgery and tamoxifen, and a combination of all three modalities. Impalpable, screen-detected, invasive lesions in general have an excellent prognosis. They are generally treated by conservative surgery, with axillary node dissection determining the use of adjuvant systemic therapy. The place of radiotherapy with these very small lesions is uncertain and is currently being determined by clinical trials.

Treatment of breast cancer: advanced disease

Breast cancer metastasizes most commonly to lymph nodes, the skeleton, lungs, and liver, but may spread to any organ. Local infiltration or ulceration of the chest wall may occur, and is very distressing to the patient. Treatment may be local, systemic, or both. Treatment of advanced disease has two objectives: palliation of symptoms and prolongation of life, with the main emphasis being to improve the quality rather than the length of the patient's remaining life (Baum *et al.* 1994).

Systemic therapy can be used to produce remission and prolong life. Simple endocrine therapy can produce good results. For pre-menopausal women this could be either by surgical removal of the ovaries or, more commonly, by the use of an LHRH agonist or tamoxifen; and for post-menopausal women, tamoxifen. Approximately 30% remission rates can be achieved. If a patient has demonstrated that her tumour has responded to tamoxifen but then relapses, it is worth trying a second-line hormonal treatment such as medroxyprogesterone acetate as the response rate is likely to be in the order of 25%. As with early breast cancer, other forms of hormonal manipulation include LHRH agonists and, more recently, specific aromatase inhibitors. The use of single agent cytotoxic therapy (for example, cyclophosphamide) produces a similar order of remission but with greater toxicity. The combination of three or more cytotoxic drugs, each with different modes of action, can produce far higher remission rates in terms of the temporary reduction of the tumour bulk, but with potentially much greater side-effects. In general it is better therefore to attempt simple endocrine therapy first, and only proceed to combination chemotherapy if this fails.

Both local surgery and radiotherapy have a useful role to play in advanced disease although appropriate systemic treatment should also be given in order to achieve maximum control of the disease. For painful bony lesions complete relief of symptoms can be achieved by a short course of localized radiotherapy. If the bone pain is more generalized, adequate analgesia is essential and treatment with biphosphonates may be of use. Dyspnoea secondary to a malignant effusion can be improved by paracentesis followed by the introduction of cytotoxic drugs into the pleural cavity. Shrinkage of liver metastases can be achieved by giving either high doses of corticosteroids or widefield radiotherapy to the liver. Cerebral metastases can be shrunk by dehydration therapy or corticosteroids, in particular dexamethasone. Radiotherapy to the brain may also achieve palliation. For anaemia, blood transfusions may be required in the short term, and pathological fractures will require fixation.

Adverse effects of treatment

Surgery to the breast

However a woman reacts to hearing her diagnosis, most hope to keep their breast. In general, the choice of initial treatment for the affected breast does not influence outcome in terms of survival. The 1980s have seen a move towards more conservative treatment with an increase in cosmetic acceptability but also an increase in the need for radiotherapy, which for some patients is as debilitating as the surgery. Since psychological problems afflict women whatever surgery they have, it is essential that adequate counselling and support is available as soon as treatment begins to be planned. It is often useful to include the partner in these discussions in order to diminish fears and dispel myths about the final cosmetic result.

The length of stay in hospital varies according to the type of surgery performed, but all women should be visited by the specialist nurse counsellor before discharge. Their feelings about the treatment so far, particularly their reaction to the scar, can be elicited and answers given to any queries they might have about further therapy. This is also the time to discuss their views about a prosthesis. While the sutures are still *in situ* or the wound is not fully healed, a permanent external prosthesis is not usually possible but a lightweight temporary prosthesis to be worn inside the bra can help women regain their confidence more quickly. Choosing the right type of permanent prosthesis is extremely important and women need to be given all the available information about what is available, both on the NHS and from private suppliers, before they make their final choice. It is not uncommon for women to feel very dissatisfied with their prosthesis – worries that it will fall out or slip and make them look uneven, that it is too hot and heavy, so that it can result in significant morbidity in terms of body image. In some women, breast reconstruction may be available but this does not always result in a satisfactory cosmetic appearance and certainly is not a panacea for women who are not coping with a prosthesis.

Damage to the intercostobrachial nerve is not uncommon after breast surgery as a result of the axillary dissection and may leave the patient with either numbness, parasthesia, or hyperasthesia in the axilla and the upper inner arm. This is usually self-limiting as the nerve regenerates but is sufficiently common as to justify warning the patient about the symptoms pre-operatively. Before discharge from hospital, all patients should be taught simple, post-operative exercises to help regain normal arm movements, but occasionally physiotherapy is needed to limit post-operative oedema and to reduce muscle stiffness and wasting from disuse. If lymphoedema develops as a consequence of either treatment or recurrent disease, discomfort can be lessened with the use of elasticated arm stockings or, in more severe cases, with a special intermittent flow pump, the Flowtron.

Radiotherapy

Most women who have radiotherapy get some side-effects. They vary from patient to patient. Explanation of what radiotherapy involves and the possible side-effects with good support during the radiotherapy can only help to reduce the fear and anxiety associated with the treatment. Skin reactions of some type are almost universal. In some, particularly those women with bigger breasts, the skin may actually break down leaving a raw area which can take some time to heal. It should not be washed or covered with cream but baby powder can be used to help diminish irritation. The breast may also swell and become sensitive. After treatment finishes the skin can remain thickened and darker, with crusting around the nipple. After treatment, zinc and caster oil cream may be used to soothe or soften the skin. The skin can take 6 months or longer to settle down.

Fatigue and tiredness is another major symptom that is almost universal. It usually gets worse towards the end of the treatment. It may not start until the end of treatment and can continue for several months after completion.

Depression is common and, like fatigue, tends to get worse as the treatment progresses. It may not even start until after its completion. There are some later side-effects which fortunately affect fewer women and are now less frequent. Costochondritis can give pain several months after treatment finishes but is helped by NSAIDs.

Brachial plexus neuropathy as a result of axillary radiotherapy has been reported and received recent attention with the formation of a pressure group (Radiotherapy Action Group Exposure (RAGE)). It is not known how common the problem is, although it may be more common than originally thought. An extensive review laid the blame for the neuropathy on patient's positioning during radiotherapy to the axillary and supraclavicular nodes, with high dose being a secondary course. Since 1986 there appears to have been a decline in incidence, possibly because of the way in which the radiotherapy is now delivered (Spittle 1995).

Hormonal therapy

Compared to chemotherapy, hormonal treatment has fewer side-effects and there is the added advantage of not needing to attend the hospital for its administration. Tamoxifen is the most commonly-used hormonal treatment. Only 3% of women on it for breast cancer stop using it because of side-effects though it may have an effect on quality of life. Hot flushes, occurring in about 50%, are most marked and unpleasant in pre- and peri-menopausal patients. These often settle with time, but if they persist an improvement can be obtained with the addition of a progesterone (e.g. Megace 40 mg once daily).

Vaginal dryness and vaginal discharge can also be a problem, as is loss of libido. Depression occurs in a small percentage of women whilst weight gain is a more common complaint. Visual disturbances and hair thinning are less common side-effects but are well-described.

The most serious side-effect of tamoxifen is induction of uterine (endo-metrial) cancer, presumably because of tamoxifen's oestrogenic effect. It is this feature of the drug that has received most attention. The risks and benefits of the effects of tamoxifen on prevention of breast cancer and induction of uterine cancer need to be put in perspective. It has been calculated that if 1000 ER-positive women with stage II breast cancer are treated with 5 years of tamoxifen, approximately 160 recurrences of breast cancer are prevented, of which at least 80 would have died. On the negative side, between 5–10 endometrial cancers would be induced, of which one would be fatal (R Peto, personal communication). Women should be alerted to report any abnormal vaginal bleeding which should then be investigated promptly with vaginal ultrasound and possibly biopsy. While the medical benefits from tamoxifen clearly outweigh the risk in women who already have breast cancer, used as a preventive measure for women at high risk, the benefits are less certain (see p. 113). There are some other positive 'side-effects' of tamoxifen: it improves HDL levels and therefore may reduce risk from heart disease and may help protect against osteoporosis.

Progestogens are more likely to cause fluid retention and weight gain compared with tamoxifen but this is not seen to be a problem with the aromatase inhibitors. Aminoglutethamide is used less frequently than previously but side-effects include skin rashes, fever, and lethargy and a third of patients require mineralocorticoid replacement.

Chemotherapy

With good reason, chemotherapy has the worst reputation of all the treatments available for breast cancer since it invariably produces at least some side-effects in all patients. However, these vary from woman to woman and depend on the drugs being used. The most common side-effects experienced are fatigue and lethargy, nausea and vomiting, diarrhoea, mouth ulceration, hair loss, cystitis, menstrual irregularities in pre-menopausal women, infections due to a lowered white cell count, reduced resistance to infection, weight gain, and depression. Hair loss is responsible for much of the psychological morbidity associated with chemotherapy, and the provision of a suitable wig is mandatory. Good social support is essential if a woman is to have the resources to complete a course of chemotherapy which involves many visits to the hospital over 6 months to a year, as well as days on end of feeling systematically unwell. The psychological sequelae of chemotherapy is such that the very thought of the next injection is enough in some women to bring on a bout of nausea and vomiting. Careful assessment of the needs of each woman is required to ensure that she is offered appropriate help to counteract any adverse reactions to chemotherapy. Relaxation therapy and desensitization have both been used with some success in this context.

CMF (cyclophosphamide, methotrexate, and 5-fluorouracil) is the commonest chemotherapy cocktail used in breast cancer in the UK. Six doses are given at 3–4 week intervals. As yet, it is not known whether other regimens containing anthracyclines, e.g. doxorubicin and cyclophosphamide, are superior. At least 80% report fatigue and lethargy. Nausea and vomiting are commonly experienced but can be controlled in most patients by appropriate antiemetic drugs. Younger patients are more at risk of nausea and vomiting and are also more likely to get extrapyramidal side-effects from standard antiemetic regimens including metoclopramide. Some units use serotonin 3(5-HT3) antagonists routinely in younger patients as first-line treatment and this should be offered to those in whom other antiemetics are not controlling the symptoms. Cannabis, which can be prescribed by the hospital specialists as nabilone, is effective in controlling the nausea but often patients are not offered it. Ten per cent will experience hair loss (whereas for those taking adriamycin it will always occur). Twenty per cent will experience weight gain of between 5–15 lb. The short-term morbidity from chemotherapy is well-documented from clinical trials. The long-term morbidity is only starting to be addressed and such information needs to be available to women when making the choice about which treatment to have.

Psychological aspects of breast cancer

The woman with newly-diagnosed breast cancer has to cope with a multitude of problems. Cancer is regarded with almost universal dread and surveys have shown that it is perceived with more alarm than any other disease. Despite the fact that breast cancer has had such a high media profile, myths and misconceptions about the disease are still very common. A study in a south London breast screening clinic (Fallowfield *et al.* 1990*a*) found that women severely underestimated the risk of getting breast cancer but also thought that most breast lumps were due to cancer. Although most women realize the significance of finding a breast lump, a surprisingly high number delay in seeking medical advice. Having made the decision to consult a doctor and been referred to the hospital, most women find the period of waiting for the result of the biopsy the most stressful (Maguire 1976; Fallowfield *et al.* 1987). The reason given for the very high levels of anxiety seems to be more associated with the fear of having cancer than the potential loss of a breast (Fallowfield *et al.* 1990*b*). Women may display five different types of response on hearing the diagnosis: denial, fighting spirit, stoic acceptance, anxious/depressed acceptance, and helplessness/hopelessness. In addition, the reaction to discovering that she has breast cancer will be determined for each woman by her own health beliefs as well as her personality and personal circumstances. Her beliefs about the role of heredity, infection, lifestyle, trauma to the breast, stress, or punishment for earlier misdemeanours in life (divine retribution) will need to be elicited by those involved in breaking the bad news. She may well have personal experience of the disease from a friend or relative and have particular fears about the loss of a breast, recurrence, the toxicity of chemotherapy, pain, or the effect of the diagnosis on family and friends. These are all important considerations when deciding on management of her disease and need to be explored in order to be able to counsel her appropriately. The manner in which the diagnosis is relayed to the woman is obviously extremely important in determining her immediate reaction; it is also likely to have more long-standing effects on the way she views her disease. Although the hospital consultant is most likely to have the major role here, nurse counsellors and psychologists with a special interest in breast cancer are increasingly being appointed in specialist breast clinics.

At the time of diagnosis many women are in such a state of shock that they are unable to take in very much of what has been told to them apart from the fact that they have cancer. The presence of a relative or a close friend during the bad news consultation not only helps in recall of facts but may lessen the subsequent anxiety and depression. Clear and concise communication from the hospital to the GP as soon as possible after the diagnosis is known is extremely important. The GP is likely to be visited either by the patient herself asking for further information about what is going to happen to her, or by members of her family asking for help. This help will be necessary in order to cope with their own distress as well as to support the patient. The GP is in an ideal position to provide continuing care to women with breast cancer, particularly on the psychological front. However, there will also often be a need to answer questions to do with the treatment that is to be undertaken at the hospital, such as the pros and cons of lumpectomy versus mastectomy. GPs need to keep up to date with the current treatment regimens at their local breast unit and to have good communication networks with the hospital team.

With the trend towards more conservative surgery it was hoped that the psychological morbidity associated with breast cancer would diminish. However, several studies have all found that the levels of anxiety and depression are about the same regardless of which treatment has been given (Fallowfield *et al.* 1986; Maunsell *et al.* 1989). Women seem to be more concerned with the fear of cancer itself and the possibility of recurrence rather than the fear of losing a breast. One area where the type of surgery does seem to have an effect on psychological well-being, with breast conservation being superior, is body image. This is not surprising but more important is the subsequent effect on sexual functioning. There is very little data available on this specific topic as most studies have combined questions on body image and sexual functioning. Kemeny *et al.* (1988) found that women who had undergone mastectomy were less likely to feel sexually attractive than women who had undergone segmentectomy, but that both groups denied problems in sexual relations. A common trap to fall into is to assume that it is only married women or younger women who worry about their sexual attractiveness. It should be routine to enquire about these feelings in *all* women having breast surgery.

Since at the present time there is no clear advantage in terms of survival between the different surgical treatments, nor are there any major differences in psychosocial functioning, it would seem reasonable to offer women greater involvement when deciding on management. The results from studies trying to demonstrate the benefits of this approach are so far inconclusive, with no long-lasting advantage in terms of psychological morbidity in women who choose their treatment (Morris and Royle 1988; Fallowfield *et al.* 1990*b*). Whatever treatment is given there are certain risk factors which predispose to significant psychological distress: inadequate information, adjuvant chemotherapy, complications of treatment, pre-existing psychological problems, lack of social support, and poor personal coping strategies. It is estimated that at least 25% of women treated for breast cancer suffer from significant psychological morbidity and that the majority of these will benefit from either simple counselling or, occasionally, referral for more specialized help. The GP and other members of the primary care team are in an ideal position to recognize these particularly vulnerable women and to offer suitable intervention.

Breast cancer genetics

Cancer genetics is concerned with the identification and management of persons at risk of an inherited form of cancer. With respect to breast cancer, 90–95% of all cancers are sporadic but approximately 5% of all cases are due to the inheritance of a dominant predisposing gene, which may result in a lifetime risk of breast cancer of almost 90%. This compares with a lifetime risk of breast cancer in the general population of 9%. Box 5.4 shows characteristics of the breast cancer susceptibility genes, BRCA1 and BRCA2. There is some indication that with the isolation of the BRCA1 gene, interest in genetic testing for cancer susceptibility is likely to be great. There are, however, significant problems associated with the widespread use of genetic testing, and it is premature to

Box 5.4 *Breast cancer susceptibility genes*

BRCA 1
- Located on chromosome 17q
- Autosomal dominant mode of inheritance
- 2–4% of all breast cancer in women under 70
- Up to 30% of all breast cancer <45 years
- >100 mutations identified to date
- Each mutation may carry a different risk
- Known mutations confer:
  – 85% lifetime risk of breast cancer
  – 44% lifetime risk of ovarian cancer
  – greater part of the risk falls at ages 30–50
  – ?colon cancer risk (4x)
  – ?Prostate cancer risk (3x)
- Mutation 185 del AG has 1% frequency in the Ashkenazi Jewish population

BRCA 2
- Located on chromosome 13q
- Autosomal dominant mode of inheritance
- 2% of all breast cancer in women under 70
- Each mutation likely to carry a different risk
- Known mutations confer:
  – 85% lifetime risk of breast cancer
  – greater part of the risk falls at ages 30–50
  – male breast cancer risk (% uncertain)
  – prostate cancer risk
  – ocular melanoma risk
  – larynx cancer risk

consider testing on a population basis. Even restricting testing to women with a strong family history poses considerable problems. There are no guidelines on how best to communicate information about cancer susceptibility to those at high risk or how best to inform women of the potential benefits or limitations of genetic testing. The appropriate management of identified gene carriers, some of whom may be at only moderately-increased risk, is uncertain as screening for ovarian cancer and for breast cancer in women under 50 are of unproved efficacy. The role of prophylactic surgery in such women is also unclear.

Most genetic services now offer counselling for family members predicted to be at high risk of developing breast cancer (Murday 1994). This includes discussion of the genetics and calculation of the genetic risk to that individual. Appropriate screening measures can be discussed and organized. Molecular diagnostic tests to determine whether a family member has inherited a predisposing gene are currently only available for a very small proportion of

---

Box 5.5 *Family history of breast cancer: suggested referral criteria*

- Three first or second-degree relatives (same side of the family) with breast or ovarian cancer (any age)
- Two first or second-degree relatives (same side of the family) with breast cancer under 60
- One first-degree relative (mother or sister) with breast cancer under 40
- A father or brother with breast cancer
- A first-degree relative with bilateral breast cancer
- Three or more first or second-degree relatives (same side of the family) with breast and other cancers under 50
- A history of both breast (under 50) and childhood cancer (same side of the family)

Need to discuss locally as there may be local variation

---

women. This proportion is likely to increase over the next few years. Because of the ethical implications in such genetic testing it is important to structure discussion and organization of testing thoroughly and consistently and this can be done by the cancer genetics clinic.

Preliminary referral guidelines, identifying women who are at three times (or more) the population risk of developing breast cancer, are shown in Box 5.5 (J. Mackay, personal communication).

Factors which suggest an inherited susceptibility to breast cancer are:

(1) a large number of affected family members;

(2) young age of onset of cancer: particularly pre-menopausal onset;

(3) the pattern of inheritance in the family;

(4) clustering of other cancers in the family such as ovarian, colon, prostate, melanoma;

(5) bilateral breast cancer;

(6) male breast cancer.

The following examples serve to illustrate some of these factors.

Case report 1

A 30-year-old woman wished to know whether she should obtain regular mammograms before the age of 50 because of her family history of cancer. Her mother had died at the age of 46 having developed breast cancer 2 years previously. Her maternal aunt had also been diagnosed with breast cancer at the age of 58. The maternal grandmother had developed ovarian cancer at the age of 69 and died 6 months later.

In families where a disposing gene is clearly segregating, the risk of inheriting the gene is 50%. Since the penetrance of the gene (i.e. the chance of developing cancer if one carries the gene) is almost 90%, the lifetime risk of developing breast cancer is therefore approximately 45%. In many families there is some family history, but it is not clear whether the clustering of cancers is due to chance

Fig 5.4 *Case Report 1*

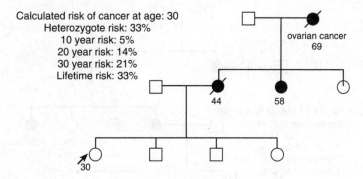

Calculated risk of cancer at age: 30
Heterozygote risk: 33%
10 year risk: 5%
20 year risk: 14%
30 year risk: 21%
Lifetime risk: 33%

ovarian cancer
69

44   58

30

(since the incidence of sporadic breast cancer is high) or due to the segregation of a dominant gene. The risk to offspring therefore lies somewhere in between the background population risk (~9%) and 45%. The risk can be calculated with a knowledge of the number of affected relatives, the degree of relatedness, and the age of onset. Using figures from data by Claus *et al.* (1991, 1994), and a computerized calculation, the risk of being a gene carrier in this case was 33%, and her lifetime risk of developing breast cancer (taking into account the background population risk and the penetrance of the gene) was also 33%.

The evidence that mammography in the under-50 age group is of benefit is inconclusive to date and the results of further trials are awaited. However, cancer genetics clinics are, in general, recommending mammography in women who are at higher risk of developing pre-menopausal breast cancer on the basis of family history. In this case therefore the recommendation is that the woman should be screened every 1 or 2 years from the age of 35 (local protocols for mammography vary). Annual breast examination by an experienced practitioner or breast surgeon may also be recommended (although breast examinations are also of unproven benefit). It would be possible to take blood from any live affected relatives for storage, to await possible future genetic tests, in this case if the maternal aunt were willing.

For at least one of these dominant predisposing genes (BRCA1) there is also an associated risk of ovarian cancer. The penetrance for ovarian cancer is lower (50–60%) than for breast cancer. The lifetime risk of ovarian cancer in this case would be approximately 15%, which is significantly higher than the general population risk of approximately 1%. Discussion of ovarian screening measures is therefore also appropriate. Screening by ultrasound scanning and CA125 markers are currently of unproven benefit but the results of studies into their value in high-risk groups are awaited.

Case report 2

G.W. is a 35-year old with the woman with the following family history: her mother had been diagnosed with breast cancer at the age of 37. The mother had had a mastectomy and radiotherapy, but had died the year after diagnosis. G.W. had two maternal aunts, one who was still alive at the age of 78 but the other had developed bilateral breast cancer and died at the age of 58. A maternal great aunt had also had breast cancer diagnosed at the age of 45.

In this case there is a first-degree relative diagnosed below the age of 40 and

Fig 5.5 *Case Report 2*

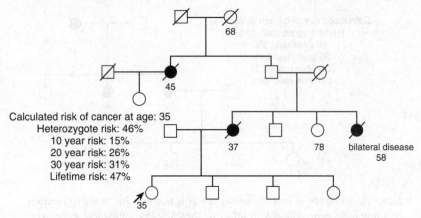

Calculated risk of cancer at age: 35
Heterozygote risk: 46%
10 year risk: 15%
20 year risk: 26%
30 year risk: 31%
Lifetime risk: 47%

a close relative with bilateral breast cancer. These factors make it very likely that there is a dominant gene segregating in this family. The chance that G.W. has inherited this gene is therefore almost 50%. Current recommendations are that she should receive annual breast examination by an experience practitioner or breast surgeon and annual or biennial mammography (local protocols may vary).

Case report 3

A 41-year-old woman presented to the cancer genetics clinic with a family history of breast cancer. Her older sister had been diagnosed with breast cancer at the age of 42 and died from disseminated carcinoma 1 year later. Her maternal aunt also had breast cancer diagnosed at the age of 52 and the sister of her maternal grandmother was said to have had breast cancer in her seventies.

Construction of her family pedigree revealed that she had another sister who was unaffected at the age of 51, her mother had died from a heart attack at the age of 60, and two further maternal aunts had lived into their seventies and eighties. Her maternal grandmother had died from an accident aged 42.

Fig 5.6 *Case Report 3*

Calculated risk of cancer at age:
Heterozygote risk: 2.5%
10 year risk: 2%
20 year risk: 4%
30 year risk: 7%
Lifetime risk: 11%

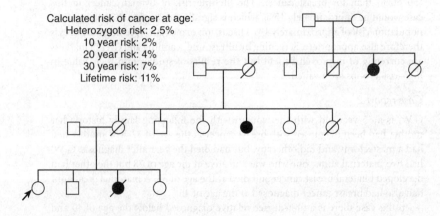

Fig 5.7 *Case Report 4*

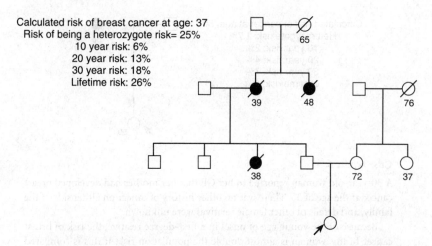

Calculated risk of breast cancer at age: 37
Risk of being a heterozygote risk= 25%
        10 year risk: 6%
        20 year risk: 13%
        30 year risk: 18%
        Lifetime risk: 26%

Although this family has an affected relative in three successive generations, there is a wide distribution in the age of onset and there are several other female relatives who have lived to a relatively old age without being affected. Calculations of the risk of developing breast cancer to the consultant using figures from Claus *et al.* (1991, 1994) revealed that the chances of being a carrier of one of the dominant breast cancer predisposing genes was in the order of 2.5% (one in 40). Her lifetime chance of developing cancer was therefore not much elevated above the background population risk (11% versus 9%) and in this case screening would not be indicated before the age of 50.

Case report 4

A 37-year-old woman had no history of breast cancer on her mother's side of the family, but there were several affected members on her father's side. Her father had had one sister, who developed breast cancer at the age of 38. The paternal grandmother and her sister had both inherited breast cancer aged 39 and 48 respectively.

This case shows how breast cancer susceptibility can also be inherited through the male line. Since the penetrance of the dominant susceptibility genes is much lower in males, the fact that her father is unaffected does not rule out the possibility of the patient inheriting a susceptibility gene. In this case, the estimated chance of her being a heterozygote for such a gene is 25%. At the age of 37 she therefore has an approximately 26% lifetime risk of developing breast cancer. As this is significantly higher than that for the general population (9%), earlier screening by examination and mammography as discussed above is recommended.

Case report 5

A 50-year-old woman had commenced screening on the national breast screening programme, and mentioned at her appointment that her mother had had breast cancer at the age of 55. She was concerned that there might be increased risk of breast cancer to her 29-year-old daughter. She did not know of any further family history of breast cancer, nor did she know any details about her mother's family.

Fig 5.8 *Case Report 5*

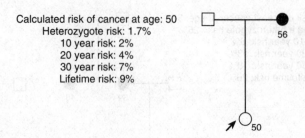

Calculated risk of cancer at age: 50
Heterozygote risk: 1.7%
10 year risk: 2%
20 year risk: 4%
30 year risk: 7%
Lifetime risk: 9%

Case report 6

A 30-year-old woman reported to her GP that her mother had developed breast cancer at the age of 35. There was no other history of cancer on either side of the family, and details of other female relatives were unknown.

Because of the young age of onset in a first-degree relative, the risk of breast cancer to this woman is almost double the population risk. If this is compared to Case 5, where the lifetime risk is approximately equal to the population risk, one can observe how important the age at diagnosis is in determining the risk of familial breast cancer.

Case report 7

A 28-year-old woman presented with a strong family history of breast and ovarian cancer. Her mother had developed breast cancer at the age of 35 and a maternal aunt had developed ovarian cancer at the age of 56. The maternal grandmother had developed breast cancer at the age of 45 as had one of her sisters at the age of 49, but another sister was still alive and unaffected at the age of 76.

With such a strong family history of both breast and ovarian cancer, it is very likely that a dominant predisposing gene, for example BRCA1 (since there is also ovarian cancer in the pedigree) is segregating in this family. Current recommendations are that this woman should receive annual breast examination. Some clinics may suggest she should have mammography now, and then annually or biennially from the age of 35. She should also be offered entry into the UKCCCR National Familial Ovarian Cancer Screening Study when it commences.

Since there are four affected family members and at least one of them is still alive, the patient might also wish to consider a gene test for BRCA1 (Eeles 1996). The maternal aunt would have to be willing to donate blood. A mutation screen

Fig 5.9 *Case Report 6*

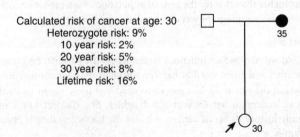

Calculated risk of cancer at age: 30
Heterozygote risk: 9%
10 year risk: 2%
20 year risk: 5%
30 year risk: 8%
Lifetime risk: 16%

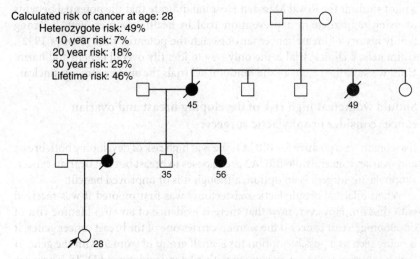

Fig 5.10 *Case Report 7*

Calculated risk of cancer at age: 28
　Heterozygote risk: 49%
　　10 year risk: 7%
　　20 year risk: 18%
　　30 year risk: 29%
　Lifetime risk: 46%

could be performed on her, and if a mutation found this could be looked for in the patient. Currently this is not a sensitive test, and carries only a 30% probability of being able to give an informative result. However, if such a result is available, then there is a 50% chance the woman could be reassured that she has not inherited the gene and her risk is therefore no higher than that of the general population. The remaining 50% chance would inform the woman that she has inherited the gene and therefore has an approximately 90% chance of developing breast cancer and a 50–60% chance of developing ovarian cancer. She might then wish to consider surgical removal of both these organs to reduce these risks.

Controversies in breast cancer management

What is the risk–benefit ratio of using tamoxifen to prevent breast cancer in young women at high risk?

Studies are now underway in the UK and US to look at prevention of breast cancer, administering 5 years of tamoxifen at a dose of 20 mg a day prophylactically, in young women (35–44 years) at high risk and older women (45–65) at moderate risk, of developing the disease. The possibility of using tamoxifen to prevent or delay development of breast cancer is the subject of continuing debates on the balance of potential risks and benefits (Jordan 1993). A gloomy view expressed by DeGregorio and Weibe (1994) in their calculations of risk/benefit illustrate the issues involved: 'Taking the US trial, in which 8000 women will receive tamoxifen, the figures look like this. Out of 8000 women, 62 may avoid breast cancer. But 1300 may have hot flushes, 1136 may have vaginal discharges, 272 may have skin rashes, between 31 and 53 may get endometrial cancer, 24 may have deep vein thrombosis requiring hospitalization, and 24 may develop life-threatening blood clots in the lungs'. Others take a more positive view and see it as offering a possible way of preventing many thousands of breast cancers in young women with relatively few side-effects. Results from a pilot study at the Royal Marsden Hospital indicate that the potential benefits of using tamoxifen in a prevention trial in healthy women with a strong family history of breast cancer far outweigh the potential risks (Powles 1992). Ultimately, a clinical trial is the only way to identify overall benefit and harm. Until we have the results of the randomized trials the answer remains unclear.

Should women at high risk of developing breast and ovarian cancer consider prophylactic surgery?

If a woman tests positive for BRCA1, she is at high risk of developing both breast and ovarian cancer, while BRCA2 predisposes to breast but not ovarian cancer. Prophylactic surgery is an option, although it is of unproved benefit.

When bilateral prophylactic mastectomy was first mooted it was received with disdain. However, now that there is evidence of an 80% lifetime risk of developing breast cancer if the woman carries one of the breast cancer genes, it is being seen as a possible option for a small group of women with the gene. It is also sometimes chosen by women with bilateral widespread DCIS. There are two options: bilateral mastectomy or subcutaneous mastectomy which leaves the nipple and outer breast skin intact. This latter is better cosmetically but leaves more breast tissue, though with the former it is very difficult to remove every bit of breast tissue even with the most radical operation, and therefore breast cancer can still develop. If a woman carries the BRCA1 gene, she is also at high risk of developing ovarian cancer, and may therefore wish to consider prophylactic oophorectomy as well as mastectomy. Preliminary data suggests that prophylactic oophorectomy does reduce the risk of ovarian cancer (Struewing et al. 1995), but ovarian cancer can still occur in the lining of the abdominal cavity even when the removed ovaries are tumour free.

Should all women with breast cancer have chemotherapy and/or hormonal therapy?

Over half of women with operable breast cancer who receive locoregional treatment alone will die from metastatic disease, indicating that for most women the cancer has already spread by the time of presentation. More and more women with breast cancer are thus being advised to have chemotherapy and or hormonal treatment. Not all women who have this treatment will benefit from it and for some women it will be a difficult choice to weigh up the possible benefits against the known and unknown side-effects – short term and long term.

Choice of treatment depends on the risk of relapse, the potential benefit of different forms of treatment, and the acceptability of the treatment to the patient.

Should women found to be node positive always have chemotherapy?

If a woman is pre-menopausal, most people would recommend chemotherapy (with or without tamoxifen). If the patient is at low or intermediate risk and if the tumour is oestrogen receptor positive, ovarian oblation (with or without tamoxifen) should be considered. If she is post-menopausal and ER negative, chemotherapy may be considered – the maximum benefit will be 3–9%. If she is 80, a woman may decide the possible benefit from chemotherapy is not worth the side-effects she may suffer. Tamoxifen (20 mg per day) produces a partial response in 75% of elderly patients with oestrogen receptor positive tumours and a complete clinical response in 15%.

Should women found to be node negative have chemotherapy?

With no chemotherapy, 20–30% of these women will get metastatic breast cancer and sooner or later die from it but, 70–80% will never have a recurrence. Chemotherapy appears to improve outlook by 30%. The worse the prognosis the bigger effect chemotherapy will have. For some of these women, and we do not know which, chemotherapy will improve the chance of a recurrence by possibly only 3–10%. This is worked out on the basis that if the likelihood of recurrence is 9% – which is true for the average node-negative woman with a tumour of less than 2 cm – then the improvement can only be 3%. Against this, the woman has to weigh up the side-effects of the chemotherapy, short and long-term quality of life, outcomes, etc. Post-menopausal, node-negative women should have tamoxifen. Pre-menopausal, node-negative women of low or intermediate risk should also have tamoxifen, but those at high risk will require chemotherapy or ovarian ablation (with or without tamoxifen) if the tumour is oestrogen receptor positive. There is no evidence that tamoxifen is effective for pre-menopausal women with oestrogen receptor negative tumours.

What is the role of high-dose chemotherapy and stem cell rescue in women with metastases?

Protocols of intensive treatment are being assessed in patients at very high risk. Women with 10 or more positive axillary lymph nodes (10–15% survival without relapse after 5 years) are being offered high-dose chemotherapy with autologous bone marrow transplantation, or harvesting and subsequent rescue of peripheral stem cells. Some of the trials look promising, but there is a 3–5% mortality related to the treatment and morbidity is high. Comparison with historical controls suggests a prolongation in time to relapse, and preliminary evidence suggests a survival benefit. Randomized controlled trials are currently under way and, because of the serious side-effects, results from these trials are required before this treatment is introduced into practice.

Who should conduct follow-up and what should it involve?

About half of all women with breast cancer will suffer some form of recurrence, and one half of all patients will eventually present with distant metastases and die from their disease. Two-thirds of all recurrences occur during the first 5 years after treatment. A recent study found that general practice follow-up of women with breast cancer in remission was not associated with increase in time to diagnosis, increase in anxiety, or deterioration in health-related quality of life (Grunfeld *et al.* 1996). Most recurrences were detected by women as interval events and presented to the GP, irrespective of continuing hospital follow-up. However, the possibility that hospital clinics were better at eliciting metastatic symptoms could not be excluded by the study design. In general, it appears that GPs would like to provide follow-up if their concerns about increased workload can be met, clear guidelines for follow-up be provided, and assurances given that patients will be seen urgently by the specialist on an open access basis. GPs would require training in relevant aspects of breast cancer. Patients would require access to a breast care nurse for at least 1 year after surgery (McArdle *et al.* 1996), and access to mammography for the treated breast when conserved, yearly during the first 5 years after surgery, and every 2 years thereafter (the ideal frequency for mammography has not been established). Some patients would prefer to be seen in specialist clinics for routine follow-up. The majority of specialists prefer routine follow-up in hospitals as currently practised (Grunfeld *et al.* 1995). Breast surgeons argue that local recurrence in mastectomy flaps and distant metastases are both difficult to recognize, and that the GP will, on average, see only one new patient with metastatic disease from breast cancer every 3–4 years (Breast Surgeons Group 1995). Also, clinical examination of a breast which has undergone conservative surgery and radiotherapy is not straightforward.

What role for MRI in follow-up of breast cancer patients?

MRI to the breast is under evaluation as a means of follow-up after breast cancer treatment, as an alternative to mammography which misses 5–10% of cancers and is more difficult to interpret in young women and after surgery. Early reports are promising and indicate the possibility of higher specificity and sensitivity than mammography.

What about breast cancer in women who are pregnant or lactating?

There is inadequate information as to the effect of pregnancy on breast cancer. It was wisdom that the prognosis was worse but there is conflicting evidence whether breast cancer occurring during pregnancy is more aggressive than other breast cancer or not. One to 2% of breast cancers present in pregnancy or lactation and 25% of those who develop breast cancer under 35 do so either during or within one year of pregnancy. They often present late because of the difficulty in knowing whether there is or is not a lump in the breast at this time – about 65% have involved axillary nodes. Treatment in pregnancy also presents difficulties and these two factors may, in part, account for the worse prognosis. Treatment in the first two trimesters is by mastectomy and axillary node clearance, and those presenting in the third trimester usually have treatment delayed until after early delivery of the baby (at 30–32 weeks). Radiotherapy is contraindicated in any trimester. Chemotherapy can be given but is associated with a small risk of fetal damage.

What is the role of complementary treatments? (see Chapter 20)

Many women who have breast cancer diagnosed turn to complementary therapies as an adjunct to routine medical treatment. Whether these affect outcomes is not known but it is likely that they help women through a difficult time especially as, despite recent improvements, many women still feel they get insufficient holistic support from the breast unit whilst attending for treatment. Some women also feel they are doing something active to help themselves in seeking complementary treatment. An attempt was made to evaluate complementary treatments by organizing a comparison of women receiving routine medical treatments only with those attending the Bristol Cancer Centre for complementary therapy. The study can only be described as a disaster and has probably set the whole interface between complementary and scientific medicine back years. The results were published in the *Lancet* in September 1990 (Bagenal *et al.*) with much sensational publicity (Richards 1995) and appeared to show that women being treated at the Bristol Centre were twice as likely to die and three times more likely to relapse than those who were treated with conventional medicine. There was much criticism of the study design and methods of analysis: women treated with complementary medicine had had more severe disease at the outset than the controls. The consensus view was that the results were inconclusive. The cancer charities involved in financing the study publicly apologised for their role in the débâcle. After publication of the study, the number of patients attending the Bristol Centre fell dramatically and the Centre nearly went into receivership. In 1994, the Charity Commission censured the charities for inadequacies in their mechanisms for supervising research (Smith 1994). Controversy still surrounds the study, but it did focus thinking on how patients can best be involved in research (Goodare and Smith 1995).

At what dose and for how long should women take tamoxifen?

There is no evidence that 40 mg of tamoxifen is better than 20 mg a day. Two years of tamoxifen is better than 1 year. There is increasing evidence that 5 years is better than 2 years. On current evidence the use of tamoxifen for more than 5 years may be justified but a definitive conclusion about long-term survival will not be available until current studies are completed after the year 2000 (Peto 1996).

Can women who have had breast cancer take HRT?

With regards to HRT and breast cancer, it is conventional advice to stop oestrogen-containing preparations on the diagnosis of malignancy and to avoid subsequent systemic oestrogen administration. Although this is safe advice, there is little evidence that short-term treatment, especially with combination HRT, has an adverse effect on prognosis. Disabling hot flushes and night sweats may be controlled with a progesterone (see above), but conventional HRT may be needed. If this is the case it is important that the patient understands that this is not conventional treatment and she may be best monitored in a specialist clinic. Many women feel they do not want to take any oestrogen given that many tumours are oestrogen dependent. For patients with breast cancer and a family history of osteoporosis and/or ischaemic heart disease, tamoxifen is the ideal 'HRT' as it has oestrogenic effects on bone and lipid metabolism.

Should women with a family history of breast cancer have ovarian screening?

A small percentage of women carry the gene BRCA1 which places them at high risk for both breast and ovarian cancer, but this does not apply to all women with breast cancer. Questions to consider are whether we should be offering population-based screening for ovarian cancer and if so for what age group, or whether it is more appropriate to target those at higher risk. Recent advances in molecular genetics have made it possible to identify women with a positive family history of ovarian and/or breast cancer who carry the susceptible gene. On the basis of current evidence, how good are ovarian screening tests in terms of reducing mortality, and should these women be offered annual ovarian screening or even prophyactic bilateral oophorectomy?

Ovarian cancer is the fifth commonest cancer in women in the UK, with an incidence of one in 5000. Ninety per cent of cases occur over the age of 45. It accounts for 6% of all deaths from cancer in women. Early disease tends to be asymptomatic, with the result that approximately 70% of cases are at an advanced stage at presentation. The overall prognosis is poor: the 5-year relative survival rate is 28%, while the 5-year survival rate of stages III and IV combined is 10% (Cancer Research Campaign 1991). However, if disease is confined to the ovary at diagnosis, the 5-year survival rate is over 90%.

Possible screening tests for ovarian cancer include measurement of the antigen marker serum CA 125, ultrasound scans (abdominal and transvaginal), bimanual pelvic examination, intraovarian Doppler flow mapping and radio-immunoscintigraphy (which may have the advantage of being able to distinguish between benign and malignant masses). None of these screening tests alone has a high enough sensitivity and specificity to be acceptable, in view of the low overall incidence of ovarian cancer and the need for surgery should the test be positive. The positive predictive value can be improved by targeting women at high risk, i.e. those with identified hereditary ovarian cancer syndromes.

There have been several prospective studies over the last 10 years to evaluate these different screening techniques, but these have been uncontrolled (Wald 1994). The combination of CA 125 and abdominal ultrasound scan is the only strategy that has been shown to achieve an acceptable positive predictive value on screening post-menopausal women in the general population. The lack of sensitivity of CA 125 in detecting early stage disease is, however, a problem. Another study suggests that transvaginal ultrasound, with colour flow imaging as a secondary test, can effectively detect early ovarian cancer in women with a positive family history (Bourne *et al.* 1993). A multi-centre randomized trial is currently being conducted in Europe to evaluate this procedure in the general population.

For the future, both specificity and sensitivity may be improved by using a combination of several tumour markers as an initial screening test, with transvaginal ultrasound and colour Doppler imaging as secondary tests.

In summary, there is no evidence to date from large, randomized controlled trials that ovarian screening reduces mortality from ovarian cancer, and the balance of potential benefits and possible harm for the individual, as well as costs for the NHS, have not been assessed. Until such evidence is forthcoming, screening for ovarian cancer should not be offered routinely to asymptomatic women. There is a stronger argument in favour of screening for those with a family history of ovarian cancer, especially if they carry the susceptible gene, but it has to be remembered that there is no evidence of effectiveness for such a strategy. At present, it is recommended that for the few women with a strong family history or inherited predisposition, annual ultrasound screening and/ or CA 125 estimation should be conducted from age 25 years or from 5 years before the earliest age of ovarian cancer in the family (Jacobs 1994). A protocol for a UKCCCR National Familial Ovarian Cancer Screening Study has recently been prepared. This study aims to develop an optimized screening procedure for ovarian cancer in women at high risk of ovarian cancer and to evaluate the performance of the screening strategy.

Are silicone implants safe?

Silicone implants have been used for a number of years in the UK for breast reconstructions. Saline prostheses are also available but do not have the same doughy consistency of silicone gel and breast tissue. Over the past few years there has been widespread concern, coupled with sensational media coverage, concerning the safety of silicone implants. Implant fatigue and rupture can lead to leakage of silicone gel. Published studies of implant failure have suggested a prevalence of failure ranging from 5–70% (Silverman *et al.* 1996). The estimate of 5% from a study of mammographic screening is thought to be the absolute minimum. Leakage of silicone breast implants has been linked to the development of a variety of systemic illnesses, though this has been controversial and a causal link denied. Most common systemic effects are fatigue, early morning stiffness, severe myalgia, arthralgia, joint swelling, and polyneuropathy. Some patients developed a multiple sclerosis-like syndrome, others motor neurone disease. The variety of symptoms is thought to be due to autoimmune disorder.

In 1992, the US FDA recommended limited availability for silicone breast implants under carefully controlled clinical protocols, and regular monitoring for those with implants. In 1994, Dow Corning Corporation, Bristol-Myers Squibb Company, and Baxter International reached agreement to create a US$3.7 billion compensation fund to settle actions brought by women claiming to have been injured by their silicone implant. To qualify, a woman has to be diagnosed with one of eight conditions alleged to be linked to implants, including scleroderma, systemic lupus erythematosus, mixed connective tissue disease, Sjogren's syndrome, and a number of neurological syndromes. She is not required to prove that her condition was caused by the implant.

At the same time, in the UK, the Department of Health set up a medical advisory panel which reported that the 'evidence is overwhelming that silicone is safe'. In reviews published in 1993 and 1994, the Medical Devices Agency concluded that there was 'no evidence of increased risk of connective tissue disease in patients who have had silicone gel breast implants, and therefore no scientific case for changing practice or policy in the UK with respect to breast implantation'. The MP, Ann Clwyd, is mounting a vigorous challenge to this finding, accusing the DoH of a failure to conduct adequate research. British patients who used American implants will receive some compensation (substantially less than their American counterparts) under a proposed worldwide class-action settlement.

Conclusion

There is a substantial morbidity and mortality associated with disorders of the breast. Breast cancer constitutes a major public health problem in the UK. Early diagnosis by the national breast screening programme for women aged 50 and over may prove of benefit in reducing population mortality from breast cancer. Improvements in the treatment of breast cancer are now becoming apparent as the mortality from breast cancer has begun to decline, and the recent results from trials of adjuvant therapy offer real prospects for improving prognosis. All breast disease, both benign and malignant, is associated with significant psychological symptoms. The GP has a major role to play in the detection, treatment, and long-term care of breast disease. When a woman presents with a breast symptom, however trivial, the GP should reassure her that she was right to attend. Some women have an obvious abnormality which requires referral, others appear to have no significant change. For those women where the position is less clear, it is best to refer for a consultant opinion, or to ensure that the patient keeps an early follow-up appointment with the GP. If there is any doubt, the woman should be referred, if only to put her own mind at rest. Before referral to hospital, the GP should discuss with the woman the possible diagnostic and treatment options.

Acknowledgement

This chapter is updated from the original chapter on Breast Cancer and benign breast disease by Joan Austoker and Deborah Sharp in the third edition of *Women's Problems in general practice*.

Useful addresses

BACUP (British Association for Cancer United Patients),
3 Bath Place, Rivington Street, London EC2 A3JR.
Tel: 0171 613 2121

Breast Care and Mastectomy Association (BCMA),
7–26 Harrison Street, Kings Cross, London WC1H GJG.
Tel: 0171 837 0908

CancerLink,
17 Britannia Street, London WC1X 9JN.
Tel: 0171 833 2451

CRC Primary Care Education Group,
University of Oxford, Department of Public Health and Primary Care,
65 Banbury Road, Oxford OX2 6PE.
Tel: 01865 310457

Health Education Authority,
Hamilton House, Mabledon Place, London WC1H 9TX.
Tel: 0171 383 3833

References and further reading

Austoker, J. (1995a) Screening and self-examination for breast cancer. In *Cancer prevention in primary care* (J. Austoker), pp. 75–94. BMJ Publishing Group, London.

Austoker, J., *et al.* (1995b) *Guidelines for referral of patients with breast problems.* NHS breast screening programme.

Bagenal, F.S., Easton, D.F., *et al.* (1990). Survival of patients with breast cancer attending Bristol Cancer Help Centre. *Lancet,* **336** (8715), 606–10.

Baum, M. Saunders, C. (1994) *Breast cancer: a guide for every woman.* Oxford University Press, Oxford.

Benson, E.A. (1982). Breast abscesses and breast cysts. *The Practitioner,* **266,** 1397–1401.

Beral V., *et al.* (1995). Sudden fall in breast cancer death rates in England and Wales. *Lancet,* **345,** 1642–3.

Bourne, T.H., *et al.* (1993) Screening for familial ovarian cancer with transvaginal ultrasonography and colour blood flow imaging. *British Medical Journal,* **306,** 1025–9.

Boyd, N.F., *et al.* (1993) A meta-analysis of studies of dietary fat and breast cancer risk. *British Journal of Cancer,* **68,** 627–36.

Breast Surgeons Group of the British Association of Surgical Oncology. (1995). Guidelines for surgeons in the management of symptomatic breast disease in the United Kingdom. *European Journal of Surgical Oncology* **21,** 1–13.

Bulbrook, R.D. (1996). Long-term adjuvant therapy for primary breast cancer: more than five years of tamoxifen is no longer justified. *British Medical Journal,* **312,** 389–90.

Bundred, N.J. Morgan, D.A.L., and Dixon, J.M. (1995) Management of regional nodes in breast cancer. In *ABC of breast diseases* (ed. J.M. Dixon), pp. 30–3. BMJ Publishing Group, London.

Byers, T., Graham, S., Rzepka, T., *et al.* (1985). Lactation and breast cancer. *American Journal of Epidemiology,* **12** (5), 664–74.

Cancer Research Campaign (1991). Factsheet 17, *Ovarian cancer.*

Cancer Research Campaign (1991). Factsheet 6, *Breast cancer.*

Cancer Research Campaign (1996). Factsheet 6, *Breast cancer.*

Claus, E.B., Risch, N., and Thompson, W.D. (1991). Genetic analysis of breast cancer in the cancer and steroid hormone study. *American Journal of Human Genetics,* **48**(2), 232–42.

Claus, E.B., Risch, N., and Thompson, W.D. (1994) Autosomal dominant inheritance of early-onset breast cancer. Implications for risk prediction. *Cancer,* **73**(3), 643–51.

Cockburn, J., *et al.* (1994). Psychological consequences of screening mammography. *Journal of Medical Screening,* **1,** 7–12.

Colditz, G.A., *et al.* (1995) The use of estrogens and progestins and the risk of breast cancer in postmenopausal women. *New England Journal of Medicine,* **332,** 1589–93.

Collaborative Group on Hormonal Factors in Breast Cancer (1996). Breast cancer and hormonal contraceptives: collaborative reanalysis of individual data on 53 297 women with breast cancer and 100 239 women without breast cancer from 54 epidemiological studies. *Lancet,* **347,** 1713–27.

Collins, F.S. (1996) BRCA1–Lots of mutations, lots of dilemmas. *New England Journal of Medicine,* **334,** 186–8.

Day N., *et al.* (1995) Monitoring interval cancers in breast screening programmes: the East Anglian experience. *Journal of Medical Screening,* **2,** 180–5.

Day, N. E. (1991). Screening for breast cancer. *British Medical Bulletin,* **47,** 500–15.

DeGregorio, M.W. and Wiebe, V.J. (1994) *Tamoxifen and breast cancer.* Yale University Press, New Haven.

Dent, D.M. and Cant, P.J. (1989). Fibroadenoma. *World Journal of Surgery,* **13,** 706–10.

Department of Health (1996). Statistical Bulletin. *Breast screening programme, England 1994–95.*

Dixon, J. (1995). Surgery and radiotherapy for early breast cancer. *British Medical Journal,* **311,** 1515–16.

Dixon, M. and Sainsbury, R. (1993). *Handbook of diseases of the breast.* Churchill Livingstone, Edinburgh.

Dupont, W.D. and Page. D.I. (1991). Risk factors for breast carcinoma in women with proliferactive breast disease. In *The breast: comprehensive management of benign and malignant diseases* (ed. K.I. Bland and E.M. Copeland), pp. 292–8. W.B. Saunders, Philadelphia.

Early Breast Cancer Trialists' Collaborative Group (1992). Systemic treatment of early breast cancer by hormonal, cytotoxic, or immune therapy. *Lancet,* **339,** 1–15, 71–85.

Early Breast Cancer Trialists' Collaborative Group (1995). Effects of radiotherapy and surgery in breast cancer: an overview of the randomized trials. *New England Journal of Medicine,* **333,** 1444–55.

Eeles, R. (1996). Testing for the breast cancer predisposition gene, BRCA1. *British Medical Journal,* **313,** 572–3.

Elwood, J.M., Cox, B., and Richardson, A.K. (1993). The effectiveness of breast cancer screening by mammography in younger women. *Online Journal of Current Clinical Trials,* **doc no. 32.**

Fallowfield, L.J. (1991). *Breast cancer.* Tavistock/Routledge, London.

Fallowfield, L.J., Baum, M., and Maguire. G.P. *(1986).* Effects of breast conservation on psychological morbidity associated with diagnosis and treatment of early breast cancer. *British Medical Journal,* **293,** *1331–4.*

Fallowfield, L.J., Baum, M., and Maguire, G.P. *(1987).* Addressing the psychological needs of the conservatively-treated breast cancer patient: a discussion paper. *Journal of the Royal Society of Medicine,* **80,** *696–700.*

Fallowfield, L.J., Rodway, A., and Baum, M. *(1990a).* What are the psychological factors influencing attendance, non-attendance and reattendance at a breast cancer screening centre? *Journal of the Royal Society Medicine,* **83,** 547–51.

Fallowfield, L.J., Hall, A., Maguire, G.P., *et al.* (199*b*). Psychological outcomes of different treatment policies in women with early breast cancer outside a clinical trial. *British Medical Journal,* **301,** 575–80.

Fisher, B., *et al.* (1995). Reanalysis and results after 12 years of follow-up in a randomized clinical trial comparing total mastectomy with lumpectomy with or without irradiation in the treatment of breast cancer. *New England Journal of Medicine,* **333,** 1456–61.

Ford, D., Easton, D., Peto, J. (1996) Estimates of the gene frequency of BRCA1 and its contribution to breast and ovarian cancer incidence. *American Journal of Human Genetics,* **57,** 1457–62.

Gillis, C.R. and Hole, D.J. (1996). Survival outcome of care by specialist surgeons in breast cancer: a study of 3786 patients in the west of Scotland. *British Medical Journal,* **312,** 145–8.

Goodare, H. and Smith, R. (1995). The rights of patients in research. *British Medical Journal,* **310,** 1277–8.

Gott, D. and Tinkler, J.J.B. (1994). Silicone implants and corrective tissue disease. Medical Devices Agency, London.

Grunfeld, E., *et al.* (1995) Specialist and general practice views on routine follow-up of breast cancer patients in general practice. *Family Physician,* **12,** 60–5.

Grunfeld, E., *et al.* (1996) Routine follow-up of breast cancer in primary care: randomised trial. *British Medical Journal,* **313,** 665–9.

Haagensen, C.D. *(1986). Diseases of the breast* (3rd edn). W.B. Saunders, Philadelphia.

Hakama, M., *et al.* (1995) Aggressiveness of screen-detected cancers. *Lancet,* **345,** 221–4.

Hemminki, E. (1996) Oral contraceptives and breast cancer. *British Medical Journal,* **313,** 63–4.

Henderson, B.E., Pick, M.C., and Casagrande, J.T. *(1981).* Breast cancer and the oestrogen window hypothesis. *Lancet,* **ii,** *363–4.*

Henderson, B.E., Pike, M.C., and Ross, R.K. *(1984).* Epidemiology and risk factors. In *Breast cancer: diagnosis and management* (ed. G. Bonadonna). John Wiley, New York.

Hoskins, K.F., *et al.* (1995) Assessment and counselling for women with a family history of breast cancer: a guide for clinicians. *Journal of the American Medical Association,* **273,** 577–85.

Hughes, L.E., Mansel, R.E., and Webster, D.J.T. (1987). Aberrations of normal development and involution (ANDI). A new perspective on pathogenesis and nomenclature of benign breast disease. *Lancet,* **ii,** 1316–19.

Hughes, L.E., Mansel, R.E., and Webster, D.J.T. *(1989). Benign disorders and diseases of the breast: concepts and clinical management, pp. 75–92.* Baillière Tindall, London.

Hulka, B.S. and Stark A.T. (1995). Breast cancer: cause and prevention. *Lancet,* **346,** 883–7.

Jacobs, I. (1994) Screening for epithelial and ovarian cancer. *Lancet,* **343,** 337–8.

Jordan, V.C. (1993). How safe is tamoxifen? *British Medical Journal,* **307,** 1371–2.

Kaufman, Z., *et al.* (1991). The mammographic parenchymal patterns of women on hormone replacement therapy. *Clinical Radiology,* **43,** 389–92.

Kemeny, M., Wellisch, D.K., and Schain, W.S. *(1988).* Psychological outcome in a randomised surgical trial for treatment in primary breast cancer. *Cancer,* **62,** *1231–7.*

Kerlikowske, K. *et al.* (1995) Efficacy of screening mammography. A meta-analysis. *Journal of the American Medical Association–r,* **273,** 149–54.

Lerman C., *et al.* (1991) Psychological and behavioral implications of abnormal mammograms. *Annals of Internal Medicine,* **114,** 657–61.

McArdle, J.M.C., *et al.* (1996) Psychological support for patients undergoing breast cancer surgery: a randomised study. *British Medical Journal,* **312,** 813–16.

McIlwaine, G. (1993). Satisfaction with the NHS breast screening programme: women's views. In *Breast screening acceptability: research and practice* (ed. J. Austoker and J. Patrick), pp. 14–16. NHSBSP Publications, Sheffield.

McPherson, K. (1995). Breast cancer and hormonal supplements in postmenopausal women. *British Medical Journal,* **311,** 699–700.

McPherson, K., Steel, C.M., and Dixon, J.M. (1995). Breast cancer – epidemiology, risk factors and genetics. In *ABC of breast diseases* (ed. J.M. Dixon), pp. 18–21. BMJ Publishing Group, London.

McTiernan, A. and Thomas, D.B. (1986). Evidence for a protective effect of lactation on the risk of breast cancer in young women. *American Journal of Epidemiology*, **124** *(3), 353–8.*

Maguire, G.P. *(1976).* The psychological and social sequelae of mastectomy. In *Modern perspectives in the psychiatric aspects of surgery (ed.* J. Howell), pp. *390–421.* Brunner/ Mazel, New York.

Mant, D. (1992) Should all women be advised to practice retular breast self-examination? *The Breast,* **1:** 108.

Maunsell, E., Brissoll, J., and Daschanas, L. (1989). Psychological distress after initial treatment for breast cancer: a comparison of partial and total mastectomy. *Journal of Clinical Epidemiology,* **42,** 765–71.

Miller, W.R., Ellis, I.O., and Sainsbury, J.R.C. (1995). Prognostic factors. In *ABC of breast diseases* (ed. J.M. Dixon), pp. 49–52. BMJ Publishing Group, London.

Morris, J and Royle. G.T. (1988). Offering patients a choice of surgery for early breast cancer: a reduction in anxiety in patients and their husbands. *Social Science and Medicine,* **26,** 583–5.

Murday, V. (1994) Genetic counselling in the cancer family clinic. *European Journal of Cancer,* **30A,** 2012–15.

NHS breast screening programme (1996). *Review 1996.* NHSBSP, Sheffield.

Nichols, S., Waters W.E., and Wheeler, M.J. (1980). Management of female breast disease by Southampton general practioners. *British Medical Journal,* **281,** 1450–3.

Nichols, S., Waters, W.E., Fraser. J.D., *et al.* (1981). Delay in the presentation of breast symptoms for consultant investigation. *Community Medicine,* **3,** 217.

Page, D.L., *et al.* (1981). Intraductal carcinoma of the breast: follow-up after biopsy only. *Cancer,* **49,** 751–8.

Peto, R. (1996). Five years of tamoxifen – or more? *Journal of the National Cancer Institute,* 88, 1791–3.

Phelan, M., Dobbs. J., and David, A.S. (1992). 'I thought it would go away': patient denial in breast cancer. *Journal of the Royal Society of Medicine,* **85,** 206–7.

Powles, T.J. (1992) The case for clinical trials of tamoxifen for prevention of breast cancer. *Lancet,* **340,** 1145–7.

Quinn, M. and Allen, E. (1995) Changes in incidence of and mortality from breast cancer in England and Wales since introduction of screening. *British Medical Journal.* **311,** 1391–5.

RCGP and OPCS. (1995) *Morbidity statistics from general practice 1991–92.* Fourth national study. HMSO, London.

Richards, T. (1995) Death from complementary medicine. *British Medical Journal,* **301,** 510–11.

Sacks, N.P.M. and Baum, M. (1993). Primary management of carcinoma of the breast. *Lancet*, **342**, 1402–8.

Sainsbury, R., *et al.* (1995). Does it matter where you live? Treatment variation for breast cancer in Yorkshire. *British Journal of Cancer*, **71**, 1275–8.

Sainsbury, R., *et al.* (1995) Influence of clinician workload and patterns of treatment on survival from breast cancer. *Lancet*, **345**, 1265–70.

Silverman, B.G., *et al.* (for the US FDA) (1996). Reported complications of silicone gel breast implants: an epidemiologic review. *Annals of Internal Medicine*, **124**, 744–56.

Sloane, J.P. (1991). Changing role of the pathologist. *British Medical Bulletin*, **47**, 433–54.

Smart, C.R. *et al.* (1995). Benefit of mammography screening in women aged 40 to 49 years. *Cancer*, **75** (7), 1619–26.

Smith, R. (1994) Charity Commission censures British charities. *British Medical Journal*, **308**, 155–6.

Spittle, M.F. (1995) Brachial plexus neuropathy after radiotherapy for breast cancer. *British Medical Journal*, **311**, 1516–17.

Stewart, H.J. (1991). Adjuvant systemic therapy for operable breast cancer. *British Medical Bulletin*, **47**, 343–56.

Struewing, J.P., *et al.* (1995). Prophlactic oophorectomy in inherited breast/ovarian cancer families. *International Journal of the National Cancer Institute*, **17**, 33–5.

Struewing, J.P., *et al.* (1995) The carrier frequency of the BRCA1 185 del AG mutation is approximately 1% in Ashkenazi Jewish individuals. *Nat. Genet.* **11**, 198–200.

Tabar, L., *et al.* (1992) Breast cancer treatment and natural history: new insights from screening. *Lancet*, **339**, 412–14.

UK National Case Control Study Group (1991). Oral contraceptive use and breast cancer risk in young women: subgroup analysis. *Lancet*, **355**, 1507–9.

Vd Mooren, M.J., *et al.* (1993). *Effects of hormone replacement therapy on mammographic breast pattern in postmenopausal women.* Proceedings of *Lancet* conference on Breast Cancer, Brugge, 1993, No. 41.

Wald, N. (1994). Ovarian cancer: screening brief. *Journal of Medical Screening*, **1**, 135.

Wald, N.J., *et al.* (1995). UKCCCR multi-centre randomised controlled trial of one and two view mammography in breast cancer screening. *British Medical Journal*, **311**, 1189–93.

Walker, L.G., *et al.* (1994). How distressing is attendance for routine breast screening? *Psycho-Oncology*, **3**, 299–304.

Watson, J.D., Sainsbury, J.R.C., and Dixon, J.M. (1995). Breast reconstruction. In *ABC of breast diseases* (ed. J.M. Dixon), pp. 65–9. BMJ Publishing Group, London.

Williams, E.M., Baum, M., and Hughes, L.E. (1976). Delay in presentation of women with breast disease. *Clinical Oncology*, **2**, 327–31.

Woodman C.B.J., *et al.* (1995). Is the three-year breast screening interval too long? Occurrence of interval cancers in NHS breast screening programme's north western region. *British Medical Journal*, **310**, 224–6.

Wright, C.J. and Barber Mueller, C. Screening mammography and public health policy: the need for perspective. *Lancet*, **346**, 29–439.

Yelland, A., Graham, M.D., Trott, P.A., *et al.* (1991). Diagnosing breast carcinoma in young women. *British Medical Journal*, **302**, 618–20.

CHAPTER SIX

Contraception

John Guillebaud

It is only in recent years that the subject of family planning has been included in basic medical training. In the past, most women sought help from Family Planning Association (FPA) clinics, or their successors after 1974 within the National Health Service. Now over 80% of women choose to consult their general practitioner (GP), although some still prefer the anonymity and specialization of the FPA clinic. General practitioners are potentially in the most favourable position to offer good advice, being already familiar with the patient's health and circumstances. But some practices lag behind the standards of the best, often perpetuating the myth that contraception equates to 'the Pill' (like vacuum cleaners equate to 'Hoovers') and so depriving their patients of other choices, or devoting too little time and skill to counselling. Research shows that not being given enough information about contraceptive methods is associated with women being dissatisfied, with not using methods correctly, and with abandoning contraception even if they do not want to get pregnant (Contraceptive Education Service 1996).

It is clear that consumer choice needs to be preserved. Although most advice is provided by the doctor, a very important contribution can be made by nurses, though they are often under-utilized. The midwife, health visitor, or other domiciliary nurse is well-placed to motivate and guide those in need. Much of the routine counselling and follow-up can be fruitfully delegated to a fully family planning-trained (ENB Course 901 or equivalent) practice nurse – with usually a gain rather than a loss in standards. Cap-fitting, pill-teaching, IUD-checking, and cervical smear-taking are all duties which can be appropriately delegated to the practice nurse, as well as the supervision of those who choose methods based on fertility awareness.

For GPs, the postgraduate training for the Diploma of the Faculty of Family Planning and Reproductive Health Care (DFFP) includes theoretical teaching and practical experience in all the methods. Since 1991, the training for IUD insertion and the management of problems such as 'lost threads' has been placed within a separate course, so that the relevant certificate will, in future, signify a higher level of training in the necessary practical skills.

Everyone involved in this work should also be equipped to receive the (maybe hidden) signals about related, often complex, psychological and emotional factors in any family planning consultation. Further training is available through the Institute of Psychosexual Medicine.

Doctors should formulate their own assessment of the risks and benefits of each method for the individual patient, based on up-to-date opinion and information, and then back their counselling with good literature. The latest UK FPA leaflets are ideal in this respect, user-friendly (in contrast to most package inserts) yet accurate and adequately comprehensive, thereby providing strong medico-legal backup for practitioners who may later be asked to justify their actions in the increasingly likely event of litigation. FPA leaflets may thus be regarded as an essential supplement to, but by no means as a replacement for, the counselling time by doctor and/or nurse, who must also routinely keep accurate and contemporary records.

Trends in contraceptive usage

The methods of contraception used by couples have changed over the years and there have been changes within the social classes. Oral contraceptive usage declines periodically in response to intermittent 'pill scares', but remains at around 3 million users (FPA figures 1996). Sterilization rates in the UK are the highest in Europe; maybe too high in the young (p. 204), and by the mid-forties as many as 50% of women rely on their own or their partner's sterilization. Newer choices such as injectables, improved copper IUDs, and the levonorgestrel intrauterine system (LNG-IUS) are proving slow to 'catch on' in the numbers that their many advantages would support. But further inroads into the supremacy of the pill must be expected.

Choice of method

The practitioner needs to assess the strength of motivation of all women who request contraception. In choosing a method to match their circumstances and needs, most women prioritize both high contraceptive effectiveness and avoidance of adverse effects and health risks (Fig 6.1). Success with the methods which are free of all systemic risk, like the condom, depends greatly upon correct and consistent use, and this is not a common commodity.

Yet condemnation of, for example, coitus interruptus, does not guarantee either adoption of or successful use of a theoretically more effective method. Indeed, it may lead to non-use even of this method in 'emergency' situations. With 'so far successful' users it may instead be worth exploring with the couple the use of a simple contraceptive pessary as an adjunct to the withdrawal method. It is safe to say that 'any method is better than none, but some are better than others'.

Fashions also change. During the last 20 years male barriers and the Pill have been the most widely-used reversible methods. Actually, both these, like the

Fig 6.1 *Current contraceptive use in the UK*
(*Source: Adapted fromContraceptive Education Service (1996). Contraceptive choices. Family Planning Association.
Used with permission*)

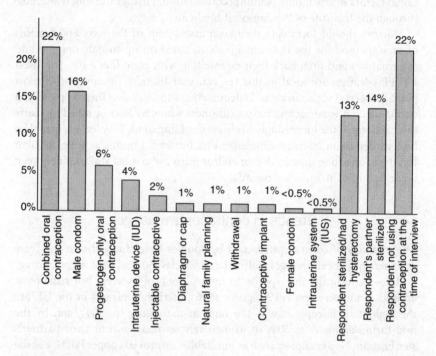

fertility awareness methods in which there is currently a growing interest, are less than ideal for many by virtue of having the wrong 'default state' – meaning the state of conception if there is a significant user-error (default)! Methods like injectables, implants, IUDs, and the LNG-IUS have the more appropriate default state of continuing contraception until a defined action is taken to reverse them.

There are also important related problems which may confront the doctor. They may be physical, psychological, or psychosexual, and unless they are considered in an understanding and flexible manner, the couple may have great difficulty with the use of contraception and unwanted pregnancies may then occur. In one chapter it is possible to highlight only the more common and most important problems.

Table 6.1 gives an updated (1996) indication of reliability ranges which can be quoted to couples. Widely varying limits are frequently quoted because the results of any study are bound to be influenced by the age, motivation, and sexual activity of the population concerned, and by the enthusiasm of the investigator and the degree and duration of follow-up achieved.

Since the first edition of this book there is a new and urgent additional concern, to advise people of all ages who are sexually active on how they may minimize their personal risk of sexually-transmitted infections, especially with the Human Immunodeficiency Virus (HIV). Monogamy is a behaviour

Table 6.1 *User-failure rates for different methods of contraception per 100 woman-years (1996)*

	Range in the world literature[1]	Oxford/FPA Study[2] – all women married and aged above 25		
		Overall (any duration)	Age 25–34 (≤2 years use)	Age 35+ (≤2 years use)
Sterilization				
Male	0–0.2	0.02	0.08	0.08
Female	0–1.0	0.13	0.45	0.08
IUS				
Levonorgestrel–IUS	0–0.2			
Injectable (DMPA)	0–1.0			
Levonorgestrel implant (Norplant)				
Combined pills				
50 µg oestrogen	0.1–3	0.16	0.25	0.17
<50 µg oestrogen	0.2–3	0.27	0.38	0.23
IUD				
Ortho-Gyne T200	>2			
Nova-T/Multiload Cu 250	1–2			
Cu-T 380 (Slimline)	0.3–0.5			
Multiload Cu 375	0.3–1.0			
(375 designed for longevity appears marginally more effective than (250)				

Table 6.1 *Continued*

	Range in the world literature[1]	Oxford/FPA Study[2] – all women married and aged above 25		
		Overall (any duration)	Age 25-34 (≤2 years use)	Age 35+ (≤2 years use)
Progestogen-only pill	⎱ 1-4	1.2	2.5	0.5
Levonorgestrel vaginal ring	⎰			
Diaphragm	4-8	1.9	5.5	2.8
Condom	2-15	3.6	6.0	2.9
Female condom	5-15			
Coitus interruptus	8-17	6.7		
Spermicides alone	4-25	11.9		
Fertility awareness	2-20	15.5		
No method, young women	80-90			
No method at age 40	40-50			
No method at age 45	c. 10-10			
No method at age 50 (if still having menses)	c. 0-5			

[1] Excludes atypical studies giving particularly poor results and all extended-use studies. Mainly based on rates of FPA leaflets – most recent (1996)

[2] Vessey et al. (1982)

Notes: 1. Ranking of efficacy, but overlap of ranges in the first column
2. Influence of age: all the rates of the fourth column being lower than those in the third column. Lower rates still to be expected above age 45
3. Much better results obtainable in other states of relative infertility, such as lactation (see below)

pattern always worthy of encouragement (on medical grounds); but this must be supplemented, in the real world, by enthusiasm for the condom – for best results often in addition to a recognized, non-barrier contraceptive (the 'double Dutch' approach). There should also be no embarrassment about taking a good sexual history, especially regarding recent partner change.

Hormonal contraception

The combined oral contraceptive (COC)

The following subjects demand brief discussion:

(1) benefits versus risks;
(2) choice of users ('safer women'), considering separately the risk factors for venous and arterial thrombosis;
(3) choice of pills ('safer pills'), taking account of:
   (a) what is known about their side-effect profile;
   (b) biological variation in the pharmacology of contraceptive steroids;
   (c) endometrial bleeding as a possible 'threshold bioassay' of their blood levels;
(4) supervision and follow-up, including implications of the monthly pill-free week.

Benefits versus risks

Capable of providing virtually 100% protection from unwanted pregnancy and taken at a time unconnected with sexual activity, the pill provides enormous reassurance by the associated regular, short, light, and usually painless withdrawal bleeding at the end of the 21-day pack. Inevitably, most of this section will be on possible risks and hazards associated with taking the pill, but the positive aspects should not be forgotten; they are listed in Box 6.1. Although some of these findings await full confirmation, such good news is rarely mentioned while the suspected risks are widely publicized and often over-stressed.

    Understanding of potential unwanted effects is based mainly on the reported findings and analyses of three valuable prospective studies, two in this country, that of the RCGP and the Oxford FPA Study which both commenced in 1968, and the American Nurses Health Study. The first compares morbidity, mortality, and pregnancy outcomes in users and non-users while the second has either IUD-users or diaphragm-users as controls. The third uses data collected from over 121 000 nurses, among whom are users of the pill and all alternatives available in the US, starting from 1976 to the present. The main findings have been confirmed by numerous case-control studies. Space does not allow full discussion of all the work which has been published in the 35 years during which the pill has been available in this country. Practitioners should form their own opinion of the risks and benefits by more extensive reading, but

---

Box 6.1 *Beneficial effects of the combined pill*

Contraceptive
 (1) Highly effective
 (2) Highly convenient, non intercourse related
 (3) Reversible

Non-contraceptive
 (4) A reduction in the rate of most disorders of the menstrual cycle:
    (a) less heavy bleeding; therefore
    (b) less anaemia
    (c) less dysmenorrhoea
    (d) regular bleeding, and timing can be controlled (for example, no pill-taker need have 'periods' at weekends)
    (e) less symptoms of premenstrual tension overall
    (f) no ovulation pain
 (5) Less functional ovarian cysts – since abnormal ovulation prevented
 (6) Less extrauterine pregnancies – since normal ovulation inhibited
 (7) Less pelvic inflammatory disease (PID)
 (8) Less benign breast disease
 (9) Possible reduction in the rate of endometriosis
 (10) Less symptomatic fibroids
 (11) Reduced incidence of severe rheumatoid arthritis – now established
 (12) Possibly less thyroid disease (both overactive and underactive syndromes according to RCGP study)
 (13) Less sebaceous disorders (oestrogen-dominant COCs)
 (14) Possibly less duodenal ulcers – this effect is not well established and could be due to anxious women avoiding COCs
 (15) Possibly less *Trichomonas vaginitis*
 (16) Possibly less toxic shock syndrome
 (17) Beneficial effect on risk of cancer of the ovary and endometrium – see text
 (18) No toxicity if overdose is taken
 (19) Obvious beneficial social effects

---

the following may help to summarize present medical opinion upon which contemporary prescription of the pill is based.

Tumours

No medication continues to receive so much scrutiny and investigation as the Pill. For some time fears have been expressed about its possible connection with breast, cervical, and liver cancers.

Breast cancer. The incidence of this disease is high and therefore it must inevitably be expected to develop in women whether they take COCs or not. Since the recognized risk factors include early menarche and late age

Table 6.2 *The increased risk of developing breast cancer while taking the pill and in the 10 years after stopping (Collaborative Group on Hormonal Factors in Breast Cancer 1996)*

User status	Increased risk
Current user	24%
1–4 years after stopping	16%
5–9 years after stopping	7%
10 plus years an ex-user	No significant excess

of first birth, use by young women was rightly bound to receive scientific scrutiny.

The literature to date is copious, complex, confusing, and contradictory! Research is complicated by the problems related to *latency, changes in formulation, time of exposure, and high risk groups*. A major cause of discrepancies may be the fact that long-term use of the COC by young women is a relatively recent and variable phenomenon between populations.

The 1996 publication by the Collaborative Group on Hormonal Factors in Breast Cancer reanalyses original data which relate to over 53 000 women with breast cancer and over 100 000 controls from 54 studies in 25 countries. This is 90% of the world epidemiological data. It has changed the 'model' described in the last edition of this book, in which the pill-associated increased risk was for breast cancer occurring at a young age, and that it diminished or disappeared at older ages, i.e. a transient risk. The new model still shows disappearance of the risk in ex-users, but now recency of use of the COC is the most important factor: with the odds ratio unaffected by age of initiation or discontinuation, use before or after first full-term pregnancy, or duration of use. The main findings are summarized in Table 6.2 and below.

COC pill-users can be reassured that:
(1) while the small increase in breast cancer risk for women on the pill noted in previous studies is confirmed, the odds ratio of 1.24 signifies an increase of 24% only while women are taking the COC, diminishing to zero after discontinuation, over the next few years;
(2) beyond 10 years after stopping there is no detectable increase in breast cancer risk for former pill-users;
(3) the cancers diagnosed in women *who use or have ever used* COCs are *clinically less advanced* than those who have never used the pill, and are less likely to have spread beyond the breast;
(4) this re-analysis shows that these risks are not associated with duration of use, the dose or type of hormone in the COC, and there is no synergism with other risk factors for breast cancer (e.g. family history).

However, if the background risk for the individual is larger, whether because of increased age or a family history, the applicable increase in Table 6.2 necessarily means more attributable cases (than in younger women without an added risk factor). Irrespective of the use of hormonal contraception the cumulative risk of breast cancer in young women is very small, being one in 500 in women up to age 35. But the cumulative risk increases with age thereafter to one in 100 at age 45 and one in 12 by age 75. The increase in attributable cases as age of last use increases has been calculated and is shown in Table 6.3.

Most importantly, for a given age at last use the excess risk is little affected by a women's prior duration of oral contraceptive use. In this reanalysis the risks for progestogen-only contraceptives (POP and injectable) failed to reach statistical significance.

The collaborative group concede that their findings in ever-takers of the pill, of less advanced cases being identified but more of them at a given age, could be explained wholly or in part by surveillance bias (pill-takers both during and after the years of use of the method perhaps being more 'breast aware' than non-takers). However, the present consensus interpretation is that the pill is a weak co-factor for this cancer, but that for some reason the resulting tumours are less aggressive.

Clinical implications

The Faculty of Family Planning has concluded that pill-users should be in-formed of the new data but reiterates the advice given by the Committee on Safety of Medicines (CSM) that there need be no change in prescribing practice.

1. The breast cancer issue should now normally be addressed, in a sensitive way, as part of routine pill counselling for all women. This discussion should be initiated opportunely, and not necessarily at the first visit if not raised by the woman, along with encouragement to report promptly any unusual changes in their breasts at any time in the future ('breast aware-ness'). The balancing protective effects against at least two malignancies (ovary and endometrium – see below) should also be mentioned. The known contraceptive and non-contraceptive benefits of COCs may seem so great to many (but not to all) as to compensate for almost any likely lifetime excess risk of breast cancer.

2. In explaining the new model to a pill-taker, I use the fourth column of Table 6.3, dividing the numbers by 10, and ask her to visualize two concert halls each holding 1000 women. Imagine that the first is filled with 1000 pill-takers, all now aged 45, but all having used the COC for varying durations of time then stopping when they reached age 35 (a common scenario). The (cumulative) number of cases of breast cancer would be 11 in Concert Hall 1. However, in Hall 2, filled with never-takers of the pill also all currently aged 45, there would be 10 cases; i.e. there is only one extra case in Hall 1. Moreover, if the pill acts as a co-factor (see above) it is possible that she was a woman who would have developed the disease without the pill at a later age anyway. And the remaining 989 women in Hall 1 will from this time on have only the same risk of breast cancer as the women of Hall 2, i.e. no ongoing added risk because it is over 10 years since their last pill. This is a very important finding, with the overall risk rising so much with age. Finally, the cancers diagnosed among the pill-takers in Hall 1, already and in future, will tend to be less advanced than those in Hall 2.

Table 6.3 Cumulative risk of breast cancer by recency of use. Showing usage in different age groups, the cumulative numbers of breast cancer cases per 10 000 women in never-users of oral contraception and the cumulative number per 10 000 women who had used oral contraception for 5 years and who were followed up for 10 years after stopping

Pill use for 5 years, or any duration[1] Breast cancers diagnosed by	To age 20 Age 30	To age 25 Age 35	To age 30 Age 40	To age 35 Age 45	To age 40 Age 50	To age 45 Age 55
Never-users	4	16	44	100	160	230
Users who stopped 10 years earlier	4.5	17.5	49	110	180	260
Excess number of cases of breast cancer per 10 000 women	0.5	1.5	5	10	20	30

[1] Since the researchers state that for a given age at last use the excess risk is little affected by a woman's prior duration of oral contraceptive use

3. *What about pill use by the older women?* As Table 6.3 shows, there is no change in relative risk but an increased attributable risk (30 extra cases per 10 000 for 10th year ex-users now aged 55). This must be explained and may be acceptable to many with the balancing (see below) from the established protection against cancer of the ovary and endometrium. But to my mind these new data will increasingly lead to more older women choosing other options (including the new IUS) (see pp. 193–98, 207).

4. *Women with benign breast disease* (BBD) or with the family history of a *young first-degree relative with breast cancer under age 40* have a larger background risk than the generality of women. The 24% increment of risk will mean more attributable cases, so that these are *relative contraindications.* If the woman chooses the COC as she is entitled to do, given its benefits, it should be a low dose formulation, for a limited duration, with specific counselling and extra surveillance.

5. If a woman develops carcinoma of the breast, COCs should be discontinued, and women with a history of this cancer should normally avoid COCs (p. 147).

We can be sure that the last word has not yet been spoken on this issue, especially in regard to the cohort of women who started the COC as teenagers and have not yet reached the ages of maximum incidence of breast cancer in large numbers. But the available data are reassuring.

Cervical cancer. A prospective study (Vessey *et al.* 1983) showed a twofold increase of cervical neoplasia in long-term users of the pill compared with IUD users. This finding was to some extent confirmed by the World Health Organisation (WHO) study of invasive disease (WHO 1985). Studies on cervical cancer are complicated by the problem of getting accurate information relating to different patterns of sexual activity, both for women and their partners. Some authorities maintain that the pill is more likely to be a true co-factor for adenocarcinoma. The prime carcinogen for the commonest (squamous) cancer is clearly sexually transmitted, and probably a virus or combination of viruses.

The COC may act, at worst, as a weak co-factor, certainly weaker than cigarette smoking; possibly speeding transition through the pre-invasive stages (Drife and Guillebaud 1986). Long-term users of oral contraceptives should have regular cervical smears, but three-yearly is still considered adequate unless there are other risk factors. The COC may continue to be prescribed in cases under treatment and/or monitoring for pre-invasive lesions (see relative contraindications below).

Liver tumours. The benign *liver tumours* are rare conditions but do occur more frequently in COC users – with an extremely low incidence estimated at around one in 100 000 users (Vessey 1989). The risk is believed to increase with duration of use of older high-dose products and all cases had significant liver enlargement. Rarely, long-term use of the pill may also be associated with primary liver cancer, the association being strongest where there is no cirrhosis or Hepatitis B infection (Vessey 1989) – and with, helpfully, no evidence of synergy with the latter.

Carcinoma of the ovary and of the endometrium. These two cancers are *less* frequent in COC-users (Drife and Guillebaud 1986). Numerous studies have shown that, in round terms, for both cancers there is a reduction to one half in the incidence among all users; to one-third in long-term users; and a protective effect can be detected in ex-users for up to 10–15 years. Suppression of ovulation and of normal menstruation in COC-users probably explains the similarity of the findings.

Choriocarcinoma. This was more common among women given the pill in the presence of active trophoblastic disease (with elevated hCG) in some studies – but not in others from the US. The COC may be used once trophoblastic activity is undetectable by hCG measurement. Other cancer links have been mooted but not confirmed, and women who are apparently cured by local surgery for neoplasia of the ovary, cervix, and for malignant melanoma may use COCs. For further discussion, see Vessey (1989). The 'bottom line' when counselling women is as follows: *Populations using the Pill may develop different benign or malignant neoplasms from control populations, but there is no proof that the overall risk of either type of neoplasia is increased.* (It could even be reduced, though there is no proof of that either.)

Cardiovascular disease

Venous thromboembolism. Now that the dust has settled somewhat since the letter from the CSM on 18 October 1995, is it possible to produce some reasonably rational and evidence-based guidelines for prescribing?

There is a range of expert views about the four main publications (references in Mills *et al.* 1996) of December 1995 and January 1996, on the combined oral contraceptive and venous thromboembolism (VTE). They were highly congruent, describing a doubling of the odds ratio for users of desogestrel/gestodene products (DSG/GSD) in comparison with the remainder (here termed non-DSG/GSD pills). Many authorities, especially in continental Europe, think that the whole of the association might be explained, not by cause and effect but by:

(1) prescriber bias (prescribers being selectively more likely, prior to October 1995, to use DSG/GSD products for first-timers and women thought to be at risk of VTE);

(2) the 'attrition of susceptibles' or 'healthy-user effect' (non-DSG/GSD pills being more commonly used by longer-term users and parous women who would be less likely as a population to suffer a VTE since those who had would no longer be using the method);

(3) diagnostic bias resulting from prescriber bias, in that women on DSG/GSD pills, because of a perceived higher risk, might then be more likely to be referred for accurate investigations leading to this easily-overlooked diagnosis.

Evidence for these has been presented by Lewis *et al* (1996*b*), who show a significant trend of increasing risk of VTE for the progestogens in COCs related solely to the recency of their introduction to the market. This is not biologically plausible, but may be readily linked to prescriber bias and the healthy-user effect. It has since been challenged, on the basis of inappropriate data selection (Vandenbroucke, personal communication, 1997).

At the time of writing, the CSM still appears to take the evidence at face value. Personally, I am sure the apparent doubling is a 'worst case scenario', because of the exaggerating effects of the above biases and confounders. But even allowing for the latter I am prepared to accept some difference of VTE risk when comparing the DSG/GSD pills with the levonorgestrel (LNG) ones (the main comparison in the studies). There is a degree of biological plausibility, since we have known for years that LNG behaves as an anti-oestrogenic progestogen. A dose of 30 µg of ethinyloestradiol (EE) raises sex hormone binding globulin (SHBG), raises HDL-cholesterol, and tends to improve acne. If LNG 150 µg is combined with the same dose of ethinyloestradiol (EE) in Microgynon, SHBG goes up less than with EE alone, HDL-cholesterol is actually slightly lowered, and clinically acne may be worsened. Combined with desogestrel 150 µg as in Marvelon, the same dose of EE raises SHBG more, raises HDL-cholesterol (like it would on its own), and tends to improve acne. Gestodene is similar. Thus on those three criteria (among others) DSG/GSD pills are more oestrogenic than LNG ones, and since prothrombotic coagulation changes are also oestrogen-related, a difference in VTE potential has always been possible.

Which progestogens for least arterial disease risk (chiefly myocardial infarction and strokes)? Until October 1995 there was no epidemiology, and the experts in haemostasis had so far failed to show any relative difference in a VTE-promoting factor – indeed, this remains true, the changes are so very complex. This explains why the possibility of a relative benefit to the arterial walls and hence arterial disease from what appeared to be the 'good' effects on lipids – not lowering HDL-cholesterol as some of the higher-dose LNG and NET brands do – of the more oestrogen-dominant formulations of the DSG/GSD pills was given greater weight by most prescribers. This possibility still exists, on the model of oestrogen used as HRT after the menopause.

Some epidemiological data on myocardial infarction in women with no history of cardiovascular disease are also now available. Lewis *et al* (1996*a*) report no significant increase in this risk in users of DSG/GSD pills compared with women not using the pill. The threefold increased risk of myocardial infarction previously reported in users of the combined oral contraceptive was still present among users of non-DSG/GSD brands. Smokers using the latter brands had 11.1 times the risk of non-smoking women not using the pill (a significant difference), but the relative risk was 3.1 (not significant) in smokers using DSG/GSD pills. This is compatible with the hypothesis that the DSG/GSD pills have a relatively lower arterial disease risk primarily among women with risk factors like smoking. Direct comparison of the two types of pill in this study (all users) did show a statistically significant difference (Lewis *et al.*, 1997). But more studies are needed to confirm these findings.

Risks in perspective. The new studies confirm that all low-dose combined oral contraceptives carry an extremely low risk for healthy women. Even if the full doubling of the risk ratio for VTE is used in calculations, the attributable

Table 6.4 *Comparative risks – estimates 1996. Annual risks per 100 000 women*

Activity	Cases	Deaths
Having a baby, UK (all causes of death)		6
Having a baby (venous thrombosis)	60	1
Using DSG/GSD Pill (venous thrombosis)	30	0.5
Using non-DSG/GSD Pill (venous thrombosis)	15	0.25
Non-user, non-pregnant (venous thrombosis)	5–11	0.1 +
Risk from *all causes* through COC (healthy non-smoking woman)		1
Home accidents		3
Playing soccer		4
Road accidents		8
Scuba diving		22
Hang-gliding		150
Cigarette smoking (in next year, if aged 35)		167
Death from pregnancy/childbirth in rural Africa		600–1000

Sources: Dinman, B.D. (1980), Journal of the American Medical Association, 44 1226–8
Anon (1991) British Medical Journal, 302 743
Mills, A. et al. (1996). British Medical Journal, 312, 121
Strom, B. (1994) Pharmacoepidemiology (2nd ed.), pp. 57–65. Wiley, Chichester

number of cases (15 per 100 000) through using DSG/GSD brands rather than one of the others, is small. Fortunately, as Table 6.4 shows, VTE has a low mortality and the difference in risk is small enough in comparison with the risks (such as those in the Table) which are taken in everyday life for a well-informed woman to take if she so chooses: for example, because she finds a DSG/GSD brand preferable for her quality of life and so-called minor side-effects such as acne, headaches, depression, weight gain, or breast symptoms.

Prescribing guidelines. If for the time being we accept that non-DSG/GSD pills are somewhat less likely to lead to VTE – how much less likely still being uncertain – how should this affect our practice and prescribing?

See Tables 6.5 and 6.6. This section is derived and adapted from my *British Medical Journal* leading article (Guillebaud 1995c), and the statement from the Clinical and Scientific Committee of the Faculty of Family Planning, issued in December 1995 and later published as a letter (Mills *et al.*, 1996). The latter includes the VTE references from the four studies published in 1995–96. More recent studies show less or even absent differential risk.

Prescribers should take a comprehensive personal and family history to exclude absolute contraindications to the use of combined oral contraceptives. These include a personal history of venous thromboembolism.

Women with possible hereditary thrombophilia in a first-degree relative (as defined in Table 6.5) should, in my view, not be prescribed any combined oral contraceptive until thrombophilia has been excluded. The main abnormalities

Table 6.5 *Risk factors for venous thromboembolism*

	Absolute contraindication	Relative contraindication
Family history (parent or sibling under 45)	Clotting abnormality or tests not done	Clotting factors done, normal
Overweight – high body mass index (BMI)	BMI >39	BMI 30–39
Immobility	Confined to bed	Wheelchair life
Varicose veins	Past thrombosis	Extensive VVs

Notes: 1. *A single risk factor in relative contraindication column indicates use of non-DSG/GSD pill, if any COC used*
2. *NB synergism, such that more than one factor in the relative contraindication column means COC method is absolutely contraindicated*
3. *The literature on the association of smoking with venous thromboembolic disease is mostly negative*

to be sought are Factor V Leiden (the genetic cause of activated protein C resistance) which is the most prevalent; and deficiencies of protein C, protein S, and antithrombin III. Any of these absolutely contraindicate all EE-containing pills. Even if they are not found the woman cannot be totally reassured and the COC should remain relatively contraindicated, since by no means all the predisposing abnormalities of the complex haemostatic system have yet been characterized.

But all women with a single relative contraindication for venous thrombo-embolism (VTE) should receive a non-DSG/GSD pill.

Other first-time users of COCs. As a rule, prescribe initially a low-dose COC containing no more than 35 μg ethinyloestradiol and no more than 150 μg levonorgestrel or 1 mg norethisterone, except when a higher dose is specifically indicated.

Preparations containing desogestrel or gestodene may have an additional therapeutic role in women with specific medical conditions, including acne and hirsutism, and the user's choice should also be respected (p. 141).

Established users of COCs containing gestodene or desogestrel. If a risk factor for venous thromboembolism is present as in Table 6.5, the woman should be advised to change to a preparation that does not contain gestodene or desogestrel, or to another contraceptive method, as appropriate. Even if free of risk factors, if after counselling the woman finds the added risk of venous thromboembolism described above unacceptable then she should use a COC that does not contain gestodene or desogestrel.

If, however, she finds that risk acceptable and declares herself unprepared to switch brands ('predictable intolerance'), the prescriber should respect the user's informed choice if she chooses to continue to take her current pill, even if only because she is satisfied with it.

Users of COCs that do not contain gestodene or desogestrel. A woman who does not tolerate these COCs, by virtue of experiencing persistent breakthrough

Table 6.6 *Risk factors for arterial cardiovascular system (CVS) disease*

Risk factor	Absolute contraindication	Relative contraindication	Remarks
Family history (FH) arterial CVS disease in parent or sibling <45	Known atherogenic lipid profile – or tests not available	Normal blood lipid profile or first attack in relative >45	POP usually a better choice oral method in all relative contraindications + consider LNG-IUS (see text)
Cigarette smoking	?40+ cigarettes/day	5–40 cigarettes/day	
Diabetes mellitus (DM)	Severe or diabetic complications present (e.g. retinopathy, renal damage)	Not severe/labile, and no complications; young patient with short duration of DM	
Hypertension (↑BP)	BP >160/95 mmHg on repeated testing	↑BP but ≤ 160/95 mmHg (see text)	
Excess weight	BMI >39	BMI 30–39	
Migraine	Focal aura symptoms; severe, or ergotamine-treated	Migraine without focal aura; severe, sumatriptan treatment	Relates to stroke risk. Consider tricycling, if non-focal aura headaches mainly in pill-free interval

Notes: 1. **Synergism: if more than one relative contraindication applies, or if woman aged >35, do not use COC**

2. *Some of the numbers selected are arbitrary and perhaps too strict if they are the sole problem (for example, the COC might actually be allowed reluctantly to a current healthy 25-year-old admitting to two packs of cigarettes a day). They also relate to use solely for contraception. Use of COCs for medical indications often entails a different risk benefit analysis, i.e. the extra therapeutic benefits may outweigh expected extra risks*

bleeding or androgenic or other 'minor' side-effects, or for personal reasons, may be prescribed a COC containing gestodene or desogestrel, having accepted the increased risk of venous thromboembolism.

Women with a single risk factor for arterial disease as in Table 6.6, or healthy and risk factor-free but above age 35. Arterial diseases are not only commoner among smoking pill-takers, the case-fatality rate is also much higher (RCGP 1983). The risk increases with age. So because of the apparently better lipid effects and some epidemiology (see above), a low oestrogen DSG/GSD may be considered. If she has already been on *any* COC for some years without a VTE she is relatively unlikely to be one of the individuals with a hereditary (or acquired) predisposition to venous thrombosis (though this previous un-complicated use does not entirely exclude a clotting abnormality). The mirror image of this point explains why it is now usual to select a non-DSG/GSD pill for those new to the COC, who are "an unknown quantity" with respect to VTE.

Neither the RCGP study (Croft and Hannaford 1989) nor the Oxford/FPA study (Vessey *et al.* 1989) nor the American nurses study (Stampfer *et al.* 1988) have been able to detect an increased risk of myocardial infarction either in current or past pill-taking *non-smokers*. This means the risk of using the modern low-oestrogen brands must be very small if not absent for women free of risk factors. But since it remains appreciable in their presence, I do not feel the suggestive data that DSG/GSD pills might have relative advantages for arterial disease in higher-risk women should be discounted, even though not yet proven epidemiologically.

If a DSG/GSD pill is chosen, whether for this indication or because the wom-an prefers it on quality of life grounds, there must for medico-legal security always be a full contemporaneous record of:

- the risk-factor history
- the discussion
- the fact that the woman accepts a possibly increased risk of VTE (amounting at most to 15 per 100 000 per year relative to other formulations).

What about norgestimate, the progestogen in Cilest? There remains consid-erable uncertainty here, through lack of epidemiological data, and the CSM's October 1996 letter did not recommend any change in prescribing practice for Cilest. Intriguingly, one of its main metabolites is levonorgestrel (22% by weight, equivalent to about 55 µg). Since as we saw above this is a relatively anti-oestrogenic progestogen, one might expect some counteraction of the oestrogenicity and maybe therefore the thrombogenicity of the extra 17% of ethinyloestradiol (35 µg rather than 30 µg) which Cilest contains, in comparison with other monophasic low-oestrogen products. Yet in 1996 the 'Transnational study' reported an increased risk ratio of 1.85 for VTE for the norgestimate product as compared with levonorgestrel pills, and this increase approached statistical significance and was not distinguishable from the rough-ly doubled rate for DSG or GSD 30 µg products (Lewis *et al.* 1996*b*), which they had earlier shown. The authors explained away this finding on the basis of the bias/confounding problems discussed above; but at present we cannot be certain that Cilest should not be put in the 'third generation' category for VTE risk. And, applying the same argument above about 'oestrogenicity' to this product, does this simultaneously mean that *for the arterial walls* norgestimate – plus levonorgestrel 55 µg plus its other metabolites together – in combination with 35 µg EE would be relatively better than levonorgestrel 150 µg plus 30 µg EE?

We need more data, but for the time being Cilest can be considered as a useful option, with no special limitations as to its use in the new prescribing environment prevailing in the UK since October 1995.

Absolute and relative contraindications

Each packet of pills contains an insert, whose wording can cause anxiety to both women and doctors! A consensus statement (Hannaford and Webb 1996) helps to put all that small print into perspective, highlighting what really matters: 'Current scientific evidence suggests only two prerequisites for the safe provision of COCs: a careful personal and family medical history with particular attention to cardiovascular risk factors, and an accurate blood pressure measurement'. But the personal and family history may unearth a range of contraindications, which are comprehensively summarized in Boxes 6.2 and 6.3. These are, in reality, extensions of Tables 6.5 and 6.6, but now also including contraindications which are unrelated to cardiovascular disease.

Intercurrent diseases. It is impossible to list every known disease which might have a bearing on COC prescription and for many the data are unavailable. A working rule is to ascertain whether or not the condition might lead to *summation* with known major adverse effects of COCs, particularly with the risk of any circulatory disease. If not, in most serious chronic conditions the patient can be reassured that COCs are not known to have any effect, good or bad; but they should then be used only with the most careful monitoring and alertness for the onset of new risk factors. Reliable protection from pregnancy is often particularly important when other diseases are present.

Diabetes. The formulation with desogestrel and only 20 µg ethinyloestradiol can be valuable for limited periods, under careful supervision and provided that there is no arteriopathy, retinopathy, neuropathy, or renal damage (or smoking!), and preferably if the duration of the diabetes has been short. Otherwise, some diabetics manage very well with barriers, but others do not. The progestogen-only pill (POP) is acceptable and usually very reliable, but the *LNG-IUS (p. 193) is now an even better choice for most diabetics*, even if nulliparous. After childbearing, if there are no menstrual problems, the copper Cu T 380S (p. 190) is still a useful option, or sterilization whenever the family is complete (see also p. 212).

Hypertension. Hypertension is an important risk factor for heart disease and stroke. In most women on COCs there is a slight increase in both systolic and diastolic blood pressure within the normotensive range. Approximately 1% become clinically hypertensive: the rate increases with age and duration of use and when pill-induced this absolutely contraindicates the combined hormonal method in future, though not the progestogen-only methods. If women with

Box 6.2 *Absolute contraindications to combined oral contraception (Guillebaud 1995a)*

There are some conditions in which all brands of the COC are absolutely contraindicated:

Past or present circulatory disease
- Any past proven arterial or venous thrombosis
- Ischaemic heart disease or angina
- Severe or combined risk factors for venous or arterial disease (see Table 6.5 and 6.6)
- Atherogenic lipid disorders
- Known prothrombotic abnormality of coagulation/fibrinolysis, congenital thrombophilias with abnormal levels of individual factors; from at least 2 (preferably 4) weeks before until 2 weeks after mobilization following elective major or leg surgery; during leg immobilization or varicose vein treatment; and during short-term exposure to high altitude (above 4000 metres)
- Focal and crescendo migraine; migraine requiring ergotamine treatment
- Transient ischaemic attacks even without headache
- Past cerebral haemorrhage, which can be secondary to cerebral venous thrombosis (also to avoid hypertension if past subarachnoid bleed)
- Most types of structural heart disease (discuss with cardiologist), including atrial septal defect (risk of paradoxical embolism), pulmonary hypertension

Disease of the liver
- Active liver disease (whenever liver function tests currently abnormal, including infiltrations and cirrhosis); recurrent cholestatic jaundice, or history of cholestatic jaundice in pregnancy; Dubin–Johnson and Rotor syndromes
- Following viral hepatitis, COCs may be resumed 3 months after liver function tests have returned to normal
- Liver adenoma, carcinoma
- Gallstones (but COCs may be used after cholecystectomy)
- Porphyrias – hepatic (cutaneous is relative contraindication)

History of serious condition affected by sex steroids or related to previous COC use
- Chorea
- COC-induced hypertension
- Pemphigoid gestationis
- Haemolytic uraemic syndrome
- Stevens–Johnson syndrome (erythema multiforme), if causation by COC is diagnosed

---

Box 6.2 *Continued*

• Trophoblastic disease but only until βHCG levels are undetectable*

Pregnancy

Undiagnosed genital tract bleeding

Oestrogen-dependent neoplasms
• Breast cancer (some oncologists permit COCs in selected cases in prolonged remission)
• Past breast biopsy showing premalignant epithelial atypia

Woman's anxiety re COC safety unrelieved by counselling

* In the US this is not considered a contraindication even when HCG present, partly because chemotherapy is given to so many cases of trophoblastic disease anyway

Note that several of the above are not necessarily permanent contraindications. Moreover, over the years many women have been unnecessarily deprived of COCs for reasons now shown to have no link, such as thrush, or positively benefited by the method, such as fully-investigated secondary amenorrhoea with hypo-oestrogenism

---

essential hypertension and no history of exacerbation in a past pregnancy are successfully treated with antihypertensives, the COC may be used under careful supervision (Box 6.3).

Past pregnancy-induced hypertension does not predispose to hypertension during COC use, but it is a risk factor for myocardial infarction, very markedly so if the women also smokes (Croft and Hannaford 1989). The COC is therefore best avoided in such cases.

Sickle-cell disorders. Sickle-cell trait has no bearing on the COC. The situation regarding the homozygous conditions (SS and SC genes) is more uncertain. Both sickle-cell disease and the COC individually lead to an increased risk of thrombosis, possibly superimposed during the arterial stasis of a crisis. Hence, many authorities and most manufacturers have for many years included the frank sickling diseases among the absolute contraindications to the COC. However, Serjeant (1985) reviewing studies in West Africa and the West Indies suggests that sickle-cell disease should only be considered a weak relative contraindication – especially when balanced against the particularly serious risks of pregnancy. In this country, injectables (see p. 171) or the POP are normally better choices.

Choice of pills and users

Initial choice of preparation. Having excluded those women with abso-lute contraindications (Box 6.2), and proceeding with due caution/extra monitoring in the presence of relative contraindications (Box 6.3), the prac-titioner is faced with a variety of formulations (Table 6.7). Which should be chosen?

For a start, there are in reality only five groups or 'ladders' of progestogens,

Box 6.3 *Relative contraindications to COCs*

The following conditions are relative contraindications, signifying that the COC method is usable in context with: the benefit-risk evaluation for that individual; the acceptability or otherwise of alternatives; and sometimes with special advice (e.g. in migraine, to report a change of symptomatology) or monitoring (e.g. more frequent blood pressure measurements). In cases with excess risk of venous thrombosis, if the pill is used at all it should be a non-DSG/GSD variety

- Risk factors for arterial or venous disease (Table 6.6) provided normally that only one is present, and not to a marked degree. Which formulation to choose is discussed on p. 141–5
- Homozygous sickle cell disease (see text)
- Long-term partial immobilization, e.g. in a wheelchair (use non-DSG/GSD pill)
- Sex steroid-dependent cancer (most specialists permit COCs after treatment for malignant melanoma)
- Oligo-/amenorrhoea (COCs may be prescribed after investigation, to supply oestrogen in a woman needing contraception or to control the symptoms of the polycystic ovary syndrome)
- Hyperprolactinaemia (relative contraindication for patients under specialist supervision)
- Very severe depression, if likely to be exacerbated by COCs (but unwanted pregnancies can be very depressing)
- Some chronic diseases: inflammatory bowel disease, which produces prothrombotic changes especially in exacerbations, including Crohn's disease (one form can also be brought on by COCs); diabetes; essential hypertension, well-controlled; otosclerosis (some authorities permit supervised COC use). See also text re 'Intercurrent disease'
- Diseases that require long-term treatment with drugs which might interact with COCs (see text)

Weak relative contraindications
- If a young first-degree relation has breast cancer (p. 138)
- The presence of established benign breast disease (p. 138)

since norethisterone acetate and ethynodiol acetate are converted *in vivo* with great efficiency to norethisterone. Secondly, although much has been written about matching pills to particular hormonal profiles, the systems have no practical value for the initial selection of the low-dose pills now in use. Few would disagree with the general recommendations of the National Association of Family Planning Doctors (NAFPD), the predecessor body to the Faculty of Family Planning and Reproductive Health Care (FFPRHC) which are as follows:

Table 6.7 *System of summarizing pills according to progestogen content ('ladders')*

Pill	μg	μg
	Levonorgestrel	*Ethinyl oestradiol*
1. Ovran (Wyeth)	250*	50
Eugynon 30 (Schering)	250	30
Ovran 30 (Wyeth)	250	30
Ovranette (Wyeth)	150	30
Microgynon 30 (Schering)	150	30
Microgynon 30ED = Microgynon 30 + 7 inert tablets		
Trinordiol (Wyeth) (triphasic) 6 tablets	50	30
Logynon (Schering) (triphasic) 5 tablets	75	40
10 tablets	125	30
Logynon ED = Logynon + 7 inert tablets		
	Norethisterone	*Mestranol*
2. Norinyl-1 (Searle)	1000	50
Ortho-Novin 1/50 (Janssen-Cilag)	1000	50
	Norethisterone	*Ethinyl oestradiol*
Norimin (Searle)	1000	35
BiNovum (Janssen-Cilag)	7 × 500; 14 × 1000	35
TriNovum (Janssen-Cilag)	7 × 500; 7 × 750; 7 × 1000	35
Synphase (Searle)	7 × 500; 9 × 1000; 5 × 500	35
Ovysmen (Janssen-Cilag)	500	35
Brevinor (Searle)	500	35
	Norethisterone acetate	*Ethinyl oestradiol*
3. Loestrin 30 (Parke-Davis)	1500	30
Loestrin 20 (Parke-Davis)	1000	20
	Ethynodiol diacetate	*Ethinyl oestradiol*
4. Conova 30 (Searle)	2000	30
	Desogestrel	*Ethinyl oestradiol*
5. Marvelon (Organon)	150	30
Mercilon (Organon)	150	20

Contained in 500 μg dl norgestrel

Table 6.7 *Continued*

Pill	μg	μg
	Gestodene	*Ethinyl oestradiol*
6. Femodene (Schering)	75	30
Minulet (Wyeth)	75	30
Femodene ED = Femodene + 7 inert tablets		
Triadene (Schering)/	6 × 50; 5 × 70;	6 × 30; 5 × 40;
Tri-Minulet (Wyeth)	10 × 100	10 × 30
	Norgestimate	*Ethinyl oestradiol*
7. Cilest (Janssen-Cilag)	250	35

Note:s A new preparation containing levonorgestrel 100 μg combined with ethinyl oestradiol 20 μg is due to be marketed by Wyeth and Schering during 1997–8

'The pill of choice should be the one containing the lowest suitable dose of oestrogen and progestogen which:

(1) provides effective contraception;
(2) produces acceptable cycle control [a concept expanded below];
(3) is associated with fewest side-effects;
(4) has the least-known effect on carbohydrate and lipid metabolism and haemostatic parameters' (NAFPD 1984).

To number 4 should now be added 'the type of pill chosen (DSG/GSD or non-DSG/GSD) being determined according to the guidelines of the Faculty of Family Planning' (Mills *et al.* 1996). As shown above (pp. 139–45), the main change from earlier editions of this book is the new need to distinguish between the risk factors for venous as opposed to arterial disease, and choose the type of COC in relation to these, in full consultation with the woman herself.

Each doctor needs to be familiar with the composition of the available preparations. Women may react unpredictably and several types may have to be tried before a suitable one is found. Some women are never suited. This is hardly surprising. Individual variation in motivation and tolerance of minor side-effects is well recognized. But there is also marked individual variation in blood levels of the exogenous hormones and in responses at the end organs, especially the endometrium (Guillebaud 1994). Thus it is a false expectation that any single pill will suit all women.

After initial selection according to the guidelines, prescribers should try to identify, if necessary over a series of initial visits as about to be described, the lowest dose for each woman which is effective – (1) in list above – and does not cause the annoying symptom of breakthrough bleeding (BTB) – (2). It is believed that this will minimize adverse side-effects – (3) – both serious and minor, and should also reduce the measurable metabolic changes – (4).

During follow-up, the aim is to give, long term, the *lowest acceptable* amount of both hormones. To achieve this, the following important concepts need to be brought together:

1. *Individual* variation in absorption and metabolism causes blood levels of all contraceptive steroids to vary tenfold, or more accurately the area-under-the-curve varies approximately threefold (Back *et al.* 1981). There are also variable end-organ responses.

2. It is hypothesized that those with the highest blood levels are likely to be the most affected metabolically, and also more at risk of both major and minor side-effects from abnormal bleeding patterns.

3. It is also probable that women with the lowest blood levels tend to manifest this by BTB – as do women whose blood levels are lowered by enzyme-inducers.

4. Absence of BTB signifies either high or adequate blood levels of the administered steroids.

How then can we avoid giving to any woman who tends to have the highest blood levels a stronger formulation than she requires? Pending the availability of direct measurements in the clinic or surgery, we can 'titrate' the dose given against the occurrence of BTB, using the endometrium as an approximate 'threshold bioassay'. The aim should be that each woman receives the least long-term metabolic impact that her uterus will allow, i.e. the lowest dose of contraceptive steroids which is just, but only just, above her own bleeding threshold. In practice this means:

1. *If there is good cycle control* at the time of repeat prescription, the possibility of trying a lower-dose brand (if available) should always be considered. On the other hand;

2. *If BTB occurs* and is unacceptable or persists beyond two cycles, provided that none of the important alternative explanations applies (Box 6.4), the next strongest brand up the 'ladder' in Table 6.7 should be tried. Especially if the complaint is absent withdrawal bleeding, phased pills may be particularly useful for purposes of cycle control. Despite the new emphases since the CSM's letter of October 1995 (p. 139), I still prefer to avoid the excessively progestogen-dominant brands Eugynon 30, Ovran 30, and Conova 30, since they markedly lower HDL-cholesterol, especially in smokers, unless indicated for therapeutic reasons, e.g. in the treatment of endometriosis (see Table 6.8). But if cycle control can only be achieved by a 50 µg oestrogen pill, for that particular woman the latter need not be considered a 'strong' brand.

Obviously this 'titrating' process is not helped by the lack of provision by the manufacturers of a good range of doses, especially for the newer progestogens.

Second choice if there are non-bleeding side-effects. The use of contemporary pills has reduced the reporting of so-called 'minor' side-effects. When symptoms do occur it is generally bad practice to give further prescriptions such as diuretics, anti-migraine treatments, or antidepressants for weight gain, headaches, or depression respectively. For the last of these, pyridoxine 50–100 mg daily may be beneficial. Otherwise there are two preferred, if empirical, courses of action namely:

Box 6.4 *Check-list in cases of possible 'breakthrough bleeding' (BTB) in pill-takers*

A note of caution: first eliminate other possible causes! The following check-list is modified from Sapire (1990):

- *Disease* – Examine the cervix. It is not unknown for bleeding from an invasive cancer to be wrongly attributed to BTB. *Chlamydia* can cause a bloodstained discharge
- *Disorder of pregnancy* causing bleeding (e.g. abortion, trophoblastic tumour)
- *Default* – missed pill(s) Remember that the BTB may start 2 or 3 days later and be very persistent thereafter
- *Drugs* – especially enzyme-inducers (see text)
- *Diarrhoea with* **vomiting** – diarrhoea alone has to be very severe to impair absorption significantly
- *Disturbance of absorption* – likewise, has to be very marked to be relevant, e.g. after massive gut resection. Coeliac disease does not pose a significant absorption problem
- *Diet* – gut flora involved in recycling ethinyloestradiol may be reduced in vegetarians. Could sometimes be a factor in BTB, but a very unlikely cause
- *Duration too short* – minimal BTB which is tolerable may resolve after 2–3 months' use of any new formulation. The opposite problem may sometimes apply during 'tricycling' (see text); the duration of continuous use may be too long in that individual for the endometrium to be sustained. If so, 'bicycling' of two packets in a row may be substituted

Finally, after the above have been excluded:

- *Dose* – if she is taking a monophasic, try a phasic pill
  - increase the progestogen component
  - try a different progestogen
  - consider using a 50 μg pill, such as Ovran

(1) decrease the dose of either hormone, if still possible – in the limit, oestrogen can be eliminated by a trial of the progestogen-only pill;

(2) change to a different progestogen (Table 6.7).

Some more specific guidance for side-effects and conditions associated with a relative excess of either steroid may be obtained from Tables 6.8 and 6.9. Note the cautions in the important notes at the bottom of each table.

Cervical ectopy ('erosion') is common and may be pill-related. It can be treated by cryocautery if, and only if, it is the cause of excessive discharge. Remember *Chlamydia* if any cervix bleeds readily. But modern pills have been shown not to cause an increase in the incidence of monilial infection, which is common in all women.

Dianette. This is an anti-androgen/synthetic oestrogen combination

Table 6.8 *Which second choice of pill? Relative oestrogen excess*

Symptoms	Conditions
Nausea	Benign breast disease
Dizziness	Fibroids
'Premenstrual tension' and irritability	Endometriosis
Cyclical weight gain (fluid)	
'Bloating'	
Vaginal discharge (no infection)	
Some cases of breast pain	

Treat with progestogen – dominant COC, such as Loestrin 30, Eugynon 30 (but with caution regarding lipids, and risk of arterial disease in those with the relevant risk factors, see p. 143). Loestrin 20, the new LNG 20 μg product (Footnote to Table 6.7) and Mercilon 20 are oestrogen-deficient options

(cyproterone acetate (CPA) 2 mg with ethinyloestradiol (EE) 35 μg) for the oral treatment of moderately severe acne and mild hirsutism in women. These are its indications; but it is also a reliable anovulant like other combined oral contraceptives, and has similar backup mechanisms, rules for missed tablets, interactions, absolute and relative contraindications. However, it is likely from animal research to cause feminization of male fetuses and is absolutely contraindicated in pregnancy and lactation.

Otherwise, practically everything in this section on the COC applies to Dianette, but bearing in mind that it is an oestrogen-dominant product and prone to the side-effects listed in Table 6.8. Since it permits EE to raise SHBG and HDL-cholesterol, it might potentially also allow the oestrogen to have relatively greater effects in a prothrombotic direction than a levonorgestrel product would (see pp. 139–40 above). Although there are no clear epidemiological data, my current working hypothesis is therefore to put it in the same category as a 'third generation' desogestrel/gestodene product and follow the prescribing guidelines on pp. 141–4 excluding those specifically related to the CSM letter of October 1995 (which made no mention of Dianette).

Duration of treatment with Dianette needs to be individualized. In the data sheet it is 'recommended that treatment is withdrawn when the acne or hirsutism is completely resolved', but 'repeat courses may be given if the condition recurs'. There is a concern that prolonged high-dose treatment with CPA can cause benign and malignant liver tumours in rats, and the much higher 50 mcg dose used by dermatologists has caused these in humans. There is no certainty that the 2 mcg dose increases the risk of such tumours or of cholestatic jaundice significantly more than all other COCs, which are (rarely) also implicated. In my experience patients develop a very strong 'brand loyalty', but I encourage them to switch (commonly to Marvelon) when their condition is controlled, usually after 1–3 years – but sometimes much longer, assuming they accept the possible hepatic and prothrombotic risks.

Table 6.9 *Which second choice of pill? Relative progestogen excess*

Symptoms	Conditions
Dryness of vagina	Acne/seborrhoea
Some cases of	Hirsutism
Sustained weight gain	
Depression	
Loss of libido	
Breast symptoms	

Treat with oestrogen-dominant COC, such as Ovysmen/Brevinor, or
Marvelon; then Dianette, an acne treatment which is also contraceptive,
containing 35 μg of ethinyloestradiol combined with 2 mg of the anti-
androgen cyproterone acetate (see text, p. 152). (Caution necessary in
that oestrogen-dominance may correlate with a slightly higher risk of
venous thrombosis, especially if relevant risk factors present, see p 142)

Supervision and long-term follow-up

Each woman needs individual teaching, backed by a good instruction leaflet
(ideally the one produced by the UK FPA). Starting on day 1 (or by day 3)
avoids the requirement to take extra precautions (see Table 6.10). It is important to remind the woman that pills must be taken in the correct order and
the packet completed regardless of bleeding. Protection is afforded during the
7 tablet-free days provided another packet follows. If taken correctly, each new
pack is started on the same weekday.

Blood pressure should be recorded before starting the pill and checked
after 3 months (1 month in a high risk case), and subsequently at intervals
of 6 months. After about 2 years if there is no significant change this interval
can be increased to annually, but the risk of hypertension never entirely
disappears. A moderate increase in blood pressure may also act as a marker
for an increased risk of thrombosis, especially in the presence of an arterial
risk factor.

Breast awareness should be taught, and checked by nurse or doctor annually. Cervical screening should be performed regularly according to local
guidelines. However it is essential to appreciate and to explain to women that
such procedures are part of well-woman care, and completely unrelated to
safe pill-management. The only items which are relevant to longer-term COC
follow-up are:

(1) *blood pressure* monitoring – put first and foremost;
(2) updating of *family history* (e.g. since both are older, the sister of a young
    client may now have had the VTE under 45 to which she was always
    predisposed);
(3) management of *new risk factors, diseases,* and *relevant drugs,* i.e. updating
    past history

Table 6.10 *Starting routines*

	Start when?	Extra precautions for 7 days?
1. Menstruating	At or after 5th day of period	Yes
	1st day/before day 3	No[1]
2. Post-partum		
(a) No lactation	Day 21 ideal (low risk of thrombosis by then, first ovulations reported day 28+)	
(b) Lactation	Not normally recommended at all (POP or DMPA preferred)	
3. Post-induced abortion/miscarriage	Same day	No
4. Post trophoblastic tumour	One month after no hCG detected	As 1
5. Post-higher or same dose COC	Instant switch[2]	No
6. Post-lower dose COC	After usual 7-day break	No
7. Post-POP	First day of period	No
8. Post-POP with secondary amenorrhoea	Any day (end of packet)	No
9. Other secondary amenorrhoea (pregnancy risk excluded)	Any day	Yes

[1] *Except in the case of Logynon ED and Femodene ED – here the starting routine entails the taking of a variable number of placebos; hence extra precautions are recommended, for 14 days in fact*

[2] *This advice is because of reports of rebound ovulation occurring at the time of transfer, if the usual 7-day break is taken. Alternative: normal 7-day break plus extra contraception for first 7 days of the new packet*

(4) current *symptom monitoring*, possibly pill-related side-effects – see Tables 6.8, 6.9, and related text;

(5) *headache* monitoring – the most important symptom to check.

The last of these is perhaps most often neglected and will now be considered in some detail.

Migraine

Studies have shown an increased risk (risk ratio about 2) of ischaemic stroke in COC-users. There is some evidence that this risk is independently increased in migraine sufferers. In Lidegaard's valuable study from Denmark, reported in 1993 and 1995, the risk through having any kind of migraine more than once a month without the Pill was increased by a little less than threefold, with the COC fivefold compared with the background risk. And there is the usual further multiplication of risk ratios if the woman has other arterial risk factors like smoking.

Because thrombotic strokes are rare in young women (two per 100 000 at age 20, or almost six per 100 000 for young women with migraine), the absolute (attributable) risk remains small. Using the above COC-linked risk ratio of two, there would be four attributable cases at 20. Unless there are other arterial risk factors this is fewer than the number of venous thromboembolism cases per 100 000 attributable to either 'generation' of COCs in Table 6.4 (p. 141), but the morbidity in survivors is potentially more serious and long term. Also, the background risk at age 40 is 20 per 100 000, so all the attributable risks are 10 times greater, meaning about 40 extra cases through migraine (>1 attack per month) and about 40 more if 100 000 sufferers also took the COC.

It is also believed, though here the data are more scanty, that certain features of the headaches in migraine with aura focus the risk of this rare catastrophe in a pill-taker. Hence the advice which follows (Clinical and Scientific Committee of Faculty of Family Planning and RHC & Medical Advisory Committee, FPA 1997).

Absolute contraindications to commencing or continuing the COC:
1. Migraine with aura during which there are focal neurological symptoms (usually asymmetrical and typically preceding the headache itself). The significant associated symptoms during an aura or the headache itself are:
   (a) disturbance of speech (nominal dysphasia);
   (b) loss of sight, or of part or whole of field of vision on one side (homonymous visual disturbance). Teichopsia is one variety, in which a bright scintillating angulated line surrounds the area of lost vision (scotoma);
   (c) numbness, severe paraesthesia, or weakness on one side of the body (e.g. one limb, side of the tongue).

Note the absence of photophobia or *symmetrical* blurring or 'flashing lights'; the main feature the relevant symptoms share is asymmetry, meaning that they are 'focal' or interpretable as due to (transient) cerebral ischaemia. Should relevant symptoms be described, the *artificial oestrogen* of the COC should normally be stopped and thereafter avoided to minimize the risk of superimposed thrombosis causing permanent ischaemia, i.e. a thrombotic stroke.

It may be difficult to distinguish such relatively common, migraine-associated transient ischaemia from rare organic episodes – true transient ischaemic attacks or TIAs (e.g. due to paradoxical embolism which is an established risk of an atrial septal defect). Upon suspicion these of course mean the same in practice, i.e. stop the pill immediately. But neurological investigation should also follow, particularly for the following focal symptoms which are *not* typical of migraine:

156

(a) focal epilepsy or severe acute vertigo, ataxia, monocular blindness, aphasia, unilateral tinnitus;

(b) a severe unexplained drop attack or collapse.

TIAs are also more sudden in onset than migraine aura and last over an hour, without other migraine symptoms like nausea.

2. Migraines which are unusually frequent/severe. 'Status migrainosus' describes attacks lasting more than 72 hours, which contraindicate the COC absolutely – *unless* they resolve after treatment for medication misuse (see below).

3. Migraines requiring ergotamine treatment, due to its vasoconstrictor actions.

NB. In any of the above, any of the progestogen-only, oestrogen-free hormonal methods may be offered immediately: similar headaches may continue, but now without the potential added risk from prothrombotic haemostatic effects of the ethinyloestradiol. HRT with *natural* oestrogen is also not contraindicated, if oestrogen deficiency is later suspected.

Relative contraindications. This term means that the COC may be used, but always with specific instruction to the woman regarding those changes in the character or severity of her symptoms which mean she should stop the method and take urgent medical advice. These are listed as the first six items in Box 6.5. Moreover, an alternative contraceptive (e.g. the IUS) would still be preferable in the cases below if, due to the synergism highlighted in Table 6.6, there are added arterial risk factors such as heavy smoking, or diabetes or older age above 35. Such factors would usually contraindicate the COC if the migraines occur more than monthly.

1. Migraine without focal aura. This includes migraine with photophobia, phonophobia, or any other prodromal or within-headache symptoms so long as none are localizable to the cerebral cortex or brain stem. If these or other 'ordinary' headaches occur, particularly in the pill-free interval, tricycling the COC may help (see p. 159–60).

2. Distant past history of migraine with focal aura; i.e. a history of the last attack being more than 5 years before commencing the COC. The COC may be given a trial with the caveats above.

3. The occurrence of a woman's first-ever attack of migraine of any type while on the COC. This should be stopped if she is seen during the attack, but can be later restarted with the usual forewarning about focal symptoms.

4. Use of sumatriptan in the absence of any other contraindicating factors.

5. Severe/frequent attacks in the past which have become moderate and 'live-withable' after treatment for medication misuse.

Reasons to stop the pill

Box 6.5 lists the reasons that should be understood by all well-counselled women from their first visit, for immediately discontinuing COCs and obtaining

---

Box 6.5 *COCs should be stopped immediately pending investigation and treatment, if the following occur:*

(1) Unusual or severe and very prolonged headache
(2) Disturbance of speech (nominal dysphasia)
(3) Loss of sight, or of part or whole of field of vision on one side (homonymous visual disturbance). Teichopsia is one variety (see p. 156)
(4) Numbness, severe paraesthesia or weakness on one side of the body (e.g. one limb, side of the tongue); indeed, any symptom suggesting cerebral ischaemia
(5) Focal epilepsy or severe acute vertigo, ataxia, monocular blindness, asphasia, unilateral tinnitus
(6) A severe unexplained fainting attack or collapse
(7) Painful swelling in the calf
(8) Pain in the chest, especially pleuritic pain
(9) Breathlessness or cough with blood-stained sputum
(10) Severe abdominal pain
(11) Immobilization, as after orthopaedic injury or major surgery (do not demand that the COC be stopped for any minor surgery such as laparoscopy) or leg surgery: stop COC and heparinize. If elective procedure and Pill stopped more than 2 weeks ahead, anticoagulation usually unnecessary

All the above could be caused by an actual or imminent thrombotic or embolic event, though other explanations may well apply. They mean that the artificial oestrogen should be stopped, but any progestogen-only method could be started immediately pending the diagnosis. Other reasons for stopping are usually less urgent

(12) Acute jaundice
(13) Blood pressure above 160/95 on repeated measurement
(14) Severe skin rash (e.g. erythema multiforme)
(15) Detection of a new risk factor, e.g. onset of diabetes or SLE, diagnosis of a structural heart lesion such as ASD, detection of breast cancer

---

urgent further advice. They appear in lay terms in the FPA's recommended leaflet, which is one reason why, in my view, it should be given to all prospective pill-takers. Note that the first six focus on the risk of stroke in relation to migraine with focal aura and TIAs – see above.

Importance of the pill-free week

This promotes a reassuring withdrawal bleed (WTB) – and indeed, if this does not occur in two successive cycles, it is best to exclude pregnancy. However, its importance might be greater than that, in allowing some degree of recovery from systemic effects of the pill. In one study, for example, HDL-cholesterol suppression by the COCs studied was eliminated by the end of the pill-free interval (Demacker *et al.* 1982). Hence it is probably wise only to cut out the gap between packets either in the short term (upon request to avoid a 'period' on special occasions) * or for special indications such as the occurrence of regular hormone-withdrawal headaches. The *tricycle regimen* is often used, in which three or four packets of a monophasic pill are taken in succession, followed by a pill-free gap. This leads to 10-week or 13-week cycles, only four or five WTBs per year and, in this example, only that number of headaches annually. Other important indications are given in Box 6.6 and discussed further below.

Biochemical and ultrasound data also demonstrate return of pituitary and ovarian follicular activity during the pill-free time in about one-fifth of pill-takers, in some women to a marked extent (Guillebaud 1994). Therefore breakthrough ovulation is most likely to follow any lengthening of the pill-free (meaning contraception-free) interval. Such lengthening may result from omissions, malabsorption, and drug interaction involving pills either at the start at the of a packet.

Clearly the advice to the woman who has missed pills which is still given in some package inserts, to take extra precautions to the end of her packet, is wrong since it fails to allow for ovarian activity returning in the pill-free time. Smith *et al.* (1986) showed, admittedly in a study involving small numbers, that even if only 14 or even as few as seven pills had first been taken, no women ovulated after seven pills were subsequently missed – implying at the very least that three or four pills may be missed mid-packet with impunity! This and other work may be summarized:

- seven consecutive pills are enough to 'put the ovaries to sleep' (therefore pills 8–21 in a packet simply 'keep them asleep')
- seven pills can be omitted without ovulation, as in the regular pill-free week
- more than seven pills missed *in total* increases the conception risk.

The 7-day 'rule', as now used by the UK FPA and also the UK manufacturers, states (wording adapted slightly):

If you are more than 12 hours late in taking any pill, or miss more than one, the pill may not work. As soon as you remember, continue to take your pills normally, but you may not be protected for the next 7 days so either avoid sex or use another method (the condom for example). In addition:

- If you have more than seven pills left in the pack, continue taking them and start the next pack as you would normally do after the usual gap between packs.
- If you have less than seven left, so your packet of pills runs out during the next 7 days, this means you should start the next pack as soon as you have finished the present one – in other words, do not have a gap between packs (and skip any dummy 'reminder tablets').

The last part of the advice is critically important and can be explained 'It would be silly to let your ovaries have another break from the effect of your contraceptive so soon after the break you made by mistake (by the pills you

---

* Note: Phasic pill-users who wish to postpone withdrawal bleeds must use the final phase of a spare packet, or pills from an equivalent formulation to that phase (e.g. Norimin, in the case of TriNovum)

Box 6.6 *Indications for the tricycle regimen (using a monophasic pill)*

(1) Headaches, including non-focal migraine, and other bothersome symptoms occurring regularly in the withdrawal week
(2) Unacceptably heavy or painful withdrawal bleeds
(3) Paradoxically, to help women who are concerned about absent withdrawal bleeds (this concern therefore arising less often!)
(4) Epilepsy: this benefits from relatively more sustained levels of the administered hormones (see also below for another reason related to the anti-epileptic treatment)
(5) Endometriosis – a progestogen-dominant monophasic pill may be tricycled for maintenance treatment after primary therapy (e.g. Eugynon 30, Conova 30)
(6) Suspicion of decreased efficacy
(7) At the woman's choice

Note: In view of the possibility that the monthly pill-free interval is beneficial (see p. 158–9), one of these special indications should normally apply

---

missed)'. The woman should of course be asked to return if she has no bleeding in the next pill-free break.

Fig 6.2 gives a useful flow diagram for patients: note the footnote re emergency contraception. Emergency contraception is only indicated if pill-omissions lead to a lengthening of the pill-free time to 9 days (or more), *or* if any combination of pills from the first seven have been omitted such as to amount effectively in the prescriber's view to a 9-day interval since effective pituitary/ ovarian suppression. Otherwise, unless very many pills are missed (arbitrarily four or more), the studies, including Smith *et al.* quoted above, indicate that the advice in Fig 6.2 will maintain normal or above-normal efficacy, mid-cycle and at the end of a pack.

Vomiting and diarrhoea. Extra contraceptive precautions should start from the onset of the illness and continue for 7 days after it ends, with elimination of the pill-free interval as indicated by the above advice. Diarrhoea alone is not a problem, unless it is of cholera-like severity!

Women who have had a previous combined pill failure. They may claim perfect compliance or perhaps admit to omission of no more than one pill. Either way, since surveys show that most women miss tablets quite frequently but very few conceive, the ability to do so selects out those women who are likely to have low levels of hormones, or ovaries with above average return to activity in the pill-free interval. So all women in this group should, in my view, be advised to take three (or four) packets in a row, the so-called *tricycle regimen*, followed by a shortened pill-free gap. Often 6 days is a good choice in these cases since it is easy to remember, with each tricycle's start day now being identical to the finish-day – but the gap may be shortened further, supplemented by a diary card, in a 'high risk' case.

Fig 6.2 *Advice for missed combined oral contraceptive pills (21-day packaging)*

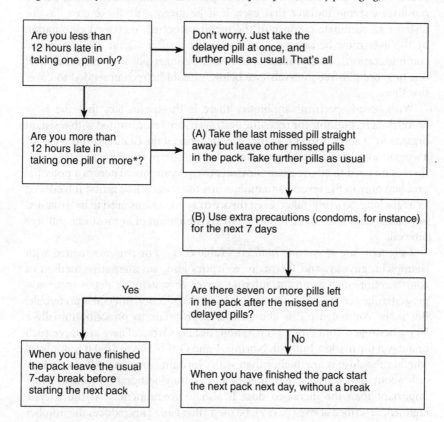

*If two or more pills missed AND if they were all from the first seven in your pack, and if you have had unprotected intercourse since the end of your last pack, talk promptly to your doctor. You may need emergency pills AS WELL AS continuing with instructions A and B above.

Drug interactions

See Back and Orme (1990) or Guillebaud (1994) for more details.

These may reduce the pill's efficacy mainly in two ways. The first and by far the more important is by induction of liver enzymes, which leads to increased elimination of both oestrogen and progestogen. Alternatively, disturbance by certain antibiotics of the gut flora which normally split oestrogen metabolites arriving in the bowel, can reduce in a very small – but unknown – minority of women the reabsorption of reactivated oestrogen. (Note: this effect on the enterohepatic cycle is not a factor in the maintenance of progestogen levels and so is irrelevant to the progestogen-only pill.) See Table 6.11 for the most important drugs and the clinical implications.

Short-term use of any interacting drug/long-term use of broad spectrum antibiotic. Extra contraceptive precautions are advised for the duration of the treatment followed by the '7-day rule' as above, according to when in the pill packet the last potentially less-effective pill was taken. Rifampicin is such a powerful enzyme inducer that even if it be given only for 2 days (as for instance to eliminate carriage of the meningococcus), increased elimination by the liver must be assumed for 4 weeks thereafter (Orme 1991, personal communication). Extra contraception or a stronger pill with elimination of one or more pill-free intervals (see below) should be recommended to cover that time.

With broad spectrum antibiotics there is the useful fact that the large bowel flora responsible for recycling oestrogens are reconstituted with resistant organisms in about 2 weeks. In practice therefore, if the COC is commenced in a woman who has been taking a tetracycline long-term (for acne, for example), there is no need to advise extra contraceptive precautions. There is a potential problem only in the reverse situation, when the tetracycline is first introduced to treat a long-term pill-taker. Even then, extra precautions need to be sustained only for a maximum of three weeks, with elimination of at most one pill-free interval.

Long-term use of enzyme inducers (Table 6.11). For patients treated with rifampicin, anyway, and for many epileptics also, an alternative method of contraception such as an intrauterine device or system, or depot medroxy-progesterone acetate with a shortened (10 week) injection interval is preferable. But if the combined pill is chosen it is appropriate to prescribe initially a 50 μg oestrogen-containing preparation, usually Ovran. There are three such brands on the market, but with Norinyl-1 and Ortho-Novin 1/50 it is doubtful whether the dose is any higher than with Norimin, since there is on average only about 70% conversion of mestranol to ethinyloestradiol. Probably more important than the increased dose is also to recommend that the tricycle regimen, described above (p. 159), be used (Box 6.6). This reduces the number of contraceptively 'risky' pill-free intervals (PFIs). It is particularly appropriate for epileptics since the frequency of attacks is often reduced by the maintenance of steady hormone levels. At the Margaret Pyke Centre we recommend that the PFI is also shortened at the end of each tricycle, usually to 4 days, and so far I am not aware of any breakthrough pregnancies with this regimen, despite numerous referrals who had had one or more such previously through enzyme induction.

If the preferred progestogen is not marketed as a 50 μg pill, an entirely logical if expensive alternative is to use combinations of tablets, e.g. one Mercilon and one Marvelon daily. If so, very careful records are essential (following the full routine described on p. 197) since this is outside the current recommendations of the Data Sheets.

Breakthrough bleeding (BTB) may be the first clue to a drug interaction; and should also be used as an indication to make appropriate alteration to the pill prescription, or to advise a change of method. If the long-term user of an enzyme-inducer develops BTB, after first checking against the 'D' checklist of Box 6.4, the first step is to give two or more tablets a day, if necessary to provide a combined oestrogen content of 80 or 90 μg (maximum), titrated against the BTB.

Table 6.11 *The more important drug interactions with COCs*

Class of drug	Approved names of important examples	Main action	Clinical implications for COC use
Drug which may reduce COC efficacy			
Anticonvulsants	Barbiturates (esp. phenobarbitone) Phenytoin, Primidone, Carbamazepine, Topiramate	Induction of liver enzymes, increasing their ability to metabolize *both* COC steroids	Tricycling preferred, as in text, using 50 µg oestrogen COCs, increasing to max 100 µg if BTB occurs. Sodium valproate, gabapentin, lamotrigine, vigabatrin and all the benzodiazepines are anticonvulsants *without* this effect
Antibiotics			
(a) Antitubercle	Rifampicin	*Marked* induction of liver enzymes	Short term, see text. Long term, use of alternative contraception is preferred. e.g. Depo-Provera with 10 week injection intervals
(b) Antifungal	Griseofulvin	Enzyme inducer	As for anticonvulsants. Beware, griseofulvin is a teratogen. Short courses – wisest to use additional contraception during illness and follow 7-day rule. No problem with
(c) Other antibiotics	Penicillins, especially Ampicillin and relatives	Change in bowel flora, reducing enteroheptic recirculation of ethinyloestradiol (EE), only, after hydrolysis of its conjugates	co-trimoxazole, sulphonamides, or erythromycin Long-term, low-dose tetracycline for acne – no apparent problem, probably because resistant organisms develop, within about 2 weeks. POP is unaffected by this type of interaction
	Tetracyclines		

Table 6.11 *Continued*

Class of drug	Approved names of important examples	Main action	Clinical implications for COC use
Hypnotics	Glutethimide, Dichloral phenazone, Meprobamate	Induction of liver enzymes probable	Avoid these drugs in COC-users (alternatives available)
Tranquillizers			
Drugs which may increase COC efficacy			
	Co-trimoxazole, Sulphonamides	Inhibit EE metabolism in liver	None, if short courses given to low-dose COC user

Note: Recent studies show no significant effect of mega-dose ascorbic acid in raising blood levels of ethinyloestradiol (as previously reported)

In this way the usual policy, giving the minimum dose of both hormones to finish just above the threshold for bleeding, can be followed. The woman can be reassured that she is metaphorically 'climbing a down escalator'. In other words, her increased liver metabolism means that her system is still basically receiving a low-dose regimen. She is exposed to more metabolites, but this is not known to be harmful (and for some women the available alternatives are just not acceptable).

Discontinuing enzyme-inducers. Enzyme induction may take numerous days to reach its peak when the drug is introduced and it may be 4–8 weeks before the liver's level of excretory function reverts to normal when it is withdrawn. Hence if any enzyme inducer has been used for a month or more (or *at all* in the case of rifampicin) it is therefore recommended (Orme 1986, personal communication to NAFPD) that there is a delay of about 4 weeks before the woman returns to a standard low-dose pill regimen. This should be increased to 8 weeks after more prolonged use of rifampicin or barbiturates; and logically there should then be no gap between the higher- and the low-dose packets.

Effects of COCs on other drugs. COC steroids are weak inhibitors of hepatic microsomal enzymes. They thus slightly lower the clearance of, for example, tricyclic antidepressants and diazepam. This theoretically increases the risk of side-effects – seriously in the case of the drug cyclosporin – but otherwise the change is very unlikely to be noticed clinically.

As COCs tend to impair glucose tolerance, sometimes cause depression, and raise the blood pressure, they naturally tend to oppose the action of anti-diabetic, antidepressant, and antihypertensive treatments. See p. 147–8 for the criteria for COC-use during (successful) antihypertensive treatment.

Practitioners who detect possible interactions (of any type) are asked to complete a yellow card for the Committee on Safety of Medicines.

Congenital abnormalities and fertility

There are many conflicting reports in the world literature, not helped by small numbers studied and confounding factors such as smoking, alcohol, and other drugs which have not always been considered. Two per cent of all full-term fetuses have an important malformation. The conclusions of a WHO scientific group (1981) have not been materially challenged subsequently. These were:

(1) no established evidence for any adverse effects on the fetus of oral contraceptives used prior to the conception cycle;

(2) with regard to oral contraceptive use after conception, the evidence for an increased risk of congenital malformations is unclear; but if such a risk exists, it must be very small.

It is always wise to warn women against taking any medication if they believe themselves to be pregnant. If the GP is asked the question 'Should I come off the pill for 2–3 months before getting pregnant?' there is no dogmatic answer. It should certainly do no harm and most metabolic changes studied have indeed returned to normal within that timescale. But there is no objective evidence that it is worth the effort. Certainly any woman finding herself pregnant less than 3 months after stopping the COC should be strongly reassured.

There is no benefit to be achieved by taking short breaks of 6 months or so every few years, as was once recommended. One quarter of young women taking such short breaks had unwanted conceptions in one study. Moreover, a pill-taker can be reminded she has regularly given her body 'breaks' from the COC totalling 13 weeks in each year (see p. 158–9).

The first period after stopping the Pill is often delayed for some weeks. However 'post-Pill amenorrhoea' is not a valid diagnosis and amenorrhoea for 6 months should always be investigated (Chapter 10), whether or not it occurs after stopping this method. With or without amenorrhoea, conception may be delayed by a few months on average on stopping the Pill, but there is no evidence that the Pill causes long-term irreversible infertility.

Duration of use

Though still uncertain it remains possible that increased duration of use may adversely affect the risk of circulatory disease in some current users, though reassuringly it clearly now does not do so in ex-users (Stampfer *et al.* 1989). Recency of use, not duration, was important in the latest analysis of the world data on breast cancer (see p. 135).

Pending more information it remains prudent to restrict total *accumulated* duration of use to a maximum of 15 years in those with definite arterial or venous risk factors. For the remaining healthy, risk factor-free women, if they want to use this method there is no strict upper limit. Some women may therefore choose to continue to age 50 with over 30 years' use – and even then switch to HRT. This is difficult to oppose when so many of the benefits (especially the protection from ovarian cancer) are also clearly enhanced as duration of COC use increases.

Summary

The combined pill provides highly acceptable contraception for many. Individuals vary, however, and some are only suited to one formulation. Presentation of multiple side-effects in spite of the prescription of low doses would indicate the need for a different method, but excessive anxiety about consequences should first be suspected and possible psychosexual aspects discussed. No matter how carefully those with contraindications are excluded, a few women will experience adverse effects. Supervision is essential, monitoring above all blood pressure and headaches, and it is important that the woman feels able to report back at any time; often to the practice nurse.

The first visit for this method is by far and away the most important and should never be rushed; there is a lot of ground to cover (see Box 6.7).

Progestogen-only pill (POP)

There are six varieties available in the UK (Table 6.12).

This is an underused and often abused method which requires maximum motivation by both patient and doctor. Taken absolutely regularly each day

---

Box 6.7 *Take-home messages for a new pill-taker*

1. Your FPA leaflet: this is not to be read and thrown away, it is something to keep safely in a drawer somewhere, for ongoing reference
2. It only works if you take it correctly: if you do, each new pack will always start on the same weekday
3. Even if bleeding like a 'period' occurs (breakthrough bleeding), carry on pill-taking. Ring for advice if necessary
4. Lovemaking during the 7 days after any packet is only safe if you do go on to the next one: otherwise start using condoms after the last pill in the pack
5. Never start your next packet late. This is because the pill-free time is obviously a time when your ovaries are not getting the contraceptive, so might anyway be beginning to escape from its actions. [This simple explanation should always be given – it greatly improves compliance]
6. What to do if any pill(s) are more than 12 hours late [p. 161]
7. Other things that may stop the pill from working, include vomiting and some drugs [p. 160, 163–4]
8. See a doctor at once if ... [p. 158]

And, finally:

9. As a one-off manoeuvre you can shorten one pill-free gap to make sure your withdrawal bleeds avoid weekends

---

within a couple of hours, without breaks, and regardless of bleeding patterns, it can provide protection from pregnancy not far short of the combined pill, especially above age 30 (for comprehensive review, see McCann and Potter 1994). The Oxford/FPA study reported a failure rate of 3.1 per 100 woman-years at age 25–29, but this improved to 1.0 at 35–39 and as low as 0.3 for women over 40 (Vessey *et al.* 1985).

Its efficacy is also enhanced during breast-feeding (but beware the young, highly-fertile woman at the time of weaning, p. 169).

NB. Existing databases suggest but do not prove the possibility that the failure rate is higher in heavier women, as already established for progestogen rings and a research version (not marketed) of Norplant implants. Women who weigh above 70 kg (irrespective of height, BMI is not thought relevant here) should in my view be warned of this possibility. Until the risk is refuted by future studies it remains practice at the Margaret Pyke Centre to offer two POPs daily – but *not* when conception risk is already low (e.g. through breast-feeding or around the climacteric).

Mechanism of action and maintenance of efficacy

Except during full lactation (when the combination regularly inhibits ovulation), there is a complex and variable interaction between the ad-

Table 6.12

				Number of tablets
Noriday	(Searle)	350 µg	norethisterone	28
Micronor	(Janssen-Cilag)	350 µg	norethisterone	28
Femulen	(Searle)	500 µg	ethynodiol diacetate	28
Neogest	(Schering)	75 µg	dl norgestrel	35
Microval	(Wyeth)	30 µg	levonorgestrel	35
Norgeston	(Schering)	30 µg	levonorgestrel	35

(NB. 75 µg dl norgestrel is equivalent to 37.5 µg levonorgestrel)
The choice of POP is largely empirical, though Neogest has been superseded (by the last two in Table)

ministered progestogen and the endogenous activity of the woman's ovary (Guillebaud 1994). Fertile ovulation is prevented in about 60% of cycles. In the remainder there is reliance mainly on progestogenic interference with mucus penetrability, backed by some anti-nidatory activity at the endometrium. Regularity of POP-taking is crucial to success with the method, but any regular time – without regard to the time of intercourse – appears to be satisfactory.

The starting routines are summarized in Table 6.13. Where there is interference with contraceptive activity due to missed pills, vomiting, or drug interaction, this is believed to start within as little as 3 hours. From mucus studies, contraception seems to be adequately restored if renewed pill-taking is combined with extra precautions for just 48 hours. However, in the UK since 1993 condom use or the equivalent has been recommended by the FPA and other bodies for 7 days, partly based on the POP having an anovulatory effect in over half of any population of POP-users; which effect by analogy with the COC might be expected to take a week to be restored. As always with the POP there is a paucity of good data. At the time of writing, this matter is still under active discussion by the FPA and the Faculty, but no change to the 7-days advice in the current leaflets has yet been advised.

Antibiotics do not interfere with the effectiveness of the POP – apart from the enzyme-inducing antibiotics rifampicin and griseofulvin. Another contraceptive method would normally be advised for users of interacting drugs in that category; though a trial of two POPs per day has also been proposed if nothing else is acceptable.

There is no scientific basis on which to decide which POP to choose. The choice depends mainly on the doctor's (and the woman's) preference, plus empirical changing to another product if side-effects develop with the first one tried. Though with all POPs the dose to the infant is believed to be harmless, it appears that the least amount of administered progestogen gets into the breast milk if a levonorgestrel preparation is used.

Table 6.13 *Starting routines with the POP*

	Start when?	Extra precautions?
Menstruating	1st day of period	No
	2nd day or later	7 days
Post-partum		
(a) No lactation[1]	Usually day 21	No
(b) Lactation[1]	Usually 21–42 days after delivery, later if LAM[2] is the initial method	No
Induced abortion/ miscarriage	Same day	No
Post-COC	Instant switch	No
Amenorrhoea	Any time[3] (e.g. post partum)	7 days

[1] *Bleeding irregularities minimized by not starting immediately after delivery*
[2] *LAM the lactational amenorrhoea method (p. 209)*
[3] *Provided the prescriber is confident that there is neither sperm nor blastocyst in the upper genital tract*

Indications

1. Side-effects with, or recognized contraindications to, the combined pill, in particular those believed to be oestrogen-related.
2. Older women – especially smokers above age 35.
3. Diabetes – see p. 143, 145.
4. Obesity – but assessing the advisability in the particular case of giving two tablets daily (see p. 167).
5. Hypertension – either COC-related, *or* other varieties controlled on treatment.
6. Migraine, including varieties with focal symptoms. The woman may continue to suffer the migraines but the fear of an oestrogen-promoted thrombotic stroke is eliminated.
7. Lactation – the combination is anovulatory. During full breast-feeding therefore – but not during or after weaning – the advice for missed pills etc. can be based on that for the COC. At the Margaret Pyke Centre we say 12 hours overdue before 7 days, added condom use is advised – but even this is probably overcautious. For young women very anxious to avoid conception the COC or an injectable should be started when breast-feeding frequency first diminishes or no later than the first bleeding episode.
8. Sickle-cell disease.
9. At the woman's choice.

Contraindications

Absolute contraindications are few (and the last four are not necessarily permanent):

(1) Past or current *severe* arterial disease, or very high risk thereof;

(2) any serious side-effect on the COC not certainly related solely to the oestrogen, e.g. progestogen allergy, liver adenoma;

(3) undiagnosed genital tract bleeding;

(4) actual or possible pregnancy;

(5) recent trophoblastic disease – until HCG is undetectable in blood as well as urine, since there is no certainty it is not the progestogen that increases the likelihood of chemotherapy being required, in some studies. In US practice this would not be seen as a contraindication (see p. 147).

(6) the woman's unrelieved anxiety about the POP method.

To these can be added two 'strong' relative contraindications specific to the POP, namely:

(1) previous ectopic pregnancy, especially in nulliparae;

(2) past *symptomatic* functional ovarian cyst formation.

The first of these is more significant, since the POP sometimes allows ovulation with the risk of implantation in the possibly already-damaged remaining fallopian tube. An anovulant method (e.g. injectable) would be preferable. The frequency of symptomatic cysts is also greater, leading to a problem in differential diagnosis among POP-users with abdominal pain. NB. asymptomatic persistent follicles, which are very commonly picked up on a routine ultrasound scan, do not have this relevance.

The remaining *relative contraindications*, which are weak and the POP may certainly be used with supervision, are:

(1) risk factors for arterial disease, including as above under 'indications'. The presence of more than one risk factor can be permissible, unlike with the COC;

(2) sex steroid-dependent cancer. Seek the agreement of the relevant hospital consultant;

(3) current liver disorder with persistent biochemical change;

(4) enzyme-inducer drugs (see above);

(5) chronic severe systemic diseases (see p. 212). If pregnancy is known to cause deterioration, the POP has the disadvantage of lesser efficacy than the COC. But if hormones were one day shown to aggravate the particular condition the tiny dose in the POP should have less effect.

(6) Past history of thromboembolism. Because it does not significantly affect blood-clotting mechanisms the POP may be used for such women. As confirmation: when norethisterone is taken as Primolut, no less than 45 times the daily dose in Micronor is advised – yet there is no mention in the data sheet of this past history as a contraindication! Good counselling and record-keeping are of course essential, as described on p. 197 for unlicensed indications.

Problems and management

Negligible changes to most metabolic variables have been reported, presumably because of the low dose coupled with the counteracting effect of endogenous oestrogen still produced by the woman's incompletely-suppressed ovaries. This may not be true in POP-users with long-term amenorrhoea, and the concern that this might cause adverse lipid effects or osteoporosis is still debated. If plasma oestradiol tests are available it is reasonable to follow the protocol described later for DMPA (p. 172–3) and also consider FSH measurements (p. 208).

Prolonged spells of amenorrhoea occur most often in older women. Once pregnancy is excluded, the amenorrhoea must be due to anovulation so signifies very high efficacy. Unless there is evidence of hypo-oestrogenism the method can be continued. Diagnosing the menopause in older women poses a difficulty discussed on p. 208.

Apart from the occasional complaint of breast tenderness, which is usually transient but may be recurrent and can sometimes be overcome empirically by changing from one progestogen to another, the main problem presented is that of menstrual irregularity. With advance warning this is usually well-tolerated. It is often helpful to keep a record chart in early months, as this quickly highlights the type of problem and usually demonstrates improvement. Premenstrual symptoms are often relieved. More than half the women will have a cycle between 25 and 35 days.

Even when cycles are short, between 21 and 24 days, complaints are rare provided the bleeding is not too heavy. Two or three days' light bleeding twice a month is another common and acceptable pattern. A few women will experience prolonged and heavy bleeding and if not relieved by changing the brand of pill another method should be selected.

Blood pressure needs to be regularly monitored but where raised during administration of the combined pill, it usually reverts to normal on the POP. Indeed if it does not do so the woman most probably has essential hypertension.

The acceptability of the POP depends largely on the practitioner's attitude and confidence, based on experience.

Injectables

There are two injectable agents available: Depo-Provera (depot medroxy-progesterone acetate or DMPA) 150 mg every 12 weeks, and Noristerat (norethisterone oenanthate) 200 mg every 8 weeks, both given by deep intra-muscular injection within the first 5 days of the menstrual cycle. If given later the FPA leaflets advise 7 days' extra precautions.

In the UK, the only injectable currently licensed by the Committee on Safety Medicines for long-term use is Depo-Provera, and it now has additional approval as a first-line contraceptive. It has been repeatedly endorsed by the expert committees of prestigious bodies, such as the International Planned Parenthood Federation (IPPF) and WHO and finally, in 1992, was fully approved by the US Food and Drug Administration. Its effectiveness is extremely high among reversible methods (0–1 failure per 100 woman-years), primarily because it functions by causing anovulation. DMPA was comprehensively reviewed by Lande (1995).

Anxiety about this method was generated by animal research of very doubtful relevance to humans. The latest WHO data imply that DMPA users have a reduced risk of cancer, with no overall increased risk of cancers of the breast, ovary, or cervix, and a fivefold reduction in the risk of carcinoma of the endometrium (relative risk 0.2). There is still the possibility of a weak co-factor effect on breast cancer similar to that suggested for COCs (see p. 136). However, this is unproven and in the WHO study the association might well have appeared because of surveillance bias in early years of use by the younger women (Lande 1995).

The effects, whether wanted (contraceptive) or unwanted, are not reversible for the duration of the injection and this must always be explained to prospective users, backed by the approved manufacturer's leaflet. It can be stressed that most experts consider DMPA to be a safer drug than COCs, despite the adverse publicity it often receives.

After the last dose conception is commonly delayed (median delay 9 months, which is of course only 6 months since stopping use of the method). A study in Thailand (Pardthaisong 1984) showed that within 24 months of discontinuation (i.e. from the first missed injection) 91% of DMPA users had conceived, compared with 93% of ex-IUD users, and 95% of ex-COC users. These differences were not statistically different, refuting allegations of permanent infertility caused by the drug.

Side-effects

In many users there are side-effects (and in a few cases these are very marked); they include:

- irregular bleeding
- weight gain
- amenorrhoea

Preliminary warning prevents anxiety about these. Menstrual abnormalities remain the greatest obstacle to any large increase in the method's popularity. Excessive bleeding may resolve if the next injection is given early (but not less than 4 weeks since the last dose). Alternatively, giving additional oestrogen may be more successful: either as ethinyloestradiol 20–30 μg (usually within a pill formulation) or, if there is a past history of thrombosis or focal migraine, as natural oestrogen (e.g. Premarin 1.25 mg). Either is given daily for 21 days, after which there is a withdrawal bleed, and such courses may be repeated if an acceptable bleeding pattern does not follow. Post-partum bleeding is minimized if the first dose is delayed for 3–6 weeks, but much earlier use is permissible.

Amenorrhoea is usually very acceptable with counselling and occurs in about one-half of long-term users. As with the POP there is concern that prolonged amenorrhoea might lead to hypo-oestrogenism. Pending more data, therefore, I now recommend that after 3 years of complete amenorrhoea (or earlier as indicated by relevant symptoms like loss of libido, hot flushes, or dry vagina) it is reasonable to *discuss* with the individual DMPA-user the option of checking her blood oestradial level prior to the next injection. The result is often perfectly acceptable, above 150 pmol/l. If it is lower it should be repeated. Repeated low levels, especially if below 100 pmol/l, usually indicate a change of method; or the alternative of cyclical 'add-back' natural oestrogen HRT by any chosen route. Adding oestrogen in this way is not licensed and still controversial, so the 'named patient' routine described on p. 197 must be followed.

Contraindications

The absolute contraindications are those listed earlier for the POP. The relative contraindications are very similar, except that there needs to be more caution because the dose is larger; some studies show a reduction in HDL-cholesterol levels and there is a built-in lack of immediate reversibility.

The frequency of ectopics and ovarian cysts is reduced, unlike with the POP.

If enzyme inducers are being taken long term, the injection interval is usually shortened to every 10 weeks, this being a better manipulation than increasing the dose.

Indications

The main indication for an injectable is the woman's desire for a highly-effective method which is independent of intercourse, when other options are contraindicated or disliked. Injectables may be used despite past thrombosis (see earlier comments for the POP), and are ideal in lactation since they have no unwanted effects on breast-milk flow and in contrast to the POP efficacy is not detectably altered by weaning. The method is appropriate for women who require effectiveness while waiting for major or leg surgery (p. 158). Injectable agents are positively beneficial in endometriosis, in sickle-cell anaemia, and in women at risk of pelvic inflammatory disease and are welcomed by many forgetful pill-takers.

Monitoring and management

Blood pressure is normally checked before each dose although most studies fail to show any hypertensive effect. Since (it has to be admitted) most users have a battle to avoid weight gain, the user herself usually asks to be weighed.

Overdue injections – i.e. patient presents beyond 12 weeks with DMPA. For this common problem the Margaret Pyke Centre follows the following protocol. Since the failure rate is so low up to 13 weeks (91 days) we will give the due dose, advising added precautions for 7 days. Beyond that, the chances of a blastocyst being in the genital tract increase. Assuming intercourse has been continuing, if the next dose is late by a further 3 days (94 days) the usual PC4 post-coital contraceptive can be given plus an immediate DMPA injection. Up to 96 days, if the earliest ovulation is assumed to be at 13 weeks a copper IUD can be inserted in good faith, plus an immediate injection – unless the woman chooses to switch to the IUD as her future method. In all these cases added precautions for a further 7 days are advisable, plus 100% follow-up with exclusion of pregnancy about 3 weeks later. Counselling must include discussion of the (very low) potential of harm to any fetus and be fully recorded.

Contraceptive implants

Norplant

This consists of six polydimethylsiloxane implants, each the size of a match-stick, implanted subdermally via a dedicated 11-gauge trocar under local anaesthesia (Newton 1996 – a useful review of all implants). Trained clinicians can insert them in around 10 minutes, and remove them upon request in about twice that time – though this can be technically much more difficult in cases where the original implants were inserted too deeply. After the first few weeks, the implants release about 40–50 μg levonorgestrel (LNG) per day, dropping to 30–35 μg per day after the first year through to 5 years of use.

The recommended site for insertion is the flexor surface of the upper arm, since implants at other sites tend to migrate under the skin, posing problems for removal.

Advantages of Norplant. The method combines most of the best attributes of the POP and of injectables. In comparison with DMPA it has the same or better efficacy, but a smaller biological effect, more comparable to the POP:

(1) absence of daily pill-taking routine, hence freedom from 'fear of forget-ting'. This leads to high acceptability and excellent continuation rates. The failure rate of the polymer 372 *marketed* version is about 0.2/100 woman-years and appears to be almost unaffected by increasing body weight;

(2) long action with one treatment (5 years: efficacy greatest in the first 3 years as the method relies more on the cervical mucus effect thereafter);

(3) absence of the initial peak dose to the liver when pills given orally;

(4) blood levels are steady rather than fluctuating (as the POP) or initially too high (as injectables). This reduces metabolic and most clinical side-effects;

(5) no changes have been seen in blood pressure and metabolic changes are small, similar to those in users of LNG-containing POPs;

(6) the implants are removable, reversing the method. The half-life of the LNG after implants are removed is about 2 days. In one study conception occurred within 1 year in 86% of women.

Main adverse effects and problems. Ovulation occurs in only 10% of cycles in the first year, but more frequently once the release rate declines to 30 ug/day. Similar problems result as with the POP:

(1) irregular and prolonged bleeding – the chief cause of requests for removal (involving 10% of women at 1 year);

(2) functional ovarian cysts are reported, but these are as usual mostly asymptomatic or can be managed conservatively. The Population Council estimates the need for surgical intervention at 0.03/100 woman-years of use;

(3) the ectopic pregnancy rate is very low, about 0.08/100 woman-years. Since ovulation is blocked more often, pregnancies are probably even less likely to be ectopic than with the POP;

174

(4) minor side-effects such as acne, nausea, headaches, and either hair loss or hair growth are also described, but these are usually transient.

Specific problems:

(5) there is inevitably some discomfort at insertion and removal;

(6) infection of the site, migration of an implant, and difficult removal. Though removal of well-inserted implants is simple, a few cases posing great difficulty due to being inserted far too deeply have received much adverse publicity.

Contraindications. These are few and similar to those for the POP.

Insertion/removal of Norplant. This requires special training, organised through the Faculty of Family Planning.

Indications. It shares most of these with DMPA and may be used during lactation and when there has been a past thrombosis.

Management. The main practical problem (apart from its price of about £170 per set) is frequent bleeding and spotting. Treating this is difficult: a course of the combined pill may be tried as with DMPA, in preference to 'add-back' natural oestrogen; owing to the theoretical risk of losing the progestogenic cervical mucus block to sperm.

Norplant itself is now rarely requested: we await *Norplant 2* which is similar but with only two capsules; a practical advantage. *Implanon* releases 3-ketodesogestrel over 3 years from a single implant injected very simply through a wide-bore needle. Both of these are expected on the market before 2000.

Post-coital contraception or emergency contraception

The use of large doses of oestrogen is outmoded as it was associated with severe nausea and vomiting. Aside from mifepristone, not yet available for this indication, three methods have now been shown to be effective: the combined hormone pill, insertion of an IUD, and recently, a *levonorgestrel-only (LNG-only) method* is showing particular promise (see Table 6.14).

Levonorgestrel-only method

This requires a 0.75 mg dose of LNG stat, repeated in 12 hours. One of its main advantages is minimal nausea, and there are virtually no contraindications to it aside from existing pregnancy. Unfortunately, the 0.75 mg dose, available in a single tablet in some countries, can only be given currently in the UK as 25 tablets of Microval/Norgeston or 20 tablets of Neogest! This means that for the present a potentially very useful new development may be reserved chiefly for women with contraindications to the combined hormone method.

Note that the Hong Kong study of this method (Ho and Kwan 1993) which showed no efficacy difference compared with the standard combined hormone method was based on use within no more than 48 hours of exposure. LNG is

Table 6.14 *Choice of methods for postcoital contraception*

	Combined hormone method	Levonorgestrel method	Copper IUD
	PC4 or Ovran two pills stat, two pills 12 hours later	Levonorgestrel 0.75 mg stat, 0.75 mg 12 hours later	Nova T, Cu T 380 Slimline or Multiload
Timing after intercourse	Up to 72 hours	Up to 48 hours	Up to 5 days after calculated date of ovulation
Efficacy	98%	97.6% in one study	Almost 100%
Side-effects	Nausea and vomiting		Pain, bleeding, risk of infection
Contraindications	Pregnancy, *Current* focal migraine, jaundice, known active porphyria, sickle-cell crisis, or serious past thrombosis (see text)	Pregnancy	Pregnancy and as for IUDs generally

also not yet licensed for this indication, though it may be prescribed by any doctor whose opinion is that it is in the best interests of his/her patient (see 'named patient prescribing' p. 197).

Combined hormone method

A 50 µg oestrogen-combined pill containing 250 µg levonorgestrel, taken as two pills stat and repeated after 12 hours, prevents implantation in about 98% of cases overall, or 95–96% at midcycle. This equates to stopping 75% of the conceptions which would otherwise occur. Though the therapy is licensed for up to 72 hours after the *earliest* act of unprotected intercourse, it may also be used later, like the IUD, though with diminishing chance of success – and see p. 197.

Incidentally, the lay term 'morning-after pill' causes pregnancies and should be abandoned. We prefer 'the emergency pill'.

Contraindications

Absolute contraindications to the combined hormone method are very few and rarely applicable: current focal migraine attack, current jaundice or sickle-cell crisis, current established arterial disease, and active porphyria. Although significant prothrombotic changes from this treatment were not shown in one small study, they did not recruit women predisposed to thrombosis: hence in our practice a past history of arterial or venous thromboembolism indicates use of the levonorgestrel – only method or an IUD (Table 6.14). If sufficient risk of conception is deemed to be present, there is no upper age limit to any of the methods and it can be used during breast-feeding with the option for 24 hours of discarding the (expressed) breast-milk.

If the woman is taking an enzyme-inducer drug, the doses with either of the hormonal methods should be increased by 50% (Kubba 1995). But the effect of antibiotics other than rifampicin/griseofulvin is too small to require any change of dose.

Copper intrauterine device (IUD) method

Insertion of a copper IUD *in good faith* before implantation, which is taken to be up to 5 days after the calculated ovulation day, is extremely effective and prevents implantation in almost 100% of women, even in cases of multiple exposure. The judge's summing up in a 1991 Court Case (Regina vs Dhingra) gives legal support to this policy: 'I further hold . . . that a pregnancy cannot come into existence until the fertilized ovum has become implanted in the womb, and that that stage is not reached until at the earliest, the 20th day of a normal 28 day cycle . . .'

NB. The LNG-IUS acts by mechanisms which appear to be slower than the effects of copper on sperm and blastocyst and it is not recommended for this indication.

Contraindications

There are recognized contraindications (see p. 191) and risks of pain, bleeding, or infection, as with any IUD, and this option is rarely advisable for the nulliparous woman. However, in selected cases with cervical swabs (for *chlamydia*, at least), antibiotic cover, and contact tracing if the bacteriology reports prove to be positive, it may be appropriate. The device may always be removed following the next period, especially if there is the past history of an ectopic pregnancy. (Withholding the IUD will not lower the risk of a tubal ectopic in the current cycle – see below – but an anovulant method would be better long term.)

Indications

Indications for the IUD method are as follows:

(1) when maximum efficacy is the woman's priority;

(2) when exposure occurred more than 72 hours earlier, or, in cases of multiple exposure, insertion may be up to 5 days after ovulation (see p. 176);

(3) in many parous women it can be ideal to solve the immediate problem and for the device to be retained as their long-term method (but it may be right in young women to remove it after they are established on a new method such as DMPA or the COC);

(4) presence of absolute contraindications to oestrogen (which are very few with so short a course, and the LNG-only oral method could be offered instead);

(5) after vomiting of either dose before full absorption anticipated (see below) in a case with particularly high pregnancy risk.

Counselling – ideally delegated to a nursing colleague

1. Careful assessment of menstrual/coital history and hence of the appropriateness of treatment is required.

2. The mode of action sometimes (not always) being post-fertilization may pose an absolute contraindication to some individuals. But most modern ethicists (and this author) believe that blocking of implantation is contraception, not abortion.

3. Medical risks should be discussed, especially:

   (a) the failure rate (2–3% for both hormone methods or up to 5% with midcycle exposure – but close to nil for the IUD method);

   (b) teratogenicity (believed to be negligible – although there is no proof – since before implantation the hormones will not reach the blastocyst in sufficient concentration to cause any adverse effect). Follow-up of women who have kept their pregnancies has so far not shown any increased risk of major abnormalities above the background 2% rate;

   (c) tubal ectopic pregnancy. If the latter occurs it is due to a pre-existing damaged tube and the blastocyst would almost certainly have settled there anyway, with or without this pre-implantation intervention. Indeed, earlier in the cycle both types of method may, if anything, reduce the risk of an ectopic, the hormonal options by interfering with ovulation, and the copper of the IUDs by its toxicity to sperm. However, a past history of ectopic pregnancy or pelvic infection remains a reason for caution and forewarning with any of the methods.

4. If the combined hormone method is used, advice should be given regarding nausea and vomiting (the latter has an incidence of 20%, usually once).

   (a) If an antiemetic is requested, a phenothiazine is commonly chosen. At the Margaret Pyke Centre we rarely give preventive treatment, since phenothiazines and related drugs may all cause acute dystonic reactions ('oculogyric crises'). Metoclopramide is particularly prone to cause these, specifically in teenage girls, whereas domperidone (Motilium) at the recommended dose of 10 mg with each dose of emergency contraception has the lowest risk. Being free of that problem hyoscine 300 mg (e.g. Kwells) has also been suggested: but it causes drowsiness, is not licensed for this indication, and there have been no good comparative trials.

   (b) If either dose is vomited within 2 hours, the woman may be given two more tablets definitely with an antiemetic, or vaginally (good data on this route are available for oral contraception but none as a post-coital method, so see p. 197). In a particularly high-risk case, an IUD might be inserted.

5. Contraception both in the current cycle (in case the hormonal method merely postpones ovulation) and long term should be discussed. The IUD option covers both aspects. If the COC is chosen it should be started as soon as the woman is convinced her next period is normal, usually on the first or second day, without the need for additional contraception thereafter (see Table 6.10, p. 155).

The above makes clear the importance of a good rapport in order to obtain an accurate coital and menstrual history and to promote effective arrangements for follow-up.

What about the vaginal examination?

This is not routinely necessary and there are very good reasons to omit it in an anxious teenager. It should be done only in the individual case if indicated on clinical grounds. At the first visit these might be to exclude overt infection or concealed clinical pregnancy and to establish a baseline size and shape for the uterus. At follow-up, examination is mainly indicated if there is clinical uncertainty because the next period is delayed, or in the presence of any pain.

Follow-up

A routine appointment is not necessary, but the woman should be advised to return if she has abdominal pain or if her next period is overdue, or if further discussion about contraception is indicated.

How often may the PC4 method be used?

The total dose is unimpressive, only the same as 4 days of normal pill-taking with a standard pill of the early seventies, or 7 days of Microgynon. So we have occasionally given it as often as three times in the same cycle, in the case of a couple with a major condom rupture problem! A woman who relied on it every month could do a lot better, contraceptively, but would be risking pregnancy (a cumulative failure rate of up to 24 per 100 woman-years) more than directly risking her health.

Special indications

Special indications apply to coital exposure when there has been:

(1) omission of two or more COC tablets after the pill-free interval (PFI, see above), or of any combination of pills from the first seven in the packet which in the prescriber's judgement amounts to the same thing as lengthening the PFI to 9 or more days. After the emergency regimen the woman may return immediately to the COC, and subject to a 100% undertaking to return for follow-up 4 weeks later – and to use added precautions for the next 7 days. As explained on pp. 159–60, midpacket pill omissions after 7 tablets have been taken never indicate emergency treatment unless at least 4 have been missed. Towards the end of a packet, omission of the next pill-free interval will suffice;

(2) delay in taking a POP for more than 3 hours, implying loss of the mucus effect, followed by exposure during the 48 hours before that would be expected to be restored. Again the POP is restarted immediately after the emergency regimen, 7-days added precautions are advised, and follow-up agreed. The above would be an over-reaction if the POP-user is fully breast-feeding and amenorrhoeic, particularly during the first 6 months post-partum (see LAM, p. 209);

(3) removal or expulsion of an IUD prior to the time of implantation, if another IUD cannot be inserted for some reason.

Research continues and alternatives may supersede the current methods in due course.

Intrauterine contraception

Copper-bearing intrauterine devices (IUDs)

These have many established advantages, listed in Box 6.8. Women who are happily suited by this method love it, the rest hate it and sadly their views are more vigorously expressed. Women in their thirties have not been requesting them because they were told in their twenties to avoid that method. Yet for a parity 2+ 30-year-old, the devices have not changed but she has; especially if she is not yet sure that her family is complete, she is the ideal user. Currently some doctors are complying too readily with requests for male or female sterilization which originate partly out of myths about this alternative. Too few women know that the latest copper (IUDs) are, in practice, more, not less, effective that the COC (WHO 1987). And then there is the IUS with its added value in medical gynaecology: but more about that later.

It cannot be overemphasized that *the effectiveness and acceptability of this method depends primarily on the skill of the practitioner who inserts it.* This cannot be learnt from books: see p. 193 re the Faculty of Family Planning's 'apprenticeship' training scheme. Considerable and maintained experience is an absolute essential for good technique. Among other sequelae, inadequately inserted devices are prone to be expelled or malpositioned (a cause of failure, or of 'lost threads'). Perforation of the uterus may occur, especially when it is soft (post-partum or post-abortion), during lactation, or if its acutely anteverted or retroverted position is not identified and allowed for with use of atraumatic holding forceps during insertion (see Table 6.15, column H).

Effectiveness

The first-choice copper IUD for a parous woman in this country is the Copper T 380 Slimline. It is more than twice as effective as the Nova T, and unlike that largely outdated option it retains or even seemingly improves its efficacy with the passage or time – and for up to at least 10 years (see p. 190).

Box 6.8 *Advantages of Copper IUDs*

(1) Safe: Mortality 1:500 000
(2) Effective: Highly (p. 190)
                   Immediately
                   Post-coitally
                   At pregnancy termination
(3) No link with coitus
(4) No tablets to remember
(5) Continuation rates high
(6) Reversible – even when removed for one of the recognized complications

---

The Multiload Cu 375 is preferable to the Multiload 250 but has no established advantages over the CuT 380 S.

Mechanism of action

In studies, fertilized ova are almost never retrievable from the genital tract of copper IUD-users, hence they must operate mainly by preventing fertilization. Their effectiveness when put in post-coitally indicates they can also act to block implantation. However, this seems to be primarily a backup mechanism when devices are *in situ* long term.

Nevertheless, in any given cycle it might be working by blocking implantation, so there is a small risk of 'iatrogenic' conception if a device is removed after mid-cycle. Ideally, therefore, women should use another method additionally from 7 days before planned device removal or this should be postponed until the next menses. If a device must be removed earlier (e.g. when treating infection) then hormonal post-coital contraception may be indicated.

Influence of age

Copper IUDs, like all contraceptive methods, are more effective in the older woman because of declining fertility. Above age 30 there is also a reduction in rates of expulsion and of pelvic inflammatory disease (PID). The latter is not believed to be because the older uterus resists infection but because the person bearing an older uterus is in general less exposed to risk of infection (through her own lifestyle or that of her only partner).

In situ conception

If the woman wishes to go on to full term, the device should be removed. This is counter-intuitive: one would think this would increase the miscarriage risk. In fact, the data for all devices studied show that the miscarriage rate is at least halved by removal of the device in the first trimester. The woman should, of course, be warned that it is impossible to remove completely the IUD-associated miscarriage risk. Obviously the device should be left for removal in

---

Box 6.9 *Adverse effects of copper IUDs*

(1) Intrauterine pregnancy, hence miscarriage risks
(2) Extrauterine pregnancy
(3) Expulsion – risks of pregnancy
(4) Perforation – risks of pregnancy
(5) Malposition – risks of bowel/bladder adhesions
(6) Infection
(7) Pain
(8) Bleeding – increased amount
        – increased duration

Note: All the first five problems listed have the risk of impairing future fertility

---

theatre if the woman is going to have a termination of pregnancy. If the threads are already missing when she is seen and other causes are excluded (see below), then the pregnancy must be flagged as one of increased risk for second trimester abortion (which could be infected) and also antepartum haemorrhage and premature labour.

If the woman goes on to full term it is essential to identify the device in the products of conception, and if it is not found to arrange a post-partum X-ray, in case the device is embedded or has perforated (see Table 6.16). There have been medico-legal cases when this was not done; leading either to symptoms from an undiagnosed perforation or to unnecessary tests and treatments for 'infertility' when only one device was later removed for a wanted pregnancy but a much earlier embedded device remained.

There is no evidence of associated teratogenicity with conception during or immediately after use of copper devices, or indeed of cancer developing in the uterus of long-term users.

Adverse effects of copper IUDs

These are listed briefly in Box 6.9. The first five problems in the Box share a single risk, namely of impairing future fertility. Moreover, they must be excluded as diagnoses before pain and bleeding are ascribed to the method as 'side-effects'. Table 6.15 expands on this summary, which is actually a remarkably short list as compared with the COC. It also draws attention to the important interrelationships of the problems. Selection and adequate instruction of potential users is emphasized by columns E–G of the Table; and the paramount importance of correct insertion is re-emphasized by column H.

IUDs with 'lost threads'

The threads are often in fact present, perhaps short or drawn up into the canal. Women should be taught how to check the strings, and if not felt, there are several other possible explanations. Looking at Table 6.15, this symptom of 'lost threads' links together numbers 1, 3, 4, and 5 in the list. As Table 6.16 shows there are at least six causes of this condition, three with and three without

Table 6.15 *Problems and complications of IUDs – a summary*

Main hazards	A. Directly or indirectly threatens fertility?	B. Linked with symptomatic pain?	C. Linked with symptomatic bleeding?	D. May present as 'lost threads'?	E. Special problem in the young nullipara?	F. Frequency with increasing age	G. Frequency with increasing duration of use	H. Can be caused by poor insertion technique?
1. Intrauterine pregnancy (device *in situ*) Miscarriage Infection, see 6	Yes	Yes	Yes	Yes	Yes	→	→	Yes, as result of 5
2. Extrauterine pregnancy Significant mortality Loss of tubal function	Yes	Yes	Yes	No	Yes	↑ (Little effect)	↑	Yes[1]
3. Expulsion Pregnancy then as 1, 6	Yes	Yes	Yes	Yes	Yes	→	→	Yes
4. Perforation Pregnancy Adhesion formation Risks of IUD removal	Yes	Yes	No	Yes	No	=	—	Yes
5. Malposition Predisposes to 1,3,7,8. A cause of 'lost threads'	Yes	Yes	Yes	Yes	Yes	=	—	Yes

Table 6.15 *Continued*

	Main hazards	A Directly or indirectly threatens fertility?	B Linked with symptomatic pain?	C Linked with symptomatic bleeding?	D May present as 'lost threads'?	E Special problem in the young nullipara?	F Frequency with increasing age	G Frequency with increasing duration of use	H Can be caused by poor insertion technique?
6. Pelvic infection	Loss of tubal function	Yes	Yes	Sometimes	No	Yes	↓	↓	Yes[1] (See text re STDs as main cause)
7. Pain	Real underlying cause may be overlooked, see column B	–	–	Often	No	Yes	=	↓	Yes as result of 5
8. Uterine bleeding	Underlying cause may be overlooked, see column C; also uterine cancer	–	Often	–	No	No	←	↓	Yes, as result of 5

[1] If insertion introduces or exacerbates (pre-existing and undiagnosed) pelvic infection, leading to tubal damage

Table 6.16 *Differential diagnosis of 'lost threads' with IUDs*

Main diagnoses A. Not pregnant	Clinical clues	B. Pregnant	Clinical clues
1. **Device in uterus** Threads cut too short, or caught up around device during original insertion or avulsed at a previous removal attempt; or device itself malpositioned	(a) Periods likely to be those characteristic of IUD *in situ* (b) Uterus normal size	4. **Device *in situ* + pregnancy**	(a) Amenorrhoea (b) Pregnancy test likely to be positive, with clinically enlarged uterus (sufficient to pull up thread)
2. **Unrecognized expulsion**	(a) Recent periods as woman's normal pattern (b) Uterus normal size	5. **Unrecognized expulsion + pregnancy**	(a) Amenorrhoea, following one or more apparently normal periods (i.e. unmodified by IUD) (b) Signs of pregnancy variably present (may be too early on first presentation)
3. **Perforation of uterus**	As 2 plus (rarely) mass or actual IUD palpated on bimanual examination	6. **Perforation of uterus + pregnancy**	As 5 plus (rarely) mass or actual IUD identified on bimanual examination

pregnancy. An intra-abdominal IUD is as useless at stopping pregnancy as one that has been totally expelled. More often there is an *in situ* pregnancy (the threads having been drawn up) or the device is rotated/malpositioned. So the slogan is: '**The woman with "lost threads" is either already pregnant or at risk of becoming pregnant**'. All such women therefore need to be advised to use an alternative contraceptive method until the protective presence of an IUD has been established.

Lost strings: expulsion and perforation

Expulsions most commonly occur during bleeding, soon after insertion, and less than one-third are beyond the first year. Even with accurate insertion some women seem prone to expulsion, especially at reinsertion with immediately preceding removal. See p. 193 below for a useful test for partial expulsion at follow-up.

For lost threads I recommend the following very practical scheme. Diagnosis and treatment are simultaneous in most cases, with minimum use of hospital facilities:

1. *Exclude implanted pregnancy.* Take a careful menstrual history, do a bimanual examination, and as indicated perform the most sensitive pregnancy test available. If the woman is pregnant, the management is primarily that of the pregnancy itself. In the absence of pregnancy, it is entirely appropriate (even in a GP's surgery) to proceed as follows:

2. *Insert long-handled Spencer-Wells forceps or equivalent into the endocervical canal* – if the jaws are gently opened and shut the missing threads can be retrieved in about half of all intrauterine-located devices. If the IUD is judged still to be correctly located, no further action need be taken. But since disappearance of the threads may be a sign of malposition it is usually advisable to remove and replace the device. If the threads are not found, the woman should be asked whether she would prefer thread retrieval (which also should quickly establish if there actually is a device *in utero*) as below or imaging first, as at step 5 below. Early recourse to imaging partly depends on her pain threshold, but is also much kinder than chasing a device which has actually been expelled or perforated.

3. *Try the use of thread-retrievers.* In the UK the most established are the Emmett Retriever and the Retrievette, which are available presterilized and disposable, and with full instructions. Appropriate analgesia is important: as a routine mefenamic acid 500 mg should be given 20 minutes earlier, but added local anaesthesia (LA) should also be offered (see below). Most GPs will prefer to arrange hospital referral if this step fails, but if convinced after imaging by ultrasound that the device is located in the uterus some may feel confident enough to continue – now definitely with use of LA.

4. *Next try small, blunt IUD-removal hooks* (Grafenberg pattern) or various resterilizable forceps, with short jaws (crocodile-type) or claws (e.g. the IUD removing forceps supplied by Rocket), opening wholly in the uterine cavity. In skilled hands these metal devices will nearly always retrieve the device.

5. *Arrange appropriate imaging if not done earlier, and referral thereafter as appropriate.* An ultrasound (u/s) scan may confirm correct intrauterine location within a non-pregnant uterus. This can enable the woman to continue using the same device, with periodic re-scanning; but if there is any suspicion that it is malpositioned, appropriate steps should be taken for its removal as at 4 above – preferably under local, rarely under general, anaesthesia. If the u/s scan shows unequivocally that the uterus is empty, and non-pregnant, an X-ray is then required to differentiate between expulsion and perforation. A uterine marker (such as another IUD inserted before the X-ray) may often be useful. In a Margaret Pyke Centre study only 2.5% of 350 *in situ* intrauterine devices with missing threads required general anaesthesia for the removal – this should be the norm.

Perforation. The incidence is about one in 1000 insertions. They are often post-partum and always insertion-related: to quote Jack Lippes, 'Devices do not perforate; for this to occur we need a practitioner'. If perforation has occurred, removal should be arranged and this can usually be effected by laparoscopy. Copper-carrying devices provoke considerable adhesions so proceeding to laparotomy is not unusual.

Infection

This is the great fear we all have about intrauterine devices. Yet it appears that infections have been blamed on the devices when they have really been acquired sexually. Much of the anxiety derived from the Dalkon Shield disaster – but this was a unique device with a polyfilament thread, increasing the risk of transfer of potential pathogens from the lower to the upper genital tract. Modern copper devices have a monofilament thread. They provide no protection against PID and the infections that occur may perhaps be more severe through the foreign body effect; but they do not themselves cause infection.

The WHO study by Farley *et al.* (1992) reinforces the above view. There were more than 23 000 insertions, worldwide. In every country the same pattern emerged. There was an IUD-associated increased risk of infection for 20 days after the insertion. Significantly, the weekly infection rate 3 weeks after insertion went back to the same weekly rate as before insertion, i.e. the norm for that particular society. In China there were no infections diagnosed at all despite 4301 insertions.

These findings are interpreted as follows: the post-insertion infection bulge cannot be because of bad insertion technique, restricted to the doctors outside China. Much more probably, although the doctors in all the centres were searching for bilaterally monogamous women, they were only truly successful in this search in China (in the 1980s: success would be less probable now). In the other countries PID-causing organisms (especially *Chlamydia trachomatis*) can be presumed to have been present in a proportion of the women. The process of insertion interfered with protective mechanisms and enabled the infection to spread from the lower genital tract where it had previously resided into the upper genital tract including the fallopian tubes. The conclusions therefore are:

(1) the greatest risk is in the first 20 days, most probably caused by pre-existing carriage of sexually transmitted diseases (STDs);

(2) risk thereafter, like pre-insertion, relates to the background risk of STDs (high in Africa, but virtually absent in the mainland China study population).

In practical terms this implies that for best practice:

1. Except where the prevalence of *Chlamydia* is too low to justify it, all prospective IUD-users should be screened at least for *Chlamydia* prior to all IUD insertions or re-insertions.

2. Evidence of a purulent discharge from the cervix indicates more detailed investigation, ideally at a genitourinary medicine clinic.

3. If *Chlamydia* is detected it should be treated vigorously (e.g. doxycycline 100 mg twice daily for 7-14 days, according to severity of infection), contact tracing arranged, and IUD insertion postponed. If the IUD has already been inserted (emergency cases) treat when the report is received and consider device removal, especially in nulliparae.

4. The cervix should be very thoroughly physically cleansed before the device is inserted, following the manufacturer's instructions, with minimum trauma.

5. Arrange a first post-insertion visit after 7 days in addition to the routine 6-week follow-up visit. This is designed to pick up any women with post-insertion infection (during the 20-day 'surge' of such infections described by Farley) and in my view is essential if there has not been preliminary screening for cervical infection.

An acceptable alternative *provided* pre-insertion screening is routinely performed is to explain to the woman that she must telephone the practice nurse about a week post-insertion if she has any of the relevant symptoms.

As an alternative to screening, questioning about recency of partner change is of relevance but never sufficient: in a Margaret Pyke Centre study during the mid-1980s the background rate of *Chlamydia* carriage was 2.4% in the general clinic population, but *higher*, 8.2%, in the pre-IUD group who had first been sensitively questioned about their likely exposure! Given the prevalence of *Chlamydia* infection in many cities of the UK today, I consider it suboptimal to fit copper devices without microbiological screening: the money for pre-insertion *Chlamydia* testing must just be found.

Blind prescription of broad spectrum antibiotics to cover all insertions is also very second-best, not only because it precludes contact tracing. In those cases who might be benefitting, re-infection (possibly worsened by the foreign body effect) will simply occur later – from the partner who must also harbour the organism.

Management of a clinical attack of pelvic infection, whether IUD insertion-related or later – and later means, according to Farley, that the case must be 'coincidental' to the IUD (i.e. occurring at the same incidence as the background rate for that society) – will depend on the circumstances of the individual case. In parous women it may be possible to retain the device. It is, however, usual to remove the device, ideally after first establishing the antibiotic therapy. Reinsertion should be delayed until at least 6 months, or indefinitely in most nulliparae.

Severe cases or those where there is a diagnostic problem (especially in excluding ectopic pregnancy or pelvic appendicitis) should be referred for probable laparoscopy. *Chlamydia* is the main primary causative organism, with secondary infection often by anaerobes frequently superimposed. A broad spectrum antibiotic, preferably a tetracycline, is therefore best given together with metronidazole while laboratory reports of full genitourinary medicine screening tests are awaited.

Two 'sins of omission' are still too often committed by hospital gynae staff and the GP needs to check. Has the woman been counselled about the high risk of tubal occlusion should her lifestyle or lack of routine condom use in future lead to recurrences? Westrom (1987) showed this risk would exceed 50% with just two more hospitalized attacks. Has anything been done about contact tracing?

Actinomyces-like organisms (ALOs). These are not infrequently reported in cervical smears, more commonly with increasing duration of use. If there are relevant symptoms (excessive discharge, pain, dyspareunia) or signs (cervical tenderness, purulent discharge, adnexal swelling) then the device should be removed and sent for culture, with a low threshold for gynae referral and antibiotic treatment. This will have to be for many months with penicillin if pelvic actinomycosis is actually confirmed – potentially a life-endangering condition.

More usually, the finding occurs in asymptomatic women. It is acceptable for the asymptomatic woman simply to be fully advised with an explanatory leaflet and monitored, especially if she is using an expensive IUS (see below). If at any time in future she has or develops pelvic pain, dyspareunia, or excessive discharge, and if tenderness is noted on examination, the knowledge that ALOs are present should markedly lower the threshold for IUD removal and other interventions as appropriate.

But more usually in our practice all that is required is IUD removal, with or without immediate reinsertion. Mao and Guillebaud (1984) reported the follow-up findings in three groups of women: one group was simply monitored (and the ALO finding commonly persisted), and two groups in whom the device was removed – with or without immediate reinsertion of another copper IUD. *In both these second two groups follow-up smears were ALO free.* As a result, after explaining the options to the woman, simple removal and reinsertion, without antibiotic treatment but with repeat of a cervical smear after 3–6 months, is now the usual recommended practice.

Ectopic pregnancy

Is this problem caused by copper IUDs? This also appears to be a myth. The main cause is previous tubal infection with one or both tubes being damaged. The non-causative association with IUDs comes about because IUDs are rather more effective at preventing pregnancy in the uterus than in the tube. Therefore the ratio of extra- to intra-uterine pregnancies is higher than expected among the pregnancies. Ectopics are actually reduced in number because very few sperm get through the copper-containing uterine fluids to reach an egg, hence very few implantations can occur in a damaged tube. However, there are even fewer implantations in the uterus. Thus the denominator in the ratio is even lower than the numerator, hence allowing the *ratio* of ectopics to intrauterine pregnancies to increase while in fact both are reduced in frequency. The risk of an ectopic in users of the the Cu T 380 and its clones is now estimated as 0.02/100 woman-years, which is at least 60 times lower than the estimated rate for sexually-active Swedish women seeking pregnancy (1.2–1.6/100 woman-years).

Clinically, caution is still necessary and **any IUD user with pain and a late period or irregular bleeding has an ectopic until proved otherwise**. A past history *relatively* contraindicates the method (see below), very strongly in nulliparae.

Pain and bleeding

Pain may be an acceptable side-effect of the method; but the safe slogan is 'pain +/− bleeding has a serious cause until proved otherwise'. See Columns B and C of Table 6.15. As well as excluding conditions like infection and an ectopic or miscarrying pregnancy, malposition of the device can cause pain as the uterus tries to squeeze the device out.

Copper devices do increase the duration of bleeding by a mean of 1–2 days, and they also increase the measured volume of bleeding by about one-third. In a population of copper IUD-users haemoglobins tend to fall, and those with the heaviest losses (above 80 ml per cycle) are prone to frank anaemia.

Bleeding problems usually settle with time. If they do not it may be necessary to change the method of contraception, perhaps to the LNG-IUS (see below). The most successful therapies are mefenamic acid 500 mg 8-hourly and tranexamic acid 1–1.5 gm 8-hourly. Unfortunately, they do not seem to help the more common and often more annoying 'spotting' or intermenstrual bleeding.

Which device to choose?

The Copper T 380 Slimline (with its clones) appears to be the most effective IUD available, at least twice as effective in the first year of use and five times as effective cumulatively over 5 years as the Nova T/Novagard. Indeed, its first year failure rate was about 0.4 per 100 woman years, as effective as the oral contraceptive pill. No pregnancies at all were detected beyond 5 years use: quite unlike the Nova T where pregnancies continued to occur in each succeeding year. In my view the Nova T should only be used when the Cu T 380 S cannot be fitted, though a new Nova T bearing added copper is expected during 1998.

As good for pregnancy prevention, but even better for resistance to expulsion and also for patient comfort, it seems, will be the innovative GyneFix (Fig 6.3). This is a frameless device, licensed and now marketed in 1998. It carries six bands of copper crimped on to a polypropylene thread bearing a knot; the latter is embedded by the special stylet-introducer in the fundal myometrium. Additional training in the insertion procedure will be necessary for all: details from the Faculty of Family Planning.

Fig 6.3 *The Cu-Fix IUD (GyneFix)*

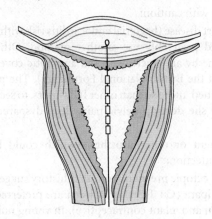

Duration of use

'Less frequent replacement would reduce the risks of pelvic inflammatory disease, uterine perforation, expulsion, and other complications that mainly occur soon after insertion . . .' (Newton and Tacchi 1990). Studies also show reduced rates of discontinuation for pregnancy, bleeding, and pain with increasing duration of use (see Table 6.15, column G). Therefore it is good news that in both the US and the UK the Cu T 380 is now fully approved for 8 years of use, and the data already support extension to at least 10 years. Moreover, **any copper device which has been fitted above the age of 40 may be that woman's last device and never needs to be changed** (Szarewski and Guillebaud 1991). However, in women under 40, the standard Nova T should normally be replaced on efficacy grounds after 5 years.

Selection of users – which user?

Main established contraindications to Copper IUDs – contrast re the LNG-IUS.

Absolute – but perhaps temporary – contraindications

(1) Suspected intrauterine or ectopic pregnancy;

(2) Unexplained uterine bleeding;

(3) Current or very recent active pelvic infection or pelvic tenderness, or purulent cervical discharge;

(4) Recent proven STD, unless fully investigated and treated;

(5) Immunosuppression (but low dose systemic steroids acceptable).

Absolute and permanent

(6) Infection with HIV;

(7) Distorted uterine cavity or cavity <5.5 cm;

(8) Wilson's disease;

(9) Known true allergy to copper;

(10) Heart valve prosthesis, or any past history of actual attack of bacterial endocarditis.

Relative contraindications

Copper IUD usable with caution:

(1) Structural heart disease (bacterial endocarditis risk without history). Such women should preferably use another method. Otherwise the fitting should be done by an expert, with full antibiotic cover (see the recommendations of the British National Formulary). The patient would also need to be warned, more so than other IUD-users, to seek prompt medical advice should she develop pelvic pain, deep dyspareunia, or excessive discharge;

(2) Hip replacement or other prosthesis which could be prejudiced by blood-borne infection;

(3) Past history of ectopic pregnancy or other history suggesting high ectopic risk in a multipara (Cu T 380 or Mirena are preferred IUDs, but even better to use an anovulant contraceptive). In young nulliparae many still consider this an absolute contraindication;

(4) Past history of definite PID;

(5) Lifestyle risking STDs;

(6) Questionable fertility for any reason;

(7) Nulliparity/young age (if any intrauterine method chosen LNG-IUS probably better on balance – p. 195);

(8) Severely scarred uterus (e.g., after open myomectomy);

(9) Severe cervical stenosis;

(10) Heavy periods/iron-deficiency anaemia;

(11) Severe primary dysmenorrhoea;

(12) Endometriosis – IUDs may worsen symptoms;

(13) After endometrial ablation/resection – risk it may become stuck in shrunken scarred cavity.

Counselling (by doctor or nurse)

After considering the contraindications, there should be an unhurried discussion with the woman of the main points above, particularly regarding her infection risk, the failure rate, and the importance of reporting pain as a symptom. It must be documented that the woman gave her informed verbal consent based on her reading and understanding the current leaflet of the UK FPA or equivalent. She must be assured that in the event of relevant symptoms she will receive prompt advice and a pelvic examination.

Timing of insertion

It is customary to insert devices in the closing days of or just after a period. The presence of a pregnancy is thereby excluded, the procedure is easier, and any associated bleeding is accepted as part of normal loss. Recent data suggest increased risks, particularly of expulsion, if IUDs are inserted during the main flow. At the Margaret Pyke Centre we normally plan to insert between day 4 and 14, but will do so later in selected cases – see p. 177 re insertion as a post-coital method.

In cases of amenorrhoea (e.g. post-partum) a very practical tip is to use the most sensitive modern pregnancy tests twice, before and after 10–14 days, during which time the couple agree to practise 'brilliantly good' birth control or abstinence.

After a recent delivery, in general practice IUDs should be inserted at 4–6 weeks, extended to 6–8 weeks after a Caesarean section. Extra care is needed, especially during lactation, to minimize the risk of perforation.

With insertion at termination of pregnancy there is no increase in complication rates if *Chlamydia* is screened for and the uterus is completely emptied. This choice (for the IUS if not an IUD) is not offered often enough, especially to parous women.

Insertion techniques

A book like this is not the right medium for teaching insertion techniques. I strongly recommend the Faculty of Family Planning's training scheme leading to the Letter of Competence in Intrauterine Contraception Techniques. This is a one-to-one apprenticeship, supplemented by videos and preliminary practice with an appropriate small pelvic model, following the illustrations in each packet. Training should include more attention than in the past to the issue of analgesia; after a randomized controlled trial showed it worked it is now our routine to offer mefenamic acid 500 mg while in the waiting room. Parenteral cervical anaesthesia should be taught, as well as the new option of 2% lignocaine jelly inserted by quill through the external cervical os.

Once learned, the skills, including management of 'lost threads', must be maintained by regular practice. It has been shown repeatedly that **insertion can be a factor in the causation of almost every category of IUD problems** (see all the "Yes's" in column H in Table 6.15). This of course is another reason to prefer long-lived devices.

Routine follow-up

Correct location of IUDs should be confirmed 4–6 weeks after insertion. Sounding the cervical canal up to the internal os with (for example) a throat swab is a valuable check for partial expulsion. Annual follow-up is then sufficient *provided* the IUD-user is fully informed of the danger-signs implied in Tables 6.15 and 6.16 and has open access to return promptly to the surgery if they occur. Devices are removed as indicated for complications, for planned pregnancy, or one year after the menopause. Otherwise, Table 6.15 column G supports a flexible policy to 'leave well alone'.

The levonorgestrel-releasing intrauterine system (LNG-IUS or 'Mirena')

This is Nova-T shaped and shown in Fig 6.4 (Andersson *et al.* 1994). It releases 20 µg/24 hours of levonorgestrel (LNG) from its polydimethylsiloxane reservoir through a rate-limiting membrane, over at least 5 years (though initially licensed in the UK for just 3 years). Its basic cost in *MIMS* is £99.25.

Fig 6.4 *The levonorgestrel intrauterine system (LNG-IUS)*

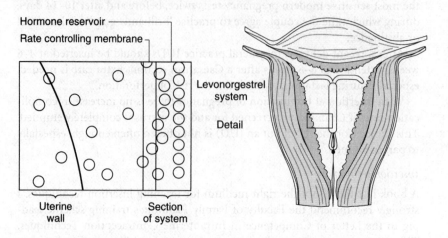

Hormone reservoir
Rate controlling membrane
Levonorgestrel system
Detail
Uterine wall
Section of system

Mechanisms

Its main contraceptive effects are local, by endometrial suppression and by changes to the cervical mucus and uterotubal fluid which impair sperm migration (and may also inhibit germ migration, see below) to the upper genital tract. The blood levels of LNG are about one-quarter of the peak levels in users of the POP, and so ovarian function is altered less: most women continue to ovulate with or without amenorrhoea (this is primarily a local end-organ effect) and in the anovulant women sufficient oestrogen is produced from the ovary despite the amenorrhoea. Contrast pp. 171 and 172–3 above.

Clinical advantages and indications

Every one of the advantages listed on p. 181 for the copper IUD apply to the IUS, except for the one about use as a post-coital contraceptive. It has unsurpassed efficacy, around 0.15 per 100 woman-years. Return of fertility is rapid and appears to be complete. It is highly convenient, has few adverse side-effects, and some beneficial effects on the menstrual cycle. It has the correct 'default state' (p. 130), unlike pills and condoms.

The above advantages are, of course, shared with the Cu T 380 S and the GyneFix, the best current copper IUDs. However, that is where the similarity ends, since the LNG-IUS has a range of gynaecological benefits which 'rewrite the textbooks' about IUDs. The user can expect a dramatic reduction in amount and, after the first few months (discussed below), in duration of blood loss. Dysmenorrhoea is also generally improved. *This is the contraceptive method of choice for non-Pill-takers with heavy or painful menses or who are prone to iron-deficiency anaemia.*

Menorrhagia

(See Chapter 10.) In an 'Effective health care' bulletin – *The management of menorrhagia* – funded by the Department of Health (1995), the value of this method of treating menorrhagia was acknowledged: 'Evidence from Scandinavian countries points to the effectiveness of the hormone-releasing intrauterine device as a first line of treatment of menorrhagia'. This is true, but it was undermined by the ensuing words: 'However, it is not yet licensed for this indication in the UK . . .'

Yet what is menorrhagia? Like amenorrhoea, it is not a disease. It is a symptom: the woman describes her menstrual periods as 'excessive'. Like any other symptom this requires a careful history, examination, and appropriate investigations. If the diagnosis is 'dysfunctional bleeding', and even if fibroids are present – so long as they do not distort the cavity (p. 196) – what is the difference between prescribing the contraceptive pill for its beneficial side-effect on heavy or painful periods and similar use of this IUS? Indeed, the data sheet states: 'Mirena^R may be particularly useful for contraception in patients with excessive menstrual bleeding'.

In short, an LNG-IUS may be used now to treat menorrhagia, *within the terms of the current licence*, by any woman who is potentially fertile; even if there is not currently a sexual relationship with a fertile partner but this is something which might come about in the future. 'Not licensed for menorrhagia' applies, therefore, only to women who are themselves sterilized. Even for them there is a recognized mechanism for 'named patient prescribing', described below (p. 197).

Infection

Although existing IUDs do not themselves cause pelvic inflammatory disease (PID), they fail to prevent it. There are now good data suggesting, but not proving, that this IUS really does reduce the frequency of clinical PID below the background rate, particularly in the youngest age groups who are most at risk. This and the very low ectopic rate make it possible to offer the device to some young women requesting a default state contraceptive who would not be good candidates for conventional copper IUDs. However, the protection is not 100%, and because:

- the superimposed foreign-body effects of an IUD or IUS may worsen an attack
- bilateral monogamy is not common in most modern societies, overall the intrauterine method remains *ideally* best avoided in the young and nulliparous woman (and with it or without it, most should use condoms anyway)

Ectopic pregnancy

The Progestasert and an experimental WHO device which released only 2 μg per day of levonorgestrel were both associated with an increased risk of extrauterine pregnancies. The data on file and published for this device show a definite reduction in that annual risk to about 0.06 per 100 woman-years.

Main problems/adverse effects of the LNG-IUS (Mirena)

.1. *Insertion* can be more difficult than the Nova T as it has a wider diameter insertion tube (see below).

2. Like any intrauterine device, *expulsion* occurs.

3. There is the usual small (approx one in 1000) risk of *perforation*, minimized by its 'withdrawal' technique of insertion.

4. A more important problem is the high incidence in the first post-insertion months of *uterine bleeding/spotting*, which through greatly reduced in quantity may be very frequent or continuous and can cause considerable inconvenience. Later in the use of the method amenorrhoea is very commonly reported. For both of these effects, particularly the first, 'forewarned is forearmed', implying good counselling in advance of the fitting. Many women can accept the early weeks of frequent light bleeding as a worthwhile price to pay for all the other advantages, if they are well informed in advance, and coached and encouraged as appropriate while it is occurring. The prognosis that the 'dribbling' will stop is actually better than for other progestogen-only methods like DMPA, but the time for resolution varies between 1–6 months (rarely longer).

5. *Amenorrhoea* should be explained and interpreted to a woman as a positive advantage of the method – not an adverse side-effect, since there is no hypo-oestrogenism.

6. *Hormonal side-effects* – women should be advised that though this method is mainly local in its action it is not exclusively so. Therefore there is a small incidence of steroidal side-effects such as mastalgia, acne, and depression.

7. *Functional ovarian cysts* are also more common, but are usually asymptomatic, and if not they should be monitored as they usually resolve spontaneously.

Main absolute contraindications

(1) Sensitivity to a constituent (e.g. levonorgestrel);

(2) Suspected intrauterine or ectopic pregnancy;

(3) Unexplained uterine bleeding;

(4) Current active or recurrent pelvic infection or marked pelvic tenderness, or purulent cervical discharge;

(5) Recent proven STD, unless fully investigated and treated;

(6) Severely distorted uterine cavity on u/s scan (congenital or through submucous fibroids – consider referral for resection);

(7) Heart valve prosthesis, or in woman with a structural heart defect, any past history of actual attack of bacterial endocarditis or severe pelvic infection;

(8) Current active arterial disease (this is arguable, probably a relative contraindication in most cases);

(9) Established immunodeficiency (not low-dose systemic steroids);

(10) Recent trophoblastic disease with continuing high hCG levels (p. 170).

In addition:

(11) The IUS should not be used as a post-coital intrauterine contraceptive (a failure has been reported). Though so effective, the mechanisms of

action, unlike copper, take time to be established. This explains the recommended *insertion timing*, no later than the seventh day of a spontaneous cycle in a currently sexually-active woman. (If there has been believable abstinence, later insertion with condom use for the rest of the cycle would be acceptable.)

Almost all the relative contraindications listed above (p. 192) for copper IUDs apply but are weaker; and heavy or painful periods constitute an indication.

Insertion of the LNG-IUS

(Re timing, see above and also pp. 192–3 for points which apply to both IUDs and the IUS.) The technique is almost identical to that for the Nova-T. However, the insertion tube is wider (4.8 mm rather than 3.7 mm), meaning that dilatation to Hegar 5 (rarely 6) is often required in nulliparae. All women should be offered premedication and local anaesthesia as described above (p. 193), though the latter is rarely needed by multiparae (outside of the peri-menopausal years).

Other uses and the issue of unlicensed indications (for licensed products)

Several times in this chapter unlicensed uses have been proposed – including here, namely the use of Mirena to treat heavy periods in sterilized women. Another unlicensed but increasingly popular use is to provide localized progestogenic protection of the endometrium during oestrogen replacement therapy by any chosen route (with contraception as well, unlike standard HRT regimens, see p. 206–7).

In the UK, if doctors wish to use this or any other medicinal product for an unlicensed indication, they may do so legally on their personal professional responsibility. 'Named patient prescribing' is an established process (Mann 1991) in which the doctor should ensure that he/she:

(1) is adopting a practice that would be *endorsed by a responsible body of professional opinion* and that all practices regarding the product are acceptable to those responsible for the doctor's professional indemnity;

(2) has *explained to the patient* that this is an *unlicensed* prescription and provides a dedicated written handout, as appropriate;

(3) has explained clearly the perceived risks and benefits, so that *informed consent can be obtained and recorded* (this does not require the patient's signature);

(4) *keeps a record* of the patient's details and the prescription.

These arrangements should be familiar; many of us regularly use other products for indications which are not yet licensed.

Conclusion

This is an excellent new choice in contraception, particularly for the older woman (especially but not exclusively if she also needs supplementary natural oestrogen) and when there is intercurrent chronic disease (see pp. 206–7, 212); also for the control of menorrhagia and/or dysmenorrhoea, and as part of the treatment of the premenstrual syndrome. In some ways its very brilliance as a contraceptive has blinded many doctors to its promising roles in medical gynaecology and endocrinology.

Barrier methods

See Table 6.1 (p. 131–2) for quoted efficacy rates for all these methods. 'Old fashioned' they may be, but they are once again in fashion. In spite of well-known disadvantages they all (notably the condoms) provide useful protection against sexually transmitted diseases.

All users of this type of method should be informed in advance about emergency contraception, in case of lack of use or failure in use.

It is also not widely enough known that vegetable and mineral oil-based lubricants, and the bases for prescribable vaginal products, can seriously damage rubber: baby oil, for example, destroys up to 95% of a condom's strength within 15 minutes. The Durex Information Service (1991) has produced a useful leaflet listing common vaginal preparations which should be regarded as unsafe to use with condoms and diaphragms. See updated lists in Table 6.17, but they are not exhaustive. Many other everyday oils can damage rubber, as found in the bathroom or kitchen, and even suntan oils are under some suspicion . . .

Male and female condoms

These are the only proven barrier to transmission of HIV and are being used increasingly with another contraceptive ('Double Dutch'). It still remains impossible for many couples to obtain this life-saver free of charge through their GP surgery. Readers are urged to lobby for this facility, and in the interim to find some means, as some practitioners have done, to utilize the AIDS budget to this end.

Male condoms are everyone's second choice, second in usage to the pill under 30 and to sterilization above that age. Most couples have had some experience of their use. Failure can practically always be attributed to incorrect use, mainly because of escape of a small amount of semen either before or after the act. One GP was able to report a failure rate as low as 0.4 per 100 woman-years, but 5–15 is more representative. The print on the packet is too small for the learner to read in the heat of the moment and a clear explanation of the basics is always appreciated. Particularly when the COC has to be stopped after many years on medical grounds, couples need to be taught just how 'dangerous' a fluid semen will now become.

Some couples are entirely satisfied with the sheath, others use it as a temporary or a backup method. For some men and some women, however, 'spoilt' by non-intercourse-related alternatives, it is completely unacceptable, but they do not always volunteer this information. Some older men, or those who have any sexual anxiety, complain that its use may result in loss of erection. In the past, 'allergy' could also be real, but it is now claimed that the whole range of the best-known brand is entirely hypo-allergenic, and the manufacturer has therefore ceased to produce the 'Durex allergy' condoms. For those women who dislike the smell or messiness of semen, the sheath solves their problem.

Table 6.17 *Vaginal preparations which are safe/unsafe to use with barrier methods*

Safe	Unsafe
Aqueous enemas	*Arachis Oil Enema*
Aci-Jel	*Baby Oil*
Betadine	*Cyclogest*
Canesten	*Dalacin cream*
Clotrimazole	*E45 (and similar)*
Delfen Foam	*Ecostatin*
Double Check	*Fungilin*
Durex Duracreme	*Gyno-Daktarin*
Durex Duragel	*Gyno-Pevaryl*
Durex Lubricating Jelly	*Monistat*
Durex Senselle	*Nizoral*
Glycerine	*Nystan Cream*
Gynol II	*Petroleum Jelly*
KY Jelly	*OrthoDienoestrol*
Nystan Pessaries (not cream)	*Ortho-Gynest*
Ortho-Creme	*Premarin cream*
Ortho-Forms	*Sultrin*
Ortho-Gynol	*Vaseline*
Ovestin Cream	*Witepsol-based products*
Pevaryl	
Replens	
Travogyn	

Source: Durex Information Service for Sexual Health (1991), updated. See text

Research is in progress into loose-fit, internally-lubricated plastic male condoms, intended to overcome the most intractable problem of the method, that undeniable interference with penile sensation during the penetrative phase of intercourse. The objective is the first truly 'user-friendly' male condom.

Femidom

Femidom is a female condom comprising a polyurethane sac with an outer rim at the introitus and a loose inner ring, whose retaining action is similar to that of the rim of the diaphragm, though the user does not have to locate the cervix. It thus forms a well-lubricated, secondary vagina. Available over the counter along with a well-illustrated leaflet, it is considerably less likely than the male condom to rupture in use. It is also completely resistant to damage by any chemicals with which it might come into contact. Using it, the penetrative phase of intercourse can start before the man's erection is complete, and many men prefer the sensation of 'freedom' as compared with male condoms. It can be especially useful post-partum in the presence of lochia or soreness.

Reports about its acceptability are mixed, and a sense of humour (with perhaps some background music!) certainly helps. But there is clear evidence of a group of women (with their partners) who use it regularly; sometimes alternating with the male equivalent ('his night' then 'her night'!). As the first female-controlled method, with high potential for preventing HIV transmission, it must be welcomed.

The cap or diaphragm

Many women express surprise at the simplicity of this method when first tried. Some who found it unacceptable early in their lives find it much easier after experience with tampons and when sexual activity takes on a relatively regular pattern, perhaps with a long-term partner and anticipating childbearing in the not too distant future. Protecting the cervix from infection, neoplasia, and semen, and inserted as a routine well ahead of coitus, it can be used without spoiling spontaneity. There is little reduction in physical sexual sensitivity as the clitoris and introitus are not affected and cervical pressure is still possible.

Spermicide is essential as no mechanical barrier is complete. The jelly vehicles (gels) may provide useful lubrication for the older woman, for those in the postnatal period and others slow to lubricate as a result of sexual arousal. Although many substances are well-absorbed from the vagina there is no proof of systemic harm from the use of current spermicides, chiefly using Nonoxynol-9 or its close relatives. Experience now spans over 70 years. A review by Bracken (1985) of 14 studies published to date concludes that, in particular, no association with congenital malformations or spontaneous abortion has been demonstrated. Occasionally, a sensitivity to spermicide arises but rubber allergy is exceptionally rare. Direct local irritation does also occur, particularly if Nonoxynol-9 is used very frequently, as by prostitutes: this effect has recently ended the advice to use it as an adjunctive virucide, though in normal use it remains entirely acceptable as a spermicide.

The acceptability of the diaphragm depends upon the manner in which it is offered. Its failure rate (now quoted as 4–8 failures in the first year, even among consistent users) makes it an unsuitable choice for most young women who would not accept a pregnancy. But it is capable of excellent protection, especially over the age of 35 (Table 6.1), provided it is correctly and consistently used. Correct fitting is important and can only be learnt by practical 'apprenticeship'. The complaint of discomfort implies wrong fitting. But even more important is skill in teaching placement and the vital secondary check that the cervix is covered. As for the IUD, there is no substitute for one-to-one training in this process of fitting and teaching, in which one can perhaps learn most from the older generation of skilled, family planning-trained nurses. The FPA leaflet should be provided as it includes all the (somewhat arbitrary) 'rules' of the method.

When it is apparent that a woman has great difficulty in inserting anything into her vagina, be it tampon, pessaries, or her own finger, obviously the method is not suitable. Sometimes this problem may be connected with some psychosexual difficulty and this may first present during the examination (p. 129). Permission to discuss associated fears and anxieties may prove helpful. Simple lack of anatomical knowledge is often involved. When any barrier is rejected on account of 'messiness' this also may be due to such a problem. The offer of a less wet-feeling alternative for the spermicide, such as Delfen foam, may help.

If either partner complains that they can feel the barrier during coitus the fitting must be urgently checked. It could be too large, or too small, or the retropubic ledge is insufficient to prevent the front slipping down the anterior vagina, or most seriously, the diaphragm may be being regularly placed in the anterior fornix. The arcing-spring diaphragm is particularly useful when this last problem is identified.

Chronic urethritis/cystitis may be exacerbated by pressure from the anterior rim and sufferers may do better with a vault or cervical cap, though spermicide-related changes to the vaginal flora may also be a factor. The smaller non-diaphragm caps are now rarely used, and should be, for this indication or because some women find them more comfortable to use than the ordinary diaphragm.

Diaphragms should be checked annually, post-partum, and if there is a 4 kg change in weight gain or loss. If the size remains constant, how often a new one is needed will vary. Some get misshapen, very discoloured, and worn by 1 year, and some appear pristine after 2 years.

Female barriers can be used happily and very successful by many women, but high motivation is essential. Once again a good sense of humour helps. 'Lea's shield' and 'Femcap' are two new plastic barrier devices invented in the USA, and both are likely to reach the UK market in the near future. Lea's shield has a floppy plastic 'valve' for cervical secretions and is intended as an over-the-counter, 'one size fits all' product. Femcap comes in two sizes (initially it is intended that a health-care provider will assist in choosing the size) and has a curved circumferential rim designed to locate in the fornices. Both devices are to be used with adjunctive spermicide, and both have loops for removal. Aside from promotional hype, preliminary efficacy data suggest that both are likely to be 'in the same ball park' for efficacy as a consistently-used diaphragm (first year failure rate 4–8 per 100 woman-years). However, either or both may be preferred on grounds of acceptability and convenience.

Spermicides

While invaluable as adjuncts to caps and condoms, by themselves creams, jellies, pessaries, and foams are usually not acceptably reliable; though there have been occasional reports of pregnancy rates under 10 per 100 woman-years. Delfen foam is very useful for women whose natural fertility is reduced, namely age over 45 and perhaps suffering vasomotor symptoms or with a high FSH reading (since that alone should not be relied upon as signifying infertility), or during lactation or secondary amenorrhoea. Spermicides in any acceptable form may also be a good supplementary method for couples who consider their only contraceptive option to be the withdrawal method; or for child-spacing.

Recently, and not before time, there has been an upsurge in research interest because of the vital need worldwide for effective, non-irritant vaginal virucide – which might well also (but not necessarily) be spermicides. Many candidate compounds and carrier vehicles are being screened but we still await the licensing of a product for this important indication. The contraceptive sponge, which was a useful carrier for spermicide, may perhaps reappear for virucide delivery.

Fertility awareness:
new methods for the natural regulation of fertility

At one time, the rhythm or safe period method was generally despised and only adopted by staunch Roman Catholics. Modern multiple index versions are increasingly demanded by those who prefer to use a so-called 'natural' method. They are more reliable, with perfect use, but in Trussell's phrase they remain 'very unforgiving of imperfect use'. The latter is common in the real world, where the highest possible cooperation from both parties is often lacking – especially from the male whose motivation may well be suspect. (In one study the failure rate was noted to be higher when the man rather than his partner was the one in charge of interpreting the temperature charts!) To be fair to these methods, failures also commonly result from poor use of other contraceptives, such as the condom, during 'unsafe' days.

Because of variable sperm survival (averaging 3–4 days but achieving 6–7 days in rare individuals or rare cycles) maximum reliability requires many days of abstinence, especially early in the cycle. Unprotected intercourse should preferably be confined, following good evidence of ovulation, to the days after the ovum is non-fertilizable (now ascertained as only 12 hours post-ovulation).

A rise in basal temperature which has been sustained for 72 hours at least 0.2°C above the preceding six days' values is the first recognized marker of the onset of the second infertile phase. This is best combined with observations of the mucus as detected at the vulva. This becomes increasingly fluid, glossy, transparent, slippery, and stretchy, like raw egg-white, under the influence of follicular oestrogen. The peak mucus day can be recognized retrospectively as the last day with such features before the abrupt change to a thick and tacky type (under the influence of progesterone). The infertile phase is defined as beginning on the evening of the fourth day after the peak mucus day, provided this is also after the third-higher morning temperature reading.

Reliance only on the later of both the above signals for the onset of the post-ovulatory infertile phase for unprotected intercourse can give very acceptable failure rates of 1–3 per 100 woman-years. Accurately identifying the pre-ovulatory infertile phase is more difficult. The indicators are:

(1) the first sign of any mucus, detected either by sensation or appearance;

(2) calendar calculation of the shortest cycle minus 20, where at least six cycle lengths are known; and the woman noted a high temperature phase in the preceding cycle to indicate that ovulation did occur in that cycle.

Whichever of these two indicators comes first indicates the requirement to abstain.

Use of both phases is only to be recommended to 'spacers', since calculations and mucus observations do not reliably predict ovulation far enough ahead to eliminate over many months or years the capricious survival of sufficient sperm to cause a pregnancy. Temperature and mucus estimations are unreliable and/ or give numerous 'false alarms' when some cycles are anovulatory, especially in the post-partum period and in the climacteric years. Yet lactation within certain guidelines does constitute an excellent 'natural method' – see LAM method.

Any who wish to use these methods deserve careful explanation and teaching. An invaluable book for prospective users is by Anna Flynn and Melissa Brooks (see Further reading for patients). Useful instruction leaflets and further advice can be obtained from:

(1) The FPA, 2–12 Pentonville Road, London, N1 9FP;

(2) The Fertility Awareness and Natural Family Planning Service of Marriage Care, 1 Blythe Mews, Blythe Road, London W14 ONW (Tel. 0171 371 1341);

(3) The Natural Family Planning Centre, Birmingham Maternity Hospital, Queen Elizabeth Medical Centre, Edgbaston, Birmingham B15 2TG.

Personal teaching may be arranged through nos. (2) and (3) above.

'PERSONA^R' – the Unipath personal contraceptive system

'PERSONA[R]' – the Unipath personal contraceptive system

This innovative product, first marketed in 1996, consists of a series of disposable test sticks and a hand-held, computerized monitor. As instructed by the monitor, the test sticks are dipped in the user's early morning urine samples and transferred to a slot in the device where the levels of both oestrone-3-glucuronide (E-3-G) and luteinizing hormone (LH) are measured by a patented immunochromatographic assay, utilizing an optical monitor. When a significant increase in the E-3-G level is detected, the fertility status is changed to 'unsafe', i.e. a red light replaces the green one on the monitor. After subsequent detection of the first significant rise of LH, the end of the fertile period is not signalled by a green light until 4 further days have elapsed. The system also stores and utilizes data on the individual's previous six menstrual cycles.

Preliminary efficacy information suggests a failure rate in consistent users around 6 per 100 woman-years comparable to the best previous results using fertility awareness, though higher than would be acceptable to those accustomed to the efficacy of the COC. A fertile period lasting 8 days or less was signalled to 80% of users, a definite improvement on the 10–12 days' abstinence usually demanded by the multiple index methods. For greater efficacy, some couples may accept using condoms in the first "green" phase, abstinence in the "red" phase and unprotected intercourse only in the second "green" phase. This should reduce the failure rate to about 2 per 100 woman-years (p. 202).

Sterilization

There is an increasing tendency for sterilizing procedures to be demanded at too early an age. Yet marriages contracted under age 25 now have a failure rate of about 50%. Deferment or even avoidance of surgery is often possible by careful discussion and explanation of alternatives, particularly injectables or the modern IUDs and the levonorgestrel-releasing intrauterine system. Older women are often particularly unwilling to discuss the whole topic, sometimes because they are embarrassed or doubt the propriety of sex except for procreation, or its indulgence over the age of 40. Psychological and physical consequences have been reported, of both tubal ligation and vasectomy, and careful preliminary discussion with both partners is absolutely essential for ultimate satisfaction to result.

There is a tendency for couples to expect sterilizing procedures to solve all problems and to be free of any associated risk, complications, or failures. Well-documented, fully-informed consent is vital, particularly now the long-term efficacy of female sterilization has been called into question by Peterson *et al.* (1996). They found, in a remarkable 10-year follow-up study of 10 000 women in the US, that the failure rate did not, as previously thought, stabilize after 2 years. The highest failure rate for all methods was in young women under age 30. For the only clip available in the US, the Hulka (not now recommended in the UK), the cumulative failure rate at 10 years approached to 4%! In this country the Filshie clip is believed to have an overall failure rate – taking account of operator errors but with follow-up to, at most, 2 years – of considerably less than 1%, and pending more data and longer follow-up, a reasonable estimate is a lifetime risk of 5 failures per 1000 procedures.

For vasectomy, a much lower rate of one case in 2000–7000 was quoted for late failures by Philp *et al.* (1984) but is is important to recognize that these followed two azoospermic semen analyses.

It must be understood by the couple that it is their responsibility to avoid conception up to the date of the procedure; the COC does not pose an excess risk of thrombosis prior to laparoscopy. General anaesthetics carry their own very small risk, and female sterilization as well as vasectomy can be performed under local anaesthetic, with excellent pain relief.

Although sterilization should be undertaken as a permanent procedure, requests for reversal do occur. In a series published by Winston (1980) reporting on 103 women who requested reversal between 1975–76, 87% were under the age of 30; 63% had been sterilized after delivery; and no less than 75% had been unhappily married. He reported a 58% pregnancy rate after microsurgery when the 37% who had had a completely irreversible operation had been excluded. With increasing experience of such specialist surgeons and the wider use of clips and rings, reversal successes have improved. Even though modern surgical techniques can be used to reverse some sterilizations, such operations demand skill, are difficult to get, are often expensive, and are not always successful. It is still wise, therefore, to consider sterilization to be irreversible and only to proceed when both partners can accept this.

The psychological sequelae of sterilization have been looked at. Earlier studies showed considerably higher rates of psychiatric morbidity, psychosexual dysfunction, and regret than a prospective study (Cooper *et al.* 1982) in which women were interviewed 4 weeks prior to elective sterilization and followed up at 18 months. In this latter study considerable regret was felt by 2% at 6 months and by 4% at 18 months, and post-operative psychiatric disturbance and dissatisfaction were largely associated with pre-operative psychiatric disturbance. The poorer results in other studies may be, in part, related to sterilization in association with a termination or immediately post-partum. Regret is more likely if the decision is made at such a time of crisis or stress.

A small GP study (Curtis 1979) identified 61 sterilized women. A control group of patients were asked similar questions about their experiences since their last pregnancy. These questions covered the area of menstrual and libido changes, and showed little difference between the two groups. As far as patient satisfaction with the sterilization was concerned, 45 had no regrets and 16 had some regrets, but only two of these seemed to be really serious. Many other studies give similar results.

Some individuals who find it impossible to use reversible contraceptive methods may be using the fear of pregnancy as a defence against sexual activity. This defence is removed by tubal ligation or vasectomy. For most couples, however, an irreversible step is just what they want, and once this decision is reached then the most appropriate procedure needs to be identified after discussion.

As compared with vasectomy, tubal occlusion is a more invasive procedure even when performed, as it now can readily be, under local anaesthesia. It confers immediate sterility while it may be several months before the semen is clear of sperm after the male operation. More importantly, especially once she passes the age of 40, the woman is unlikely to wish for restoration of her fertility, even with any future new partner; and unlike a man she loses that option after her menopause. Following vasectomy, however, after death of the wife or marriage breakdown, the man (even if past 50) nearly always finds a new and younger partner, and she makes him then more likely to regret his sterility. So although the male procedure is very simple and safe medically, with occasional haematomas the main complication, this difference from the female operation needs to be faced by older couples during counselling.

Long-term effects

After female sterilization, the later development of menstrual problems is often reported. Since these and the operation in women are both common, and many have lost the control of menstrual symptoms given by prior use of the COC, a chance association is likely. It is never possible to anticipate any woman's menstrual future. There are many published series which refute any connection, including one that measured menstrual blood loss before and 2 years after surgery. A possible benefit shown in three studies, that tubal sterilization reduces the risk of ovarian cancer, is difficult to explain but may be real (Wilson 1996).

Over the years, vasectomy has stood accused of various long-term effects, notably accelerated arteriosclerosis and cancer either of the testes or of the prostate. So far, none of these risks has been established by a voluminous epidemiological literature, though 'the jury is still out' regarding prostate cancer. The reported relative risk from the US is close to doubling after 20 years, but this is for diagnosis of, not death from, the disease – raising the real possibility of surveillance/detection bias rather than causation to explain the link. The US National Institutes of Health in 1993 reviewed all the studies and concluded, like WHO, that there was insufficient basis to recommend any change in clinical practice (NIH Statement 1993).

Our practice is to mention this possibility with all men pre-vasectomy, pointing out that the method(s) they have expected their wives to use hitherto may also not have been risk-free! The attributable number of cases is small: the background cumulative risk of being diagnosed by age 75 is 39 per 1000, so even if the doubled risk ratio is correct, 922 out of 1000 vasectomized men will not have developed prostatic cancer by this age.

The over 35-year-old woman

Most women of this age have achieved their desired family size and/or established themselves in some form of career or working life. Conception in the fifth and sixth decades may well be catastrophic: psychosocially, and also through the ever-increasing risk of maternal mortality, perinatal mortality, and fetal abnormality. Those (relatively few) women who continue menstruating regularly are likely to be fertile. But for the remainder, during the 10 years before the menopause, menstrual cycles become irregular.

Older women are not easily convinced that episodes of amenorrhoea along with less frequent intercourse mean that conception is actually much less likely to occur. Yet as we have seen, simpler methods like the contraceptive foam have acceptable efficacy above age 45. The cap or diaphragm can be extremely reliable, though usually acceptable only if already in use since a younger age. There is now agreement that any copper IUD fitted after the fortieth birthday may be left *in situ* until the menopause. These are all good reversible options for any older woman.

Hormone methods

Until recently, many practitioners have considered these (apart perhaps from the POP) as off-limits for the older woman. This rigid view is now outdated. For a start, post-coital oestrogen–progestogen (the Yuzpe regimen) is clearly not contraindicated on the grounds of age alone, at any time up to the menopause, if conception is likely (see p. 177). But what about much longer use of an oestrogen plus progestogen regimen? In these pre-menopausal years there are many potential non-contraceptive advantages, such as the reassurance of regular bleeds and the sexual benefits: avoiding intercourse-related methods and preventing oestrogen deficiency with associated skin-ageing, poor vaginal lubrication, and loss of libido. Symptoms of the so-called 'normal' menstrual cycle (especially the pre-menstrual syndrome and frequent, heavy, painful periods) are controlled. Even more important is the reduced risk of gynaecological pathology. Pelvic infection, extrauterine pregnancy, fibroids, dysfunctional haemorrhage, endometriosis, functional ovarian cysts, and above all, carcinoma of the ovary and uterus, are all less frequent in long-term users of combination oestrogen/progestogen therapy. The principal, entirely acceptable, alternatives are either neutral (e.g. barriers, sterilization); or, *though they may in many individuals be entirely satisfactory*, they have the potential to exacerbate menstrual cycle-linked problems (e.g. intrauterine devices, progestogen-only methods). If the latter occur, the risks of some treatments (notably hysterectomy) may well be considerably greater than those of the Pill. Moreover, hot flushes and early osteoporosis may begin before the actual menopause. In short, age alone no longer rules out a modern contraceptive/ hormone replacement regimen. *In selected healthy risk factor-free non-smokers well above age 35* the many therapeutic/preventive benefits outweigh, in my view, the small though definite increased risks (mainly of venous or arterial thrombosis but now probably also breast cancer, pp. 137–8) of prescribing a modern 20 µg pill. My personal preference at this age, if the woman has previously (as most have) used the COC for years without suffering a venous thrombosis, is still to offer Mercilon, since this is the only marketed 20 µg formulation with a more 'lipid friendly' progestogen.

Scrupulously careful supervision is essential, and, pending more data, smokers above age 35 should use a progestogen-only method, such as the POP or DMPA or a copper IUD if there are no menstrual problems. But an IUS with its menstrual and other benefits might be better still (see p. 193–8), and is indeed also increasingly being chosen by non-smokers. It is a good option anyway, but especially so if there are symptoms of oestrogen deficiency, when as well as giving the reassurance of contraception it will protect the uterus from hyperplasia during oestrogen replacement (p. 197).

Though sterilization (of either party) solves the problems of many, it may prove unnecessary with good presentation of alternatives.

When to stop contraception

Despite much research, there is no simple answer to the question which many patients will ask: 'When can I stop contraception?' Long spells of amenorrhoea in women under 45 may indicate the arrival of a premature menopause, but they may be due to other spontaneously reversible or treatable causes requiring investigation (see Chapter 10). Even above that age, prolonged amenorrhoea does not rule out the chance of a later ovulation, though the risk is less if there are definite vasomotor symptoms. We now know that FSH measurements alone are most misleading – they only mean reduced feedback of ovarian hormones on the pituitary at that time, the ovaries may well still have potentially fertile ova to release. So most authorities would still advise women only to discontinue all contraception after the occurrence of complete amenorrhoea for 2 years if under age 50 (reducing to 12 months above 50).

If the combined pill is now useable in selected cases until the menopause, how may that be diagnosed? The 'standard' teaching above is impossible to follow with increasing use at this age of HRT, and, for healthy non-smokers, of Mercilon (since the withdrawal bleeds will indefinitely mask the true menopause). The former is not safely contraceptive, and if it can be avoided the latter is best not used (unnecessarily) after full natural infertility is established. A possible protocol follows. We normally use it when the woman reaches age 50.

COC-users

Measure FSH at the end of the pill-free week. If it is normal she still needs contraception – though above 50 the risks of the COC would in most cases be judged greater than the necessity for such a powerful contraceptive, so an alternative should be offered (see p. 206). If the FSH is high, above the 'menopausal' level specified by the laboratory, there are preliminary data that such a woman has begun – as a consequence of ovarian failure – to rely totally on the COC for her oestrogen. Therefore when it is stopped for just 7 days the FSH climbs rapidly. She may even report 'hot flushes' at the end of each pill-free week, the situation being comparable to sudden loss of ovarian oestrogen by oophorectomy. If she now switches to a simple barrier contraceptive (or just Delfen foam, which is adequate at this age) for about 6 weeks, and records any subsequent bleeds and vasomotor symptoms, a second high FSH result with no spontaneous bleeds after stopping the COC is suggestive of final ovarian failure above age 50 – particularly if she reports 'hot flushes'. After advice that the risk of later ovulation can even so not be completely excluded, the woman may then elect to discontinue contraception, whether or not choosing to start HRT. Ultra-caution otherwise dictates contraception for 12 more months.

HRT-users (using separate contraception)

Measure FSH, logically at the end of the oestrogen-only phase. A level above 25iu/litre, raised despite the HRT feedback on the pituitary, is suggestive of ovarian failure – but this should be confirmed, exactly as for the COC above, after stopping exogenous hormones for 6 weeks. If, however, the woman has a normal FSH result and/or ever menstruates while off either COC or HRT, she should assume some residual fertility and (continue to) use a simple contraceptive, again whether or not she decides to take HRT.

POP-users

If prolonged amenorrhoea occurs as a new phenomenon along with symptoms suggestive of the menopause, the woman may have her FSH measured while still taking the method. If it is low, she still needs the POP. If it is high, the presence and persistence of vasomotor symptoms and a repeat high FSH value 6 weeks after stopping the treatment mean that her chances of a further fertile ovulation are extremely low at 50, and possibly nil. With all the caveats above, she may therefore discontinue contraception (Guillebaud 1994). Younger women and any who want more complete reassurance may, if preferred, continue using a simple method, as usual until 1 year after the last non-hormonally-induced bleed.

We still do not have – and badly need – a simple test of complete and final ovarian failure at the menopause.

The woman who has just been pregnant

If not breast-feeding

Ovulation may occur as early as 10 days after abortion and by about day 28 after delivery. Early contraception is therefore important. In women who do not breast-feed the COC should be started no earlier than day 21 in order to minimize any extra risk of venous thrombosis. Moreover, if there has been severe pre-eclampsia the COC should be taken only after biochemical normality has been restored.

If breast-feeding

Studies have shown that ovulation is delayed among women who fully or nearly fully breast-feed their babies until an average of 34 weeks post-partum, but with considerable individual variation related to the frequency and duration of breast-feeding episodes and the timing of introduction of food other than breast-milk. In 1988 at a consensus conference in Bellagio, Italy, guidelines were produced leading to a method of family planning known as the lactational amenorrhoea method or LAM (Labbok *et al.* 1994). LAM is an algorithm, as shown in Fig 6.5, allowing a woman to determine when she can rely on her pattern of infant-feeding and menstruation or should add an additional method of contraception.

In the UK, despite efforts to encourage breast-feeding, only around 50% of new mothers breast-feed their babies beyond a few days, and two-fifths of them give supplementary bottle-feeds by 6 weeks. With current infant feeding patterns, LAM could not be used beyond about 4 months post-partum, and many women could not use it at all. In summary, successful breast-feeders who freely choose the lactational amenorrhoea method are the only reasonable candidates for it.

The COC may inhibit lactation and does enter the milk in small quantities. The POP is preferable, usually started like the COC on day 21. This does not interfere significantly with lactation and although traces may enter the milk the quantity would be so small that it has been equated to a baby getting the equivalent of one pill in 2 years. This is considerably less than the progesterone level found in dried cow's milk. Strangely, the natural childbirth movement nevertheless advises against its use.

Unwanted pregnancies are not uncommon when lactating POP-users have not been warned that their margin for error in POP-taking will diminish at weaning. If efficacy is at a premium, they should switch to the COC (or DMPA) when their infant first takes solid food, or no later than the first bleed.

The injectable, DMPA, aside from slightly higher milk levels (which seem to be harmless to the infant) may be a preferable progestogen-only method for women who might be short-term breast-feeders and unreliable POP-takers, but

Fig 6.5 *LAM – use of the lactational amenorrhoea method during the first 6 post-partum months*

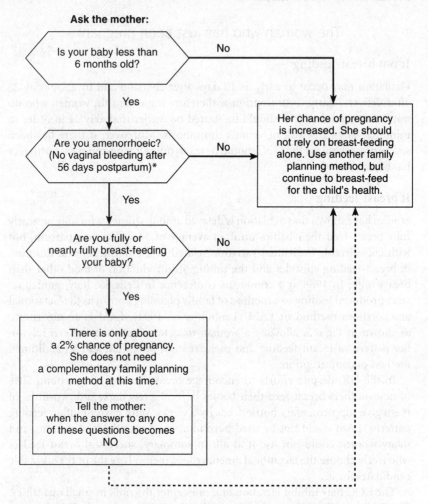

Ask the mother:

Is your baby less than 6 months old? — No → Her chance of pregnancy is increased. She should not rely on breast-feeding alone. Use another family planning method, but continue to breast-feed for the child's health.

Yes ↓

Are you amenorrhoeic? (No vaginal bleeding after 56 days postpartum)* — No →

Yes ↓

Are you fully or nearly fully breast-feeding your baby? — No →

Yes ↓

There is only about a 2% chance of pregnancy. She does not need a complementary family planning method at this time.

Tell the mother: when the answer to any one of these questions becomes NO

* Spotting that occurs during the first 56 days is not considered to be menses.

want high efficacy right through weaning and thereafter. It does no detectable harm to the quality and may even improve the quantity of the breast-milk.

The IUD or IUS are easily inserted at 4–6 weeks post-partum but the uterus is still soft and great care is necessary, particularly if the woman is lactating. Earlier insertion is more likely to lead to expulsion. If any infection (endometritis) is present, insertion is better delayed.

Condoms (especially the female condom, see p. 199) are useful until other methods are established. Caps and diaphragms may be refitted at 5–6 weeks and this is necessary even after Caesarean section. Aside from the LAM above, natural regulation of fertility is very difficult – the mucus signs give 'false alarms' and force prolonged abstinence on the couple to obtain acceptable efficacy before normal cycling resumes.

Sterilization procedures performed at abortion or in the post-partum period carry extra operative, failure rate, and emotional risks. Surgery in both sexes is usually, and preferably, delayed for a few months.

The very young

Although early cycles after the menarche are assumed to be anovulatory, very early conceptions are being reported, and surveys show that around half of the total female population under 16 years of age have had intercourse. This represents a major category of technical law-breaking, not by the girl but by all male partners.

A modern, low-oestrogen combined pill usually proves the most suitable method, initially. As far as we know, once periods are established it poses no special problems in teenagers, as compared with women in their twenties. However, like the condom, the COC has the wrong 'default state' (p. 130). With the difficulties so many young people have in their compliance we badly need methods modelled on a utopian future method, reversible vaccination against pregnancy! Those available have their own problems. Injectables (or implants) are usually preferable to IUDs through providing some protection against pelvic infection, but copper IUDs are not absolutely contraindicated; and the LNG-IUS 'opens the door' a little wider to the intrauterine method, especially for insertion at termination of pregnancy when other options have been proved wanting.

Since teenagers generally are now at greatest risk of all sexually transmitted agents, including HIV it is essential to promote use of the condom in addition, often, to the selected main contraceptive.

Any GP faced with an under-16-year-old needs first, opportunely and non-patronizingly, to raise the advantages, both psychological and physical, of delaying intercourse until later (and then of mutual loyalty). S/he must also study the revised *Memorandum of guidance* [DHSS HC(FP)86] issued after the Gillick case in 1986. Although involvement of at least one parent is vastly preferable and we are legally obliged to discuss this, the memorandum describes circumstances in which it is good practice to proceed to prescribe the Pill without it. The young person must understand the risk/benefit analysis applying in her situation. At all times the young woman must be assured 100% of confidentiality: fears about this, not always justified, but fears all the same, are established as the greatest single deterrent to obtaining contraception. The duty of the doctor and of all ancillary staff, given in respect of confidentiality to a person not yet 16, is as great as that given to any other person.

Dedicated sessions with the right ambience for young people are the ideal, the model being those run by the Brook Advisory Centres. Where these are not available some general practices have combined in a locality to develop highly successful drop-in centres, for the young of both sexes.

Women with intercurrent disease

Historically, this has mainly been a problem where the condition poses a contraindication (absolute or strong relative) to the COC: see the discussion of 'summation' on p. 212, and of contraception for some particular conditions such as diabetes, hypertension, and sickle-cell disease. Such women usually require maximum possible protection from pregnancy, which often has its own additional disease-related risks. This leads to the principle that the added risks of a contraceptive like the COC may sometimes be acceptable because of its efficacy in comparison with medically safer but less effective reversible alternatives. Female sterilization is a possibility, but not always relevant. Likewise, the woman's healthy partner's kind offer to have a vasectomy may not necessarily be rightly accepted – depending on factors like her expectation of life. Clearly, each couple has to be considered individually and discussion with the consultant in charge is often mandatory, especially in cancer cases or conditions with a highly unpredictable prognosis like multiple sclerosis.

My own lecture with this title has become much shorter since May 1995, the month that the LNG-IUS (pp. 193–8) first arrived on the UK market. Chiefly because of its efficacy and the virtual absence of life-endangering adverse effects, it is surprising how often incoming queries about difficult contraceptive problems may now be answered by suggesting this option! But the other progestogen-only methods or the Cu T 380 S or GyneFix are usually also options.

The future

In spite of the availability of a full, comprehensive contraceptive service, the requests for termination of unwanted pregnancies continue. Some women find it difficult to get contraceptive advice, and others seem unable to use any method successfully. Despite all the medico-legal obstacles, new pills, intrauterine devices and systems, injectables, implants, skin patches, new vaginal barriers, condoms, and sterilization clips are known to be ready for marketing before the year 2000; plus shortly thereafter the long-awaited injectable for men based on a long-acting testosterone ester, probably in combination with a progestogen or with cyproterone acetate. None of these is quite that utopian future method, a 100% effective and side-effect-free method akin to reversible vaccination against pregnancy!

Regardless of the hoped-for research developments, practitioners (and practice nurses) in this important field of reproductive health will always need sensitivity to understand, and allow for in their counselling, the innumerable factors which affect the acceptability of contraceptive methods. There needs to be more perception by the very young about the ease of conception and by the older woman of the persistence of fertility. As a team, whether in general practice or in local clinics, we have a responsibility to make it easy for our patients to ask for advice and then to have the skill to help them use their own choice, happily and effectively.

References and further reading

Andersson, K., Odlind, V., and Rybo, G. (1994). Levonorgestrel-releasing and copper-releasing (Nova-T) IUDs during five years of use: a randomised comparative trial. *Contraception*, **49**, 56–72.

Back, D. J., Breckenridge, A. M., Crawford, F. F., MacIver, M., Orme, M.L'E., and Rowe, P. H. (1981). Interindividual variation and drug interactions with hormonal steroid contraceptives. *Drugs*, **21**, 46–61.

Back, D. J. and Orme, M.L'E. (1990). Pharmacokinetic drug interactions with oral contraceptives. *Clinical Pharmacokinetics*, **18**, 472–84.

Bracken, M. B. (1985). Spermicidal contraceptives and poor reproductive outcomes: the epidemiological evidence against an association. *American Journal of Obstetrics and Gynecology*, **151**, 552–6.

Clinical and Scientific Committee of Faculty of Family Planning and Reproductive Health Care and Medical Advisory Committee of Family Planning Association (FPA) (1997). Joint statement: migraine and combined oral contraceptives. *British Journal of Family Planning*. (In press.)

Collaborative Group on Hormonal Factors in Breast Cancer (1996). Breast cancer and hormonal contraceptives. *Lancet*, **347**, 1713–27.

Committee on Safety of Medicines (1995). *Combined oral contraceptives and thrombo-embolism*. [Letter]. CSM, London.

Contraceptive Education Service (1996). *Contraceptive choices*. Family Planning Association.

Cooper, P., Gath, D., Rose, N., *et al.* (1982). Psychological sequelae to elective sterilization: a prospective study. *British Medical Journal*, **284**, 461–4.

Croft, P. and Hannaford, P. C. (1989). Risk factors for acute myocardial infarction in women: evidence from the Royal College of General Practitoners' oral contraception study. *British Medical Journal*, **298**, 165–8.

Curtis, D. M. (1979). The sequelae of female sterilization in one general practice. *Journal of the Royal College of General Practitioners*, **29**, 366–9.

Demacker, P. M., Schade, R.W., Stalenhoef, A. F., *et al.* (1982). Influence of contraceptive pill and menstrual cycle on serum lipids and high-density lipoprotein cholesterol concentrations. *British Medical Journal*, **284**, 1213–15.

Drife, J. O. and Guillebaud, J. (1986). Hormonal contraception and cancer. *British Journal of Hospital Medicine*, **35**, 25–9.

Durex Information Service for Sexual Health (1991). *Warning: oil-based lubricants and ointments can damage condoms and diaphragms*. LRC Leaflet, 1–4.

Effective health care bulletin (1995). *The management of menorrhagia*. Bulletin 9. University of Leeds, Leeds.

Farley, T. M., Rosenberg, M. J., Rowe, P., *et al.* (1992). Intrauterine devices and pelvic inflammatory disease: an international perspective. *Lancet*, **339**, 785–8.

Guillebaud, J. (1994). *Contraception – your questions answered*. Churchill Livingstone, Edinburgh.

Guillebaud, J. (1997). *Contraception today: a pocket book for general practitioners*. Martin Dunitz, London.

Guillebaud, J. (1995*b*). When do you need to give emergency contraception for missed pills? *Fertility Control Reviews*, **4**, 18–20.

Guillebaud, J. (1995*c*). Advising women on which pill to take. *British Medical Journal*, **311**, 1111–12.

Hannaford, P. and Webb, A. (1996). Evidence-guided prescribing of combined oral contraceptives: consensus statement. *Contraception*, **54**, 125–9.

Ho, P .C. and Kwan, M. S. (1993). A prospective randomized comparison of levonorgestrel with the Yuzpe regimen in post-coital contraception. *Human Reproduction*, **8**, 389–92.

Kubba, A. (1995). *Emergency contraception guidelines for doctors*. Contraceptive Education Service, London.

Labbok, M. H., Perez, A., Valdez, V., *et al.* (1994). The lactational amenorrhoea method (LAM): a postpartum introductory family planning method with policy and program implications. *Advances in Contraception*, **10**, 93–109.

Lande, R. E. (1995). *New era for injectables*. Population reports, Series K, No. 5. Population Information Program of Johns Hopkins School of Public Health, Baltimore.

Lewis, M. A., Spitzer, W. O., Heinemann, L. A., *et al.* (1996*a*). Third generation oral contraceptives and risk of myocardial infarction: an international case study, *British Medical Journal*, **312**, 88–90.

Lewis, M. A., Heinemann, L. A., MacRae, K. D., *et al.* (1996*b*). The increased risk of venous thromboembolism and the use of third generation progestagens: role of bias in observational research. *Contraception*, **54**, 5–13.

Lewis, M. A., Heinemann, L. A., Spitzer, W. O. (1997). The use of oral contraceptives and the occurrence of acute myocardial infarction in young women. *Contraception*, **56**.

Lidegaard, O. (1993). Oral contraception and risk of a cerebral thromboembolic attack: results of a case-control study. *British Medical Journal*, **306**, 956–63.

Lidegaard, O. (1995). Oral contraceptives, pregnancy and the risk of cerebral thromboembolism: the influence of diabetes, hypertension, migraine and previous thrombotic disease. *British Journal of Obstetrics and Gynaecology*, **102**, 153–59.

Loudon, N., Glasier, A., and Gebbie, A. (ed.) (1995). *Handbook of family planning*. Churchill Livingstone, Edinburgh.

Loudon, N. B., Barden M. E., Hepburn W. B., and Prescott R. J. (1991). A comparative study of the effectiveness and acceptability of the diaphragm used with spermicide in the form of C-film or a cream or jelly. *British Journal of Family Planning*, 17, 41–44.

McCann, M. F. and Potter L. S. (1994). Progestin-only oral contraception: a comprehensive review. *Contraception*, **50** (1), S9–S195.

Mann, R. (1991). Unlicensed medicines and the use of drugs in unlicensed indications. In *Pharmaceutical medicine and the law* (ed. A. Goldberg and I. Dodd-Smith). pp.103–10. Royal College of Physicians, London.

Mao, K. and Guillebaud, J. (1984). Influence of removal of intrauterine contraceptive devices on colonization of the cervix by actinomyces-like organisms. *Contraception*, **30**, 535–45.

Mills, A. M., Wilkinson, C. L., Bromham, D. R., *et al.* (1996). Guidelines for prescribing combined oral contraceptives. *British Medical Journal*, **312**, 121.

National Association of Family Planning Doctors (NAFPD) (1984). Interim guidelines for doctors following the pill scare. *British Journal of Family Planning*, **9**, 120–2.

Newton, J. (1996). New hormonal methods of contraception. In *Bailliere's clinical obstetrics and gynaecology* (ed. A. Glasier), pp.87–101. Bailliere Tindall, London.

Newton, J. R. and Tacchi, D. (1990). Long-term use of copper intrauterine devices. *Lancet*, **336**, 182.

NIH: National Institute of Child Health and Human Development. Final statement from vasectomy and prostate cancer conference (March 2, 1993). NIH, Bethesda.

Pardthaisong, T. (1984). Return of fertility after use of the injectable contraceptive, Depo-Provera: updated analysis. *Journal of Biosocial Science*, **16**, 23–34.

Peterson, H. B., Zhisen, X., Hughes, J. M., *et al.* (1996). The risk of pregnancy after tubal sterilization: findings from the US Collaborative Review of Sterilization. *American Journal of Obstetrics and Gynecology*, **174**, 1161–70.

Philp, T., Guillebaud, J., and Budd, D. (1984). Late failure of vasectomy after two documented analyses showing azoospermic semen. *British Medical Journal*. **289**, 77–9.

RCGP (1983). Incidence of arterial disease among oral contraceptive users. *Journal of the Royal College of General Practitioners*, **33**, 75–8.

Sapire, K. E. (1990). *Contraception and sexuality in health and disease*. McGraw-Hill, London.

Serjeant, G. R. (1985). Pregnancy and contraception. In *Sickle-cell disease* (ed. G. R. Serjeant), pp. 287–8. Oxford University Press, Oxford.

Smith, S. K., Kirkman, R. J., Arce, B. B., *et al.* (1986) The effect of deliberate omission of Trinordiol (R) or Microgynon (R) on the hypothalamo-pituitary-ovarian axis. *Contraception*, **34**, 513–22.

Stampfer, M. J., Willett, W. C., Colditz, G. A., *et al.* (1989) A prospective study of past use of oral contraceptive agents and risk of cardiovascular diseases. *New England Journal of Medicine*, **19**, 1313–17.

Szarewski, A. and Guillebaud, J. (1991). Regular review: contraception, current state of the art. *British Medical Journal*, **302**, 1224–6.

Vessey, M. P. (1989). Oral contraception and cancer. In *Contraception, science and Practice* (ed. M. Filshie and J. Guillebaud), pp. 52–68. Butterworths, London.

Vessey, M. P., Lawless, M., and Yeates, D. (1982). Efficacy of different contraceptive methods. *Lancet,* **i**, 841–2.

Vessey, M. P., Lawless, M., McPherson, K., and Yeates, D. (1983). Neoplasia of the cervix uteri and contraception: a possible adverse effect of the Pill. *Lancet,* **ii**, 930–4.

Vessey, M. P., Lawless, M., Yeates, D., and McPherson, K. (1985). Progestogen-only oral contraception. Findings in a large prospective study with special reference to effectiveness. *British Journal of Family Planing,* **10**, 117–21.

Vessey, M. P., Villard-Mackintosh L., McPherson K., and Yeates D. (1989). Mortality among oral contraceptive users: 20 year follow-up of women in a cohort study. *British Medical Journal,* **299**, 1487–91.

Weström, L. (1987). Pelvic inflammatory disease: bacteriology and sequelae. *Contraception,* **36**, 111–28.

WHO Scientific Group (1981). *The effect of female sex hormones on fetal development and infant health.* Technical report series, 657. WHO, Geneva.

WHO collaborative study of neoplasia and steroid contraceptives (1985). Invasive cervical cancer and combined oral contraceptives. *British Medical Journal,* **290**, 961–5.

WHO Scientific Group (1987). *Mechanism of action, safety and efficacy of intrauterine devices.* Technical Reports Series, 753. WHO, Geneva.

Wilson, E. W. (1996). Sterilization. In *Bailliere's Clinical Obstetrics and Gynaecology: contraception* (ed. A. Glasier), pp.103–19. Bailliere Tindall, London.

Winston, R. M. L. (1980). Reversal of tubal sterilization. *Clinical Obstetrics and Gynaecology,* **23**, 1261–8.

Reference books

Drife, J. O. and Baird, D. T. (ed.) (1993). *British medical bulletin: Contraception.* British Council, London.

Hannaford, P. C. and Webb, A. M. (ed.) (1996). *Evidence-guided prescribing of the pill.* Parthenon, Carnforth.

The IPPF (International Planned Parenthood Federation) produce much useful literature for doctors, including the bimonthly *Medical Bulletin.*

Further reading for patients

Flynn, A. and Brooks, M. (1994). *A manual of natural family planning.* Thorsons, London.

Guillebaud, J. (1997). *The Pill* (5th edn.). Oxford University Press, Oxford.

Szarewski, A. and Guillebaud, J. (1994) *Contraception – a user's handbook.* Oxford University Press, Oxford.

Useful patient leaflets concerning all methods and instructions in other languages can be obtained from the FPA, 2–12 Pentonville Rd, London N1 9FP.

CHAPTER SEVEN

Unwanted pregnancy and abortion

Lis Davidson

Most general practitioners (GPs) will be familiar with the clinical situation of a woman who is unhappy about her pregnancy but some will find it arouses uncomfortable feelings. The doctor may feel uneasy at being asked to provide a service – referral for abortion – rather than being asked to exercise the classical medical skills of diagnosis or treatment. In addition, the doctor's attitude to abortion may make it difficult to respond to the woman's needs. In this chapter we hope to show that, whatever the views of the doctor, there is a great deal that can be done to help and there are useful skills that can be developed. In fact, the role of the GP in this area can be just as rewarding as in any other medical situation. But first some background.

The background

Terminology

This is not a chapter simply about abortion. To talk only about abortion would be to pre-empt the decision that the doctor and the woman with an unwanted pregnancy must make. There will, however, be a strong emphasis on abortion, not because it is always the most appropriate outcome for an unwanted pregnancy, but because it is the area that is most likely to involve the GP rather than the social services.

We have chosen the term 'unwanted' rather than 'unplanned' or 'unintended' pregnancy. A pregnancy may have been planned and intended, yet for a number of reasons may be unwanted; on the other hand an unplanned pregnancy may yet be wanted. However, the term 'unwanted' is not without problems; in particular, it hardly does justice to the ambivalence that many women feel.

Abortion legislation

History of the law in England and Wales

The 1861 Offences Against the Person Act made abortion illegal in all circumstances, although in practice an exception was made when the woman's life was in danger.

In 1938, interpretation of the law was made more liberal by Judge Macnaghten in the Bourne case when he stated that it was lawful to terminate a pregnancy not only to save a woman's life but also 'if the doctor is of the opinion ... that ... the continuation of the pregnancy would make the woman a physical or mental wreck' (*British Medical Journal* 1966).

In spite of the Bourne judgement, the limits of the law remained unclear; and the need for clarification was one of a number of factors that led to attempts to change the law. After the war there was a gradual liberalization of views on certain social issues such as homosexuality and divorce as well as on abortion. In the case of abortion this was partly due to concern about the prevalence of illegal abortion with its often dire results. During the 1950s and 1960s the demand for abortion seemed to be increasing; with more effective contraception, many women were choosing to delay or limit their childbearing and take on other roles. Many women were also less willing to accept an unplanned pregnancy than in the past, when the opportunity to control fertility had been more limited. The thalidomide tragedy in the early 1960s further underlined the need for a change in the law. Alongside these factors, the advent of new methods and the use of more effective antibiotics meant that abortion was becoming safer.

The 1967 Abortion Act. The 1967 Abortion Act was the seventh attempt to reform the law on abortion; it came into effect in April 1968.

In 1974 the Lane Committee, which was set up to report on the working of the Abortion Act, concluded that ' ... the gains facilitated by the Act have much outweighed any disadvantages for which it has been criticised' (Lane 1974).

The 1967 Abortion Act did not repeal the 1861 Act but defined exceptions to that Act in which abortion would be legal. These defined exceptions are:

if two registered medical practitioners are of the opinion, formed in good faith – (a) that the continuance of the pregnancy would involve risk to the life of the pregnant woman, or of injury to the physical or mental health of the pregnant woman, or any existing children of her family, greater than if the pregnancy were terminated; or (b) that there is a substantial risk that if the child were born it would suffer from such physical or mental abnormalities as to be seriously handicapped.

In determining the risk of injury to health the Act states that 'account may be taken of the pregnant woman's actual or reasonably foreseeable environment'.

Abortions not covered by these exceptions remained illegal and a time limit was laid down, not by the 1967 Act but by the 1929 Infant Life (Preservation) Act. This states that abortion is illegal (except to save the woman's life) once the fetus has become 'capable of being born alive' which for many years was assumed to be 28 weeks' gestation.

There have been numerous attempts to restrict the 1967 Act but the only alteration has come from the 1990 Human Fertilization and Embryology Act which reset the time limit for abortion at 24 weeks' gestation. However, it also allows that this limit does not apply where there is risk of grave permanent injury or death to the mother or a substantial risk of serious handicap in the child. In fact, the 1990 Act is an example of statute law falling in line with existing practice since very few abortions, 23 in 1989 in England (Hall 1990), were being performed after 24 weeks gestation, and these were being done for reasons permitted under the 1990 Act. It is unlikely therefore that this Act will lead to any radical change in practice.

Abortion laws in Scotland

The 1861 and 1929 Acts did not apply in Scotland. Before 1967, abortion was a common law offence but there were no prosecutions in cases of therapeutic abortion carried out without secrecy by a gynaecologist. By the 1960s a few gynaecologists were openly performing abortions on married women with many children but most gynaecologists were reluctant to test the law.

When the Abortion Act passed into Scottish law in 1968, some feared it might act restrictively but this was not the case. As in England and Wales, many doctors became increasingly willing to perform abortions. Although the absence of the 1861 and 1929 Acts from the statute books does not affect the availability of abortion in Scotland, some differences between England and Scotland remain.

Abortion laws in Northern Ireland

The 1967 Abortion Act did not extend to Northern Ireland but the 1861 Act does apply there, so abortion remains illegal except to save the woman's life. Every year more than 1000 women travel from Northern Ireland to England for a private abortion.

Abortion laws in Guernsey

Abortion is illegal on Guernsey under a law dating from 1910; a woman convicted of obtaining an abortion could face 3 years to life imprisonment. More than 100 women make the journey to Britain each year. The Guernsey Board of Health is presently considering proposals for a new abortion law.

The changing role of the GP

Before 1938, when a woman consulted her doctor about an unwanted pregnancy, the doctor had little option but to persuade her to continue the pregnancy and to help her through this and through adoption if appropriate. Doctors were rarely involved in helping women to procure an abortion and when they did so they were usually acting illegally. Yet most doctors practising at that time would have been only too familiar with the sight of an ill, infected, and partially exsanguinated woman suffering the results of a backstreet or self-induced abortion.

Over the next 30 years a few women were able to obtain a more or less legal abortion but even then the GP was rarely involved. The abortion was usually performed privately and the woman usually referred herself. Although the numbers began to increase during the 1960s, the availability of abortion depended above all on the woman's knowledge and her ability to pay.

Table 7.1 *Regional variations in NHS provision of abortion in 1994 (England and Wales only)**

Region	Percentage of abortions on women resident in that region performed in NHS hospital	Percentage of abortions on women resident in that region performed by agency for the NHS
Wales	99	0
Anglia and Oxford	98	0
Trent	90	0.01
North	85	4
South and West	69	12
North Thames	57	7
North West	55	9
South Thames	45	16
West Midlands	20	45

Source: OPCS abortion statistics 1994

* Figures include only those women who had an abortion within the region that they also reside in. Some women cross borders; because they live on them, because they are away from home, or because the other side is more sympathetic. However, some regions have a greater proportion of private clinics so to include women not residing in a particular area is also confusing!

Estimates of the number of illegal abortions before 1968 vary widely; inevitably we cannot know the numbers accurately as, by their very nature, illegal abortions were clandestine and usually unreported. However, there is ample evidence that illegal abortion was widespread before 1968 and has declined dramatically since (Potts *et al.* 1977).

Since 1968 the role of the GP has changed enormously. The Abortion Act leaves the decision about abortion to doctors and it gives them far more opportunity than before to help a woman decide for herself about the future of her pregnancy. Although GPs differ in their interpretation of the law, the vast majority support the 1967 Act and recognize the improved health that has resulted from it. However, gynaecologists also differ in their interpretation of the law with the result that the availability of NHS abortion varies from one part of the country to another (see Table 7.1). Thus the Abortion Act has not ensured that women can obtain help regardless of where they live and their ability to pay. But it has encouraged women to consider their situation, and to seek help, openly. The GP, who will often know the woman and her family, and who can ensure adequate follow-up, is ideally placed to offer help. The recent purchaser provider split in the NHS gives GPs greater power to demand good NHS abortion services for their patients. In April 1996, all fundholding GPs became responsible for purchasing services. The Birth Control Trust has published a leaflet *Purchasing abortion services*. It outlines the choices available to fundholders to best meet the needs of women, and includes an outline service specification to aid GPs in choosing a high-quality provider.

Statistics

It is not easy to calculate the number of pregnancies that are unwanted. Some are terminated but some are not, so that abortion statistics do not give a true indication of the scale of unwanted pregnancy. For example, Cartwright (1987) found that in 1984, 28% of women having their third child and 38% having their fourth child regretted their pregnancies (i.e. were 'sorry it had happened at all' or 'would rather it had happened later'). The proportion of women who described their pregnancy as unintended was 27% in 1975, and in 1984 was 22% of legitimate births and 27% of all births.

More precise statistics are available for legal abortions (OPCS Abortion Statistics and Scottish Health Statistics). After the implementation of the Abortion Act in 1968 the number of legal abortions rose rapidly in the late 1960s and early 1970s, finally slowing down in 1974 when the number of abortions fell for the first time. The introduction of a free contraceptive service seems to have had an important effect, the rate of abortions falling from 11.4 in 1973 to 10.4 in 1977 per 1000 women aged 15–44. Since then, the overall numbers and rates have increased slowly with only the occasional dip. Various explanations such as increased use of condoms in relation to AIDS and decreased use of the contraceptive pill following 'pill scares' have been suggested. For example, the number of abortions in England and Wales rose by 14.5% during April to June 1996 compared with the same period the year before, following the October 1995 'pill scare'. However, the full reasons are likely to be somewhat more complex.

The abortion rate in Scotland has been consistently lower than in England and Wales (Table 7.2). This is due, at least in part, to the greater difficulty of obtaining an abortion in some parts of Scotland than in England. Thus each year nearly 1000 Scottish women travel south to obtain an abortion in England.

In 1987, approximately one in five pregnancies in England and Wales and one in eight pregnancies in Scotland ended in abortion. However, Britain still has one of the lowest abortion rates of any country with a liberal abortion legislation (see Table 7.3).

Over half of all abortions are now performed on women who are single, nulliparous, and under 25 years of age. However, young single women are more likely to bypass their own doctor and go direct to the private sector, so GPs will see a disproportionate number of older, married parous women requesting abortion.

There has never been a time when the NHS has kept pace with the number of abortions requested (see Table 7.4). At best, in the first flush of the 1967 Act, and now, with increased use of buying in services from the private sector for NHS patients, 67–70% of abortions have been provided by the NHS. This leaves 30–33% being paid for by individual women. We should not assume that those paying for abortions necessarily come from more affluent sectors of the community, in fact there is good evidence to the contrary (Ubido and Ashton 1993).

The provision of NHS abortion varies greatly between regions (Table 7.1), although the overall picture has improved in the last few years. Historically,

Table 7.2 *Legal abortions in Britain (resident women) numbers and rates 1969–95[1]*

	Abortions in England and Wales (resident women)		Abortions in Scotland[2]	
	Number	Rate[3]	Number	Rate[3]
1969	49 829	5.3	3 556	3.5
1971	94 570	10.0	6 856	6.2
1973	110 568	11.4	8 566	7.4
1975	106 224	11.0	8 354	7.1
1977	102 677	10.4	7 139	7.0
1979	119 028	12.0	7 754	7.2
1981	128 581	12.4	9 007	8.3
1983	127 375	11.9	8 459	7.6
1985	141 101	13.0	9 189	8.2
1987	156 191	14.1	9 460	8.4
1989	170 463	13.4	9 460	9.1
1991	167 376	13.1*	11 068	9.9
1993	157 846	12.3	11 072	10.0
1994	156 539	†	11 376	10.3
1995	153 135	†		

[1] For clarity, alternate years only are shown
[2] Figures do not include Scottish women having abortions in England (approximately 1000 each year or one per 1 000 Scottish women aged 15–44 years)
[3] Per 1 000 women aged 15–44
* From 1991 onward rate calculated per 1 000 women aged 14–49
† Not available at time of publication
Source: OPCS Abortion Statistics 1995; Scottish Health Statistics 1995

this regional variation has been attributed to differences in the attitude of gynaecologists (Maresh 1979). In 1992, Francome and Savage used a postal survey to look at the relation between gynaecologists' opinions on the provision of abortion and the service provided by the health service in their district. At the time less than 50% of abortions in England and Wales were being preformed in the NHS; however, fewer than 40% of gynaecologists reported problems in providing abortion services. Twenty-one per cent thought they were providing over 80% of abortions for women who lived in their district whereas only 2% of districts achieved this proportion.

In Scotland, 98% of abortions are performed within the NHS but this is more a reflection of the lack of a private sector in Scotland than an indication of superior NHS resources or of a more liberal interpretation of the law.

In 1972 approximately 80% of abortions had been performed by the 12th week of pregnancy. By 1994 89% were preformed by the 12th week, and just 3.3% were performed after the 16th week.

Fig 7.1 shows that whilst the rates of women having abortions under 16

Table 7.3 *Abortion rates some international comparisons in 1987 (unless otherwise stated)*

	Rate[1]
England and Wales	14.2
Scotland	9.0
Cuba (1988)	58.0
Czechoslovakia	46.7
China	38.8
Singapore	30.1
US (1985)	28.0
Sweden	19.8
Australia (1988)	16.6
Finland	11.7
The Netherlands (1986)	5.3

[1] *Rate per 1000 women aged 15–44*
Source: Henshaw (1990)

has not risen nearly as much since the early 1970s as those in the age range 16–19, the 20–24 year group has increased the most. The teenage abortion rate fell from 17.3 per 1000 in 1992 to 16.5 in 1993 (HMSO 1995). NHS priorities guidance for 1995–96 requires health authorities to achieve further improvements in this area in line with the *Health of the Nation* target which calls for a reduction in 'unwanted pregnancies' (HMSO 1992). Smith (1993) has shown that the rate of teenage pregnancy is three (women under 16) to six (women under 20) times as high in the most deprived areas as in the most affluent areas of Tayside Scotland. The proportion of teenage pregnancies ending in abortions was higher in the affluent areas, where two out of three ended in abortion

Table 7.4 *NHS provision of abortion in England and Wales 1969–95*

Year	Total abortions on resident women	Percentage of total in NHS hospitals	Percentage of total as agency (for NHS)	Percentage of total paid by NHS
1969	44 829	67	–	67
1974	109 445	51	–	51
1979	119 028	46	–	46
1984	136 388	47.5	3.6	51
1989	170 463	41	5	46
1994	156 539	54.5	12.5	67
1995	153 135	54.5	15.8	70.3

Source: OPCS Abortion Statistics 1995

Fig 7.1 *Age-specific abortion rates, residents of England and Wales, 1968–92*
(Source: OCPS Abortion Statistics, AB No. 20)

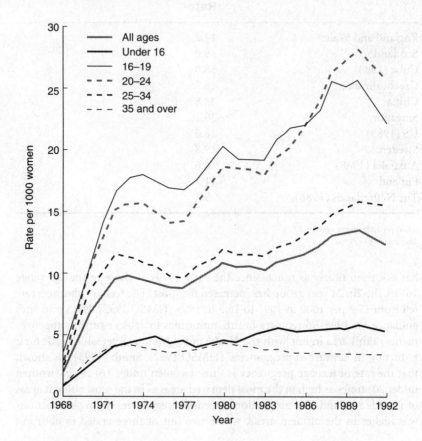

compared with one out of four in the deprived areas. As Peckham (1993) points out, to prevent unintended teenage pregnancy good sex education and access to contraceptive services need to be provided alongside a commitment by central and local government to tackle the adverse socio-economic factors which are associated with teenage pregnancy.

Methods of abortion

Traditionally, methods used in performing abortions divide into those used in the first trimester and those used later in pregnancy (see Fig 7.2). The arrival of mifepristone (RU 486) will widen the choice of methods available for abortion, especially very early abortion, and this will be described first.

Mifepristone (RU 486; Mifegyne)

Progesterone plays a key role in maintaining pregnancy. Mifepristone, an anti-progesterone, binds to progesterone receptors in the uterus, thus blocking the

Fig 7.2 *Methods of abortion according to gestation of pregnancy*

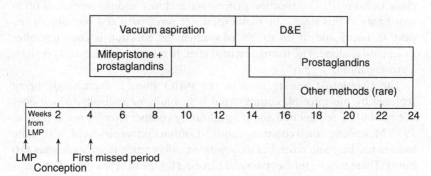

effect of progesterone. Its mode of action also involves increased production of prostaglandins, increased sensitivity of the uterus to prostaglandins, and increased myometrial contractility. Mifepristone has potential as a post-coital contraceptive, to enhance the effects of prostaglandins in second trimester abortions, and to induce abortion in early pregnancy. It was licensed in July 1991 and its main use has been for early medical abortions. Given to women in early pregnancy (up to 9 weeks), mifepristone on its own produces abortion in 40% of pregnancies.

A recent WHO (1993) randomized, double-blind, multi-centre trial compared the abortificant efficiency and side-effects of three single doses of mifepristone (200 mg, 400 mg and 600 mg), followed 48 hours later by a vaginal pessary of 1 mg Gemoprost. There were no significant differences between the doses of mifepristone. The combined results for 1182 women with an early pregnancy (menstrual delay 7–28 days) was of 95.5% complete abortion, 3.7% incomplete abortion, and 0.8% missed abortion and continuing live pregnancies. Apart from breast tenderness, there was no significant difference between the doses of reported side-effects. The use of analgesia varied considerably between the centres involved; in Aberdeen, Edinburgh, and Stockholm 50–60% of women received analgesia, one-half to two-thirds of them were given an opioid preparation. Antibiotics were given to 16 women (1.3%) for suspected pelvic or upper genital tract infection.

At a conference organized by the Birth Control Trust (Williams 1990) it was estimated that 5% of women would need curettage and that the complication rate (pain or bleeding) would be about 3%, that is, similar to conventional methods.

Women need to be screened for contraindications and precautions. The contraindications are: suspected ectopic pregnancy, chronic adrenal failure, long-term corticosteroid therapy, known allergy to mifepristone, haemorrhagic disorders, treatment with anticoagulants, and smokers over the age of 35. It should be used with caution in women with cardiovascular disease or risk factors, women with renal or hepatic failure, women with prosthetic heart valves, and women with pregnancies of 56–63 days gestation.

Mifepristone in the form of 200 mg tablets is taken initially at an approved clinic or hospital. The abortion process starts slowly and the woman is often sent home at this stage. She may experience some pain and bleeding in the next 48 hours and in up to 2% of women the abortion is complete after mifepristone alone. The woman returns after 48 hours and if necessary is given a prostaglandin.

The Gemoprost pessary used in the WHO study is increasingly being replaced by misoprostol, administered both orally or vaginally, which does not need to be refrigerated and is significantly cheaper (Joo Thong and Baird 1992; M. Rees, personal communication). Contractions are induced, with some women needing pain relief; but most women will be ready to go home after 4–6 hours. There may be further pain and bleeding for the next few days. As there is a small chance that abortion will not be induced, follow-up is very important, and this is usually under taken 5–12 days later.

Henshaw (1994) looked at both the efficacy and the acceptability of medical abortion (172 women) compared with surgical abortion (190 women). He found that there was a 98% complete abortion rate for both procedures, but a surgical abortion at this gestation carries an 11 times greater risk of the sac being missed. At 50–63 days the complete abortion rate for medical abortions went down to 92%, whereas surgical abortion retained its 98% rate. Acceptability was greatest in women who chose medical abortions. Women who could not decide and were randomized to either medical or surgical abortion were much more likely to find the method acceptable if they were under 50 days gestation (close to 100%). Of those over 50 days 22% said they would opt for surgery next time.

The law and mifepristone/Gemoprost. At present both mifepristone and the prostaglandin must be administered in an NHS hospital or approved premises. The law does not require the woman to stay during the abortion process but it is likely that regulations will insist on a bed being available for some hours after prostaglandin administration and that there is immediate access to specialist help and theatre facilities. The 1990 Act allows the Minister of Health to recognize premises for medical abortion and it is possible that GPs may be able to administer mifepristone in the future.

Women's experience of mifepristone. As previously cited (Henshaw 1994), the women's choice of method is of major importance to the outcome of her experience, together with the ability to have the procedure before 50 days gestation. A patient information leaflet (see end of chapter for details) is useful backup to give *after* explaining the procedure fully.

Medical termination involves a changing role for doctors and nurses with more active participation by the woman: with surgical termination the operating doctor is terminating the pregnancy; with medical termination the woman is technically initiating the termination when she swallows the mifepristone; however, the medical and nursing team is still needed to supervise and troubleshoot problems.

For mifepristone to become part of abortion provision in this country, an organized early abortion service needs to be implemented. A fast referral system is vital with speedy referral by GPs, (by telephone or fax) and a minimal wait for appointments on the part of the service.

Other methods of first-trimester abortion

Menstrual aspiration. This is the name given to very early abortion performed, usually without anaesthetic, using a fine cannula and vacuum source (large syringe) to evacuate the uterus without dilating the cervix. Before very early pregnancy tests were introduced, this method was sometimes used to evacuate the contents of the uterus at or just after menstruation (Savage and Paterson 1982). With the advent of early testing, menstrual aspiration has a role in the development of a service for very early abortions. There is a small risk at this stage that the fetus will be missed because of its small size, so follow-up is vital. Unfortunately, this method is not widely available today.

Vacuum aspiration. This has been used successfully for some years and can be performed safely until 13 weeks gestation. The cervix is dilated if necessary and the contents of the uterus are evacuated by suction. Early in pregnancy (up to 6 weeks) this can be done with minimal dilation, and even without anaesthetic if the setting is supportive and the woman wishes it. A vacuum aspiration can be carried out under local anaesthetic up to 13 weeks but traditionally most are performed under general anaesthetic. (It is easier for the operator and there is less need to select women carefully.) The procedure is safe and with appropriate arrangements it can be carried out as a day case on women at low risk of complications. When referring women for day care, it is important to know the protocol of the local service to avoid the possibility of refusal. GPs should indicate their willingness, if appropriate, to provide after-care for women undergoing day-care abortions. It may be worth approaching individual gynaecologists on a woman's behalf.

Second-trimester abortion

Dilatation and evacuation. From 13–16 weeks, dilatation and evacuation is the safest method of abortion but is still more widely used in the private sector than in the NHS. It can be unpleasant for staff and is time-consuming to teach. Vaginally-administered prostaglandins have recently been introduced to aid cervical dilatation, and mifepristone has also been used experimentally. This technique in skilled hands is recommended up to 18–20 weeks gestation (Savage 1990).

Prostaglandins. The commonest second trimester method of abortion used in Britain today entails the use of prostaglandins. These are used either extra-amniotically, by instillation through the cervix; or more recently, by inserting prostaglandin pessaries into the vagina; or intra-amniotically via the abdominal wall. Mifepristone is now being used in conjunction with prostaglandin pessaries and appears to shorten the induction/delivery interval and lessen pain and discomfort, as a smaller dose of prostaglandin can be used.

In most medical abortions the uterus starts to contract within a few hours and the fetus is expelled within 8–18 hours. In about 50% of cases the abortion is not complete and evacuation of the uterus under anaesthetic is required.

Other methods. Methods such as hysterotomy are now very rarely used as the side-effects are too great.

Risks of abortion

There is an enormous literature on this subject, much of it difficult to interpret. Research into the long-term consequences of abortion is particularly fraught with difficulties (Savage and Paterson 1982). However, there is agreement on certain matters.

The risks of abortion depend above all on the gestation of pregnancy when the abortion is performed (RCGP/RCOG 1985); and at any gestation the risks also depend on the method used, the age, health, and parity of the woman, and the experience, skill, and attitude of the operator. Thus the incidence of complications will vary from one gynaecological unit to another.

In the RCGP/RCOG attitudes to pregnancy study (1985) of over 6000 women undergoing induced abortion, some morbidity relating to the abortion occurred in 10% of women but in only 2% was this considered to be major. When the requirement of blood transfusion was used to define severe blood loss, major morbidity was reduced to 0.7%, which corresponds closely to figures of 0.7% from two large studies in the US.

The impact of abortion on subsequent fertility has been extensively studied, and a review of the literature (Hogue 1986) reveals that women whose first pregnancy is terminated have no increased risk of subsequent infertility unless their abortion is complicated by pelvic infection. This also applies to risk of ectopic pregnancy. *Chlamydia trachomatis* has been found to have a prevalence of 2–12% in general practice and is higher in inner city populations. Oakeshott and Hay (1995) suggest that where the prevalence is over 6% it may be cost-effective to screen all sexually-active young women. Certainly, prior to abortion it may alert the doctor to preventing a possible cause of later infertility.

Other long-term risks (e.g. recurrent spontaneous abortion or premature delivery due to cervical incompetence) are rare and are less likely with first-trimester abortion. Long-term risks may increase with recurrent abortions and this should be discussed if appropriate.

First-trimester abortion

First-trimester abortion by vacuum aspiration is safe. Major early complications (e.g. perforation of the uterus, haemorrhage, and infection) are uncommon (RCGP/RCOG 1985) and the mortality is very low indeed (one per 100 000 compared to a maternal mortality of eight per 100 000). Retained products can cause bleeding and pain some days after the procedure and this may necessitate readmission to hospital and re-evacuation of the uterus. If a woman has not been screened for sexually-transmitted diseases the possibility of pelvic infection should also be considered.

Second-trimester abortion

There is no doubt that immediate complications of abortion (trauma, haemorrhage, infection, retained products) are more common as gestation of

228

pregnancy increases. With more widespread use of prostaglandins the complication rate has decreased, but it could probably be reduced still further by more use of D & E in skilled hands (Savage 1990). There is no large study of pregnancy outcome in women subsequent to late vaginal terminations but MacKenzie and Fry (1988) found that 104 out of 105 women who had had a previous second trimester prostaglandin abortion succeeded in conceiving.

The lessons for GPs are that women should be referred as soon as possible, that the service should provide minimal delay, and that GPs should get to know which local gynaecologists and agencies can provide a skilled and caring service for their patients.

Psychological risks

Gilchrist *et al.* (1995) published a large prospective study which compares the rate of subsequent psychiatric problems in women who had a termination and those with other outcomes to their unplanned pregnancy. Anonymized comprehensive information was obtained for 13 261 women from 1509 volunteer GPs by the RCGP and RCOG joint study of induced abortions, which began in 1976. There was no difference in rate of reported psychiatric disorder between the two groups.

Many women experience feelings of guilt and sadness immediately after an abortion but these feelings are usually transient and are often accompanied by a marked feeling of relief. Although women having late abortions are more likely to find the procedure distressing, they do not seem to be at greater risk of severe psychological consequences (Brewer 1978). However, women who have been advised to have an abortion for medical reasons are more likely to experience long-term depression (Donnai *et al.* 1981). A retrospective study by Elder and Laurence(1991) of women who had had a second-trimester termination for fetal abnormalities found 77–80% of women described an acute grief reaction. Forty-six per cent of 48 women had not resolved their grief 6 months after the termination. This compared with 25% of 69 women who had had the intervention of skilled support from a genetic fieldworker. Clearly, this is a group of women who underwent abortion for what had been a wanted pregnancy and they obviously need very different support.

Interpreting the 1967 Abortion Act (amended 1990)

The 1967 Abortion Act requires two doctors to decide whether a woman has grounds for abortion. However, doctors vary enormously in their interpretation of the Act and this has been a cause of much controversy. We offer here a liberal view as a basis for discussion.

Doctors who have a conscientious objection to abortion do opt out of signing blue forms (certificate A in Scotland). The BMA regards this as ethically acceptable but legally it is not entirely clear whether it would be carried in a court of law. Their policy (1993) is that 'a patient seeking termination of pregnancy has a right to receive balanced medical counselling from her chosen doctor and a second opinion if she wishes . . . in any circumstances where an individual doctor is unable to do this the patient should be referred to a

Table 7.5 *Grounds for abortion 1993*

Statutory grounds	Mention of each as percentage of all grounds mentioned
(A) Risk to life woman	0.09
(B) To prevent grave permanent injury to physical or mental health of woman	2.2
(C) Risk of injury to physical or mental health of woman (pregnancy **not** more than 24 weeks)	87.6
(D) Risk of injury to physical or mental health of existing child(ren) (pregnancy not more than 24 weeks)	8.8
(E) Substantial risk of child being born seriously handicapped	1.1

Source: OPCS Abortion Statistics 1993

colleague who can'. Any doctor who does not have a conscientious objection to abortion is required by the Abortion Act to make a *clinical* decision concerning, in most cases, the comparative risks of having an abortion or continuing the pregnancy. This decision should not be concerned with whether the woman 'deserves' an abortion or not.

From Table 7.5 it can be seen that most abortions are performed using grounds C and D which require the doctor to make a clinical decision concerning the risk to the physical or mental health of continuing the pregnancy compared to having the pregnancy terminated. If the woman has children already, how will their physical or mental health be affected if the pregnancy continues? What risks will be entailed for **her** if she continues this pregnancy? Here it is important to consider the psychological implications to the woman of having to continue with a pregnancy that is unwanted. How will her circumstances, both 'actual' and 'reasonably foreseeable' be affected if she were to continue with the pregnancy?

Having assessed the risks of continuing the pregnancy, these must be compared to the risks of having an abortion. This will depend, above all, on the stage at which abortion is performed. Nine out of 10 women who request an abortion consult their GP by nine weeks of pregnancy (Cartwright and Lucas 1974); thus nearly all women who request an abortion will be within the first trimester. As discussed earlier, the physical and psychological risks of an abortion performed during the first trimester are very small. Taking into account the risk entailed in having a general anaesthetic, one can say that, for any woman in good health, the risk to her physical and mental health of an abortion during the first trimester is less than the risk of continuing with an unwanted pregnancy. Thus it might be argued that most women requesting an abortion would have grounds under the law. This argument has not been ventilated in court but as Kennedy comments, 'there is no logical answer to it' (Kennedy and Grubb 1989).

However, a few women do not consult their doctor until the second trimester. As pregnancy advances the psychological risks of abortion do not increase but by 10–18 weeks the physical risks probably outweigh those of continuing the pregnancy (see 'Risks of abortion' above). This will vary from unit to unit.

Later in pregnancy the decision is more difficult. However, very few women request an abortion after 20 weeks and there are usually serious reasons for the delay. The law does not make special reference to late abortions but in deciding whether or not to refer a woman for an abortion after 20 weeks, it is worth noting the BMA ethical guidelines on this matter: 'The doctor should recommend or perform termination after 20 weeks only if he is convinced that the health of the woman is seriously threatened, or if there is good reason to believe that the child will be seriously handicapped' (BMA 1984).

The role of the GP today

When a woman consults about an unwanted pregnancy, the emotions felt on both sides sometimes make it difficult for the doctor to offer the help that would be appropriate. The woman may be upset and full of self-blame; her distress may make communication difficult. Or she may appear to be irritatingly over-casual and off-hand. She may try to convince the doctor of her case for abortion or she may talk unrealistically of her plans to care for the child. The doctor may feel annoyed that the woman has conceived so unwisely, perhaps in spite of the contraceptive advice that the doctor has given.

If the emotions on both sides can be accommodated, there is a great deal that the doctor can do to help by:

(1) confirming the pregnancy;
(2) helping the woman to make a decision about the future of her pregnancy;
(3) carrying out the decision;
(4) follow-up.

Each of these will be dealt with in turn.

Confirming the pregnancy

Many women who consult about an unwanted pregnancy are already certain that they are pregnant; some are not. All need to have the pregnancy confirmed and the gestation assessed but this should not be a cause of delay.

It is now possible, using radio-immunoassay techniques, to detect beta-subunit human chorionic gonadotrophin (hCG) in the serum or urine within a few days of conception. Tests detecting β-hCG are now available both for home tests and for use in GPs' surgeries. Most will confirm pregnancy within a few days of a missed period. The older (and cheaper) latex agglutination inhibition test detects hCG in urine at 6 weeks or more amenorrhoea and is more commonly used by hospital laboratories. To make best use of early abortion services, GPs need to offer the newer radio-immune assay techniques in their surgery. The latex agglutination inhibition test can always be used for amenorrhea of more than 6 weeks, although a negative result may then need repeat testing with the newer test.

Although a positive pregnancy test is reliable and false positives are uncommon, a pelvic examination is worthwhile to check gestation. Examination is also worthwhile if the test is negative, as tests can remain negative for some time in a few women, and in some cases can become negative in the second trimester of pregnancy. Examination also helps to exclude other causes of amenorrhoea.

If the test is negative but there is a possibility of pregnancy, the woman should be asked to return for a repeat test after 1 week (bringing an early-morning urine sample), rather than waiting for the next period to be missed. Hormonal preparations designed to induce a withdrawal bleed should never be used. They often produce a withdrawal bleed even if the woman is pregnant, and they may cause congenital abnormalities.

One pitfall for the unwary is the danger of making assumptions. It should not be assumed that a happily married woman will be pleased or that an unmarried teenager will be unhappy to be pregnant. Even before the pregnancy is confirmed it may be worthwhile to ask, 'How would you feel if you were pregnant?'

Helping the woman to make a decision

Once the pregnancy is confirmed, a decision must be made about the future of the pregnancy. Any woman who is pregnant has three possible courses of action: she may continue the pregnancy and keep the baby, she may continue the pregnancy and have the baby adopted, or she may request an abortion. Who should make the decision? This is a controversial area where the needs of the woman, the views of the doctor, and the intention of the law often become confused.

It is possible to untangle these three sometimes conflicting strands by dealing with the decision-making process in two stages. Whatever the views of the doctor and whether or not the law will allow her to carry out the decisions she has made, it is important for the woman to make a realistic decision for herself about what she wants. A woman will gain more self-understanding from making such a decision even when it cannot be carried out than if her decision is dictated by the views of her doctor or by the law. Once the decision has been made, she and her doctor can explore the possibility of carrying out this decision within the limits of the law or the resources available.

In practice, some women seem unwilling to make this decision but seem to want it made for them. They may need positive encouragement to take responsibility for their future. The doctor may be tempted to make a decision for the woman but this should be resisted.

Despite possible initial relief, people feel ultimately demeaned if responsibility is taken from them; they also have a way of undermining decisions that they feel have been imposed on them (Cheetham 1977).

A woman persuaded to have an abortion or to give up her baby for adoption may seem to comply readily with the arrangements made for her but then she may become pregnant again very soon afterwards. A woman who is apparently easily persuaded that she must continue with a pregnancy that she does not want may seek and obtain an abortion elsewhere.

It should be possible for any doctor to help a woman to decide the future of her pregnancy, even if the doctor's views make it difficult to pursue certain courses of action once the decision is made. In order to decide the future of her pregnancy a woman needs:

(1) information about the alternatives available, what they entail and their risks, if any;

(2) an opportunity to explore the implications of these alternatives in the light of her own feelings and attitudes.

In practice, most women have made a decision, sometimes with great difficulty and often with regret, before they consult their GP. Although they may need only information and support, they may also welcome the opportunity to discuss their situation further. Others consult when they are still undecided or they may feel they are being pressured into a decision by someone else. Or there may be other problems that have been brought to light by this pregnancy. Thus, although all women will need information, they will vary greatly in how much other help they need.

Helping a woman in this way is often described as 'pregnancy counselling' (as opposed to 'abortion counselling' which implies that only women requesting an abortion need this help). The need for such counselling was emphasized by the Lane Committee in its report in 1974 and was confirmed by the Department of Health and Social Security in a circular to all health authorities in 1977 (DHSS 1977), where counselling is described as follows:

Counselling should aim to ensure that the pregnant woman has a full opportunity to make a reasoned assessment of her own wishes and circumstances, to obtain any advice she may need in reaching her own decision, and to secure that any after-care facilities including social work help which she may need can be made available. In helping the woman to understand the implications of termination or the continuation of pregnancy, it is essential that counselling should be both non-judgemental and non-directional. It is in no sense a way of putting pressure on the woman either for or against abortion.

The *aims* of pregnancy counselling are:

(1) to enable the woman to reach an informed decision that she will not regret;

(2) to lessen the risk of emotional disturbance whatever decision is reached;

(3) to lessen the risk of a further unwanted pregnancy.

However, counselling can sometimes achieve far more than this. The situation of crisis may help the woman to come to a better understanding of herself and her behaviour, not only about her use of contraception but also about her attitudes to her own sexuality and about difficulties she may have had with relationships. This understanding may help her to learn something from her experience and gain for the future. She may find herself not only better able to avoid a repetition of the circumstances that led to the unwanted pregnancy but also better able to plan and control other aspects of her life. Thus an unwanted pregnancy can be the trigger which leads to positive change and personal growth. Although such gains may rarely be achieved, the potential of such counselling makes it very worthwhile.

Too often, pregnancy counselling is seen as a barrier that a woman must pass through before she can have an abortion. To see counselling in this way is to diminish its purpose and worth.

Discussing the alternatives

However certain a woman seems of her decision, it is important to consider the alternatives with her as this may be the only opportunity that she will have to do this. Most women will have discussed their situation with one or more other people before consulting the doctor and their opinions may be strongly influencing how the woman feels about her pregnancy. Perhaps the most useful role the doctor can play is to offer information and support in an atmosphere free of pressure and free of the constraints that may have limited the woman's ability to think clearly and decide for herself.

Although this chapter is concerned mainly with abortion, we shall deal briefly with some of the factors that will need to be considered by those who wish to continue the pregnancy or at least wish to consider this option.

Keeping the baby. Many women who consult the GP about unwanted pregnancy are married or partnered and already have children; they may have little need of factual information about pregnancy itself but may require information about childcare, child benefits, or housing.

A single woman may have more questions to consider. Is she in a relationship? Is there mutual agreement about a future together? Is there pressure from outside to make it work (to 'get married')? Is this pregnancy a bid to hold a relationship together? Are her parents her main form of support? What form does this take? Perhaps her parents are offering to adopt the child. How would this feel? Can she see it working in the long term?

She will need factual information about finance, housing, and childcare. This is a complicated and specialized area but the doctor may wish to become acquainted with the basic information, especially as it relates to the local situation. The rules concerning benefits change rapidly and up-to-date information is best obtained from leaflets published by the DSS, obtainable from benefit offices, social services departments, or Citizens Advice Bureaux. Information about housing is best obtained from the local housing department, social services department, or from a Shelter Housing Aid Centre. The availability of childcare varies from area to area; there may be day nurseries, private nurseries, or child-minders. A health visitor attached to the practice may have much of this information or it is usually obtainable from the social services department. The National Council for One Parent Families and its Scottish counterpart, one Parent Families, Scotland, are excellent sources of information, support, and sometimes practical help. Gingerbread is a national self-help organization for one-parent families which has many local groups operating day care projects or drop-in information centres. In some areas there are other voluntary organizations which may have some help to offer.

It may be appropriate for the GP to share antenatal care with the hospital so that contact with the woman can be maintained throughout pregnancy; the health visitor should also be involved at an early stage. It is perhaps worth emphasizing the difficulties that still face single mothers today, two-thirds of whom will remain dependent on income support (DSS 1989).

Adoption. In recent years there has been a move away from adoption and, for most women, the choice now lies between abortion and caring for the child themselves. However, some women will choose adoption; often they are women who are morally opposed to abortion but are unable to care for the child themselves, or occasionally they are those who have opted for abortion but this has been refused. Women who wish to have their child adopted should be referred to the local social services department or to an adoption agency. Information about these agencies can be obtained from the British Agencies for Adoption and Fostering. Under the terms of the Child Care Act 1980, adoptions can only be arranged by registered adoption societies, including social services departments, except when the proposed adopter is a relative of the child.

Some women, especially young women, who are forced to leave home may need temporary accommodation during the last few months of pregnancy and for a few weeks after the baby is born. Although they are declining in number, mother-and-baby homes still exist. For example, the Life Care and Housing Trust (set up in 1977 by the anti-abortion organization, Life) offers accommodation to young pregnant women in over 40 areas of the country. However, this accommodation is only temporary and there may be little or no continuing support for the mother even if she decides to keep the baby.

When a woman is considering adoption it is important to remember the risk of depression after the birth. The doctor may feel it appropriate to warn her of this risk and should be aware that she is likely to need support at this time and may not ask for it.

Abortion. A woman who is considering an abortion should be offered information about what the operation involves and the risks entailed (see pp. 230); using models or diagrams, it should be possible to do this in a few minutes. When discussing the risks, it is important to discuss their implications.

The woman should be told how long she will need to be in hospital and what kind of anaesthetic she will have (if this is known). It is helpful to mention the possibility that she may feel sad and weepy or even full of regrets after the abortion and that it will be worthwhile to arrange for someone close to her to be available to offer support at this time.

Exploring feelings and attitudes

Up to this point the doctor has had to concentrate on asking questions and giving information to the pregnant woman. Now a change is needed. The woman needs the opportunity to explore her feelings and attitudes and to discuss any problems that this pregnancy may have brought to light. The purpose is not to offer advice nor to try to make her change her mind but to listen and interpret.

When counselling a pregnant woman, it may help for the doctor to have a check-list of points to cover. Although the majority of women will have few problems, and the discussion may be quite brief, some women may have worries, that they find difficult to express and a check-list may help to reveal these. These are the main points to cover:

1. *Why is this pregnancy unwanted?* If this question is not asked, the wrong assumption may be made. There may be practical difficulties that need to be resolved. Or the woman may have unrealistic fears – about fetal abnormalities or about pain in labour, for example. She may even be seeking reassurance about these worries so that she can continue the pregnancy.

2. *Has she been able to talk to others about her predicament?* Some women may welcome help in discussing their situation with others. For example, a young woman may wish her parents to know but may find it difficult to tell them herself; she may wish the doctor to broach the subject with them. Other women will remain unable to talk to anyone else and they need extra support in tackling whatever they decide to do.

3. *When she first suspected that she might be pregnant, what was her attitude to the pregnancy?* Here one is concerned about the woman's own view of this pregnancy. She may reveal a degree of ambivalence about being pregnant and may need help in understanding this to avoid the danger that whatever decision she makes, she may subsequently feel that it was wrong. If the pregnancy was motivated by a need to change her environment in some way (e.g. by a need for attention or a desire to leave home) she may need help in understanding this and help to deal with her difficulties in other ways.

4. *If she has talked to others, how did they react and what did they suggest she might do?* It is important to check that she is not being pressured into a decision by others. Although she may be influenced by the views of those close to her, ultimately she will need to make her own decision independently of them.

5. *Before she found herself pregnant, what was her view of abortion, of illegitimacy, of adoption, of single parenthood – both in general and for herself?* If she finds herself having to make a decision which does not fit in with her previous views, she may need extra help in coming to terms with her decision. For example, a woman may have strong feelings against abortion, even believing it to be murder, and yet may still request an abortion.

6. *What is the nature of the relationship she is in, if any?* When an unwanted pregnancy occurs in a stable relationship, there may be support available from the partner. However, even the most stable relationship can be threatened by an unwanted pregnancy. Sometimes the pregnancy is used to test the relationship, which is then found to be wanting. If a relationship that was previously seen to be secure has suffered as a result of the crisis, the woman may need help in coming to terms with this.

7. *What is the worst aspect of her present situation?* It is useful to ask this at some stage. She may have worries or fears about her situation that she

finds difficult to express. For a young woman it may be fear of her parents' reaction. Or she may have decided on a course of action but may have some remaining doubts. For example, she may want an abortion but may be worried about the operation or the risk of sterility afterwards. If such doubts and worries can be expressed and dealt with at this stage, they may be less likely to trouble her later.

8. *Has this crisis come out of the blue or does she have other problems with which she needs help?* For many women an unwanted pregnancy is a crisis which upsets an otherwise settled existence; once the crisis has been resolved she may need no further help. For other women an unwanted pregnancy may be just one more disaster in a life full of difficulties of an emotional or practical kind. Such women need ongoing practical help and support after the present crisis is over.

9. *How did this pregnancy happen and how can a further unwanted pregnancy be avoided?* Was this pregnancy the result of contraceptive failure, risk-taking ambivalence, or possibly even a desire to be pregnant? Sometimes her motives will not be clear to the woman herself and she may need help in understanding them. Can she learn from this self-understanding for the future so that she is less likely to find herself in this situation again? Does she need to reconsider her method of contraception or her reasons for not using any? Although these questions need to be tackled at some stage, it may not be appropriate to do so in detail until the immediate crisis has been resolved; this will depend on the woman's feelings and immediate needs. For example, she may find it difficult to consider her need for future contraception if she is not in a relationship. She should not be pressured into making a decision at this stage, particularly not a decision about sterilization (see p. 244).

Who else should be seen?

If the woman agrees to this, it is often appropriate to see others who are involved, such as the woman's partner or parents. This may be helpful to the woman as it may enable her to express feelings to them which she found difficult to do on her own; it may allow her to understand more clearly how these others view her situation. It may also help the others to work through their own distress about the situation or to accept the woman's decision when it is in conflict with their own wishes. Thus it may be useful to see the other(s) both alone and with the woman, but it is always essential to spend some time with the woman alone so that her own views can be aired rather than being overridden by others.

Difficulties with counselling

Although the GP is ideally placed to counsel a woman with an unwanted pregnancy, such counselling is not without difficulties.

Time. On average a GP will see five or six women with an unwanted pregnancy in a year. For the majority of women a discussion of the alternatives is unlikely to take longer than 20–30 minutes. But sometimes this discussion reveals the need for further help which may need to be extended over two or three sessions. It is worthwhile making time for such extended counselling for the few who need it, as it may help them to cope more easily with the decision they make, as well as in the future. But a busy doctor may not be able to make time for this and referral elsewhere may be necessary.

The doctor's attitude. It is difficult to offer help to a woman in reaching her own decision if one hopes to persuade her of one course of action rather than another. Not only can factual information be presented in a misleading way but it is also difficult to encourage a woman to explore her feelings if the doctor cannot accept them. Doctors are usually aware of their attitudes: they may be against abortion in all circumstances or they may feel it is wrong for a young girl to have a baby and care for it herself. Sometimes, however, such attitudes are less easy to recognize as they may not apply in all circumstances. One particular woman may induce a response in the doctor who may then find it difficult to offer her help. For example, a doctor may be irritated by a woman who seems very casual about her request for abortion. In fact, a casual manner often conceals considerable distress; women do not often request an abortion lightly.

Although such negative feelings cannot be avoided altogether, it is important to be aware of the extent to which they affect one's ability to help. It may be helpful to discuss such cases with colleagues.

The woman's response to the doctor's role. Some difficulties with counselling arise from the doctor's role and how the woman perceives this. When the pregnancy is confirmed the woman may feel angry with herself for what has happened and sometimes this anger will be directed at the doctor – the messenger bringing the bad news. The doctor must establish how the pregnancy occurred, an enquiry that may be perceived as criticism, and then must give factual information about the options open and their risks. The next stage is quite different. The doctor will try to create an atmosphere in which the woman can talk freely. But sometimes the woman's anger and the atmosphere created during the early stages of the consultation may make this difficult. It is important to make a clear change from the didactic approach involved in giving information. It may sometimes be appropriate to break off after giving the necessary information and arrange another appointment to discuss things further. This will also give the woman time to absorb the information and to talk to others who may be involved.

Another problem stems from the fact that the doctor is the final arbiter as to whether a woman may have an abortion or not and the woman usually knows this. She may feel that she needs to convince the doctor of her case and this may make it difficult for her to express any doubts that she may have. If the woman is requesting an abortion, it may be appropriate to make a hospital appointment at an early stage. Once an appointment has been made 'a woman will probably be more able to look at her situation calmly, and to acknowledge any doubts she may have, without fearing that the expression of ambivalence will lead to the doctor's refusal to consider abortion any further' (Cheetham 1977). Some women may be so preoccupied with the question of whether they can *get* an abortion that they are quite unable to consider whether they *want* an abortion until the first question has been resolved.

If, in spite of these precautions, a woman still finds it difficult to talk freely to the doctor yet would welcome the opportunity for further discussion, it may be appropriate to refer her elsewhere for help, especially to someone who is not required by law to make the decision.

Special groups

Teenagers. Counselling a teenager with an unwanted pregnancy may present special difficulties.

1. Teenagers are more likely to present late having denied the possibility of pregnancy to themselves or because they fear the reaction of their parents or the doctor (Bury 1984).

2. Abortions, especially late abortions, in young teenagers have an increased risk of causing cervical damage and thus difficulties in future pregnancies (Bury 1984). But pregnancy and childbirth in this age group also carry substantial risks, quite apart from the difficulty that a young woman may have in coping with a child (Huntingford 1981).

3. A young woman may be quite unable to assess realistically her ability to cope with a child and she may even look forward to having a baby whom she believes will offer her the unconditional love that she may have lacked herself.

4. She may wish to have an abortion but without her parents' knowledge. This is always a difficult situation but especially if she is under 16 years. As the legality of performing a termination without parental consent is uncertain, such consent is always advisable and in practice few gynaecologists will perform an abortion on an under-16-year-old without such consent. Conversely, 'a termination should never be carried out in opposition to the girl's wishes even if the parents demand it' (Medical Defence Union 1974).

5. If a teenager comes with her mother it is essential to spend some time with the young woman alone to find out what *she* wants to do; she may have no opportunity to express this while her mother is there. In practice the young woman, her boyfriend, and her parents are often in agreement about the best course of action. But even here it is important that the young woman should be able to feel that she has made this decision for herself. Being given the responsibility for determining her future can then be a stage in her developing maturity rather than a confirmation of her immaturity and dependence.

6. A young woman may have difficulty in accepting her need for contraception even if she is in a stable relationship. This may be partly due to fear of parental disapproval and this should be explored.

Repeat abortion

Women who have had a previous abortion often cause considerable concern. In fact, repeat abortions account for 21 out of every 100 abortions performed (OPCS 1989). In some instances it will be found that the woman has been particularly careless in her use of contraception or that she is particularly ambivalent about pregnancy and she may need help in coming to terms with this. However, such women often differ from other women with an unwanted pregnancy only in that they have more difficulties with contraception – they are often just unlucky (Brewer 1977). The decision about whether a woman has grounds for abortion should depend on her present circumstances and not on whether she has already had an abortion. Although some studies have shown a slightly greater risk of long-term complications after repeat abortions, the significance of this is doubtful (Savage and Paterson 1982).

Some doctors express concern that the increased availability of legal abortion has encouraged women to rely on abortion as an alternative to using contraception, but there is no evidence for this.

Abortion for fetal abnormality

Abortions performed because of a risk of the child being born seriously handicapped (Ground E of the amended 1967 Act) account for only 1.1% of all abortions. They present quite separate problems. The pregnancy is usually planned and wanted; the woman has often undergone an amniocentesis which is, in itself, often associated with anxiety; and the abortion is often performed late in pregnancy, after fetal movements have been felt. It is not surprising therefore, that the risk of long-term depression is greater after such abortions (Elder and Laurence 1991).

Such women need careful counselling, including full information before the abortion and support afterwards. Unfortunately, the GP is not always involved in the decision to abort, nor in the immediate follow-up. However, the GP is in an ideal position to offer long-term support, particularly around the time that the baby would have been born and during a subsequent pregnancy.

Other counselling services

If the doctor does not feel able to counsel the woman, who else can do this? If the practice has an attached counsellor who can accommodate a 'crisis slot' this can be a great asset to everyone. An attached health visitor may be willing to undertake it. She may need some training and, like the doctor, she would need to be aware of her attitudes, but her role in health education and her contact with mothers and young children in the community may make her a very good counsellor. Alternatively, a social worker attached to the practice, at the local gynaecology unit, or social services department may be willing to offer counselling to pregnant women.

In some areas there are other sources of counselling help available; the charitable pregnancy advisory services (BPAS and PAS) have over 30 agencies throughout the country. They offer counselling for a small charge (which for women in some areas is met by the local health authority). There are also Brook Advisory Centres in some areas where pregnancy counselling may be available free of charge. Other voluntary agencies such as Relate, although not specializing in this field, may offer counselling to pregnant women. However, some organizations (e.g. Lifeline) offer 'counselling' which may seek to persuade women to continue with their pregnancy. It is therefore essential to find out what kind of help is offered before referring a woman.

Carrying out the decision

We have already referred to the support that is available for those women who decide to continue their pregnancy. Here we shall be concerned with those women who, after counselling, decide on abortion.

Whom to refer

If a woman wants an abortion it is necessary to consider whether she has grounds within the law. This has already been discussed in the section on interpreting the 1967 Abortion Act (see p. 229).

If the doctor considers that the woman does not have grounds for abortion, this should be explained to her, together with the reasons for this decision. If she is still adamant that she wants an abortion, the doctor may decide to refer her to a gynaecologist for a second opinion. Such a referral should not be used as a means to delay her and she should be warned if the gynaecologist is unlikely to accept her request. Alternatively, the doctor may offer her information about other services where she can seek advice. If, on the other hand, she accepts the doctor's opinion and decides to continue the pregnancy, she may need extra help and support.

Where to refer

If the woman has grounds for an abortion, referral should be made to a gynaecologist who will consider her request sympathetically, and ideally this referral will be to an NHS gynaecologist in a local hospital. So it is essential to know the views of the local gynaecologists. One way to ascertain this on moving to a new area is to telephone the gynaecologist about a woman who is being referred.

The likelihood of a successful NHS referral will vary very much from one region to another (see above, Table 7.1), and in any region will depend on the gestation of pregnancy. For example, some gynaecologists who adopt a fairly liberal policy during the first trimester, will perform no abortions after 12 weeks. Where an NHS referral is unlikely to be successful, the GP may feel it appropriate to refer the woman elsewhere; indeed, the woman herself may prefer this. Few NHS gynaecologists accept referrals from women outside their catchment area, so a referral to the private sector may be necessary.

Within the private sector, the non-profit-making pregnancy advisory services, BPAS and Marie Stopes, have clinics in a number of areas. They are the main contractors of agency work for the NHS and extra contractual referrals can be organised with them. Where there is no charitable clinic nearby, it is necessary to investigate the profit-making services available. Before making a referral to a private clinic, doctors should satisfy themselves about the standard of care offered. In some cases it may be preferable to travel further to obtain a better service.

For women who can afford to pay, referral to the private sector may be speedier (see 'Delays', below), as well as safer. In the RCGP/RCOG study (1985) women having terminations in the private sector encountered a lower morbidity from the operation than women having NHS terminations. This applied particularly to women having an abortion at 13–16 weeks gestation.

How to refer

Some areas (e.g. Newcastle and Edinburgh) operate a centralized referral service (Lawson *et al.* 1976; Glasier and Thong 1991) and others have regional day care units, but in many areas appointments have to be made with individual consultants. Time can be saved by making an appointment by telephone, especially if she wants mifepristone, is close to 12 weeks, or is late in pregnancy; direct contact with a consultant by telephone may be helpful. Appointments should always be made with a named consultant whose views are known. (The consultant with the shortest waiting list for appointments may not do abortions.)

The referral letter should indicate the woman's circumstances, the grounds for abortion, the gestation of pregnancy, and how far counselling has been pursued. If the referring doctor is supporting the request, an abortion certificate (blue form in England and Wales, certificate A in Scotland) should be signed and enclosed. If the request is not being supported, the doctor should say so. While the woman is waiting for her appointment or is awaiting admission to hospital she may welcome further support and this should always be offered.

If the request for abortion is refused, the desirability of another referral should be discussed with the woman; this will often be to the private sector. At any stage some women will change their minds and they may need help in coming to terms with their new decision.

Delays

In general, the earlier an abortion is performed the safer it is; even when a woman consults at 6 weeks, a delay will increase the risks (Roe 1988). Yet women requesting an abortion are often delayed unnecessarily by the medical services. Cartwright and Lucas (1974) found evidence of GPs who delayed deliberately 'in the hope that the pregnancy would be accepted or that it would be too late to get an abortion'. This still happens (Pro Choice Alliance 1991).

Most delays are not deliberate and there are many ways in which they can be avoided, while still allowing ample time for the woman to make a decision. In the RCGP/RCOG study (1985) of over 6000 women undergoing induced abortion, 27% of women having an NHS abortion had to wait at least 3 weeks from first consulting their GP to their operation, compared to 14% of those having their operation in the private sector. The main cause of delay in the NHS was in the wait for an appointment with the gynaecologist, rather than in waiting for the operation.

Follow-up

Careful follow-up is important whatever the outcome of the pregnancy. If a woman is continuing with a problem pregnancy or has had an abortion she may welcome the opportunity to talk further about her feelings. After an abortion or after giving up a child for adoption there may be a period of acute distress when much support will be needed and may not be provided by friends and family.

Although some hospitals and clinics see the woman again for a post-abortion check, some do not. It is advisable that the woman be examined between 2–4 weeks after the abortion to confirm that the abortion has been successful and that she does not have retained products or an infection.

Most women do not experience pain after an abortion. Bleeding usually becomes no more than a pink or brown loss within 1–2 weeks of the abortion, although this loss may continue until the first menstrual period. If the woman has previously had a regular cycle, this period usually comes within 4–5 weeks of the abortion.

Further bright red bleeding with or without clots, approximately 1 week after an abortion and especially if associated with pain and fever, is suggestive of retained products and infection. If the uterus is enlarged, re-admission to hospital for re-evacuation is advisable; alternatively a course of antibiotics may suffice; for example, co-amoxiclav for 1 week as first choice, add metronidazole if especially worried. Use cefuroxime if the woman is allergic to co-amoxiclav.

The pregnancy test sometimes remains positive for a few days after an abortion but should always be negative by 2 weeks afterwards.

At follow-up it is important to consolidate the gains made during counselling. Has this crisis given the woman any insights into her behaviour? Does she need to make any changes in her life to avoid repetition of the circumstances? This may be no more than a need for more efficient contraception but it may involve a more profound exploration of her attitudes and behaviour, requiring several consultations.

The follow-up appointment is often an appropriate time to establish a woman on contraception and most women will be highly motivated to consider contraception at this time. However, some women may not accept their need for contraception and they will require particularly careful follow-up.

It is sometimes appropriate to start contraception earlier than this, at the time of the abortion. An IUD can be inserted immediately after the procedure. Insertion at this time is associated with an increased risk of infection and of expulsion but these risks may be acceptable to the woman if she is anxious to avoid any further risk of pregnancy. Alternatively, the contraceptive pill can be started on the day of the abortion or the following day and many women prefer to do this rather than wait until the first menstrual period. The time to start contraception will often depend on the woman's ability to make a firm decision about her future contraception before the abortion; she may prefer to consider this after the procedure is over. However, it is important to remember – and to emphasize to the woman – that she could conceive within a few days of having an abortion; ovulation may occur as early as 10 days afterwards.

A GP may find it difficult to offer after-care to a woman who has referred herself for an abortion. In fact, it is quite likely that she went elsewhere for help because she did not know how the doctor would respond to her request or, for a young woman, because she feared her parents would find out. Thus the decision to bypass the doctor may reflect the woman's uncertainty and lack of confidence rather than any criticism of the doctor.

Sterilization

Some women who have completed their family and others who do not wish to have children may wish to consider sterilization. Although the unwanted pregnancy may have provoked the need to consider this option, the decision should be made quite independently of the decision about the pregnancy. They involve quite different considerations, and decisions about the long-term future are not easy to make when in a crisis.

It has been suggested that some gynaecologists have on occasion agreed to perform an abortion only on condition that the woman agrees to be sterilized at the same time (Savage 1981). This is clearly unethical. Sterilization performed at the same time as abortion is far more likely to be regretted than when it is performed as an interval procedure; combining sterilization with abortion may also increase the mortality from abortion (Savage 1981; RCGP/RCOG 1985). There are circumstances when it may be appropriate to consider sterilization at the same time as abortion (e.g. when a woman conceives while awaiting a sterilization operation) but she should be told the risks and offered the option of having the sterilization at a later date.

Prevention of unwanted pregnancy

Drife (1991) calculated that one in every three women will have at least one abortion in their lifetime at present rates. A massive problem, which, if the Dutch experience could be followed, could be greatly reduced. The GP has an important role to play here. It requires an understanding of the causes of unwanted pregnancy as well as knowledge of contraceptive practice. These subjects are dealt with in Chapter 5.

Conclusions

GPs will continue to face new ethical dilemmas as the techniques for early abortion become increasingly sophisticated. In the field of *in vitro* fertilization, fetal reduction is becoming almost routine for multiple pregnancies. Now that it is possible selectively to abort one fetus, women with twin pregnancies are occasionally requesting this for psychological reasons as well as for fetal anomalies.

Acknowledgements

I would like to thank Judith Bury, who wrote this chapter for the original edition; Katy Gardner, who worked with me on revising it for the penultimate edition; and Margaret Rees, whose comments on the mifepristone section were invaluable.

The leaflets on early surgical abortion and early medically-induced abortion were written by Margaret Rees, Ian MacKenzie, and Ray Anson, Department of Gynaecology, The Women's Centre, John Radcliffe Hospital, Oxford, and are reproduced with permission.

Useful addresses

Pregnancy testing

Organon Laboratories Ltd,
Cambridge Science Park, Milton Road, Cambridge CB4 4FZ.
(Makers of Pregnosticon.)
Unipath Ltd,
Wade Road, Basingstoke, Hants EG24 8PW.
(Makers of Clearview.)

Pregnancy counselling

Brook Advisory Centre (national office)
165 Grays Inn Road, London WC1X 8UD.
Tel: 0171 713 9000/833 8488

Pregnancy counselling and abortion

British Pregnancy Advisory Service (head office),
Austy Manor, Wootton Wawen, Solihull, West Midlands B95 6DA.
Tel: 01564 793225; Fax: 01564 794935.

Pregnancy Advisory Service,

Calthorpe Nursing Home, 4 Arthur Road, Birmingham B15 2UI.
Tel: 0121 455 7585.

Single parents

National Council for One Parent Families,
255 Kentish Town Road, London NW5 2LX.
Tel: 0171 267 1361.

One Parent Families, Scotland

13 Gayfield Square,
Edinburgh EH1 3NX.
Tel: 0131 556 3899.

Gingerbread

16–17 Clerkenwell Close, London EC1R 0AA.
Tel: 0171 336 8183.

Shelter

88 Old Street, London EC1V 9HU.
Tel: 0171 253 0202.

Adoption

British Agencies for Adoption and Fostering,
Skyline House, 200 Union Street, London SE1 0LX.
Tel: 0171 593 2000.

Fundholding

Birth Control Trust,
16 Mortimer St, London W1N 7RD.
Tel: 0171 580 9360; Fax: 0171 637 1378; (bct @ birthcontrol trust. org. uk).

References and further reading

Birth Control Trust (1980). *Abortion counselling.* Proceedings of a meeting held at the Royal College of Obstertricians and Gynaecologists in 1978.

Brewer, C. (1977). Third time unlucky: a study of women who have had three or more legal abortions. *Journal of Biosocial Science,* **9,** 99–105.

Brewer, C. (1978). Induced abortion after feeling foetal movements: its causes and emotional consequences. *Journal of Biosocial Science,* **10,** 203–8.

British Medical Association (1993) *Medical ethics today: its practice and philosophy,* pp. 103–9. B.M.J. Publishing Group, London.

British Medical Journal (1966). Report by the BMA Special Committee on Therapeutic Abortion. *British Medical Journal,* **2,** 40.

Bury, J. (1984). *Teenage pregnancy in Britain.* Birth Control Trust, London. (Obtainable from BCT, 27–35 Mortimer Street, London W1N 7RJ, price £4.50.)

Cartwright, A. (1987). Trends in family intentions and the use of contraception among recent mothers 1967–81. *Population Trends,* **49,** 31–4.

Cartwright, A. and Lucas, S. (1974). *Survey of abortion patients for the Committee on the Working of the Abortion Act,* Vol. III of the Lane Report. HMSO, London.

Cheetham, J. (1977). *Unwanted pregnancy and counselling.* Routledge & Kegan Paul, London.

Department of Health (1992). *The Health of the Nation: a strategy for health in England.* HMSO, London.

Department of Health (1995) *On the state of the public health 1994,* p. 81. HMSO, London.

Department of Health and Social Security (1977). *Arrangements for counselling of patients seeking abortion.* Health Circular. HC (77) 26.

Department of Social Security (1989). *DSS statistics.* HMSO, London.

Donnai, P., Charles, N., and Harris, R. (1981). Attitudes of patients after 'genetic' termination of pregnancy. *British Medical Journal,* **i,** 621–2.

Drife, J. O. (1991). One in three. *British Medical Journal* **303**: 653.

Elder, S. and Laurence, K. (1991). The impact of supportive intervention after second trimester termination of pregnancy for foetal abnormality. *Prenatal Diagnosis,* **11**(1), 47–54.

Francome, C. and Savage, W. (1992). Gynaecologists' abortion practice. *British Journal of Obstetrics and Gynaecologists,* **99**(2), 153–7.

Gilchrist, A., Hannaford, P., Frank, P., and Kay, C. (1995). Termination of pregnancy and psychiatric morbidity. *British Journal of Psychiatry,* **167,** 243–8.

Glasier, A. and Thong, J. (1991). The establishment of a centralised referral service leads to earlier abortion. *Health Bulletin, Edinburgh.* **49**(5), 254–9.

Hall, M. H. (1990). Changes in the law on abortion. *British Medical Journal,* **301,,** 1109–10.

Henshaw, R. (1994). The acceptability of early medical abortion. In *Mifepristone in practice: running an early medical abortion service* (ed. A. Furedi and D. Paintin), pp. 38–42. Birth Control Trust. London. (Also (1993) *British Medical Journal,* **307,** 714–17)

Henshaw, S. K. (1990). *Induced abortion: a world review.* Allan Guttmacher Institute, New York.

Hogue, C. J. (1986). Impact of abortion on subsequent fecundity. *Clinical Obstetrics and Gynaecology,* **13**(1), 95–103.

Huntingford, P. (1981). The medical and emotional consequences of teenage pregnancy. In *The consequences of teenage sexual activity.* Brook Advisory Centres, London.

Joo Thong, K. and Baird, D. T. (1992). Induction of abortion with mifepristone and misoprostol in early pregnancy. *British Journal of Obstetrics and Gynaecology,* **99,** 1004–7.

Kennedy, I. and Grubb, A. (1989). *Medical law: text and materials.* Butterworth, London.

Lane, Lord Justice (1974). *Report of the Committee on the Working of the abortion Act.* HMSO, London.

Lawson, J. B., Yare, D., Barron, S. L., *et al.* (1976). Management of the abortion problem in an English city. *Lancet,* **ii,** 1288–91.

MacKenzie, I. Z. and Fry, A. (1988). A prospective self-controlled study of fertility after second trimester prostaglandin-induced abortion. *American Journal of Obstetrics and Gynecology,* **158** (5), 1137–40.

Maresh, M. (1979). Regional variation in the provision of NHS gynaecological and abortion services. *Fertility and Contraception,* **3,** 41.

Medical Defence Union (1974). *Consent of treatment.* MDU, London.

Oakeshott, P. and Hay, P. (1995). General practice update: *Chlamydia* infection in women. *British Journal of General Practice*, **45**, 615–20.

OPCS Abortion Statistics Series. AB 1–20, 1974–94.

Peckham, S. (1993). Preventing unintended teenage pregnancies. *Public Health*, **107**, 125–33.

Potts, M., Diggory, P., and Peel, J. (1977). *Abortion*. Cambridge University Press, Cambridge.

Pro Choice Alliance (1991). *Abortion: who decides*. (Obtainable from Pro Choice Alliance, 54 Grange Road, Lewes, Sussex BN71 1TU.)

Roe, J. (ed.) (1988). *Reducing late abortions: access to NHS services in early pregnancy*. Birth Control Trust, London.

RCGP/RCOG (1985). *Induced abortion operations and their early sequelae*. Joint study of the Royal College of General Practitioners and the Royal College of Obstetricians and Gynaecologists. *Journal of the Royal College of General Practitioners*, **35**, 175–80.

Savage, W. (1981). Abortion and sterilisation – should the operation be combined? *British Journal of Family Planning*, **7**, 8–12.

Savage, W. (1990). Late induced abortion. *Contemporary Review of Obstetrics and Gynaecology*, **2**, 163–70.

Savage, W. and Paterson, I. (1982). Abortion: methods and sequelae. *British Journal of Hospital Medicine*, **28**, 364–84.

Scottish Health Statistics 1969–94. HMSO, Edinburgh.

Simms, M. (1977). *Report on non-medical abortion counselling*. Birth Control Trust, London. (Obtainable from BCT, 25–37 Mortimer Street, London W1N 7RJ, price 50p.)

Smith, T. (1993). Influence of socioeconomic factors on attaining targets for reducing teenage pregnancies. *British Medical Journal*, **306**, 1232–5.

Templeton, A. A. and Urquart, D. R. (1990). The efficiency and tolerance of mifepristone and prostaglandin in first trimester termination of pregnancy. UK multicentre trial. *British Journal of Obstetrics and Gynaecology*, **97**, 480–6.

Ubido, J. and Ashton, J. (1993). Small area analysis; abortion statistics. *Journal of Public Health Medicine*, **15**(2), 137–43.

Williams, C. (1990). *The abortion pill (mifepristone/RU 486): widening the choice for women*. Birth Control Trust, London. (Obtainable from BCT, 27–35 Mortimer Street, London W1N 7RJ, price £4.95.)

World Health Organization (1993). Termination of pregnancy with reduced doses of mifepristone. *British Medical Journal*, **307**, 532–7.

Further reading for doctors and patients

Davies, V. (1991). *Abortion and afterwards*. Ashgrove Press, Bath.

Frater, A. and Wright, C. (1986). *Coping with abortion*. Chambers, Edinburgh.

Neustatter, A. with Newson, G. (1986). *Mixed feelings: the experience of abortion*. Pluto, London.

Information leaflet on early medically-induced abortion

It is now possible to have termination of an early pregnancy without an operation rather than surgery with an operation.

The treatment involves:

(1) hospital assessment, examination completing the legal form, and counselling as appropriate;

(2) taking RU 486 tablets at the hospital;

(3) being given a vaginal prostaglandin pessary in hospital 2 days later;

(4) having a final check up 1–2 weeks later with your GP.

How the abortion pill (RU 486) works

You can take RU 486, also known as mifepristone or mifegyne, up to 63 days or 9 weeks after the start of your last period. It's essential to know you are definitely pregnant: so you need to have a pregnancy test, and sometimes an ultrasound scan is necessary. RU 486 works by blocking the action of the hormone which makes the lining of the uterus or womb hold on to the fertilized egg.

The prostaglandin pessary relaxes the cervix and makes the uterus contract: this is like a normal miscarriage.

The treatment

The RU 486 tablets are taken in the hospital; this is the first part of the treatment. You must not take the tablets unless you are completely sure about having a termination. An appointment will be made for you to return to hospital 2 days after taking the tablets.

The 2 days between visits can be spent in the normal way – at home or work. During this time you may experience a little nausea, start to bleed, or have period-like pains. There is a small chance that the miscarriage will occur during this time. If you do have bleeding you should use sanitary pads and not tampons.

At the second visit a small prostaglandin pessary (it is smaller than a tampon) is put into the vagina. This causes contractions which are usually felt as strong period-like pains. You can have painkillers if you need them. Since painkillers may take some time to be fully effective, it is best to take them early on. Bleeding will also begin and you may feel sick and have diarrhoea during this time. Most women miscarry within 4–6 hours of the pessary being given. When you miscarry you will notice largish clots of blood and tissue coming from the vagina, like a very heavy period.

It is not necessary to go to bed or lie down; you may feel more comfortable walking about. It is best to bring something with you to do and to wear comfortable clothes. You are very welcome to bring someone to stay with you while you are at the hospital. You will need to bring sanitary towels (not tampons) and toiletries.

Once the miscarriage or bleeding has settled you will be re-examined. If all is well you can go home providing that someone can take you and that there is someone to stay with you at night. A small number of women do not miscarry in hospital but do so after they have gone home.

About 5 in 100 women treated in this way need to have a minor operation (D&C or scrape) under general anaesthetic to stop continuing bleeding due to some pieces of tissue left behind in the womb.

One woman in 100 will not miscarry. If you do not miscarry, you are strongly advised to have a surgical termination since the treatment you have received may have caused harm to the pregnancy.

Medicines

Some medicines can interfere with the treatment and should not be taken after you have taken the RU 486 tablets. These include painkillers such as aspirin or ibuprofen. Please tell the doctor about any medicines you take.

Smoking/drinking

You should not smoke or drink alcohol for at least 4 days after taking the RU 486 tablets.

What happens afterwards

You may bleed for up to 2 weeks, and some women will have a slight blood loss until their next period starts.

Do not have sexual intercourse until the bleeding has stopped. Do remember to use an effective form of contraception – ask your GP or family planning clinic for advice.

You need to be seen at your GP's surgery, family planning clinic, or the hospital 1–2 weeks later to check that everything is back to normal and these arrangements will be discussed with you.

You may feel low for a short time after the termination but as your body returns to normal this will settle. Look after yourself and give yourself time to recover. If you do feel upset, it often helps to talk to someone about it. Doctors and nurses at your general practice or family planning clinic are there to help you if you need it.

Information leaflet on early surgical abortion

Surgical abortion is carried out under general anaesthetic and is undertaken up to 12 weeks of pregnancy. The operation is usually performed as a day case and does not involve any kind of cutting. The abortion involves:

(1) hospital assessment, examination, completing the legal form, and counselling as appropriate at an outpatient clinic;

(2) admission to the day services unit a few days later;

(3) a short operation under general anaesthetic;

(4) having a final check-up 1–2 weeks later with your GP or at a family planning clinic.

Admission to the Day Services Unit

The following conditions must be fulfilled otherwise it will not be possible to carry out the operation.

1. No food or drink must be taken after midnight the night before your operation.

2. If you normally take tablets or medicines or use inhalers, these should be taken as usual, with only a sip of water. Bring them with you.

3. If you are under 16 years of age you must be brought by a parent or legal guardian.

4. You need to be collected by a responsible adult to take you home by car or taxi and to look after you overnight. You are welcome to bring someone with you to the Day Surgery Unit to sit with you during the day.

What happens during the operation

After you have been admitted, when all the checks have been done, it is sometimes necessary to have a small prostaglandin pessary (it is smaller than a tampon) put into the vagina. It helps to soften the cervix which is opening into the uterus or womb, and reduces the amount of bleeding that occurs. You may experience some cramp-like pains after the pessary is inserted. If you have any doubts about going ahead with the abortion you should tell the nurse looking after you before the pessary is put in.

The general anaesthetic is usually injected through a fine needle into a vein in the back of your hand. As soon as you are asleep, the pregnancy tissue is removed by suction and D&C (dilatation and curettage). The whole procedure only takes a few minutes.

Very rarely the wall of the womb can be damaged (perforation). In most cases no further action will be necessary and the perforation will heal up on its own, but in exceptional circumstances further surgery may be required.

What happens afterwards

When the anaesthetic has worn off you may have some slight pain but this should soon disappear. You may bleed for up to 2 weeks; some women will have a slight blood loss until their next period starts. This is quite normal, but if you have a lot of bleeding, or profuse or mucky discharge, or lasting pain or a temperature you must see a doctor as soon as possible. These symptoms might suggest that you have an infection which will need treating or need to have a D&C. After the abortion you should use sanitary towels instead of tampons until your next regular period.

Do not have sexual intercourse until the bleeding has stopped. Do remember to use an effective form of contraceptive before you resume sexual relations – ask your GP or family planning clinic for advice.

You will need to be seen at your GP's surgery or family planning clinic a few weeks later to check that everything is back to normal and these arrangements will be discussed with you. Very rarely the pregnancy may still continue: if your pregnancy symptoms still persist or you have no period within 6 weeks of the abortion you will need to see a doctor to obtain further advice.

It is very unlikely that your future fertility is damaged. Most women who undergo this operation will have successful pregnancies. It is not possible to guarantee future pregnancy after termination as with any other pregnancy. Very rarely women will fail to have a successful pregnancy and this may be due to a complication of the termination.

You may feel low for a short time after the termination but as your body returns to normal this will settle. Look after yourself and give yourself time to recover. If you do feel upset, it often helps to talk to someone about it. Doctors and nurses at your general practice or family planning clinic and the medical social worker at the hospital are there to help you if you need them.

CHAPTER EIGHT

Infertility and early pregnancy loss

Gillian M. Lockwood

The 'epidemic of infertility'

To paraphrase Tolstoy, 'All fertile couples resemble one another, but all infertile couples are unhappy in their own way'. Since about one in six couples seek specialist help because of difficulty or delay in conceiving a first or subsequent child, the problem of infertility will continue to play a significant and increasing role in the general practitioner's (GP's) consultation load.

There are several reasons for this apparent 'epidemic of infertility'. The human species is relatively inefficient at reproducing itself and Nature offers a fairly narrow window in a woman's life in which she is reasonably fecund. Current demographic trends towards delayed childbearing due to career or financial pressures, in conjunction with a high rate of divorce which results in many women seeking to conceive in a new partnership and at an older age, contribute to this picture. Also the option of adoption, especially adoption of a baby, is no longer available except to a tiny minority of childless couples. This situation is due in part to the wide availability of effective contraception and the provision of legal termination for unwanted pregnancy. Social acceptance of, and financial provision for, unsupported single mothers is another factor here. The media attention given to the conspicuous success of 'state of the art' fertility treatments has also encouraged many couples, who in former years would quietly have tolerated their childlessness or claimed it was voluntary, to request access to investigation and treatment.

The prime role of counselling in infertility care

Fundamental to the treatment of infertility, whether or not 'high-tech' solutions eventually need to be adopted, is the role played by counselling of the infertile couple. It may appear, during the course of investigations, that one or other partner is primarily 'responsible' for their problem of infertility. However, it is vital that the couple's state of childlessness is seen as a 'shared' problem, and the attribution of sole responsibility should be avoided in all but the most overt cases; a position supported by recognition of the fact that in at least one-third of all cases of infertility there are mutifactorial causes predisposing to a fertility problem.

Considered overall, and given ready access to available techniques and resources, it is likely that modern fertility practice can achieve successful pregnancies for about two-thirds of all couples referred. But the appropriate audit of success lies with how the eventually unsuccessful third are treated. If counselling helps the irrevocably childless to accept their state, but makes them aware that their sorrow and disappointment are appreciated and sympathized with – if it makes them feel that all possible avenues of assistance have at least been recognized, even if not explored – then something of great value has been achieved.

Psychological morbidity of infertility

GPs are uniquely placed to recognize the powerful personal drives that operate in the field of infertilty and it is vital that they should not allow themselves to become judgemental when viewing requests for fertility assistance from apparently unpromising or undeserving candidates. In no other field of medicine is the GP so obviously acting as a gatekeeper to facilitate or deny access to medical care. Fertility patients are particularly sensitive to any implication that they are in some sense responsible for their childlessness; they are often suffering anyway from feelings of guilt or remorse, and treating this morbidity with appropriate counselling and sympathy is often just as important as is the ability to diagnose and treat their fertility problem.

Patient autonomy and infertility

Patients seeking help with a fertility problem are quite unusual in that the treatment they seek is elective, optional, and voluntary. They are not 'ill' by any usual definition of illness (although their infertility may have an underlying pathological cause) and yet a medical solution to their 'problem' is likely to have a greater impact on their lives than almost any other medical intervention. Fertility patients need a high level of information about options for investigation and treatment and are often extremely well-informed about their diagnosis and about the therapies that could help them. Fertility patients also differ from 'normal' patients in that their expectations about any course of treatment are likely to be unrealistically high. Achieving successful pregnancy is an 'all or none' event and so 'failure' in any given cycle of treatment (which even with a very successful treatment like IVF occurs in 75% of cycles) results in devastating disappointment. It is simply not possible to have infertilty 'symptoms' improved by anything other than a baby, unlike the case of a less than totally successful operation which may nevertheless provide palliation or improved quality of life.

Fig 8.1 *Graphs of the highest conception rates in a normal population of proven fertility during the first 2 years trying. 'Cumulative' refers to the total who have conceived after any particular length of time. 'Monthly' refers to the proportion conceiving in any particular month amongst those who have not already conceived*

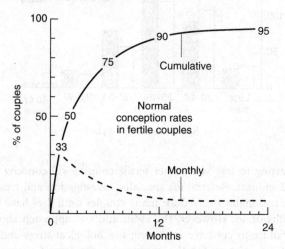

The provision of fertility services within the NHS varies enormously from region to region, reflecting a widely-held belief that fertility treatment is a low priority and scarce resources should be preferentially directed at life-saving and pain-relieving interventions. This view has led inevitably to the proliferation of private provision of fertility care. The relatively recent development of the new reproductive technologies such as *in vitro* fertilization and embryo transfer (IVF-ET) has accelerated this trend and nowadays the vast majority of units offering such treatments are private clinics where patients are fee-paying consumers rather than NHS recipients of medical services. This trend has rightly focused attention on the need for audit of fertility care provision in both the private and public sectors. Drugs for IVF and similar therapies may be prescribed by GPs, but they are expensive (typically £400–600 per treatment cycle) and many practices which do prescribe may set limits to the number of cycles provided. GPs involved in counselling and referring patients must therefore be ever conscious of the need to strike a balance between offering hope to childless couples on the one hand and on the other, not raising unrealistic expectations in the minds of a potentially vulnerable group.

Normal fertility

The graphs (Figs 8.1–8.4) show the basic parameters of fertility within which ultimately all fertility treatment including 'high-tech' treatments must operate. The implications of these data are that the vast majority (90%) of fertile couples where the female partner is aged under 35 will conceive within

Fig 8.2 *Age of women giving birth*

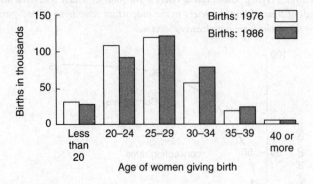

a year of starting to try. Most other fertile couples will conceive during the following 12 months. Referral for specialist investigation and treatment may therefore be reasonably delayed for many couples until they have been trying for 18 months or so. However, this 'wait and try' approach should not be adopted if failure to conceive is causing psychological stress and anxiety, if the infertility is primary for the couple and the female partner is in her mid-thirties or older, or if there are features in the medical histories of either partner (see below) which are suggestive of underlying reproductive pathology.

Causes of infertility

As the pie-chart (Fig 8.5) shows, male factor infertilty, failure to ovulate effectively, and tubal disease are by far the commonest causes of infertility in British couples. Absolute infertility is relatively rare but subfertility is common and, when two or more factors are present (e.g. oligomenorrhoea in the woman

Fig 8.3 *Statistics show that, on average, biological infertility commences 10 years before the menopause in British women*

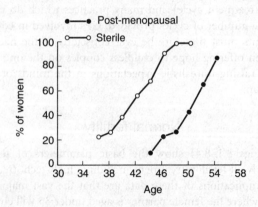

Fig 8.4 *Graph to show declining fertility in North American Hutterites (who are very fertile), Swedes (who are moderately fertile), and Chinese (who are least fertile). Studies clearly show that in each population women over the age of 40 have a sharp decline in fertility*

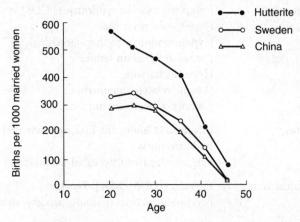

and oligospermia in the man), then the chance of a spontaneous conception occurring becomes very low indeed.

These major categories may be subdivided (as shown in Table 8.1) although, with few exceptions, making a specific diagnosis may not be particularly therapeutically beneficial.

The investigation of infertility in general practice

The problem of infertility can frequently be managed in general practice and, with appropriate investigation, advice, and treatment, many couples will achieve a successful pregnancy without recourse to the specialist fertility clinic.

Fig 8.5 *Causes of infertility in British couples*

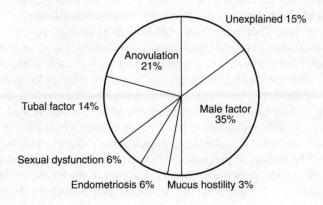

Table 8.1 *Major causes of infertility – subdivided*

Fertility factor	Causes
Anovulation	Polycystic ovarian syndrome (PCOS) Hyperprolactinaemia Hypogonodotrophic hypogonadism Premature ovarian failure Hypopituitarism Weight-related amenorrhoea Exercise-related amenorrhoea
Tubal factor	Infection (*Chlamydia*, PID, appendicitis) Endometriosis Surgical (laparotomy, tubal sterilisation)
Sexual dysfunction	Physical (IDDM, MS, β-blockers) Psychological (loss of libido, anxiety, stress
Mucus hostility	Anti-sperm antibodies Increased mucus viscosity
Male factor	Obstructive azoospermia Severe sperm dysfunction Primary testicular failure Congenital abnormality (cryptorchidism) Post-chemo/radiotherapy Endocrine disturbance Anti-sperm antibodies

General practice is the ideal setting for lifestyle advice about obesity, smoking, and alcohol consumption and for preconception advice about folic acid supplements and diet.

In general practice, the couple's medical records are readily available, often dating back to birth, with a wealth of valuable family medical history which may be highly relevant. These records will contain details of previous operations and diseases in addition to psychological factors. Psychological support is one area where the GP has a great deal to contribute, not least because fertility problems can cause severe stress in a marriage, and it is often difficult for partners to support one another.

During history-taking and routine investigation, factors related to one partner's medical or reproductive history may emerge which are not known by the other partner. For example, eliciting a history of previous undisclosed paternity, termination of pregnancy, STD, or even sterilization may involve a breach of confidence between couples. Early on in the course of infertility consultations, it is therefore vital that an opportunity is made for the partners to be seen separately; and where significant features emerge, patients should be asked if their partners are aware of these facts. In order to provide optimal care, both partners should be encouraged to register with the same GP so that any such issues may be resolved.

The initial consultation

It is frequently the female partner who first raises the issue of delay in conceiving with the GP although the fertility problem may be disguised as concerns over menstrual irregularity or pelvic pain. Ideally, both partners should be present.

It is important to provide both a proposed plan of investigation and to give an outline of the diagnostic procedures that are to be undertaken. A full medical history is then taken including:

 (1) age of both partners;
 (2) duration of infertility;
 (3) previous fertility and pregnancy outcome;
 (4) coital frequency, difficulties, and timing in relation to the 'fertile period';
 (5) medical disorders such as diabetes, thyroid problems, hypertension, anaemia;
 (6) previous history of inflammatory disease of the reproductive tract;
 (7) surgical history of the female – abdominal, pelvic, or cervical surgery;
 (8) surgical history of the male – groin or genital surgery;
 (9) drug history for both partners;
 (10) previous contraceptive use.

Investigations in primary care

Assessment of the menstrual cycle and confirmation of ovulation

It may be assumed that women with regular menstrual cycles in the range 23–35 days ovulate normally most months. Ovulation occurs approximately 14 days prior to the next menstruation and therefore women with particularly short or long cycles need to be aware of their 'fertile period' Serum progesterone will be elevated to at least 30 nmol/l in the mid-luteal phase (day 21 of a 28 day cycle) if ovulation has occurred, but timing of this test is crucial and it is only required if the infertility is long-standing in the presence of regular cycles, or if ovulatory therapy is being undertaken. Basal body temperature charting to identify the tiny rise in temperature which occurs following ovulation, and the use of LH urine testing kits to identify the pre-ovulatory surge in LH are generally both to be discouraged as they are a source of considerable stress and are prone to mistake. Most couples may be reassured that they will maximize their chances of conception by having intercourse every 2–3 days from cycle day 8 to 20. Identifying the 'fertile period' may be readily taught in general practice and the mucus changes associated with the ovulatory phase are recognized by most women (see Fig 8.6). There is little evidence to support the widely-held belief

Fig 8.6 *The ovarian cycle and the 'fertile period'*

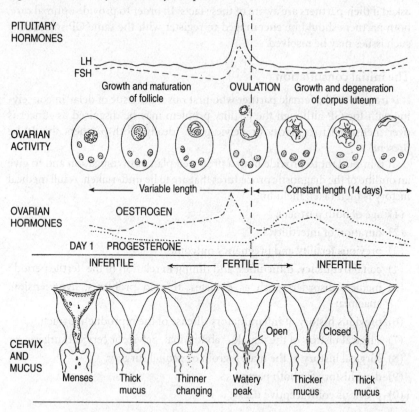

that a prolonged period of abstinence will 'strengthen' poor sperm and since it is the progressive motility rather than the concentration of the sperm that is crucial to its fertility, increasing the frequency of intercourse is likely to prove more helpful to couples with male factor infertility.

Even where the menstrual cycle is regular and normal, endocrine investigations should include serum follicle stimulating hormone (FSH), luteinizing hormone (LH), prolactin (PRL), testosterone, and an assessment of oestrogen status. These hormone assessments may be made from one blood sample taken in the early follicular (day 1–5) phase of the cycle. The main purpose of measuring FSH levels is to exclude primary or secondary ovarian failure in which case the FSH level will be significantly raised (>15 iu). If the LH:FSH ratio is >3 and especially if the testosterone is elevated the diagnosis may be one of polycystic ovarian syndrome (PCOS) and these endocrine abnormalities are most likely to occur in women with oligomenorrhoea (cycle length >42 days), amenorrhoea (absence of periods >6 months), acne, hirsutism and, obesity (Balen *et al.* 1995).

The presence of galactorrhoea may suggest hyperprolactinaemia which is an important cause of secondary amenorrhoea. The interpretation of serum prolactin levels which may be marginally raised (>800 iu/l) is difficult as PRL is a stress hormone and is often elevated by a physical examination, but in fertility patients with hyperprolactinaemia, thyroid function should be assessed as hypothyroidism is associated with this condition. Where PRL is consistently elevated, (>1000 iu/l), CT or MRI scanning of the pituitary fossa should be requested to exclude a pituitary tumour. If the serum PRL is mildly elevated, but the menstrual cycle is regular and ovulatory, there is no need for treatment.

Where a woman complaining of infertility presents with secondary amenorrhoea, a progestogen challenge test will rapidly establish her oestrogen status. The test is based on the principle that an oestrogen-primed endometrium will be shed on progestogen withdrawal. A pregnancy test should be performed first, and if negative, the patient takes 10 mg oral medroxyprogesterone daily for 7 days. The majority of patients with ovulatory dysfunction and PCOS will experience withdrawal bleeding at the end of the course of progestogen and they may then proceed to ovulation induction with oral anti-oestrogens such as clomiphene citrate (see later). A negative progestogen challenge test is suggestive of severe hypothalamic-pituitary dysfunction and this group merit early referral to a specialist unit.

Assessment of the pelvis

Tubal damage and pelvic adhesions are usually due to infection. STDs including *Chlamydia*; ascending endometritis following childbirth, miscarriage, or abortion; complications of IUCDs, etc. can all cause tubal damage. Appendicectomy and other abdominal surgery can also compromise tubal function and this was frequently the case when powdered gloves were favoured by general surgeons. Infection often causes irreversible functional damage to the ciliated tubal lining epithelium and surgical restoration of patency may not be associated with a return of proper tubal function.

Pelvic examination will alert the GP to unexpected tenderness, immobility of the pelvic organs, or swelling in the adnexae. Formal assessment of tubal patency by hysterosalpingogram (HSG), contrast ultrasonography (HyCoSy), or laparoscopy normally requires referral, but some GPs may have access to HSG and this out-patient procedure is a useful screen for 'low-risk' patients. *Chlamydia* serology is a useful screening test of past 'silent' infection indicating likely tubal damage and requiring early laparoscopy. Chlamydial antibodies are quite common in the general population and it is only when raised (immunofluorescence test or IFT titre >1/512) that there is a strong probability of finding otherwise unexpected tubal or pelvic inflammatory damage and adhesions. If a recent infection is suspected, both partners should be treated with a course of doxycycline and erythromycin.

Laparoscopy remains the 'gold standard', not only for the investigation of tubal patency but also because it offers the opportunity for treatment of a range of pelvic pathologies. Tubal patency is checked by passing methylene blue dye through the cervix, and observing its passage through the fallopian tubes. Laparoscopic examination, which is usually a day-case GA procedure, is ideally combined with diagnostic hysteroscopy to exclude intrauterine pathology such as fibroids, septae, adhesions, and polyps. These pathologies have an uncertain impact upon fertility and they are found frequently in the fertile population; however, in the infertile population they are thought to warrant treatment.

The diagnosis of endometriosis is frequently made during infertility investigations, although there is much debate about the relevance of this finding. Clearly, significant endometriosis which has caused structural damage to the fallopian tubes and ovaries can lead to infertility, but it is less clear how milder forms of endometriosis contribute to the problem. Epidemiological studies have shown an increased prevalence of endometriosis in infertile women, but these studies do not indicate whether endometriosis predisposes to infertility or vice versa (Mahmood and Templeton 1990). There is no evidence to date that proves that medical treatment is beneficial in women with mild endometriosis in terms of improving their fertility outcome. Thus, many specialists now regard fertility patients with minimal or mild endometriosis as their only diagnostic finding as having unexplained infertility (Thomas and Cooke 1987).

Investigation of the male in general practice

In a third of infertile couples there is an identifiable defect either in the production or functional competence of sperm and there is evidence of a decline in sperm quality over recent decades (Skakkeback and Keiding 1994). Investigation of the male partner of a couple complaining of infertility in general practice should aim to exclude the relatively few, but sometimes reversible, disorders that may affect sperm and also identify rare, but serious, associated conditions such as testicular tumours. The history should include past STDs, mumps orchitis, history of scrotal, inguinal, prostatic, or bladder neck surgery or testicular injury. The importance of maintaining the testicles at a temperature below body heat by wearing cool, loose-fitting underwear may be stressed, especially to men who drive long distances each year – long-distance lorry drivers have notoriously poor sperm parameters. Enquiry should be made about exposure to toxic agents such as radiation, cytotoxic drugs, chemicals, or drugs affecting spermatogenesis. Excessive smoking and alcohol consumption are well-recognized as reducing sperm quality. Physical examination should include assessment of secondary sexual characteristics, an estimation of testicular size and consistency, a search for varicocele, and assessment of the epididymes and vasa.

The semen analysis is the most important test for the diagnosis of male infertility, and the GP should stress the importance of it being produced into a sterile container after the correct period of abstinence (3–4 days), transported to the laboratory at the correct temperature (a jacket pocket is ideal), within an hour of production. Table 8.2 shows the criteria for a normal, i.e. fertile, semen sample as defined by the World Health Organization (WHO).

A DGH bacteriology laboratory will normally report volume, count, motility, and morphology. More detailed analysis, including computer assisted sperm analysis (CASA) which will provide measurements of straight line and curvilinear velocity, linearity, and lateral head displacement, can be performed by a specialist andrology service. The sperm penetration test (SpermSelect) and

Table 8.2 *WHO criteria for a normal sperm count*

Volume	2 ml or more
pH	7.2–8.0
Count	20×10^6/ml or more (Abnormal= azoospermia [no sperm] or oligozoospermia [reduced numbers])
Motility	50% or more with forward progression, or 25% or more with rapid progression (within 60 minutes of ejaculation) (Abnormal = asthenozoospermia)
Morphology	30% or more normal forms (Abnormal = teratozoospermia) (14% using Kruger strict criteria)
MAR test	Fewer than 10% of sperm with adherent particles
Immunobead test	Fewer than 20% of sperm with adherent particles

sperm preparation through a PERCOLL column can give valuable information about the fertility potential of the sperm, but would only normally be indicated if the initial semen analysis was abnormal. Given the great variability over quite short periods of time of serial analyses, it is vital that no great significance is attached to an isolated low count. Sperm function can only be properly tested in the context of appropriately receptive media such as pre-ovulatory cervical mucus and artificial culture fluids, as used in the 'swim-up' test (see below).

In the event of low or absent (azoospermia) sperm counts, endocrine assessment should include FSH, LH, PRL, and testosterone. If FSH levels are elevated, this suggests end-organ failure. Male patients who present with azoospermia, normal sized testes, and a normal gonadotrophin profile should be referred for a urological opinion, vasogram, and testicular biopsy since some of these patients may have a surgically correctable obstruction.

Antisperm antibodies

The MAR (mixed antiglobulin reaction) test may be performed as a routine part of standard seminal analysis, to screen for antibodies in seminal plasma. It should be requested if the 'sperm count' reports significant 'clumping' or if the proportion of poorly progressive or non-motile sperm is high (asthenozoospermia). This finding is far more significant than a low count (<20 million per ml=oligospermia). Specific assays to detect IgA, IgG, and IgM and their binding sites are available in specialist centres, but a positive result is only likely to be significant if sperm penetration of mucus is affected.

Fig 8.7 *Cumulative conception rates of the most and least successfully treated of the common causes of infertility compared with normal, excluding the use of donor insemination, or IVF, or surgery for reversal of sterilization. (SE=standard error, which is a statistical guide to the confidence limits of a graph)*

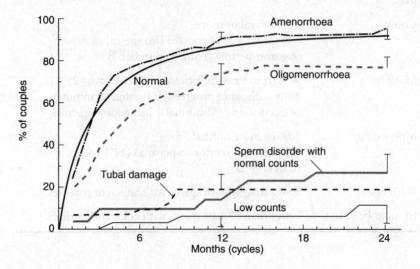

Sperm–mucus interaction

Sperm–mucus interaction can be tested *in vivo* (by the post-coital test, PCT) or *in vitro*. The post-coital test is ideally performed 1 or 2 days prior to ovulation (day 12 in a 28 day cycle) as this is the time that the mucus is well oestrogenized. The patient is instructed to have intercourse the night prior to attending for the test. A sample of cervical mucus is obtained from the cervical os and inspected under the microscope for the presence of motile sperm. A post-coital test is considered normal if the mucus demonstrates good Spinnbarkeit or stretchability, normal ferning pattern, and at least 5 sperm per high power field.

It is clear that the PCT is a particularly demanding investigation for patients and doctors alike! Many couples with a long-standing fertility problem find the stress of having to have intercourse at a particular time very difficult and for the female partner, to then attend for an intimate medical investigation without even being allowed to bathe first, is quite unacceptable. From the technical point of view, if the test is done at the wrong point in the cycle, then the results are uninterpretable. Although the post-coital test has become an integral part of fertility investigations, and may readily and more conveniently be performed in the GP surgery, nevertheless a review of the literature suggests that as an assessment of sperm function, this test is rather inadequate as it has a poor correlation with pregnancy (Covaz *et al.* 1978).

Fertility treatment: a 'ladder of assistance'

Contemporary fertility treatment is best regarded as a 'ladder of assistance', in which the lowest rungs are perhaps the most important, not least because they

Table 8.3 *The 'ladder of assistance'*

Indication	Therapy	
Premature ovarian failure (POF) Menopause Uterine anomaly or absence	'Extraordinary procedures'	Ovum donation surrogacy
Very severe male factor	Micromanipulation IVF Donor insemination (DI)	MESA, TESA* +ICSI*
Blocked tubes Cervical hostility Endometriosis Idiopathic infertility	Extracorporeal fertilization	IVF-ET*
Oglio/asthenozoospermia Anti-sperm antibodies Cervical stenosis	Extracorporeal gamete enhancement	GIFT, ZIFT*, IUI*
Anovulation Oligo-ovulation PCOS	Superovulation Ovulation induction	Anti-oestrogens Gonadotrophins
	2° investigation	Laparoscopy Hysteroscopy HSG, PCT
	1° investigation	Day 21 progesterone Hormone profile Semen analysis
	Counselling and general health advice	

* *MESA = micro-epepdydimal sperm aspiration; TESA = testicular sperm aspiration; ICSI = intracytoplasmic sperm injection; IVF–ET = in-vitro fertilization and embryo transfer; GIFT = gamete intrafallopian transfer; ZIFT = zygote intrafallopian transfer; IUI = intrauterine insemination*

offer significant opportunities for early and successful intervention. The ladder shown in Table 8.3 illustrates the heirarchy of therapies available to the infertile couple, although it must be recognized that treatment has to be guided both by the clinical findings on examination and investigation, and by the couple's own wishes.

The graph above in Fig 8.7 shows the cumulative conception rates resulting from conventional management of couples with a single cause of infertilty, compared with conception rates for the normally fertile. It is clear that the ovulatory disorders and idiopathic or unexplained infertility have the best chance of responding to relatively simple procedures such as ovulation induction and IUI. However, great progress has been made in IVF in the last 5 years, particularly since the introduction of the micromanipulating techniques such as intracytoplasmic sperm injection (ICSI); and now even patients with irremediably blocked fallopian tubes or where there are very severe sperm disorders can be offered a chance of pregnancy that is as good as normal in each cycle of treatment.

Treatment options for infertility

Anovulation and PCOS in general practice

Patients with irregular periods and persistant anovulation may be started on ovulation induction therapy prior to referral to a specialist unit. Clomiphene citrate is the most commonly used anti-oestrogen and it works by boosting endogenous FSH production. The treatment is successful in patients who are adequately oestrogenized (i.e. have a positive progestogen challenge test) but is less successful in hypo-oestrogenic states. Approximately 80% of patients respond to clomiphene with ovulation as monitored by luteal phase progesterone elevation and the onset of regular menses, but only half of these will conceive on clomiphene alone.

The starting dose is usually 50 mg daily for 5 days, beginning on the second day of a spontaneous or induced bleed. If anovulation persists the dose may be doubled, but at doses higher than this the deleterious effect of the anti-oestrogen on the cervical mucus becomes significant. The side-effects of clomiphene therapy include multiple gestation (a sixfold increase in twin pregnancies), vasomotor symptoms such as nausea and hot flushes, weight gain, and, occasionally, visual disturbance which is an indication for stopping treatment at once.

Recently, anxieties have been raised about an association between clomiphene and ovarian cancer (Rossing et al. 1994) and current guidelines restrict the prescription of clomiphene to a maximum of 6–12 cycles. Clomiphene has been quite widely used empirically in cases of unexplained infertility. There are no good studies showing a benefit over placebo for this indication and it should therefore be discouraged.

Gonadotrophin therapy, with daily injections of FSH, is indicated for women with PCOS who have been treated with clomiphene and have repeatedly failed to ovulate, show persistent hypersecretion of LH (>10 iu/l), or have a negative post-coital test due to the effect of anti-oestrogens on cervical mucus. Gonadotrophin therapy carries a significant risk of ovarian hyperstimulation syndrome (OHSS) (see below) and multiple pregnancies and in order to minimize these risks, treatment should only be undertaken at specialist units with appropriate monitoring. Monitoring should include ultrasound scanning of the developing follicles and regular assessment of oestradiol levels. The graphs in Fig 8.8 show the cumulative conception rates for 103 women with PCOS

Fig 8.8 *(a) Cumulative conception rate (CCR); (b) Live birth rate (CLBR) in 103 women with PCOS who did not ovulate with anti-oestrogen therapy. (PCO, polycystic ovaries; HH, hypogonadotrohic hypogonadism; WRA, weight-related amenorrhoea)*

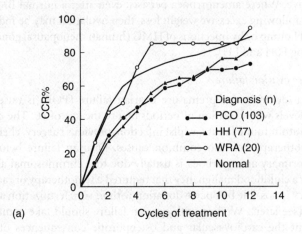

(a)

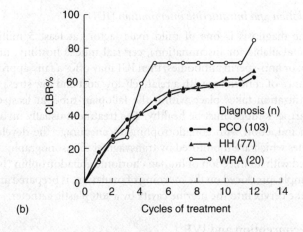

(b)

treated with gonadotrophins who did not ovulate with clomiphene (Balen *et al.* 1994).

Laparoscopic ovarian diathermy (LOD) has replaced wedge resection for clomiphene-resistant women with PCOS (Armar and Lachelin 1993). It is performed as a day-case procedure and is particularly useful where a laparoscopic assessment of the pelvis is required and when the patient is not able to attend the frequent visits required for the intensive monitoring of gonadotrophin therapy.

Weight-related amenorrhoea

Anorexia nervosa accounts for 15–35% of patients with amenorrhoea, and for these women it is essential to encourage weight gain as the main therapy, since embarking upon a pregnancy when seriously underweight greatly increases the risk of intrauterine growth retardation (IUGR). A Body Mass Index (BMI) of at least 20 kg/m^2 should be the goal of amenorrhoeic women who wish to conceive. Where amenorrhoea persists, even after a normal BMI has been regained following excessive weight loss, then ovulation may be induced using the GnRH pump or by injections of HMG (human menopausal gonadotrophin containing FSH and LH).

Premature ovarian failure

The usual definition of premature ovarian failure (POF) is raised gonado-trophin levels with cessation of periods before the age of 40. The commonest cause is autoimmune failure, whilst infection, previous surgery, chemotherapy, and radiotherapy are also common causes. Ovarian failure before puberty causing primary amenorrhoea is usually due to a chromosomal abnormality (70%) or a childhood malignancy that required chemotherapy or radiotherapy. Pregnancy is possible by oocyte donation with *in vitro* fertilization and embryo transfer (see later). Women with ovarian failure should take combined HRT to prevent the cardiovascular and osteoporotic consequences of oestrogen deficiency.

Superovulation and intrauterine insemination (IUI)

Where the diagnosis is one of mild male factor (at least 5 million motile sperm are available for insemination), cervical mucus hostility, unexplained infertility, or anti-sperm antibodies, then IUI may offer a fair (approx 10% per cycle) chance of conceiving with a relatively low cost and low stress technique. Since fertilization takes place within the fallopian tube, at least one of the female partner's tubes must be healthy. The treatment usually involves gentle ovulation induction with gonadotrophins to encourage the development of 2–3 follicles which are monitored by transvaginal ultrasonography. Ovulation is triggered with an injection of human chorionic gonadotrophin (hCG) and a sperm sample, produced on the morning of ovulation, is prepared and inserted through the cervix into the uterine cavity by a soft plastic catheter.

Assisted conception and IVF

The treatment of infertility by assisted conception is one of the most pro-gressive areas of modern medicine. Since the birth of Louise Brown, the world's first test-tube baby, in 1978, there have been enormous advances both in the success rates for assisted conception techniques and in the range of fertility disorders which they can treat. The original indication for IVF was tubal blockage, but it is now used for a wide range of disorders (see Box 8.1).

The technique of IVF

The IVF procedure involves removing one or more eggs from the ovary, fertiliz-ing them in the laboratory with sperm from the male partner and transferring

---

Box 8.1 *Indications for IVF*

- Tubal damage (minor degrees of tubal damage may be amenable to tubal surgery such as laparoscopic adhesiolysis or salpingostomy)
- Unexplained infertility (greater than 3 years duration with no apparent cause identified)
- Endometriosis (moderate and severe disease responds well to IVF although minor disease should be treated initially as 'unexplained')
- Anovulation (failure to conceive after 6–12 cycles of successful ovulation induction suggests an additional cause for the continuing infertility)
- Male factor (moderate degrees of oligo/astheno/teratozoospermia will produce normal fertilization rates of oocytes *in vitro*: men with extremely low numbers of functional sperm or obstructive azoospermia will require micro-assisted fertilization (MAF) techniques such as ICSI)
- Egg donation (POF, gonadal dysgenesis, iatrogenic, carriers of genetic disease, recurrent miscarriage, failed IVF)
- Failed donor sperm insemination (DI)

---

some of the resulting embryos to the womb for implantation and pregnancy. Box 8.2 shows the steps in an IVF treatment cycle.

Embryo cryopreservation

Embryo freezing increases the overall pregnancy rate by 5–10% per cycle. Unfortunately not all 'spare' embryos are suitable for freezing, as poorer quality ones do not withstand the freeze/thaw process. Where the concept of freezing is ethically acceptable to the couple, it should be encouraged as if the fresh cycle is unsuccessful, the use of frozen embryos permits a 'second chance' without further stimulation and oocyte recovery being required; and if the fresh cycle was successful, then the embryo quality (which oftens deteriorates markedly with age) will be frozen at the point that success was achieved. All the evidence available suggests that cryopreservation of embryos is safe for the future child.

Egg donation

Many women have fertility problems that can only be overcome by the use of donated eggs as part of an IVF programme (Abdalla *et al.* 1989). However, there is a scarcity of donors since the treatment requires, that the donor (who may be an altruistic volunteer or a friend or relative of a fertility patient who needs donor eggs) undergoes IVF treatment herself. The donor undergoes conventional IVF treatment up to the point of oocyte collection and in the meantime, the recipient's cycle is coordinated with HRT (for non-functioning ovaries) or GnRH agonist and HRT (for functioning ovaries). The oocytes collected from the donor are then fertilized with sperm from the recipient's partner and the embryos are transferred as normal. If the recipient conceives then HRT needs to be continued until luteo-placental shift has occurred (7–8 weeks).

Box 8.2 *The technique of IVF*

- Downregulation – Drug treatment with a GnRH agonist (daily injections (buserelin) or nasal spray (nafarelin) for 2–3 weeks) to desensitize the pituitary and suppress endogenous FSH and LH secretion. The agonist may be commenced at the start of the cycle (day 2) or in the mid-luteal phase (day 21)
- Ovarian stimulation – daily injections of gonadotrophin (FSH: Metrodin or Orgafol or FSH and LH: Pergonal or Humegon) are given to encourage the recruitment of multiple follicles
- Monitoring of treatment – by transvaginal ultrasound to measure the growth of the follicles and by serial assay of oestradiol to individualize dosages and minimize the risk of ovarian hyperstimulation syndrome (OHSS; see later)
- Ovulatory triggering – the average time for achieving a satisfactory follicular response is about 10 days. When approximately three follicles have reached a diameter of 16 mm, an ovulatory dose of human chorionic gonadotrophin (hCG) is given ('the late-night injection') to complete the maturation of the oocytes within the follicles
- Oocyte retrieval – this was originally carried out at laparoscopy under general anaesthetic, but now, in the majority of cases, it is carried out under ultrasound guidance using a needle passed through the vaginal vault. Intravenous sedo-analgesia is employed (customarily an opiate with a benzodiazepine). Oocyte retrieval is performed 35–36 hours after the ovulatory trigger
- Sperm preparation – the male partner produces a semen specimen and this is prepared either by swim-up into a culture medium or passage through a PERCOLL gradient and centrifugation
- Insemination and embryo culture – insemination is performed 4–6 hours after the oocytes have been retrieved, depending on their maturity. The oocytes are cultured in individual petri dishes and approximately 200 000–400 000 motile sperm are added to each dish. Overnight incubation results in fertilization rate of 65–75% for normal sperm and eggs
- Embryo transfer – a maximum of three embryos are transferred to the womb 48–56 hours after collection at the four-cell stage. 'Embryo transfer' is performed with a fine, soft plastic catheter passed through the cervix into the uterine cavity
- Luteal support – progesterone is given in the form of intramuscular (i.m.) injections (Gestone) or vaginal pessaries (Cyclogest) to overcome the luteolytic effect of the GnRH agonist during the luteal phase of the cycle. Additional oestradiol is not necessary and, if implantation takes place, embryonic hCG will rescue the corpus luteum
- Pregnancy test – relatively few women will bleed sooner than 13 days after embryo transfer (ET). Inviting patients to attend for a formal pregnancy test therefore ensures that early pregnancy monitoring can be instituted for all those with a positive test, and it is a good opportunity to discuss future plans with those couples whose cycle has not worked

Fig 8.9 *ICSI technique. Individual sperm are injected via a microneedle 12 times thinner than a human hair, directly into the centre of the oocyte. The oocyte is stabilized by a holding pipette*

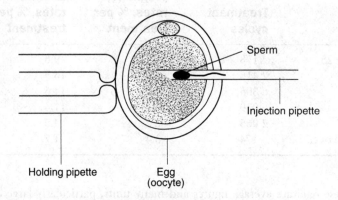

Sperm

Injection pipette

Holding pipette

Egg
(oocyte)

Micro-assisted fertilization (MAF) and IVF

Where there is a history of failed fertilization or very low fertilization rates with conventional IVF, then MAF techniques such as intracytoplasmic sperm injection (ICSI) may be employed. In ICSI, a single sperm is injected directly into the cytoplasm of the oocyte (see Fig 8.9). With this technique, fertilization rates of 70–80% may be expected, and the clinical pregnancy rates per cycle started are comparable with those of good conventional IVF.

Other treatments for male factor infertility

Where the male partner is azoospermic and no sperm can be obtained by either micro-epididymal sperm aspiration (MESA) or testicular sperm aspiration (TESA) for use in IVF with ICSI, then artificial insemination using donor sperm (AID) may be offered.

Where the female partner has normal fertility, the cumulative conception rate in accurately-timed AID cycles is close to that for normally fertile couples, and those who are not successful can proceed to IVF using donor sperm.

Donor insemination requires careful consideration and all couples should be offered counselling to discuss the legal and ethical implications of AID as covered by the Human Fertilization and Embryology Authority (HFEA). Any child conceived as a result of AID is the *legal* offspring of the social father and may be granted access to certain information (but not the identity) of the donor.

Success rates for IVF

The most important statistic for couples considering IVF is the chance that an individual couple has of having a baby following one completed cycle of treatment, the so-called 'take-home baby' rate. Table 8.4 gives the data provided by the HFEA which licenses and inspects all units providing assisted conception treatments.

Table 8.4 *IVF success rates by woman's age (all UK centres)–using own eggs*

Age	Treatment cycles	Clinical pregnancy rates, % per treatment	Livebirth rates, % per treatment
Under 25	178	16.9	9.6
25–29	2 416	22.1	16.5
30–34	6 806	19.0	14.6
35–39	6 039	15.2	11.4
40–44	2 065	8.2	4.5
45 and over	174	3.4	1.7

These data are average figures and many units, particularly large centres associated with research facilities, report much higher success rates (live-birth rates of 20–25% per cycle started). The HFEA now publishes annual 'league tables' giving the success rates for each unit in a standardized format, however not all units offer all types of treatments and many centres have upper age limits or other conditions for acceptance onto a programme. The success of IVF should not be measured by one treatment cycle alone. The cumulative conception rates give a better impression of the extent to which IVF compares favourably with spontaneous conception in the natural menstrual cycle (see Fig 8.10).

Complications associated with IVF treatment

The side-effects of the GnRH agonist treatment include headaches, hot flushes,

Fig 8.10 *Cumulative baby rate, 1987–95 (Oxford Fertility Unit)*

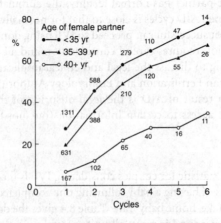

mood swings, and nasal irritation with the nasal spray. Approximately 15% of patients will develop functional follicular cysts whilst taking the agonist, especially if they had prior ovulatory dysfunction. These cysts normally disappear if the agonist administration is continued or they may be aspirated under ultrasound guidance.

Bleeding following oocyte retrieval is usually slight and the rate of infection is very low (<1%).

Ovarian hyperstimulator syndrome (OHSS)

Mild hyperstimulation is a feature of all IVF cycles but severe OHSS occurs in 1–2% of cases and is a medical emergency requiring admission to hospital. Severe OHSS is characterized by the following features in descending order of frequency:

- Gross ovarian enlargement
- ascites
- haemoconcentration
- lectrolyte disorders
- pleural effusion
- clotting disorders
- pericardial effusion.

These symptoms are prolonged if conception occurs and therefore women who appear to be at risk of developing significant OHSS prior to oocyte retrieval should either have their treatment cycle cancelled, or have all their embryos frozen so no embryo transfer (ET) is performed until the symptoms have resolved.

High order multiple pregnancy

The transfer of three embryos at ET maximizes the pregnancy rate, but gives a high (30%+) multiple pregnancy rate. The vast majority are twins, but there are many sets of triplets (see Fig 8.11). Since premature delivery is the most important cause of increased perinatal mortality (70 per 1000 live births) many of these tragedies will be amongst IVF triplets.

In 1992, the perinatal mortality rate (PNMR) in the UK for children conceived after assisted conception was 27.4 per 1000 births compared to a general population figure of 8 per 1000. This is largely attributable to the increased PNMR associated with multiple pregnancies.

Multiple pregnancies have significant consequences which can be assessed at several levels: risks to the mother and her babies, and costs to the community resulting from the distortion these pregnancies produce in the provision of obstetric and neonatal care. There are also less tangible but nevertheless significant risks associated with even successful multiple pregnancies. 'Instant' families, produced by the arrival of triplets, are subject to great psychological, emotional, and financial stress (Botting et al. 1990).

Gamete intrafallopian transfer (GIFT)

GIFT differs from IVF in that the eggs collected from the stimulated ovaries

Fig 8.11 *IVF cycle outcomes (Oxford Fertility Unit)*

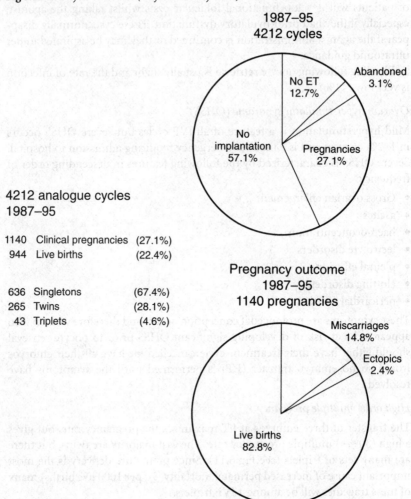

1987–95
4212 cycles

No ET
12.7%

Abandoned
3.1%

No
implantation
57.1%

Pregnancies
27.1%

4212 analogue cycles
1987–95

1140	Clinical pregnancies	(27.1%)
944	Live births	(22.4%)
636	Singletons	(67.4%)
265	Twins	(28.1%)
43	Triplets	(4.6%)

Pregnancy outcome
1987–95
1140 pregnancies

Miscarriages
14.8%

Ectopics
2.4%

Live births
82.8%

are transferred to the fallopian tubes together with a small sample of prepared sperm immediately after collection. Egg collection and transfer of a maximum of three eggs are carried out laparoscopically under general anaesthetic, so unlike IVF, fertilization takes place in its natural environment in the fallopian tube. GIFT, like IVF, has proved a very successful assisted conception technique and because no laboratory fertilization or embryo culture is required, GIFT can be performed in non-specialist units. However, the requirement for general anaesthesia can make GIFT more expensive than IVF (which generally has a better success rate), and its use is restricted to women with totally healthy fallopian tubes and where the sperm has previous proven fertilizing ability.

Zygote intrafallopian transfer (ZIFT)

ZIFT is a combination of IVF and GIFT in which stimulation and egg retrieval are carried out as for IVF, with fertilization occuring *in vitro* in the laboratory, but the resulting zygotes are replaced into the fallopian tubes at laparoscopy before cell division to the 4–6 cell pre-embryo stage has occurred. ZIFT is reserved for situations in which it is important to establish that fertilization has taken place, and where cervical transfer of the embryos is difficult.

Spontaneous and recurrent miscarriage

Reference has already been made to the relative subfertility of the human species. In fact, its seems that only about half of all successfully fertilized eggs ever result in a live birth. The weak link in the chain occurs at the stage of implantation, as is shown by IVF where two or three apparently normal embryos are transferred to an appropriately prepared uterus and yet only 30–40% of women undergoing embryo transfer will get a positive pregnancy test, let alone a baby.

Box 8.3 *Causes of spontaneous abortion*

- Chromosomal abnormalities – approx 50% of first-trimester abortions are chromosomally abnormal
- Placental abnormalities – ischaemia and retroplacental haemorrhage
- Infection – *Listeria, Campylobacter, Brucella,* cytomegalovirus, rubella, and herpes simplex
- Uterine – congenital anomalies such as bicornuate uterus, septae, DES
- Endocrine – PCOS
- Immunological – SLE, anti-phospholipid antibodies
- Cervical incompetence – cone biopsy, repeated mid-trimester terminations

---

Spontaneous miscarriage

In spontaneous conceptions, following a missed period and positive pregnancy test, approximately 15–20% will end in the early weeks with a heavier than average bleed (although some women may not be aware of the pregnancy having ended as they may have no bleeding and still 'feel pregnant' – a 'missed abortion'). If these miscarriages are very early, the woman may not even realize that she was pregnant and just report a delayed and heavier than usual period.

Early pregnancy losses are, technically, abortions, but the association of this word with deliberate termination of pregnancy is so close that clinicians should always use the term miscarriage, however early the pregnancy loss occurred. Women with PCOS and a raised LH level in the follicular phase (>10 iu) have a higher incidence of first-trimester pregnancy loss. The frequency of PCOS in recurrent aborters is 82% compared with 23% in normal pregnancies. Trials have so far failed to demonstrate that lowering the periconceptual LH level in these women improves their pregnancy outcome. Box 8.3 lists the causes of spontaneous abortion.

Whenever tissue from early pregnancy failures is available for cytogenetic analysis, as is the case where the woman is admitted for an evacuation of retained products of conception (ERPOC) because of prolonged bleeding, incomplete abortion, or 'missed abortion', the chromosomal structure of the conceptus is often very abnormal. It is obviously helpful to the couple to be able to tell them that the pregnancy was doomed from the outset and also that there is no reason to believe that it is more likely than average to occur in subsequent pregnancies.

Recurrent miscarriage

Recurrent miscarriage is defined as three consecutive miscarriages. By chance alone one in 25 women will suffer two early miscarriages in a row and one in 125 will suffer three. However, if subfertility has been an associated feature, with long delays between failed conceptions, or if there is a family history of miscarriage, it is reasonable to arrange a recurrent miscarriage screen. Most tertiary referral centres have a recurrent miscarriage clinic often associated with their fertility or high-risk pregnancy clinics and patients should be referred after three miscarriages or sooner if there is an associated fertility problem.

Numerous treatments for recurrent miscarriage have been tried including passive immunization with paternal WBCs, suppression of LH with GnRH analogues, high-dose progesterone, prednisolone, and IVF. None of these therapies has proved more successful than close monitoring with frequent hospital visits at a dedicated clinic. Low-dose aspirin and heparin combined has been shown to help in recurrent pregnancy loss due to anti-phospholipid antibodies.

Management of bleeding in early pregnancy

The management of threatened abortion (bleeding, minimal pain, closed cervix) is rest followed by an ultrasound scan (USS) to confirm viability. No treatment has been shown to be effective, but the risk of abortion following a positive USS (i.e. a beating foetal heart seen *in utero*) is a reassuring 5%.

Inevitable abortion (heavy bleeding, pain, open cervix) and incomplete abortion (bleeding with products of conception seen on USS) have historically been treated surgically with curettage; however, the evidence from a recent prospective study of expectant management (Nielsen and Hahlin 1995) suggests that in the vast majority of cases surgical intervention is unnecessary and spontaneous resolution within a few days may be expected.

Missed abortion (failure of embryonic growth in spite of placental function) may be associated with a brown discharge and reduced or minimal pregnancy symptoms. Pelvic examination will suggest a uterus smaller than expected and USS will reveal an empty gestational sac. Although spontaneous resolution will occur in the majority of cases within 2 weeks, evacuation of retained products of conception (ERPOC) is often advised because many women, but especially fertility patients, find this state of 'obstetric limbo' upsetting.

Ectopic pregnancy **must** be excluded in any woman presenting with pain and abnormal vaginal bleeding. Predisposing factors include previous ectopic pregnancy, congenital anomalies of the reproductive tract, previous tubal surgery, previous PID, progestogen contraceptives, and IVF and GIFT. A positive pregnancy test and an USS showing an empty uterus with free fluid with or without an adnexal mass is 93% predictive of an ectopic.

Rhesus isoimmunization following the sensitization of a rhesus-negative woman by fetal red cells positive for the rhesus antigen can occur after even very early pregnancy loss. All women who have bleeding in pregnancy should have serum examined for rhesus antigen and rhesus-negative women should receive anti-D γ globulin within 3 days.

Life after miscarriage

The advice often meted out to 'wait a few months for the cycle to settle' before trying again after a miscarriage is profoundly misguided. It was presumably felt that any uncertainty about the exact date of a 'last menstrual period' would complicate the obstetric management of a subsequent pregnancy. But USS can give a very precise dating of the pregnancy and there seems to be good evidence for a 'rebound' enhancement of fertility in the months immediately following an early pregnancy loss. Fertility patients inevitably find the disappointment of a miscarriage much harder to bear and this psychological stress is compounded if they are discouraged from trying soon for another pregnancy.

Current controversies in assisted conception

The very rapid developments in reproductive medicine and science made during the last two decades have resulted in a fierce debate between practitioners who wish to utilize the new reproductive technologies for the benefit of childless couples and others in society who are concerned that the existence of such techniques will lead inevitably to their application in ways that are unacceptable to the wider public.

Recent controversies have involved the fate of frozen embryos whose genetic 'parents' could not be traced by the clinics where they were being stored, the use of 'selective reduction' to reduce the number of fetuses in ongoing multiple pregnancies, the use of 'sex selection' of IVF embryos prior to transfer, and the use in treatment and research of donated ovarian tissue from cadavers and aborted fetuses.

Since 1 August 1991, all IVF and donor insemination (DI) centres have been licensed and regulated by the Human Fertilization and Embryology Authority (HFEA). The Authority was established by the Human Fertilization and Embryology Act 1990, which attempted to legislate for concerns about the creation and use of human embryos outside the body, and about the storage and use of genetic material for the treatment of others. Other aspects of the legislation were aimed at the concern for, and protection of, the interests of the patient, egg, or sperm donor and the child or children that may be born as a result of treatment, including the possible need for the child to have some knowledge of his or her genetic origins.

The legislation requires centres offering treatments such as IVF to take into account 'the welfare of any child who may be born as a result of the treatment (including the need of that child for a father), and of any other child who may be affected by the birth'. This may mean that the patient's GP will be asked to offer an opinion as to whether or not the couple should be treated. The HFEA does not preclude any particular category of patient from receiving treatment nor does it set an age limit on who should be treated, but it gives guidance on factors to be considered:

(1) the commitment of the woman and her partner to having and bringing up children;

(2) their ages and medical histories;

(3) any risk of harm to any child who may be born, including the risk of inherited disorders;

(4) the effect of a new baby on any existing child in the family.

It may be considered, that as the five-sixths of the population who do not require medical help to conceive, also do not have to convince anybody of their suitability to become parents, it is an unwarrantable intrusion to impose these conditions on treatment centres and hence on their patients. However, centres are generally considered to allow a fair and unprejudiced assessment of patients. It is more often the financial restrictions that, with few regional exceptions, limit access to assisted conception to those who can afford to purchase treatment in the private sector that are seen as a greater source of inequity.

Coming to terms with childlessness

The very conspicuous success of many of the new reproductive technologies in treating what was until recently incurable infertility has made it particularly difficult for many couples to accept that *they* are not going to succeed. Some couples doggedly pursue treatments, feeling that they cannot move beyond their infertility until they have 'tried everything', and with the rapid development of new treatments, the decision to end treatment altogether may become almost impossible to take.

Valuable work can be done in this context by specialist infertility counsellors, and the HFEA Code of Practice (1991), which applies to all fertility units offering IVF or treatments using donated gametes, specifies that three distinct types of counselling (implications counselling, support counselling, and therapeutic counselling) should be available for all fertility patients if they want it. It is difficult, however, not to empathize with the young woman whose third cycle of IVF had just failed who shouted in anguish, 'I don't want counselling, I want a baby!'

The following organizations provide useful information and support for people with fertility problems.

ISSUE (the national fertility association), Unit 9, 509 Aldridge Road, Great Barr, Birmingham B44 8NA.

CHILD, Room 219, Caledonian House, 98 The Centre, Feltham, Middlesex TW13 4BH.

The Miscarriage Association, PO Box 24, Ossett, West Yorkshire WF5 9XG.

British Agencies for Adoption and Fostering (BAAF), 11 Southwark Street, London SE1 1RQ.

References and further reading

Abdalla, H. I., *et al.* (1989). Pregnancy in women with premature ovarian failure using tubal and intrauterine transfer of cryopreserved zygotes. *British Journal of Obstetrics and Gynaecology*, **96**, 1071–5.

Armar, N. A. and Lachelin, G. C. L. (1993). Laparoscopic ovarian diathermy: an effective treatment for anti-oestrogen resistant anovulatory infertility in women with polycystic ovaries. *British Journal of Obstetrics and Gynaecology*, **100**, 161–4.

Balen, A. H., *et al.* (1994). Cumulative conception and live birth rates after the treatment of anovulatory infertility. *Human Reproduction*, **9**, 1563–70.

Balen, A. H., *et al.* (1995). Polycystic ovary syndrome: the spectrum of the disorder in 1741 patients. *Human Reproduction*, **10**, 2107–11.

Botting, B. J., *et al.* (ed.) (1990). *Three, four and more. A study of triplet and higher order births*. HMSO, London.

Covaz, G. T., *et al.* (1978). The post-coital test – what is normal? *British Medical Journal*, **1**, 8118.

Mahmood, T. A. and Templeton, A. (1990), Pathophysiology of mild endometriosis: review of literature. *Human Reproduction*, **5**, 765–84.

Nielsen, S. and Hahlin, M. (1995). Expectant management of first-trimester spontaneous abortion. *Lancet*, **345**, 84–5.

Rossing, M. D. V. M., *et al.* (1994). Ovarian tumours in a cohort of infertile women. *New England Journal of Medicine*, **331**, 771–6.

Skakkeback, N. E. and Keiding, N. (1994). Changes in semen and the testis. *British Medical Journal*, **309**, 1316–17.

Thomas, E. J. and Cooke, I. (1987). Successful treatment of asymptomatic endometriosis: does it benefit infertile women? *British Medical Journal of Clinical Research*, **294**, 1117–19.

CHAPTER NINE

Premenstrual syndrome

Katy Gardner and Diana Sanders

Premenstrual syndrome (PMS) has received much publicity, in both the lay and medical press. Although there is still debate over the syndrome's definition, aetiology, and treatment, nowadays there is a greater understanding of PMS and a range of ways of managing the problem. It is a complex and fascinating topic which raises many questions about the interactions between hormones and physiological changes and life events and stress; and it is no wonder that many women, and their general practitioners (GPs), feel bewildered as to how to deal with it. Women are taking an active and positive role in acquiring knowledge and information about health issues and many women today recognize that PMS is a problem for them and are taking steps to try to deal with it. With information, patience, and encouragement, women can work out ways of helping themselves, but may also come to seek medical advice from their GP.

Definition

Many women notice changes in their emotional and physical feelings during the menstrual cycle. While for the majority such changes are acceptable, for others they are distressing. These distressing premenstrual changes have recently been described as 'premenstrual syndrome' rather than as 'premenstrual tension', in recognition of the variable nature of the symptoms which may not always include tension. The definition of PMS has been fraught with problems, since the type of symptoms and their severity can vary enormously, both between women and between cycles for individual women. There are a number of definitions of PMS available, including Magos's (1990): '. . . distressing physical, psychological and behavioural symptoms not caused by organic disease which regularly recur during the same phase of the menstrual cycle and which significantly regress or disappear during the remainder of the cycle'; and O'Brien's (1990): '. . . a disorder of non-specific somatic, psychological or behavioural symptoms recurring in the premenstrual phase of the menstrual cycle. Symptoms must resolve completely by the end of menstruation leaving a symptom-free week. The symptoms should be of sufficient

---

Box 9.1 *Features of premenstrual syndrome*

General

1. Symptoms occur 1–14 days before menstruation begins
2. Symptoms disappear at, or shortly after, the onset of menstrual bleeding
3. The woman feels well for the rest of the cycle
4. Symptoms occur regularly, for most menstrual cycles
5. PMS causes distress and possibly other problems, such as with relationships

Symptoms

Physical changes
- Breast tenderness
- Swelling or bloated feelings, possibly with swollen face, abdomen, or fingers
- Headaches
- Appetite changes
- Carbohydrate cravings
- Acne or skin rashes
- Constipation or diarrhoea
- Palpitations
- Changes in sleep
- Muscular stiffness or aches and pains
- Abdominal pains or cramps
- Backache
- Exacerbation of epilepsy, migraines, asthma, rhinitis, urticaria

Psychological changes
- Depression or feeling low
- Feeling upset
- Tiredness, lethargy, or fatigue
- Tension or unease
- Anxiety
- Irritability
- Clumsiness or poor coordination
- Difficulty concentrating
- Changes in sexual interest

---

severity to produce social, family or occupational disruption. Symptoms must have occurred in at least four of the six previous menstrual cycles'. Over 150 symptoms have been described; common features are shown in Box 9.1. Some women notice only mood changes, others only physical symptoms, but it is more common for both to be experienced together. Although different subtypes of PMS have been defined (Abraham 1983), the distinction between types of PMS remains arbitrary and based on clinical observations, and in general individual women tend to report their own unique combination of symptoms.

Recently, a subgroup of women who have severe, predominantly mood-related symptoms has been defined in the appendix of the American Association's Diagnostic and Statistical Manual (DSM IV; 1994) as having a possible psychiatric condition requiring further study. This has been classified as 'late

Fig 9.1 *A menstrual diary*

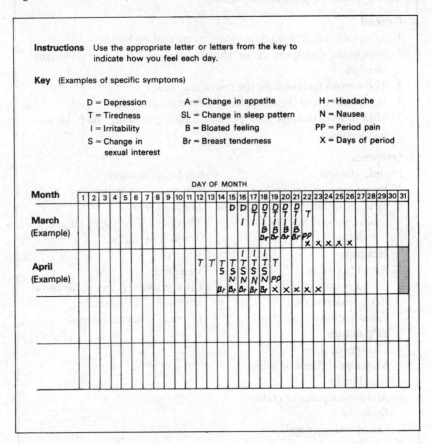

luteal phase dysphoric disorder or premenstrual dysphoric disorder'. While being yet another medical label for women, this may be helpful with regard to management approaches (see later).

Distressing changes may start up to 14 days before menstruation, although it is more common for the symptoms to last for up to a week, and disappear at or shortly after the start of menstrual bleeding. Many women say that the severity varies from cycle to cycle, depending on general life events or stresses. The most important defining feature of PMS is the appearance of symptoms in the luteal phase and disappearance at menstruation; until the timing in relation to menstruation is established, PMS can be confused with more general problems such as anxiety or depression, and may be misdiagnosed or mistreated. Hence, the first step in diagnosis is careful and regular symptom recording to establish the nature and timing of the problems. Women should be asked to complete menstrual charts, recording their moods, feelings, and symptoms for at least two cycles. Various menstrual diaries are available (Fig 9.1), or a simple practical alternative is the self-assessment disc, the PM-cator (Magos and Studd 1988).

Prevalence

It is hard to evaluate how many women experience PMS since the distinction between PMS and more common, but less severe, cyclical changes is not always clear. Epidemiological studies indicate that between 75–90% of ovulating women experience cyclical changes at least some time in their lives. For many these are in no way a problem. They can indeed be a positive part of their lives and could be regarded as normal 'physiological' aspects of the menstrual cycle. Logue and Moos (1988) found that between 5–15% of women actually feel better in the premenstrual phase, experiencing increased well-being, energy, and activities before menstruation. For other women, however, premenstrual changes are upsetting but not devastating, and Sampson (1989) refers to such changes as 'premenstrual vulnerability' rather than PMS. Severe and distressing PMS leading a woman to seek advice is less common. Johnson (1987) estimates that while about 20–30% of women experience PMS as a problem for which they have sought various kinds of self-help and may have tried treatment from their GP, for about 10% PMS is severe and disabling. This leads to a significant number of consultations for PMS in the surgery. It is likely that what brings a woman to seek medical help is the effect of PMS on her life. Women seek help when symptoms interfere with personal, home, or working life, and in particular with relationships with family, children, partner, friends, or colleagues.

Effects of PMS

PMS is undoubtedly distressing for many women, not only for themselves but also for those around them. Women with small children too young to understand PMS may feel extra stress and be worried about the effect their feelings are having on their children. Cyclical mood changes, particularly if seemingly unpredictable, may be a problem in relationships with a partner, unless PMS is discussed, understood, and accepted. Women whose colleagues at work are unsympathetic and dismiss suggestions or complaints on their part as 'it's that time of the month again' will obviously find PMS hard to bear. Women often worry that their performance at work may be impaired before menstruation but studies have shown that this is largely not the case (Johnson 1987; Cockerill *et al.* 1994), and that many women who suffer with PMS organize their work and home life so that they avoid stressful events premenstrually. Evidence suggests, however, that women who are admitted to psychiatric hospital, attempt suicide, or commit crimes are more likely to be in the luteal phase of their cycle. This is not to say that all premenstrual women are at risk of these events, but women who are likely to require psychiatric admission or commit crimes, and who experience PMS, may be more vulnerable in the premenstrual phase.

PMS may well influence women's sexuality, and there is no doubt that mood changes interact with sexual feelings. A woman who experiences severe premenstrual tiredness or breast tenderness may find this reduces her interest in sexual activities before menstruation, although sexual interest may well increase after menstruation once she feels an improvement in well-being. However, some women feel more sexually interested in the premenstrual phase. Fluctuations in sexual interest may cause worry to women, and possible problems in relationships unless links to the menstrual cycle are understood. Problems of varying sexual interest, linked to PMS, may be one reason for consulting the GP.

Who experiences PMS?

There appears to be no distinctive 'type' of woman likely to experience PMS, although in general it appears to be more common in women in their thirties and forties and in women who have children. Certain events may be linked to the onset of PMS, such as stopping the oral contraceptive pill, the birth of a child, or sterilization. The observation that PMS may often occur for the first time after the birth of a child raises the question of whether the stress of having a child precipitates or exacerbates PMS or whether there is some hormonal connection (Brush 1985). PMS can still be experienced following hysterectomy if the ovaries remain (Bäckström *et al.* 1981). Women who are experiencing severe period problems, such as menorrhagia or dysmenorrhoea, may also experience PMS in anticipation of bad times to come. Once the menstrual problems are treated, the premenstrual difficulties may reduce. PMS seems to be common across all social classes although it seems that women who seek medical help specifically for PMS are more likely to be in social classes I and II. Therefore the primary health care team should be alert to the possibility of PMS in women consulting for other problems, such as anxiety or depression. There also appears to be a general link between adverse life events and PMS. Women tend to experience PMS as more of a problem during times of stress, such as when there are problems at home or at work, or during examinations or moving house, than during holidays or when life is generally going well.

Despite some views that PMS is a complaint of 'neurotic' women, there is no consistent relationship between women's personalities and PMS. There do, however, appear to be links between PMS and general psychological health. Women who are psychiatrically ill may experience more, and more severe, premenstrual psychological symptoms than psychologically healthy women (Clare 1983). Recently, interest has focused on PMS in perimenopausal women. During the time leading up to the menopause, PMS can become more severe and blur into the menopause. It is possible that some women are more vulnerable than others to hormonal fluctuations, and are therefore at risk of problems with PMS, the menopause, and a mild form of postnatal depression, and so require extra support at these times.

PMS and the primary care team

Now that many practices have well woman and family planning clinics the 'best person' to deal with PMS may be any member of the team. It is probably helpful to have someone with some expertize in PMS in the practice because it is such a common and complex problem. Health visitors, counsellors, and nurses, as well as GPs, should be aware of PMS and how it may be affecting their clients. Primary care team members, because of their knowledge of an individual woman and her circumstances, are ideally placed to help her work out whether PMS is the main cause of her distress or whether other factors in her life are actually to blame. Groups for women with PMS – run in the surgery or in a local community centre – can be very valuable for women with PMS and their partners or families. Some women may be helped by a discussion about PMS as part of a series of meetings on women's health issues where they can obtain information and discuss their problems. Specific PMS groups have been run by GPs and psychologists, giving women a chance to air their feelings, try out self-help techniques such as relaxation, and discuss medical treatments.

Causes of PMS

There has been no shortage of hypotheses to explain PMS. The most plausible include abnormal tissue responses to normal levels of ovarian hormones, abnormalities of serotonin and other neurotransmitters including beta-endorphin. Certainly, medical suppression of the ovarian cycle with gonadotrophin releasing hormone, or surgical obliteration by bilateral oophorectomy has been proven to eliminate PMS. To these can be added nutritional theories, including deficiencies of pyridoxine, essential fatty acids, hypoglycaemia, and low magnesium or calcium levels. Cultural, psychological, and social theories have also been put forward (Rodin 1992).

PMS probably results from a combination of physical, psychological, and social factors interacting with life events. Various causes of PMS have been extensively reviewed in the literature (Bäckström 1988; Brush 1988; Sampson 1989; Mortola 1992; O'Brien 1993) and will be mentioned as relevant to treatment.

Management

PMS is a common problem which deserves sympathetic attention and appropriate management. Many women find that with support and encouragement they can work out solutions for themselves; and if problems persist, then various medical treatments can be tried. General approaches to management are summarized in Table 9.1.

Self-help

Women coming to the surgery with PMS need time to work out what the problems and solutions are, and so a number of appointments may be necessary. The woman and her adviser can both gain a great deal from a *menstrual chart* in defining and managing the problem (Fig 9.1). A chart is also very valuable in determining whether remedies or treatments are helping, and the woman should be encouraged to keep the chart for several months. Knowing in some

Table 9.1 *Approaches to management of premenstrual syndrome*

General PMS	
Mild	Discussion/talking
	Attention to general health/lifestyle
	Make allowance for PMS
Moderate	As above, but also
	Anxiety management
	Cognitive therapy
Severe	As above, plus
	SSRIs
	Oestrogen therapy
	Consider GnRH analogues
	Consider referral
For particular symptoms	
Depression/low mood	SSRIs
	Cognitive therapy
Mastalgia	Evening primrose oil
Anxiety	Relaxation
	Consider benzodiazepines in small amounts
Bloatedness	Lifestyle
	Avoid diuretics if possible

Note Any drug treatment must be accompanied by attention to lifestyle and self-help

detail how she may feel at any time of the month helps a woman to deal with her feelings, since this introduces some predictability into cyclical changes and allows her to plan for the difficult times. It is very helpful to make allowances for PMS, and many women have benefited from fairly simple rearrangements to their schedules of work and activities to reduce the stress during the premenstrual days.

Talking to her GP, health visitor, or practice nurse may open the door for a woman to talk to others, such as her partner, family, friends, or colleagues. This means that problems are brought out into the open, rather than the woman feeling isolated or 'going round the bend'. Talking to others can also reveal a wealth of remedies and strategies for dealing with PMS. These include yoga, swimming, relaxation techniques (those learnt in preparation for childbirth may be very useful), vigorous exercise, beating up cushions or having a supply of old plates to smash if she feels very angry, having a premenstrual sauna or steam bath, having a good cry, or reading a gripping novel. Many women spend their time looking after others and an important part of the strategy to combat PMS is for the woman to look at *her* needs and to nurture herself. Local women's health groups will also have information and leaflets on self-help strategies.

A check on general health is useful. A person will probably be fitter and deal better with stress if eating a balanced, 'healthy' diet and incorporating some form of exercise and relaxation into their lifestyle. There is some evidence that eating less fat will reduce breast pain in women with cyclical mastalgia (Goodwin *et al.* 1988). It is also possible that women are more sensitive to changes in blood sugar levels in the premenstrual days resulting in feelings of weakness, fatigue, and carbohydrate cravings. Careful attention to diet can help, eating frequent, small, protein-rich meals, particularly if the woman tends to skip meals or eat sugary snacks. It is well worth looking at caffeine intake, since caffeine can increase levels of anxiety and irritability. Many people drink more tea and coffee than they realize, and cutting down or cutting these drinks out completely can be very helpful. The following case history illustrates the importance of diet:

Sandra is a 29-year-old youth worker who came to the well woman clinic defining herself as having PMS and having tried vitamin B₆ and evening primrose oil with no benefits. She was interested in the nutritional theories of PMS and had heard that hypoglycaemia was a possible cause. Breast tenderness and irritability were her main symptoms and she brought along her chart showing cyclical changes. Discussion revealed that she tended to eat junk food at work, regularly drank seven or eight cups of tea and coffee each day, and that premenstrually she craved chocolate. Life in general was fine and she described herself as happy, although recent promotion at work meant more stress. Although initially she asked about vitamins and mineral supplements, talking about her diet helped her to see that it might be better to concentrate on her nutrition and cutting down on caffeine rather than buying expensive supplements. We wondered if her premenstrual treats could be, for example, a luxurious soak in the bath, rather than chocolate bars. She went away to try these strategies and report back in 2 months.

There may be links between smoking and premenstrual symptoms and cutting down or stopping smoking is part of general health advice. Exercise can help many of the physical and emotional symptoms of PMS including tiredness, anxiety, irritability, and bloating. Learning simple relaxation techniques or meditation can help too (Goodale *et al.* 1990). If breast tenderness is a problem, a well-fitting sports bra may help.

Alcohol consumption may influence PMS. A recent study suggested that women who drank more alcohol tended to have more severe premenstrual symptoms that women who drank less (Caan *et al.* 1993).

One of the most distressing symptoms of PMS is aggressive irritability which women say affects their activities and relationships. Although in our culture women are generally brought up to be more passive and nurturing than men, it is possible that PMS may bring out real anger about real problems in an otherwise easygoing woman. She and those around her may perceive this as irritability, and dismiss the underlying problems which need to be explored. The premenstrual days may not be the best time to tackle problems which are making her angry, but this is not a reason for ignoring them. Another case history follows:

A woman was brought to the well woman clinic by her husband who said she was very ill with PMS. After discussion it was clear that the woman did experience moderate symptoms before her periods, particularly anger and aggression, but that there were significant and stressful events in her life. When seen alone, she said that for many years her husband had been drinking regularly, returning home aggressive and sometimes violent. She had decided to stay with him while their two children were growing up, but now that they had left home she was debating whether and when to leave.

She was able to tolerate his drinking most of the time, but felt angry and upset about it during her premenstrual days. After several sessions with both of them, the husband came to see that he had a severe problem, and that his wife was not ill with PMS but understandably angry with the problems at home. The couple were referred to Relate.

This history illustrates the importance of taking a holistic approach to PMS and looking at every woman's circumstances, particularly before embarking on medical treatments. Books on PMS are available with sections on diet, relaxation, and exercise (see Sanders 1985; Duckworth 1990; Harrison 1991; Hayman 1996). More information can be obtained from Women's Health (see Useful Address, p. 298). If no women's health group is run in the surgery there are often local groups which women can be referred to.

Finally, women have sought help for PMS from various complementary or alternative practitioners including acupuncturists, homeopathists, and herbalists. The authors do not have experience in these fields, but in assessing any treatment for PMS the placebo effect must be remembered and women seeking these therapies should be advised of this.

Psychological approaches and cognitive therapy

There have been various psychological approaches to the management of premenstrual syndrome, including counselling, psychotherapy, and hypnotherapy, although none have been evaluated in controlled trials. Group therapy or self-help groups allows women to shared their experiences and approaches to PMS (Kirkby 1994). One promising approach is cognitive therapy (Blake 1995).

Cognitive therapy has been shown to be an effective treatment for many psychological problems, such as anxiety and depression, which are common components of premenstrual syndrome (Hawton *et al.* 1989). Cognitive therapy may be particularly suitable for premenstrual syndrome, being brief, time-limited, structured, and collaborative; therapist and patient working together to help the woman work out solutions to the problems she is facing. It is a common-sense approach that is particularly acceptable to people who are wary of psychological therapy implying that the symptoms are 'all in the mind'. The focus of therapy is on the woman's psychological response to emotional and physical changes, and the therapy aims to help the individual to examine patterns of negative thinking and her assumptions about the symptoms, and to learn more adaptive and helpful thoughts and behaviours.

The cognitive model of PMS proposes that the woman's cognitive appraisal of the premenstrual changes, in the context of the woman's circumstances and personal assumptions, determines whether she sees the changes as normal and a manageable part of her life, or distressing. For example, interpreting physiological changes in the luteal phase in a negative way is likely to lead the individual to become distressed and upset by the symptoms, thereby increasing the woman's overall level of distress. The symptoms may be magnified by vicious circles of negative thinking, thereby increasing the woman's anxiety, irritability, or low mood. In particular, the woman may find that physiological changes interfere with her normal coping mechanisms, leading her to predict that she is going to lose control. These thoughts lead the individual to feel tense

Fig 9.2 *Cognitive therapy for premenstrual syndrome. From: Fiona Blake (1995) Cognitive therapy for premenstrual syndrome, from Cognitive and Behavioural Practice, 2, 167–85. Copyright by the Association for Advancement of Behavior Therapy. Reprinted by permission of the publisher and the author*

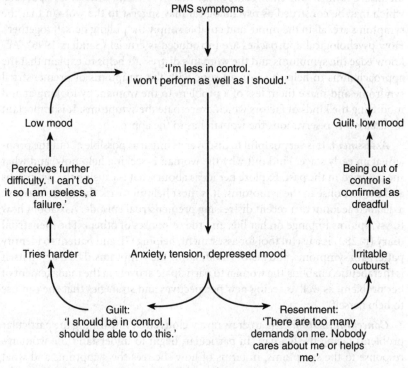

and anxious, leading to indecision and inability to concentrate. These changes are then interpreted as further evidence that she is losing control, and so on in a vicious circle (Blake 1995; Blake *et al.* 1995), as illustrated in Fig 9.2.

The rationale for cognitive therapy is that whilst psychological factors do not in their own right cause premenstrual distress, psychological factors influence the response to both psychological and physiological symptoms, thereby modifying the degree of distress. For many women, directly targeting the symptoms with physical treatments alone has proved unhelpful; therefore reducing the distress about the symptoms is a more useful strategy.

In a small controlled trial in Oxford, of cognitive therapy for severe premenstrual syndrome, the treated group had a significant relief of premenstrual symptoms (Blake 1995). The treatment involved 12 sessions of 1 hour duration, weekly on an individual basis. The method is at a very early stage of development and so it is too soon to say what aspects of the treatment might be effective, and whether it can be adapted for use in general practice. However, the common-sense nature of the approach, and clinical observations, suggest that it will prove a valuable addition to the range of treatments for premenstrual syndrome, and can be modified for use in general practice.

The steps of cognitive therapy for PMS are outlined below (Blake 1995).

Engagement. Although many women welcome the opportunity to talk to their GP about their problems, some may be unhappy about being offered a psychological approach. It is not uncommon for women to want and expect medical treatment for their symptoms; therefore being offered an approach which may be construed as psychological may suggest to the woman that the symptoms are 'all in the mind' and curable simply by 'pulling herself together'. How psychological approaches are introduced is crucial (Sanders 1996). Acknowledge the symptoms and the woman's distress. It helps to explain that the approach aims to help the woman cope with the symptoms of premenstrual syndrome and make them less of a problem to the woman, by looking at and modifying the kinds of factors which exacerbate the symptoms. It is important to discuss any reservations the woman has to the approach.

Assessment. It is very helpful to discover as much as possible about the problem at an early stage. Find out why the woman is seeking help now, and what she has tried in the past. Explore her ideas about what is causing the symptoms and her response to the symptoms. It is most helpful to ask the woman to give a detailed account of a recent distressing premenstrual episode. Ask about how the symptoms impinge on her life, and the responses of others. The **menstrual diary** (p. 282) is a useful tool for assessment, helping GP and patient to identify patterns of symptoms, and factors modulating the symptoms. The diary in itself is therapeutic, enabling the woman to participate actively in the management of her problem, as well as seeing new perspectives and strategies that she can use to help herself.

Conceptualization. Aim to draw up a vicious circle illustrating the particular problems facing the woman. In particular, begin to understand the woman's response to the symptoms, in terms of how she sees the symptoms and what she does in response to them, and how her responses may exacerbate the problem. Once patient and GP have a conceptualization, areas to target can be discussed.

Education. The assessment provides the opportunity to educate the woman about the normal range of menstrual experiences. This can help to alleviate anxiety about the meaning of symptoms. Education about general measures to improve health, outlined in this chapter, are often appropriate.

Learning alternative responses to the symptoms. Once GP and patient have identified how the woman usually responds to the symptoms, treatment aims to help the woman to identify and try out alternative responses. She may have certain *thoughts* whenever she experiences symptoms such as 'this is terrible; I can't cope; other women don't feel like me'. Cognitive therapy aims to help the individual consider reasonable alternatives to such thoughts. She may behave in certain ways; for example, working harder in response to symptoms rather than allowing herself to rest. Identifying and practising alternative responses to the symptoms is valuable; for example, a woman can be helped to predict her symptoms and plan measures to help herself, so that symptoms are no longer a catastrophe that strike her down. She can also begin to look after herself better during the premenstrual days.

Identifying assumptions. There are several assumptions which create problems for women with premenstrual changes, such as 'if I have PMS it is a hormonal imbalance and there is nothing I can do to help myself; if I have PMS I am weak and neurotic; I should be in control and cope all the time; I am responsible for everyone else's needs; it is selfish to look after myself; I must be perfect all of the time'. Treatment involves helping the woman to identify her beliefs about PMS and begin to identify and try out alternatives.

The approach may be adapted for use in several consultations for women with mild or moderate symptoms. For those with more severe symptoms, referral to specialized cognitive therapy services may be necessary.

Medical treatments

There are many different medical approaches for PMS although, as for self-help remedies, there is still a scarcity of well-conducted clinical trials. One problem in evaluating the efficacy of treatments is that most trials conducted show a very large placebo effect, particularly in the first month of treatment: in one study (Magos *et al.* 1986), 94% of the women in the placebo group showed a significant improvement. Hence any drug trial should be placebo-controlled and ideally double-blind crossover, with each phase continuing for at least 3 months (Moline 1993).

A general approach to managing PMS should start with the psychological, stress-relieving, self-help approach outlined above. Medical treatments should be reserved for women whose symptoms are severe and who have not responded to the above measures. This is because most medical treatments shown to be effective in relieving PMS symptoms have potentially harmful side-effects (Mortola 1994).

It may be possible to take a symptomatic approach if one particular symptom is a problem but in general to relieve severe PMS one either has to abolish the cycle or manipulate neurotransmitter levels. Many treatments which even a few years ago looked hopeful, for example, pyridoxine, gamma-linolenic acid, progesterone, and progestogens, have shown not to be effective on the whole (Mortola 1994). Women may still ask for pyridoxine. The evidence for its value is inconclusive but those who wish to 'take something' should be advised not to take more than 50–100 mg daily (Doll 1989) because of the possible risks of peripheral neuropathy with higher doses.

Any treatment used for PMS must be thought about in terms of its possible hazards in pregnancy, and women should be warned about these, particularly with endocrine treatments. Women should also be reminded that no treatment, except the Pill, can be regarded as contraceptively effective.

A number of hospitals run out-patient PMS clinics, and referral to a specialist clinic can be useful for very severe PMS, or when considering one of the more sophisticated treatments discussed below. Menopause clinics may also see women with PMS; it is useful to check what facilities are available locally. Simply referring women to a gynaecologist may be unhelpful unless s/he has an interest in PMS and is sympathetic to the problem.

Selective serotonin re-uptake inhibitors (SSRIs)

These drugs have had a significant impact on the treatment of depression in recent years. The symptom overlap between depression and PMS has been pointed out (Roy-Byrne *et al.* 1987) and depression itself is often exacerbated premenstrually. SSRIs increase serotonin levels by inhibiting uptake of serotonin, and serotonin may play a role in PMS, particularly the affective and mood-related symptoms (Rapkin 1992). Women who experience predominantly mood-related and affective symptoms of PMS (including tension, irritability, and derpessive symptoms) to a severe degree, enough to disrupt their daily life and social activities, have been classified as having late luteal phase dysphoric disorder (LLPDD) or premenstrual dysphoric disorder. Fluoxetine has been shown in well-conducted, randomized, double-blind, placebo-controlled trials to be effective in women with both general PMS (Menkes *et al.* 1992) and LLPDD (Steiner *et al.* 1995). At present, evidence suggests that a dose of 20 mg daily is adequate. Larger doses cause more side-effects and these, particularly nausea and heightened anxiety, can be severe in some women. Women should be closely monitored when starting these drugs. One recent study (Pearlstein *et al.* 1994) showed that fluoxetine maintained its effectiveness over 18 months and that women who stopped it in order to conceive returned to it after giving birth when PMS became a problem again. Studies are under way to look at whether fluoxetine may simply be given to women premenstrually either in a single dose or over several days. (Steiner 1994). If intermittent treatment is successful it will be a bonus for women who do not want to take medication all the time and will raise the question of how the drug is working in PMS as opposed to in depression. At present it not known whether SSRIs have a specific 'anti-PMS' action separate from their antidepressant effect. SSRIs may also be particularly useful in women who have underlying depression that is worsened premenstrually, but studies have not been carried out in this area yet.

Endocrine treatments

These either attempt to abolish the menstrual cycle or to moderate hormonal fluctuations. Women often arrive at the surgery saying 'it must be a hormone imbalance, doctor'. Some informed patients may ask for hormone measurements. Unless the GP feels the women may be menopausal or suffering from some other complaint such as a thyroid disorder, hormonal measurements are inappropriate. It is important to remember that apart from oral contraception, and the possible use of the progestogen-containing IUCD in the future as an adjunct to oestrogen therapy, endocrine therapies cannot be guaranteed to prevent pregnancy.

Oral contraception. While some women have experienced an exacerbation of premenstrual symptoms with the combined oral contraceptive pill, probably as the result of progestogens, many women, in practice, are helped. Surprisingly few trials have been done however and those that have been mainly involve cyclical pills (Bäckström *et al.* 1992). In women for whom PMS is exacerbated by the thought of terrible periods with pain and heavy bleeding, combined oral contraceptives, possibly used continuously for several months, will offer relief. More work needs to be done on the effects of COCs on PMS. A case history follows:

Laura had suffered with severe PMS and heavy periods for nearly 20 years, regularly experiencing violent tempers, severe insomnia, and what she called 'mind-numbing fear'. She had tried self-help remedies: relaxation, pyridoxine, evening primrose oil, and also progesterone pessaries, all to no avail. Four years previously she had a baby and noticed great relief during pregnancy and whilst breast-feeding. When her cycle resumed PMS became worse than ever. Although previously wary of hormonal treatments she needed contraception and decided to try the oral contraceptive pill Mercilon. Since then she has had pain-free periods with no premenstrual symptoms and has chosen to stay on Mercilon despite the recent anxieties about its safety.

Oestrogen therapy (HRT). Studd and Magos (1986) realized the potential of oestradiol implants in abolishing ovulation. They conducted a double-blind trial in 68 women using implants plus cyclical oral norethisterone versus placebo. There was a significant improvement in six symptoms including concentration, mood changes, fluid retention, and breast pain. Unfortunately, implants can cause problems with tachyphylaxis, so recently gynaecologists have been using oestradiol patches in women with PMS approaching the menopause. A study of women aged 30–45 showed that these were more effective than placebo in relieving most PMS symptoms (Garnett *et al.* 1989). Although large doses were used in the initial studies there is evidence that 100 µg patches can control symptoms (Smith *et al.* 1995). In the author's experience, lower doses (50 µg patches twice weekly) may be of just as much benefit.

Oestrogen can be helpful in women of any age with PMS and it is worth starting on conventional HRT doses and working up from there until symptoms are controlled. Cyclical progestogen must be used in women who have a uterus. Different progestogens can be tried. Currently dydrogesterone or medroxyprogesterone acetate look like being the least likely to cause PMS-type symptoms (West 1990).

Progestogen should probably be given for 10 days per month, but for women who find it really hard to tolerate, some gynaecologists working in the field are giving 7 days only. It is now possible to give oestrogen systemically while protecting the endometrium with a progestogen-containing IUCD. This has the advantage of minimal systemic absorption of progestogen, thereby circumventing the PMS-like side-effects. The levonorgestrel IUCD is licensed for contraception at present but it has great potential for use in PMS. Studies are in progress to evaluate oestrodiol patches in conjunction with the levonorgestrel IUCD for PMS.

While oestrogen is known to have many benefits for women, particularly those nearing the menopause in terms of bone preservation and prevention of heart disease, some women do experience side-effects. Oestrogen can cause breast tenderness and nausea. Patches may cause skin irritation, and there is still a worry over the risk of breast cancer with very long-term oestrogen use in menopausal women. A case history follows:

Gail is 44 and has suffered with PMS all her life. She is a single mother, working full-time in a bookshop, with two children, the youngest of whom, aged 10, is deaf. Gail's PMS appeared to worsen after each pregnancy. Her main problems were feeling bloated, severe irritability, and often severe migraines lasting several days; and she felt she treated her children unfairly premenstrually. PMS usually incapacitated her for up to a week each month, which was very difficult both at work and at home. She had tried all kinds of self-help, including yoga and relaxation techniques, and most of the remedies available from the chemist, including pyridoxine. These helped somewhat but the irritability and migraine were still hard to cope with. Five years ago her PMS became intolerable and she decided to seek medical help. Her diaries showed that although she was leading a stressful life, she definitely had PMS. She had already cut down on caffeine and because of the migraines was very careful with her diet. After discussion she decided to try progesterone pessaries.

Initially, the progesterone did seem to help the migraines but not the other symptoms, and after 9 months the migraines started to reappear; she was started on danazol, having discussed its side-effects. She took 200 mg daily for over a year with relief from both migraines and irritability. Even the bloating decreased to tolerable level. Eighteen months ago, however, her symptoms gradually started to reappear, and in consultation with a sympathetic local woman gynaecologist, her treatment was changed to oestrogen patches (100 μg twice weekly) and progesterone pessaries (200 mg twice daily for 12 days out of 28) to provide progestogen coverage.

To begin with, she had some severe breast tenderness with this regime but this soon settled and she is now doing a degree as well as working and looking after her children. She says she feels like a new woman and much more energetic.

GnRH analogues (e.g. gosenelin, buserelin, naferelin). GnRH analogues work by producing a 'medical oophorectomy' Muse *et al.* 1984) and have been shown to be more effective than placebo in several well-conducted trials (Hammarback and Bäckström 1988). Unfortunately, they produce low oestradiol levels and this makes them unsuitable for long-term use because of the risks of osteoporosis. The bone loss caused by low oestradiol has been well-documented (Dodin *et al.* 1991) but can be counteracted to a large extent by 'add back' therapy with oestrogen and progestogen, as used in HRT. So much hormonal manipulation seems drastic but it must be borne in mind that women with very severe PMS can find life so intolerable that they will try anything. The best use for GnRH analogues may, however, be in making a definitive diagnosis of PMS in women who are suffering severely but for whom treatment does not appear to be working. Treatment with GnRH analogues is usually initiated in a specialist clinic rather than in general practice.

Danazol (GnRH antagonist). The advent of oestrogen therapy has relegated danazol very much to the sidelines in PMS treatment. Danazol is an antigonadotrophin and in large doses (400–800 mg daily) inhibits ovulation, thus alleviating PMS by abolishing the cycle. Most women find this dose intolerable because of side-effects such as weight gain, acne, bloating, and hirsutism (Watts *et al.* 1987). However, danazol is effective in relieving premenstrual mastalgia at smaller doses of 200 mg daily. PMS in some women may also be helped at this dose with considerably reduced side-effects. Long-term use of danazol may adversely affect blood lipids; therefore women taking it for more than 6 months should have these monitored.

Progesterone and progestogens. Many women are still being prescribed progesterone or progestogens for PMS – Katharina Dalton has advocated the use of progesterone. Her books make interesting reading and she has done much to publicize the plight of women with PMS. However, results of well-conducted trials of progesterone (usually in the form of pessaries or suppositories) have been disappointing and a double-blind crossover study of

168 women (Freeman *et al.* 1990) showed no difference between progesterone in a dose of 400 mg or 800 mg daily from day 16 to 28 of the cycle and placebo. Although dydrogesterone has also been used in PMS, results of placebo-controlled trials are conflicting Williams *et al.* 1983; (Sampson 1988). Given that women may experience PMS-like symptoms when taking progestogen as part of HRT (Magos *et al.* 1986) the authors feel that progesterone and progestogens have little place in the treatment of PMS at present.

Oophorectomy and hysterectomy. For women with extremely severe PMS, perhaps particularly for those who also have menstrual problems, oophorectomy and hysterectomy with subsequent oestrogen replacement therapy will result in a cure for PMS. However, women and their GPs must make an informed decision about this as it is a major step; GPs may be mediators between women and gynaecologists to ensure that the best decision is made for a particular woman (Casper and Hearn 1990).

Specific problems

Mastalgia

Gamma-linolenic acid (evening primrose oil) has been shown to help this particular problem at a dose of three to four 40 mg capsules twice a day. Unfortunately, it is expensive. A randomized trial of EPO in cyclical mastalgia (Pye *et al.* 1985) found that it was effective in 45% of 291 women, but less effective than danazol or bromocryptine, although EPO caused fewer side-effects. There is no convincing evidence that it is helpful for any other PMS symptoms. See also Fig 9.3 'Guidelines for referral of patients with breast problems'.

Fluid retention

Women may request diuretics for bloating and fluid retention. If these symptoms are very severe the gold standard is to abolish the cycle (see above). Diuretics do not have a good track record in women with PMS; their effects are short-hold and non-potassium sparing diuretics may lead to severe hypokalaemia. One of the authors has seen a woman admitted to psychiatric hospital with lethargy and depression due to hypokalaemia, having received diuretics for premenstrual fluid retention. Although some trials with spironolactone have looked promising (O'Brien 1987), diuretics are probably best avoided.

Anxiety

All the psychological and self-help approaches should be tried. If, however, severe bouts of anxiety definitely precede menstruation, occasional use of small doses of benzodiazepines may be used. Work has been done with aprazolam (Harrison *et al.* 1990) but the authors feel that occasional use of well-known and cheaper drugs, such as diazepam, is safer.

Dysmenorrhoea

Prostaglandin inhibitors are used widely for dysmenorrhoea and a double-blind, controlled trial of naproxen 550 mg twice daily from 7 days before

Fig 9.3 *Protocol for treating moderate to severe cyclical mastalgia (mild mastalgia requires examination and reassurance)*

(From: NHS breast screening programme (1995). Guidelines for referral of patients with breast problems. Reproduced with permission)

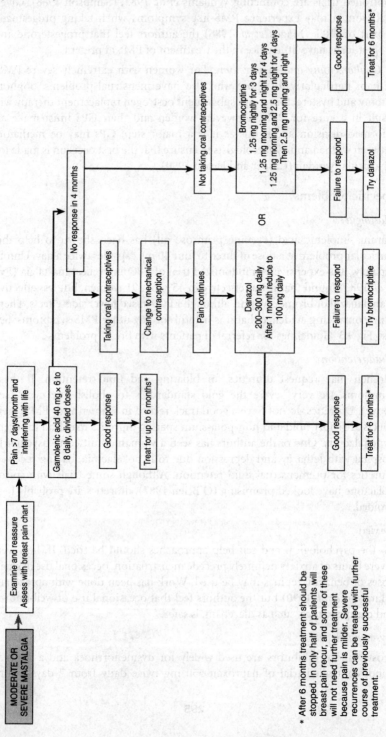

* After 6 months treatment should be stopped. In only half of patients will breast pain recur, and some of these will not need further treatment because pain is milder. Severe recurrences can be treated with further course of previously successful treatment.

menstruation until day 4 of the cycle (Facchinetti *et al.* 1989) demonstrated relief for premenstrual symptoms related to pain but not for mood-related symptoms. Mefenamic acid has also been shown in double-blind studies to relieve some PMS symptoms (Moline 1993) but symptom relief has not been shown to be consistent in different trials and more work needs to be done before recommending prostaglandin inhibitors for PMS, except where pain is the overriding problem.

Controversies

The effectiveness of SSRIs in women with severe PMS has brought the problem into the limelight once more; Runibow and Schmidt (1995) point out how little is still known about it. Which women will respond to SSRIs and how are these drugs working in PMS?

The introduction of SSRIs also raises another question for the future. Will women with moderate PMS simply take a couple of fluoxetine tablets premenstrually, or will they make efforts to cope with PMS using cognitive approaches, relaxation, talking about it, and helping themselves? The primary care team may have an important role in steering women away from a 'quick fix' approach. Cognitive therapy may well provide a long-term solution, unlike hormonal manipulation or antidepressant medication. With the advent of a new diagnostic category (late luteal phase dysphoric disorder) and the availability of more effective medical treatments, will PMS become more of an 'illness' and will we lose sight of the social and cultural factors involved (Rodin 1992)?

Conclusion

Premenstrual syndrome includes a wide range of physical and emotional changes which vary in severity, duration, and effects on a woman's life. It is unlikely that there is a single or simple cause, and any consideration of the aetiology of PMS must take into account psychological, physiological, and social factors. Management of PMS is not simple, but it is certainly aided by a greater understanding and acceptance of the problem, and the development of a range of approaches and remedies. Women need to devote time to experiment to find an appropriate solution, and may require help from the primary health care team to evaluate how they can help themselves and, if necessary, what medical treatments might be useful. In any individual woman it is essential to determine whether or not she has PMS, what her main problems are, and the circumstances which led her to seek medical help. The first steps are sympathetic discussion of the problems and reorganization of aspects of her life to cope with times of feeling low. Attention to general health and lifestyle is the key to dealing with PMS. Following this, a woman may try a variety of self-help approaches or cognitive therapy and for those women severely affected by PMS, medical treatment may also be necessary.

If a woman is not helped by any of the approaches available in primary care, even closer attention must be paid to what is going on in her life. Referral to a specialist PMS clinic may be indicated. Gynaecologists vary in their interest in PMS and menopausal problems and referral will very much depend upon what is available locally.

Acknowledgement

Thanks to Fiona Blake for her help with the section on cognitive therapy for PMS.

Useful addresses

Women's Health
52 Featherstone Street, London EC1Y 8RT.
Tel: 0171 251 6580.

References and further reading

Abraham, G. E. (1983). Nutritional factors in the aetiology of the premenstrual tension syndromes. *Journal of Reproductive Medicine*, **28**, 446–64.

American Psychiatric Association (1994). *Diagnostic and statistical manual of mental disorders* (4th ed). Washington, DC.

Bäckström, T. (1988). Endocrine factors in the aetiology of premenstrual syndrome. In *Functional disorders of the menstrual cycle* (ed. M. G. Brush and E. M. Goudsmit), pp. 87–96. Wiley, Chichester.

Bäckström, T., Boyle, H., and Baird, D. T. (1981). Persistence of symptoms of premenstrual tension in hysterectomised women. *British Journal of Obstetrics and Gynaecology*, **88**, 530–6.

Bacstrom, T., Hansson-Malmstrom., Y. Lindhe, B.A., *et al.* (1992). Oral contraceptives in premenstrual syndrome; a randomised comparison of triphasic and monophasic preparations. *Contraception*, **46**, 253–68.

Blake, F. (1995a). Cognitive therapy for premenstrual syndrome. *Cognitive and Behavioural Practice*, **2**, 167–85.

Blake, F., Gath, D., and Salkovskis, P. (1995b). Psychological aspects of premenstrual syndrome: developing a cognitive approach. In ed. R. Mayou, C. Bass, and M. Sharpe), pp. 271–84. *Treatment of functional somatic symptoms* Oxford University Press, Oxford.

Brush, M. G. (1985). The premenstrual syndrome before and after pregnancy. *Maternal and Child Health*, **10** (1), 19–25.

Brush, M. G. (1988). Vitamins, essential fatty acids and minerals in relation to the aetiology and management of premenstrual syndrome. In *Functional disorders of the menstrual cycle* (ed. M. G. Brush and E. M. Goudsmit), pp. 69–86. Wiley, Chichester.

Caan, B., Duncan, D., Hiatt, R., *et al.* (1993). Association between alcoholic and caffeinated beverages and premenstrual syndrome. *Journal of Reproductive Medicine*, **38** (8), 630–6.

Casper, R. F. and Hearn, M. T. (1990). Effect of hysterectomy and bilateral oophorectomy in women with severe premenstrual syndrome. *American Journal of Obstetrics and Gynecology*, **162**, 105–9.

Clare, A. W. (1983). Psychiatric and social aspects of premenstrual complaint. *Psychological Medicine Monographs Supplement*, **4**, 1–58.

Cockerill, I. M., Wormington, J. A., and Nevill, A. M. (1994). Menstrual cycle effect on mood and perceptual motor performance. *Journal of Psychosomatic Research*, **38** (7), 763–71.

Dodin, S., Lemay, A., Maheux, R., *et al.* (1991). Bone mass in endometriosis patients treated with GnRH agonist implant or danazol. *Obstetrics and Gynaecology*, **77**, 410–15.

Doll, H., Brown, S., Thurston, A., *et al.* (1989). Pyridoxine and the premenstrual syndrome: a randomized crossover trial. *Journal of the Royal College of General Practitioners*, **39**, 364–8.

Duckworth, H. (1990). *Premenstrual syndrome: your options*. Attic Press, Dublin.

Facchinetti, F., Fioroni, L., Sances, G., Romano, G., Nappi, G. and Genazzani, A.R. (1989). Naproxen sodium in the treatment of premenstrual symptoms: a placebo controlled study. *Gynecological and Obstetric Investigations*, **28**, 205–8.

Freeman, E., Rickel, K., Sondheimer, S. J., *et al.* (1990). Ineffectiveness of progesterone suppository treatment for premenstrual syndrome. *Journal of the American Medical Association*, **264**, 349–53.

Garnett, I., Savvas, M., Watson, N. R., *et al.* (1989). Treatment of severe premenstrual syndrome with oestradiol patches and cyclical norethisterone. *Lancet*, **8665**, 730–2.

Goodale, I. L., Domar, A. D., and Benson, H. (1990). Alleviation of premenstrual syndrome symptoms with the relaxation response. *Obstetrics and Gynaecology*, **75**, 649–55.

Goodwin, P. J., Neelam, M., and Boyd, N. F. (1988). Cyclical mastopathy: a critical review of therapy. *British Journal of Surgery*, **75**, 837–44.

Hammarrback, S. and Bäckström, T. (1988). Induced anovulation as a treatment of premenstrual tension syndrome – a double-blind crossover study with LRH agonist versus placebo. *Acta Obstetricia Gynecologica Scandinavica*, **67**, 159–63.

Harrison, M. (1991). *Self help with PMS*. Macdonald Optima, London.

Harrison, W. M., Endicott, J., and Nee, J. (1990). Treatment of premenstrual dysphoria with alprazolam: a controlled study. *Archives of General Psychiatry*, **47**, 270–5.

Hawton, K., Salkovskis, P. M., Kirk, J., and Clark, D. M. (ed.) (1989). *Cognitive behaviour therapy for psychiatric problems*. Oxford University Press, Oxford.

Hayman, S. (1996). *PMS: the complete guide to treatment options*. Piatkus, London.

Johnson, S. R. (1987). The epidemiology and social impact of premenstrual syndrome. *Clinical Obstetrics and Gynaecology*, **30**, 367–76.

Kirkby, R. J. (1994). Changes in premenstrual symptoms and irrational thinking following cognitive-behavioural coping skills training. *Journal of Consulting and Clinical Psychology*, **62** (5), 1026–32.

Leather, A. T., Studd, J. W. W., Watson N. R., *et al.* (1993). The prevention of bone loss in young women trated with GnRH analogues with 'add back' estrogen therapy. *Obstetrics and Gynaecology*, **81** (1), 104–7.

Logue, C. M. and Moos, R. H. (1986). Perimenstrual symptoms: prevalence and risk factors. *Psychosomatic Medicine*, **48**, 388–414.

Logue, C. M. and Moos, R. H. (1988). Positive perimenstrual changes: towards a new perspective on the menstrual cycle. *Journal of Psychosomatic Research*, **32**, 31–40.

Magos, A. L. (1989). Premenstrual syndrome. *Contemporary Review of Obstetrics and Gynaecology*, **1**, 80–92.

Magos, A. L. (1990). Advances in the treatment of the premenstrual syndrome. *British Journal of Obstetrics and Gynaecology*, **97**, 7–10.

Magos, A. L., Brincat, M., and Studd, J. W. W. (1986). Treatment of premenstrual syndrome by subcutaneous oestradiol implants and cyclical oral norethisterone: placebo controlled study. *British Medical Journal*, **292**, 1629–33.

Magos, A. L. and Studd, J. W. W. (1988). A simple method for the diagnosis of premenstrual syndrome by use of a self-assessment disk. *American Journal of Obstetrics and Gynecology*, **158**, 1024–8.

Menkes, D. B., Taghavi, E., Mason, P., *et al.* (1992). Fluoxetine treatment of severe premenstrual syndrome. *British Medical Journal*, **305**, 346–7.

Moline, M. L. (1993). Pharmacologic strategies for managing premenstrual syndrome. *Clinical Pharmacy*, **12**, 181–96.

Mortola, J. F. (1992). Assessment and management of premenstrual syndrome. *Current Opinion in Obstetrics and Gynaecology*, **4**, 877–85.

Mortola, J. (1994). A risk–benefit appraisal of drugs used in the management of the premenstrual syndrome. *Drug Safety*, **10** (2), 160–9.

Muse, K., Cetel, N., Futterman, L., *et al.* (1984). The premenstrual syndrome: effects of medical ovariectomy. *New England Journal of Medicine*, **311**, 1345–9.

O'Brien, P. M. S. (1987). *Premenstrual syndrome*. Blackwell, Oxford.

O'Brien, P. M. S. (1990). The premenstrual syndrome. *British Journal of Family Planning*, **15**, (suppl.), 13–18.

O'Brien, P. M. S. (1993). Helping women with premenstrual syndrome. *British Medical Journal*, **307**, 1471–5.

Pearlstein, M. D. and Stone, A. B. (1994). Long-term fluoxetine treatment of late luteal phase dysphoric disorder. *Journal of Clinical Psychiatry*, **55** (8), 332–5.

Pye, J. K., Mansel, R. E., and Hughes, L. E. (1985). Clinical experience of drug treatments for mastalgia. *Lancet*, **ii,** 373–7.

Rapkin, A. J. (1992). The role of serotonin in premenstrual syndrome. *Clinics in Obstetrics and Gynecology*, **35,** 629–36.

Rapkin, A. J. Edelmuth, E., Chang, L. C., *et al.* (1987). Whole blood serotonin in premenstrual syndrome. *Obstetrics and Gynaecology*, **70,** 533.

Rodin, M. (1992). The social construction of premenstrual syndrome. *Social Science and Medicine*, **35** (1), 49–56.

Roy-Byrne, P. P., Hoban, M. C., and Rubinow, D. R. (1987). The relationship of menstrually-related mood disorder to psychiatric disorders. *Clinics in Obstetrics and Gynecology*, **30,** 386–95.

Sampson, G. A. (1989). Premenstrual syndrome. *Baillières Clinical Obstetrics and Gynaecology*, **3,** 687–704.

Rubinow, D.R. and Schmidt, P.J. (1995). The treatment of premenstrual syndrom – forward into the past. *New England Journal of Medicine*, **332,** 1574–75.

Sampson, G. A. (1990). The boundaries of premenstrual syndrome – who defines them and how do they affect clinical practice. *British Journal of Family Planning*, **15** (suppl.), 19–22.

Sampson, G. A., Heathcote, P. R. M., Wordsworth, J., *et al.* (1988). A double-blind cross-over study of treatment with dydrogesterone and placebo. *British Journal of Psychiatry*, **153,** 232–5.

Sanders, D. (1985). *Coping with periods.* Chambers, Edinburgh.

Sanders, D. (1996). *Counselling for psychosomatic problems.* Sage, London.

Smith, R. N. J., Studd, J. W. W., Zamblera, D., and Holland, E. F. N. (1995). A randomised comparison over 6 months of 100 mg and 200 mg twice-weekly doses of transdermal oestradiol in the treatment of severe premenstrual syndrome. *British Journal of Obstetrics and Gynaecology*, **102,** 475–84.

Steiner, M. (1994). Fluoxetine in the treatment of LLPDD: a multicentre, placebo-controlled, double-blind trial. *International Journal Gynaecology and Obstetrics*, **46** (2), 122.

Steiner, M., Steinberg, S., and Stewart, D. (1995). Fluoxetine in the management of premenstrual dysphoria. *New England Journal of Medicine*, **332,** 1529–34.

Studd, J. W. W. and Magos, A. L. (1986). Hormone manipulation in the management of premenstrual syndrome. In *Hormones and behaviour* (ed. L. Dennerstein and I. Fraser), pp. 147–59. Elsevier, Holland.

Watts, J. F., Butt, W. R., and Logan-Edwards, R. (1987). A clinical trial using danazol for the treatment of premenstrual tension. *British Journal of Obstetrics and Gynaecology*, **94,** 30–4.

West, C. P. (1990). Inhibition of ovulation with oral progestins: effectiveness in premenstrual syndrome. *European Journal of Obstetrics, Gynecology and Reproductive Biology*, **34,** 119–28.

Williams, J.G.C., Martin, A.J., Hulkensberg-Tromp, T. (1983). PMS in four European countries Part 2. A double blind placebo controlled study of dydrogesterone. *British Journal of Sexual Medicine*, **10,** 8–18.

CHAPTER TEN

Menstrual problems

Margaret C. P. Rees

Introduction

Disorders of menstruation, 'the curse', 'the devil's gateway', or whatever one likes to call them, form a significant part of the general practitioner's (GP's) work. This is not surprising since women will each experience about 400 menstruations between the menarche and the menopause. In a national community survey, 1069 women aged 16–45 were interviewed in their homes (MORI 1990): 31% reported heavy periods and 38% painful periods. Of these, one-third had consulted a doctor within the past 4 months. The Fourth National Morbidity Survey in General Practice (1991–92) showed that for women aged 25–44 the consultation rates for menorrhagia and dysmenorrhoea were 65 and 40 per 1000 woman-years at risk: and 5% of women aged 30–49 consult their GP for menorrhagia in 1 year.

When it comes to hospital referral, menorrhagia is the eighth most common cause of all referrals for all ages and both sexes (see Chapter 3) and the main presenting complaint in women referred to gynaecologists. About 73 000 hysterectomies and 10 000 endometrial ablations were performed in England in 1993–94, of which about two-thirds were undertaken for women presenting with menorrhagia. By the age of 43, one in 10 women have undergone hysterectomy and 15% have had at least one D&C (Kuh and Stirling 1995).

Since ancient times the idea of menstruation has had magical and mythical connotations. In many prehistoric cultures and up to the Middle Ages, the uterus was considered as a separate creature with autonomous rights. It was regarded by some as a type of wild beast roaming through the woman's body and endangering her life. Pliny noted that while menstrual blood cured epilepsy, gout, malaria, and boils, it also caused iron to rust and copper to turn green. Menstruation has been considered to be a taboo subject. The word 'tabu' comes from the Polynesian where it means menstruation as well as things which are both sacred and unclean. In various cultures women have been prohibited from making food, tending plants, and having any contact with men; and have been banished to menstrual huts. In our own society mothers may still tell their daughters not to bath, wash their hair, or undertake physical exercise during menstruation. These attitudes have no doubt contributed to the relatively recent development of effective sanitary protection with commercial tampons only being introduced in the 1920s.

As a result of these myths it is not surprising that it can be difficult for women to distinguish between normal and abnormal menstruation. The purpose of this chapter is to try and suggest which symptomatology, as usually presented to the GP, might indicate the need for further appropriate investigation and treatment either at a primary care level or by the specialist.

At any one time women might complain that their periods are:

- too short
- too long
- too frequent
- too infrequent
- too light
- too heavy
- too painful
- too irregular
- too early (menarche)
- too late (menarche)
- too early (menopause)
- too late (menopause)
- too awful!

This is excluding the complaint that it is unfair that they should have them at all and men are remarkably lucky.

It is probably best when discussing menstrual disorders with patients to use simple, descriptive English terms such as heavy or painful periods rather than refuge behind schoolboy classical Greek. For instance, polymenometrorrhagia literally means frequent month womb rushing out rather than frequent heavy irregular periods.

This chapter will first discuss the normal menstrual cycle and then its problems, whether excessive, painful, or absent.

The normal menstrual cycle

Endocrine changes

The sequence of hormone events occurring in the menstrual cycle during which ovulation takes place is shown in Fig 10.1. At menstruation, plasma levels of the anterior pituitary hormone, follicle stimulating hormone (FSH), are already rising, stimulating the growth of several graafian follicles within the ovary. In general, the end result of this follicular development is (usually) one mature follicle and ovum. The developing follicle produces increasing amounts of oestrogens, notably oestradiol. As levels of oestradiol begin to rise early in

Fig 10.1 *Hormone changes during the menstrual cycle, showing fluctuating levels of the pituitary hormones, leutenizing hormone (LH), and follicle-stimulating hormone (FSH), and of the ovarian hormones, oestradol and progesterone*

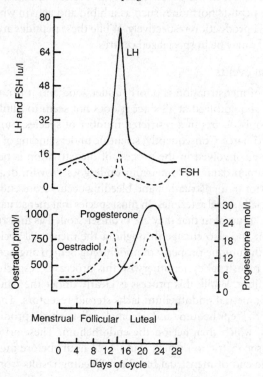

the follicular phase of the cycle, production of FSH is suppressed by negative feedback but oestradiol levels continue to increase over the next few days until a critical level is reached. Here, by positive feedback it triggers the anterior pituitary to release about 24 hours later a surge of luteinising hormone (LH) with levels up to 50 iu/l and to a lesser extent FSH with levels up to 15 iu/l; such levels only occur for one day. Ovulation follows the onset of the LH surge within about 34–36 hours and the ruptured ovarian follicle develops into the corpus luteum which secretes both oestradiol and progesterone in the second half or luteal phase of the cycle. Levels of both oestradiol and progesterone therefore rise after ovulation, reaching peak levels between days 18 and 22 of a 28 day cycle. In the last few days of the cycle, if pregnancy has not occurred, the corpus luteum degenerates and oestradiol and progesterone levels fall before menstruation ensues. Plasma levels of progesterone can be measured to assess ovulation and levels greater than 16 nmol/l on days 18–22 are indicatory. The time period from the LH surge to menses is consistently close to 14 days but may vary normally from 12–17 days. However, variability in cycle length among women is principally due to varying number of days required for follicular growth and development in the follicular phase. Menstrual bleeding can occur both in ovulatory and anovulatory cycles. In the latter the ovary produces enough oestrogen to stimulate endometrial growth and bleeding occurs when oestrogen levels fall. Bleeding in anovulatory cycles tends to be irregular, painless, and heavy. In the past decade it has been found that ovarian follicles also produce peptide hormones such as inhibin and activin which inhibit and stimulate FSH production respectively. While these peptides are not measured routinely, they may be in specialized centres.

Endometrial events

The process of menstruation is poorly understood and it is not really known why women should bleed at all since it does not seem to fulfil any biological function. It only occurs in a restricted number of species: humans and most subhuman primates. Consequently, scientific understanding of the physiological mechanisms involved in the process of menstruation is based on animal as well as human data. Endometrium undergoes growth, degeneration, and regression prior to menstruation and bleeding occurs from endometrial blood vessels, especially spiral arterioles. In most species that menstruate, endometrial arterioles are unusual in that they are profusely coiled as they run through the endometrium and also change throughout the menstrual cycle. Endometrial vessels have the unique property of undergoing benign angiogenesis (growth) during each menstrual cycle; otherwise this process is restricted to neoplasia and tissue injury. While this process is clearly under the control of ovarian steroids, endometrial endothelium lacks steroid receptors. These are present on endometrial epithelium and stromal cells, which produce angiogenic polypeptides, which then act on the endothelium. These arterioles undergo profound vasoconstriction which starts 4–24 hours before menstruation and lasts until the end of menstrual bleeding. Bleeding results from relaxation of individual blood vessels and then ceases as they constrict. If constriction did not occur it could not unreasonably be expected that women would bleed to death at the menarche.

Another phenomenon that occurs during menstruation is myometrial contraction. The myometrium contracts throughout the menstrual cycle and there is increased activity during menstruation, especially in women with primary dysmenorrhoea.

Of the pathways thought to play a major role in menstruation, the evidence for altered prostaglandin biosynthesis is the most compelling. Prostaglandins have the capacity to affect both haemostasis and myometrial contractility. Very high levels of prostaglandins are found in uterine tissues and menstrual blood and furthermore administration of prostaglandin F2alpha during the luteal phase of the cycle results in menstrual bleeding. Prostaglandin levels are further increased in women with menorrhagia and dysmenorrhoea, and clinically, inhibitors of prostaglandin biosynthesis are effective in these disorders. In menorrhagia there is also additional evidence of an altered responsiveness to the vasodilator prostaglandin E2. Increased concentrations of prostaglandin E2 receptors are present in myometrium collected from women with excessive bleeding. In dysmenorrhoea the leukotriene pathway allied to prostaglandins has also been implicated in that higher levels of leukotrienes are present

Fig 10.2 *Frequency distribution (%) of menstrual blood loss in several hundred women in Oxford before insertion of a intrauterine device. Mean menstrual loss is 33 ml; median loss is 32 ml*

(From: Unpublished data of J. Guillebaud, with permission)

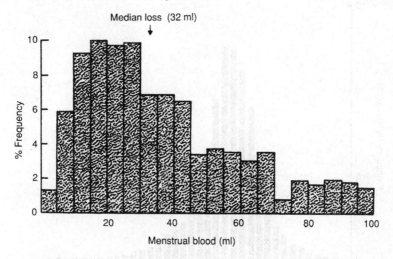

in endometrium of dysmenorrhoeic women. Finally, increased endometrial fibrinolysis has been implicated in menorrhagia, leading to the use of antifibrinolytic agents.

Variation in menstrual blood loss

The amount of blood loss at each menstruation has been measured in several population studies. In several hundred women not complaining of any menstrual problems objective measurement of menstrual blood loss (MBL) shows a skewed distribution with the mean of about 35 ml and the 90th percentile of 80 ml. MBL is considered excessive if greater than 80 ml: without treatment such a loss leads to iron deficiency anaemia and constitutes objective menorrhagia (Fig 10.2). Blood losses up to 1600 ml have been measured in some women. Despite variation in the total amount of blood lost, 90% is lost within the first 3 days, fitting in with patients' descriptions of a tap being turned on and off.

Variation in cycle length and duration of menstruation

Cyclical vaginal bleeding is known to occur at well-defined intervals from the menarche to the menopause. Since ancient times it was shown that the length of the menstrual cycle, i.e. from day 1 of one period to day 1 of the next, approximated to the phases of the moon. The Greek '*men*' means month. Women in many cultures refer to their periods as the moon and some women believe they are actually caused by the moon! As recently as 1938 a textbook for American medical students stated that the majority of women menstruated with the moon! Not surprisingly, the 28-day cycle has become the symbol of health and normality in relation to reproductive function and women begin to

Fig 10.3 *Frequency distribution (%) of length of the menstrual cycle in days from menarche to the menopause. 31 645 menstrual cycle lengths recorded by 656 women aged 11–58 years.* (Redrawn from Fig 33, p.54, in Vollman, 1977.)

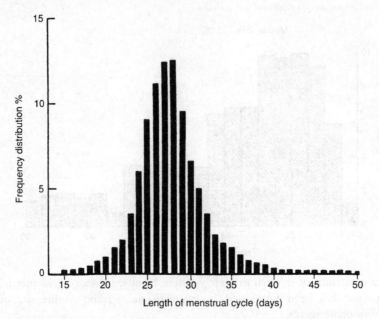

worry that something is wrong if their menstrual cycle deviates from this 28 day 'norm'. Furthermore, medications to induce artificial cycles such as the oral contraceptive and hormone replacement are also generally geared to producing 28-day 'ideal' cycles. It therefore leads to women seeking medical treatment to regulate periods if cycles become either short or long.

It is important that women should be informed that there is a large degree of variability in cycle length that is compatible with good health. Variability in cycle length was best evaluated in the classical study of Vollman (1977). The famous 28-day cycle happens to be the commonest cycle length recorded (Fig 10.3), but only just, and then in only 12.4% of cycles documented. Cycle length changes with age forming a U-shaped curve from the menarche to the menopause. Mean cycle length drops from 35 days at age 12 to a minimum of 27 days at age 43, rising to 52 days at age 55 years with an enormous range of cycle length. Clearly, there is a wide variation in normal cycle length, especially in the first few years after the menarche and in the years preceding the menopause. It is important that normal biological variation be recognized by both women and their doctors so that they do not become crippled by the 28 day 'ideal'.

Similarly, there are also misconceptions about duration of menstruation. In a series of 321 women in Oxford, average duration of menstruation was found to be 5–6 days (Fig 10.4) (Rees, unpublished observations). Furthermore, there was no difference in duration of menstruation between women with normal blood loss and objective menorrhagia.

Fig 10.4 *Duration of menstruation*
(Rees, unpublished observations)

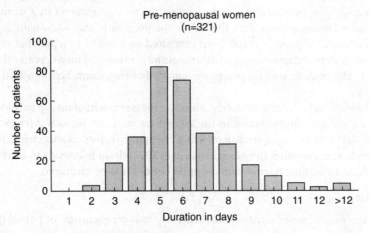

Pre-menopausal women
(n=321)

The abnormal menstrual cycle

In this chapter, menstrual cycle problems, ways of dealing with them in general practice, and indications for referral are presented.

Menorrhagia (heavy blood loss)

Menorrhagia comes from the Greek '*men*' month and '*rhegynai*' to rush out. It is a complaint of excessive menstrual bleeding, but in objective terms is a blood loss greater than 80 ml per period. While various pathologies have been implicated in menorrhagia, in 50% of cases of objective menorrhagia no pathology is found at hysterectomy. Although 'unexplained' menorrhagia is a very appropriate term, this state is often labelled less clearly as dysfunctional uterine bleeding which implies endocrine abnormalities. It must be emphasized that most cases of menorrhagia are associated with regular ovulatory cycles and anovular cycles tend mainly to occur soon after the menarche or close to the menopause. In ovulatory cycles excessive menstrual loss has been ascribed to abnormal uterine levels of prostaglandins with increased concentrations of receptors to the vasodilator prostaglandin E, and elevated levels of the fibrinolytic enzyme plasminogen activator.

Assessment of menstrual blood loss

A common presentation of a patient with menorrhagia is a complaint of increased menstrual loss requiring more sanitary protection or the passage of clots and flooding. While soaking of bed sheets and staining of clothes is suggestive of a heavy period, women find it very difficult to assess accurately the amount of blood loss. Thus some women who are losing several hundred ml consider their flow to be normal while others losing only a few ml complain bitterly of menorrhagia. Furthermore, numbers of pads and tampons as well as degree of staining, parameters often used by doctors, do not give reliable estimates. Women with true menorrhagia may not necessarily drop their haemoglobin concentration; losses of 800–1000 ml can occur without anaemia. Conversely, the presence of a hypochromic microcytic anaemia in a woman who menstruates should alert the GP to the possibility that she might have menorrhagia. At present it has been estimated in hospital practice that only 40% of women complaining of menorrhagia have measured losses greater than 80 ml. The level in general practice is currently being examined in a trial in Oxford.

Although not available routinely, objective measurement of menstrual blood loss is a valuable investigation in the assessment of heavy periods. Menstrual blood loss can be easily measured using the non-invasive alkaline haematin method, where sanitary devices are soaked in 5% sodium hydroxide to convert the blood to alkaline haematin and optical density is then measured.

Causes of menorrhagia

A diagnosis of unexplained menorrhagia depends on exclusion of pathology. Menorrhagia may be due to systemic or pelvic pathology, or iatrogenic causes. However, this widespread view perpetrated by many gynaecological textbooks is based on clinical impression without essential, objective menstrual blood-loss measurement. Disorders of haemostasis such as von Willebrand's disease and deficiencies of factors V, VII, and X, and idiopathic thrombocytopenic purpura are thought to increase menstrual loss, but blood loss was not objectively measured in the cases originally reported. When it has been measured, platelet disorders (thrombocytopenia) rather than coagulation disorders have been implicated in menorrhagia. With regard to pelvic pathology, fibroids (leiomyomas), endometriosis, pelvic inflammatory disease, and endometrial polyps are thought to cause menorrhagia. Again there is a paucity of data with objective MBL measurement. The few studies where it has been measured show that these lesions are associated with objective menorrhagia in only about half to two-thirds of cases. While iatrogenic causes such as intrauterine contraceptive devices have been shown objectively to increase menstrual blood loss there is no such data for anticoagulants.

Diagnosis of menorrhagia

History-taking and general physical and pelvic examination should allow the GP to reach a diagnosis and decide whether hospital referral is necessary. The length and interval of periods and duration of excessive bleeding as well as any intermenstrual or post-coital bleeding should be ascertained. The method of contraception should also be noted since intrauterine contraceptive devices are associated with increased menstrual blood loss. General examination, including bimanual and pelvic examination, should be performed and a cervical smear obtained. A particular search should be made for polyps protruding through the cervical os and for enlargement or tenderness of the uterus or adnexae. A routine full blood count should be performed to check for anaemia.

The next step is to decide whether the endometrium needs to be assessed. Since the incidence of endometrial hyperplasia and carcinoma increases significantly after the age of 40, a prudent guideline is that biopsy is mandatory in women over that age but may be deferred in younger women unless the bleeding is severe, does not respond to treatment, or is associated with intermenstrual bleeding. However, in a woman aged over 40 with regular periods and no intermenstrual bleeding, a trial of a prostaglandin synthetase inhibitor or an antifibrinolytic agent could be used first since blood-loss reduction tends not to occur in the presence of pathology.

While 106 146 D&Cs, were undertaken in England in 1993–94, the use of this procedure has been seriously questioned in women under the age of 40, since the prevalence of endometrial cancer is so low in these women. Based on estimates of endometrial cancer incidence of 0.66 per 100 000 women aged 30–34, it has been calculated that 3000–4000 D&Cs would have to be performed to detect one endometrial cancer in women aged under 35. D&C is not a procedure without risk and is being replaced by outpatient biopsy techniques for assessment of the endometrium. These are also cheaper since they avoid operating and hospitalization costs. Outpatient biopsy can also be undertaken at the time of the initial consultation. The minority of cases such as those who are difficult to examine, have a relatively tight cervix, or decline outpatient testing will still need biopsy under anaesthesia.

The reasons for referral can therefore be for management of pelvic pathology, endometrial assessment, or help with clinical findings if these are uncertain.

Methods of endometrial assessment

The main methods of assessment are endometrial biopsy, hysteroscopy, and vaginal ultrasound.

Endometrial biopsy

1. *D&C*. The classic method of obtaining endometrium is by D&C. This technique was first described by Recamier in 1843; he described the use of a small scoop attached to a long handle for removing intrauterine fungal growths and called this method curettage. This instrument was controversial until antiseptics were available, Recamier reported three deaths from its use as a result of perforation and subsequent peritonitis. D&C is being increasingly replaced by out-patient procedures which avoid general anaesthesia and are also less costly. D&C is not without risk. Complications include perforation, haemorrhage, cervical laceration, and even death. Despite having been considered a gold standard, D&C does not sample the whole of the endometrium. A study where curettage was performed pre-hysterectomy found that in 60% less than half of the cavity was curetted and in 16% less than a quarter. Since D&C is essentially a blind procedure it can miss lesions; in one study 6% of cases (polyps, hyperplasia, and carcinoma).

For many years D&C has erroneously been considered to be a therapeutic as well as a diagnostic procedure. The reason is that traditionally follow-up after any gynaecological procedure is at 6 weeks when most women will have only had one post-operative period. Objective menstrual blood loss measurement has shown that while the first period after D & C is lighter than previous ones, subsequent ones are no different.

2. *Aspiration curettage.* Vacuum or aspiration curettage was introduced in 1970. The first instrument was a 3 mm diameter stainless steel cannula with a curved tip and a wide slit on the concave surface attached to a plastic aspiration chamber and a vacuum (Vabra). Since then various types have been used with a plastic cannula (Rockett) which has either a 3 or 4 mm cannula. Suction can be generated either mechanically or electrically. More recently, internal piston suction devices have been devised (Pipelle, Wallach). They consist of a 3 mm plastic tube with an internal piston; its withdrawal after insertion into the uterine cavity generates suction, pulling in tissue into the cannula as it is rotated. The advantage of aspiration curettage is that it avoids general anaesthesia and has fewer complications than D&C. The technical skills required for outpatient endometrial biopsy are similar to those needed to fit an intrauterine contraceptive device and there is an argument in favour if its use in general practice after suitable training.

There have been many comparative studies of the different methods which support the use of outpatient aspiration curettage. Comparisons of Vabra, Pipelle, and D&C show equal accuracy. However, a comparison of Pipelle and Vabra as measured by endometrial denudation in hysterectomy specimens showed that the Pipelle sampled significantly less of the endometrial surface than the Vabra. Conversely, Pipelle is less painful than Vabra curettage. In general, any discomfort is mild and lasts for about 10–15 seconds as the cannula is passed and the biopsy taken. Thus each tool has advantages and disadvantages.

How to interpret endometrial biopsy reports
Proliferative and secretory changes are reported in endometrium removed from normal women. In the case of endometrial hyperplasia the situation is more complicated because there have been several classifications over the years. The only important distinction in both prognostic and therapeutic terms is between hyperplasias which are associated with a significant risk of progressing into an endometrial adenocarcinoma and those devoid of such risk. It is now generally agreed that cytological atypia is the definitive feature of an endometrial hyperplasia indicative of a potentiality for malignant change. Hence the fundamental division of endometrial hyperplasia into those with cytological atypia and those lacking this feature is as follows:
(1) cytological atypia – classed as atypical hyperplasia, which can progress to carcinoma in 30% of cases, may coexist with malignant endometrium and is considered an indication for hysterectomy;
(2) without cytological atypia – subdivided into simple and complex forms, the latter having architectural atypia where the risk of progression to malignant disease is less than 5% over 13 years, and is usually treated with progestogens. Finally, the report may say 'inadequate tissue for diagnosis'. This does not mean anything sinister, reflecting a thin endometrium, and does not warrant further biopsy.

Hysteroscopy

The hysteroscope provides direct visualization of the endometrial cavity and was introduced over a century ago. However, it has only been recently widely used. Flexible as well as rigid hysteroscopes are now available. Some women require paracervical blocks for anaesthesia. It can be undertaken as an out-patient procedure. Even hysteroscopy is not 100% accurate and rarely adenocarcinomas are missed on initial evaluation.

Although the hysteroscopic evaluation of an endometrium is better able to identify endometrial polyps and submucous fibroids than endometrial biopsy, the necessity of hysteroscopy in all women with abnormal uterine bleeding has not yet been confirmed. Its place is best reserved for women with persistent bleeding where endometrial biopsy is negative or the endometrium abnormally thickened on ultrasound.

Previous endometrial resection/ablation and endometrial assessment

We are now seeing an increasing number of women who have had a previous endometrial resection or ablation. Here the endometrial cavity may be partially obliterated, and assessment of the endometrium extremely problematic.

Transvaginal ultrasound

This technique is increasingly being used to evaluate the endometrium. A thickened endometrium or a cavity filled with fluid is suggestive of malignancy or other pathology (hyperplasia, polyps). Pre-menopausally, total anteroposterior thickness (both endometrial layers) varies from 4–8 mm in the proliferative phase and peaks at 8–16 mm during the secretory phase. Detection of endometrial polyps can be enhanced by instillation of contrast medium into the uterine cavity. It is debated whether vaginal ultrasound can replace endometrial biopsy. However, it must be remembered that ultrasound does not give a histological diagnosis and cannot replace biopsy, but it is a useful adjunct.

Who the GP should treat and how

Women under the age of 40 with otherwise uncomplicated regular heavy periods are extremely unlikely to have endometrial cancer or hyperplasia and referral for specialist opinion in the absence of clinically detectable pathology seems unnecessary. If there are no worrying signs such as bloodstained vaginal discharge, intermenstrual or post-coital bleeding, the GP can use medical therapy to try and reduce blood loss if this is what the woman wishes. The aim of therapy is to reduce blood loss to a socially convenient level and where the woman is not at risk of anaemia. In the absence of objective menstrual blood loss measurements it must be remembered that there are two sorts of treatment failures: (1) those with extremely heavy periods; and (2) those with a normal loss where therapy is only perceived to be effective if the patient is rendered amenorrhoeic. Some women are prepared to put up with their heavy loss if it is not too debilitating or socially inconvenient, and fear the side-effects of drug therapy in the long term. Anaemia should be looked for and corrected. In women over the age of 40 with menorrhagia, referral to a gynaecologist should be considered. However, not all women over 40 will need referral and the GP may try medical therapy first in women whose loss has been gradually increasing over the years. A sudden change in loss is suggestive of pathology and needs earlier referral.

Young girls with heavy periods in the years after the menarche are very unlikely indeed to have any pelvic pathology. Probably all that is required is for the GP to give reassurance by explaining to the girl and her mother that this type of menstrual upset usually settles with time. It is probably part of the maturation of the hypothalamic-pituitary-ovarian axis. GPs should be cautious about giving young girls hormonal treatment in the early years after the menarche because of possible long-term consequences. There are a very few young girls with persistent heavy irregular periods associated with anovular cycles. In these cases, sustained unopposed oestrogen levels leads to endometrial hyperplasia which may ultimately progress in later years to carcinoma. Specialist investigation is required in these young girls to consider the need for cyclical progestogens.

Drug therapy

First-line treatment should be medical. A wide variety of options are now available. Each year about £7 million is spent on primary care prescribing for menorrhagia in the UK; 822 000 prescriptions were issued to 345 225 women for this condition in 1993 (Coulter *et al.* 1995*a*). Medical therapy is indicated when there is no obvious pelvic abnormality and the woman wishes to retain her fertility. Since menstrual loss in the absence of pathology does not change markedly, treatment is long term. Thus the drug regimen chosen must be effective, have few or mild side effects, and must be acceptable to the patient.

The aims of therapy are to reduce blood loss, reduce the risk of anaemia, and improve quality of life. Menorrhagia is the commonest cause of iron deficiency anaemia in Western women and thus iron therapy is often indicated as well as the options discussed below. It could be argued that blood loss should be reduced to be within the normal range (i.e. less than 80 ml per period). However, women who are keen to avoid surgery may accept a higher loss if they can cope with the flow, and any anaemia is controlled with iron.

It is important to assess drug therapies in terms of reduction of measured menstrual blood loss, since there is poor correlation between objective and subjective assessment of menstrual blood loss. Various visual scoring techniques have been devised, however they do not provide an objective measure. Well-designed, randomized controlled trials provide the best evidence of the efficacy of any intervention, as any differences between groups can be more confidently attributed to differences in treatment. In routine clinical practice menstrual blood loss measurements are not available; studies show that over half the women complaining of menorrhagia have a blood loss within normal limits. Here it is the woman's perception and the effect of her menstrual flow on her quality of life which cause her to seek medical help. These factors must be taken into account when discussing treatment options. It must be remembered that even if the overall menstrual blood loss per cycle is less than 80 ml, if most of it occurs in a few hours it can still be a significant problem for the woman and

Table 10.1 *Results of meta-analysis (Coulter et al 1995b)*

Drug	% reduction in menstrual blood loss (95% CI)
Hormone-releasing coil	58.6(56.7–60.6)
Danazol	49.7(47.9–51.6)
Tranexamic acid	46.7(45.0–46.7)
Mefenamic acid	29.0(27.9–30.2)
Diclofenac	26.9(23.2–30.6)
Naproxen	26.4(24.6–28.3)
Ibuprofen	16.2(13.6–18.7)
Ethamsylate	13.1(10.9–15.3)
Norethisterone	−3.6(−6.1–1.1)

should not be disregarded by the GP. A trial in Oxford is currently underway to examine the reasons for consultation by women with objectively normal blood loss.

Medical treatments for menorrhagia can be divided into two main classes: non-hormonal and hormonal. The former includes prostaglandins synthetase inhibitors and antifibrinolytics, and the latter progestogens, oral contraceptives, hormone replacement therapy, danazol, gestrinone, and GnRH analogues. Non-hormonal treatment is taken during menstruation itself and should be a first line in general practice using either mefenamic acid or tranexamic acid; both can be used together, but there are no good studies of the effect of the combination. Referral should be considered if neither inhibitors of prostaglandin synthesis or antifibrinolytic agents are effective.

A meta-analysis of 31 randomized controlled trials of drug therapy for menorrhagia (Table 10.1) showed that tranexamic acid was the most effective non-hormonal treatment (Coulter *et al.* 1995*b*). This is appropriate as a first-line treatment in general practice, though side-effects may limit its use (see below). Mefenamic acid is less effective in reducing menstrual flow but has the advantage of alleviating dysmenorrhoea and women may find it more acceptable. Of the hormonal preparations, only danazol and the progestogen-IUCDs were effective. Danazol is expensive, has a high incidence of unpleasant side-effects, and is not recommended for long-term use. The levonorgestrel IUCD looks very promising, but further trials are needed to evaluate it. The effects of the combined pill on reducing blood loss come from observational studies only, and there are no randomized controlled trials of the use of hormone replacement therapy for this purpose.

Non-hormonal treatments (Table 10.2)

Prostaglandin synthetase inhibitors. Inhibitors of prostaglandin synthesis can be chemically classified into four main groups: salicylates (aspirin), indolacetic acid analogues (indomethacin), aryl proprionic acid derivatives (naproxen,

Table 10.2 *Non-hormonal treatments for menorrhagia*

Prostaglandin synthetase inhibitors	Mefenamic acid
	Meclofenamic acid*
	Naproxen
	Ibuprofen
	Flurbiprofen
	Diclofenac
Antifibrinolytics	Tranexamic acid
	Epsilon-amino caproic acid
Ethamsylate	

* Not available in UK at present

ibuprofen), and fenamates (mefenamic acid, flufenamic acid, meclofenamic acid). Of the four groups, the fenamates have been the most extensively studied for the treatment of menorrhagia.

The use of prostaglandin synthetase inhibitors is based on the observations showing that prostaglandin (PG) biosynthesis is altered in menorrhagia. As well as inhibiting prostaglandin synthesis, the fenamates have the unique property of also binding to prostaglandin receptors: PGE (a vasodilator) receptor concentrations are significantly higher in women with menorrhagia. Also, fenamates are thought to improve endometrial haemostasis. Clinically, the ability of mefenamic acid to reduce excessive menstrual bleeding was first described by Anderson *et al.* (1976). In this preliminary report, five women were treated with mefenamic acid 500 mg three times daily on the first 3 days of menstruation when heavy blood loss was anticipated by the patient. Measured menstrual loss was reduced from a pre-treatment mean of 119 to 60 ml. Subsequent studies have confirmed efficacy. With regards to long-term therapy, follow-up 12–15 months after commencing treatment showed that mefenamic acid continued to be effective.

Reductions in menstrual loss have also been documented for other PG synthetase inhibitors such as naproxen, ibuprofen, sodium diclofenac, and flurbiprofen. The percentage reduction in blood loss varied from 25–47%, depending on the agent and dose used. It has been reported that naproxen and ibuprofen were ineffective in women with leiomyomas. In general, prostaglandin synthetase inhibitors are contraindicated in women with peptic ulceration, but otherwise have few side-effects if taken for only a few days each cycle.

Thus PG synthetase inhibitors should be considered as a first-line treatment in essential menorrhagia since they are well-tolerated and suitable for long-term treatment. An added factor is that these drugs will also alleviate menstrual pain.

Antifibrinolytics. The use of antifibrinolytic agents is based on the observation of increased levels of fibrinolytic activity in endometrium in women with

Table 10.3 *Hormonal treatments for menorrhagia*

Progestogens	Norethisterone
	Medroxyprogesterone acetate
	Dydrogesterone
Intrauterine progestogens	Levonorgestrel IUCD
	Progestasert IUCD
Combined oestrogen/progestogens	Oral contraceptives
	Hormone replacement therapy
Other	Danazol
	Gestrinone
	GnRH analogues

menorrhagia. The effect of tranexamic acid was first reported in 1967. Overall tranexamic acid reduces blood loss by 40%. Thus antifibrinolytics should be considered as a first-line treatment for menorrhagia, but they do not deal with any attendant dysmenorrhoea. The incidence of side-effects is related to dose and about one-third of women receiving 3–6 g daily experience gastrointestinal symptoms. Serious side-effects were originally suggested, including cerebral sinus thrombosis and central venous stasis retinopathy. However, over a 19-year time span and 238 000 woman-years of treatment with tranexamic acid from the late 1960s, no increase of thrombotic events over and above that of the general population of the same age was observed in Scandinavia. The use of antifibrinolytics is to be encouraged among GPs in view of the evidence of its effectiveness.

Ethamsylate is though to act by reducing capillary fragility, though the precise mechanisms are uncertain. It is not widely used to treat menorrhagia. While one comparative study has shown a 20% reduction in loss, another has shown none.

Hormonal treatments (Table 10.3)

Progestogens. The use of progestogens is based on the concept that women with menorrhagia principally have anovulatory cycles and that a progestogen supplement is required. However, many studies have shown that most women with regular excessive menstrual bleeding have normal ovulatory cycles. Progestogens are the commonest prescription for women complaining of menorrhagia. The first report of its use was in 1960 in a study where menstrual blood loss was not measured, and the conclusions based on a subjective response. However, studies where MBL has been measured with luteal phase administration for 7 days of norethisterone 5 mg twice daily, show either a 20% decrease or even an increase in flow. Thus with current evidence the short-term use of norethisterone for ovulatory menorrhagia (i.e. regular heavy menstruation) cannot be justified. It is possible that if given for a longer time, say 14 or 21 days, or in higher dose it may be effective; but there are no studies to date. The use of oral progestogens should be limited to regularizing irregular menstrual cycles, postponing periods, or arresting a torrential bleed.

1. *Regularizing irregular periods* – There are no good studies about the dose or duration of progestogen that should be used; but norethisterone 10 mg daily for 2–3 weeks out of 4 is usually effective.

2. *How to postpone a period* – Sometimes women ask for something to postpone a period because of, for example, a special event such as a wedding, an examination, or a holiday. Periods can be postponed using a progestogen such as norethisterone 5 mg three times daily, starting 3 days before the anticipated period. An alternative, if given several months' warning, is to take the combined oral contraceptive pill continuously.

3. *A torrential bleed* – Very large doses of progestogens such as 30 mg daily can be used to arrest a torrential bleed. This is usually effective within 24–48 hours, when the dose can be reduced and then finally stopped over the next few days when another, usually lighter bleed will occur. Bleeding of this magnitude requires referral for specialist assessment, and may initially require emergency measures by the GP.

Intrauterine progesterone or more especially levonorgestrel are much more successful than oral progestogens in reducing menstrual loss. With the levonorgestrel IUCD reductions of MBL of 88% and 96% are found after 6 months and 12 months respectively. The levonorgestrel IUCD also provides very effective contraception. It could now be considered to be a serious candidate as an alternative to surgical management for essential menorrhagia. However, it is important to emphasize the essential difference between the levonorgestrel IUCD and other IUCDS which can increase menstrual loss. Women also need to be counselled about irregular bleeding which can occur in the first few months after insertion.

Oestrogen/progestogen. The combined oral contraceptive pill is often used clinically to reduce MBL. In general, the reduction in loss is about 50%. The mechanism of action is probably related to the induced endometrial atrophy resulting in decreased PG synthesis and fibrinolysis. Monthly cyclical oestrogen/progestogen HRT is also used to treat menorrhagia in peri-menopausal women. Although clinically it seems to work there has been to date no randomized controlled trials. However, open studies of three preparations show that their measured withdrawal bleeds are not heavier than normal periods. Data on three monthly bleed regimens are awaited.

Danazol is an isoxazol derivative of 17α-ethinyl-testosterone which acts on the hypothalamic pituitary ovarian axis as well as on the endometrium to produce atrophy. Studies have shown MBL reductions ranging from 50–85%. However, the clinical use of danazol is limited by its androgenic side-effects which include weight gain and skin rashes. The use of danazol is probably best restricted to women awaiting surgery.

Gestrinone is a 19-nortestosterone derivative which has antiprogestogenic, anti-oestrogenic, and androgenic activity. In a placebo controlled study, gestrinone was given 2.5 mg twice weekly for 12 weeks to 19 women with proven menorrhagia. Ten women became amenorrhoeic and a marked reduction in MBL was seen in five; placebo had no effect. In three of the non-responders submucous fibroids were found at subsequent hysterectomy. The therapy was well-tolerated since all women completed the trial. However, gestrinone's androgenic side-effects preclude long-term therapy.

GnRH analogues can be used to reduce MBL by pituitary down regulation and subsequent inhibition of ovarian activity resulting in amenorrhoea. However, the induced hypo-oestrogenic state with its adverse effects on bone metabolism limits its use beyond 6 months. When cyclical oestrogen/progestogen hormone replacement therapy has been used in conjunction with GnRH analogues, median MBL after 3 months' treatment in the women with objective menorrhagia was 74 ml. This treatment combination is expensive and should not be used as a first line. Specialist advice should be sought before using such regimes.

Other treatments

Acute bleeds have been stopped with intravenous infusions of conjugated equine oestrogens; however this therapy is not a suitable strategy in general practice. Some women may be keen to avoid drug therapy altogether. Diet and exercise have been proposed as influencing blood loss, but no controlled trials have been undertaken.

Treatment failures

Several options have to be considered when the patient says that the treatment has failed. First, her loss may be so excessive that, unless the treatment produces amenorrhoea, it has been insufficiently controlled. For example, with tranexamic acid where pre-treatment blood loss is less than 200 ml per menstruation, 92% of women will have their blood loss reduced to less than 80 ml on therapy. However, if blood loss exceeds 250 ml, tranexamic acid is very unlikely to achieve a loss within normal limits. A similar pattern would be expected with PG synthetase inhibitors. Second, she may have a pre-treatment blood loss less than 80 ml and the perceived reduction in loss on therapy is not sufficient for her. This was illustrated in a study including women with normal MBL where therapy with mefenamic acid did not reduce loss and actually increased it. Lastly, the patient may have unsuspected uterine pathology such as a submucous fibroid or endometrial polyp which makes medical treatment ineffective. It is unfortunate that many studies do not follow up their treatment failures with hysteroscopy to check for such pathology.

Surgical treatment

GPs need to state clearly in their referral letters what the question is and to discuss treatment options with the patient beforehand so that she can make an informed decision. Surgical treatment may be necessary to deal with pelvic abnormalities such as polyps, fibroids, chronic pelvic inflammatory disease, or endometriotic masses. Operations should be as conservative as possible in women who wish to retain their fertility. Referral letters need to state what the problem is and what has been discussed with the patient. Surgical treatment is also indicated when medical treatment has failed. Surgical treatment includes removal of cervical or endometrial polyps, myomectomy, and ultimately, hysterectomy. Over recent years there has been increasing use of minimally invasive surgery options using laparoscopic or hysteroscopic approaches, which have the potential of shorter hospital stay and recovery times. These techniques will be discussed in some detail so that GPs can explain them to their patients.

Hysterectomy

Hysterectomy is offered more often to younger women whose families are complete because many are reluctant to take treatment for several years until the menopause. Although 100% effective, hysterectomy is accompanied by significant morbidity (pyrexia, haemorrhage, infection) but fortunately a low mortality rate. Estimates of the risk of operative mortality vary from 0.4–2 per 1000 women, depending on the definition of operative mortality and type of study. Mortality in women under the age of 50 for hysterectomy for non-cancer indications has been estimated as 4.2 per 10 000. Short-term morbidity is high with complication rates of 25% for vaginal and 43% for abdominal hysterectomy; similarly mortality for vaginal hysterectomy is half that of abdominal hysterectomy. The reason is unclear but may reflect selection of healthier women for the vaginal operation.

Concern exists with the long-term sequelae which may include premature onset of ovarian failure even when ovaries are conserved, psychosexual dysfunction, urinary tract and bowel symptoms. In general, hysterectomy has a beneficial effect on mental well-being. However, while some studies show increased sexual enjoyment, other show reduced libido. There is currently a vogue for subtotal hysterectomy, conserving the cervix, with the understanding that sexual function is better preserved than with total hysterectomy. The down side is that cervical smears have to be continued. Similarly, the evidence of the effects of total or subtotal hysterectomy on urinary tract and bowel function is conflicting.

Ovaries and hysterectomy

Until relatively recently, it was naively thought that if ovaries were conserved at hysterectomy they continued to function normally. However, there is increasing evidence that ovarian function is compromised and the age of menopause is brought forward by several years. This increases the risk of developing cardiovascular disease and osteoporosis. The diagnosis of ovarian failure is more difficult in the absence of menstrual function. It is important that women who have had a hysterectomy in their thirties are not told they are too young to be menopausal if they develop symptoms of ovarian failure a few years later, and undergo a premature menopause.

Oophorectomy is often performed prophylactically at the time of abdominal hysterectomy in order to avoid the risk of ovarian cancer. Its use is highly debated in women not at risk of developing the disease, where it has been estimated that about 200 oophorectomies would need to be undertaken to avoid one case of ovarian cancer. Oophorectomy results in a surgical menopause with marked menopausal symptoms, and increased risk of cardiovascular disease and osteoporosis. It must be remembered that in Western societies cardiovascular disease is the major cause of death in women. Oophorectomy reduces average life expectancy in younger women by at least 5 years if they do not take oestrogen HRT. It is of concern that compliance with long-term HRT is low, with most women in the UK only taking it for a few months. Thus, prophylactic oophorectomy in women at low risk of ovarian cancer cannot really be justified. In women with a family history of ovarian cancer who are considered to be at high risk, prophylactic oophorectomy is justifiable when their family is complete and after thorough counselling. It must be remembered however that familial ovarian cancer may be a generalized field change disease in the peritoneal cavity and some doubt exists about the efficacy of oophorectomy, since cases of intraabdominal carcinomatosis have been reported, following surgery in which subsequent review of the ovarian specimen revealed a small focus of ovarian cancer.

Laparoscopic hysterectomy

The laparoscope can be used in a variety of ways to assist in performing a hysterectomy. If the uterine vessels are defined and secured by laparoscopic techniques, the procedure is considered to be a true laparoscopic hysterectomy. If the laparoscopic portion of the operation is discontinued at any stage before the uterine vessels are secured, the procedure is described as a laparoscopically-assisted vaginal hysterectomy. The uterine tissue is either removed from the abdominal cavity vaginally or through the umbilical port instruments. There is interest about retaining all or part of the cervix, or coring out the centre of the cervix, including the transformation zone. A Belgian national survey of laparoscopic hysterectomy shows that the major complications are urinary tract injury and haemorrhage. The VALUE hysterectomy study is currently underway in the UK to evaluate this approach.

Endometrial ablative techniques

The concept of endometrial ablation as a treatment for menorrhagia is based on the observation that destruction of the endometrium led to amenorrhoea, and is called eponymously Asherman's syndrome. Because of the significant regenerative capacity of the endometrium it is essential to destroy its basal layer for the techniques to be successful. The methods employed are resection of the endometrium, or ablation of the endometrium by laser, rollerball diathermy, radiofrequency, cryoablation, microwaves, and thermal balloons. Like hysterectomy, these treatments should only be offered to women who desire no further children. However, although the risk of pregnancy is minimal, patients cannot be assured it is a sterilization procedure. Pregnancies both intrauterine and ectopic have been reported: there are also concerns about the potential risk of placenta accreta (where the placenta becomes embedded in the myometrium) in view of the altered endometrium. Some gynaecologists offer laparoscopic sterilization at the time of resection.

Transcervical resection of the endometrium (TCRE) is a hysteroscopic method of endometrial ablation similar in concept to transurethral resection of the prostrate. It aims not only to remove the basal layer of the endometrium but also the first few millimetres of myometrium, thereby ensuring endometrial destruction with the electrocautery loop of a resectoscope. The resectoscope can also be used to remove submucous fibroids which alone may be a cause of menorrhagia. The resected endometrium can be examined histologically for unsuspected abnormalities. A recent variant of this technique, transuterine mucosal ablation (where a cylinder of uterus containing the endometrial cavity is cored out), is being piloted in some countries.

The rollerball or ball-end electrode destroys the endometrium thermally using unipolar cautery as it is rolled along the uterine lining. The rollerball has a blunt contact area which potentially lessens the probability of perforation which is of concern with the resectoscope, and has improved access for the uterine cornua.

The neodynium, yttrium aluminium garnet (Nd: YAG) laser is the most suitable laser for endometrial ablation since it can be transmitted through flexible quartz fibres and liquid distension media and can penetrate and destroy tissue to a controlled depth of 4–5 mm. The laser energy can be applied by either the touch or the non-touch technique or by a combination of the two. The original description used the touch technique where the quartz fibre is allowed to be in actual contact with the endometrium, while in the non-touch technique the end of the fibre is brought as near to the lining of the uterus as possible without touching it, and is generally considered to be the faster method.

Radiofrequency-induced thermal endometrial ablation relies on hyperthermia induced by an electric field that is generated around an intrauterine conductive probe. Tissue lying within the electric field becomes heated by locally generated currents. Since direct contact between the probe and the tissue is not necessary, irregularity of the endometrial cavity does not preclude whole cavity heating. A vaginal guard is used to avoid thermal vaginal damage.

Microwaves, thermal balloons, and cryosurgery have been used to a lesser extent. Thermal balloons are currently being assessed in an international multi-centre trial.

In the last techniques no tissue is obtained for histological examination, and therefore abnormality should be excluded by previous endometrial biopsy. Many hysteroscopists recommend pre-operative medical therapy to render the endometrium atrophic in order to simplify surgery and thus maximize the possibility of complete resection. The most frequently-used agents are progestogens, danazol, and GnRH analogues, with the last providing the most promising approach.

Efficacy and complications. Success of endometrial ablative techniques has been generally measured in terms of induced amenorrhoea or significantly reduced menstrual flow; few studies have more than 12-month follow-up and most emphasize the learning curve with each method. Amenorrhoea rates vary from 20–64% and reduced flow from 30–93%. It has been suggested that endometrial ablative techniques are not suitable where there is significant dysmenorrhoea. Women where treatment has failed are variously managed by a repeat procedure or hysterectomy. Reoperation rates vary from 6–23%, with higher rates found in studies with longer follow-up. Regardless of the techniques used, complications can only be minimized once the surgeon has gained sufficient expertize. The most common complications are haemorrhage, perforation, and absorption of distending medium (radiofrequency-induced thermal ablation, microwaves, and thermal balloons do not use a distending medium). A national UK study (MISTLETOE) of 10 700 hysteroscopic procedures between April 1993–October 1994 showed that the incidence of operative complications associated with resection was 6.4%, compared with 2.1% for rollerball and 2.7% for laser. Haemorrhage may occur during or after the procedure, with the majority of cases being post-operative when the tamponade effect of the pressurized distending medium is released and vessels not fully coagulated start to bleed. Two types of uterine perforation may occur: those occurring during the insertion of the rigid surgical instruments and more seriously, that caused during the ablation itself which can lead to damage of other pelvic organs (bladder, ureter, bowel, major vessels). The rate of uterine perforation is higher with resection (1.6%) than with laser ablation (0.3%). Vesicovaginal fistulae have been reported after radiofrequency ablation when the vaginal guard was insufficiently protective. Absorption of abnormally large volumes of distension medium, presumably through open blood vessels, can occur, resulting in fluid overload and pulmonary oedema. Careful monitoring of fluid balance is essential and can be aided by the use of automatic infusion systems.

Apart from failure, a variety of late complications have been reported which include haematometra, pelvic pain, and necrotizing granulomatous endometritis. Another long-term complication is masking an adenocarcinoma of the endometrium, which could develop in theory in small endometrial cavities created by synechial formation. However, the incidence of carcinoma of the endometrium is low, and thus large long-term studies are required to assess this.

Comparison of endometrial ablative techniques with hysterectomy

Endometrial ablative techniques cannot really be considered to replace hysterectomy since they do not render all women amenorrhoeic or sterile: but they can be considered as an alternative strategy. Furthermore, when HRT is given after endometrial ablation the oestrogen must be opposed with progestogen to prevent development of hyperplasia and carcinoma in any remaining endometrium. Three randomized trials have been undertaken to compare abdominal hysterectomy and resection/ablation. Operating time, hospital stay, return to daily activities, and work were shorter after resection/ablation than after hysterectomy. Recovery times after hysterectomy and resection/ablation are estimated to be 8–11 and 2–3 weeks respectively. While patient satisfaction is high after both approaches, it is higher after hysterectomy. Initially, endometrial resection appears to be less costly than hysterectomy, however this advantage decreases with longer follow-up because of the need for repeat surgery.

Counselling

It is of concern that only 40% of women complaining of menorrhagia actually have objective menorrhagia. Thus the majority of women could be considered to have inappropriate treatment, and counselling would be a better option in these cases. A study of 17 women referred for hospital treatment for menorrhagia, in whom blood loss was less than 80 ml, showed that counselling is effective (Rees 1991). A 3-year follow-up of these women showed only one woman had opted for hysterectomy, two had taken drug therapy, and the remainder had accepted the advice. The effectiveness of reassurance and counselling is not known; it is currently being examined in primary care in a randomized controlled trial in Oxford.

What happens in current practice

Current management in primary care has been recently examined in Oxford and in a national survey (Coulter *et al.* 1995 *a* and *b*). In the Oxford study of six general practices with 4977 registered female patients in the 30–49 age group, 6.5% consulted during 1991 for menorrhagia. Only 15% had a pelvic examination and 13% a blood test. Sixty-three per cent were given drug therapy and 30% referred to a specialist. In those given drug therapy 41% were prescribed norethisterone, 35% mefenamic acid, and 1% tranexamic acid. A similar pattern was found in the national survey of 518 GPs. It is of concern that the most frequently prescribed drug is norethisterone, when scientific evidence shows that it is the least effective therapy.

The effect of fundholding on patterns of referrals in 11 specialties has recently been examined. While four of the 11 specialities showed an increase in referral (general medicine, dermatology, psychiatry, plastic surgery), the only significant decrease was in gynaecology, a trend not found in non-fundholding practices. This suggests that fundholders may be persisting more with medical treatments before referral.

The role of patients' preferences and the decision to treat by GPs is another important issue. Women are more likely to continue medical treatment long term if they have explored the treatment options and come to an informed decision. In a recent survey in primary care only 36% of patients indicated that they had a strong treatment preference (Coulter *et al.* 1994). The best predictors of having a treatment preference were higher education and previous consultation for gynaecological problems. Women with higher education were more likely to choose medical treatment; and female GPs were more inclined than their male counterparts to instigate drug treatment rather than refer for surgery. A history of prior surgery and a male GP increased the likelihood of referral to a gynaecologist. Similarly, a national survey showed significant socio-economic variations in admission for D&C and hysterectomy (Kuh and Stirling 1995). There were significant inverse educational gradients, the risk of admission increasing more than twofold between the most and least-educated women. Only 1% with the highest educational qualifications compared to 19% of those with minimal qualifications had been admitted to hospital. There was a significant educational gradient in hysterectomy rate from 1% to 15%, and a twofold difference in risk of D&C; and an increased risk of admission and surgery in lower social class groups. The precise reasons for these trends have not been fully established, but would suggest that better-educated women from higher social groups may get more discussion and reassurance about their menstrual symptoms, which makes them less likely to opt for surgical treatment.

In this context, it is interesting that a comparison of treatment decisions made in gynaecological clinics in the NHS and private sector were similar, but the decision-making styles appeared to be different. Private patients were more likely to participate in treatment decisions than NHS patients, a difference persisting after adjustment for educational status. The authors of this study concluded that gynaecologists were better at involving women in decision-making in their private than their NHS clinics (Coulter et al. 1995c).

In conclusion, there is a need to make good information packages (video, information leaflets) to help women make informed decisions. A multi-centre study is currently underway to evaluate this approach.

The ideal management of menorrhagia

Firstly, the GP needs to find out how much of a problem menstrual bleeding is to the woman concerned. Objective menstrual blood-loss measurement is not available routinely.

The ideal management of complaints of menorrhagia should be based on objective menstrual blood loss measurements; tailoring treatment to loss. In women with a normal pelvic examination and blood loss, reassurance and counselling would be the most appropriate option. If blood loss is less than 200 ml, effective drug therapy such as tranexamic acid or mefenamic acid should be employed. Norethisterone should not be used as it is ineffective in reducing blood loss. A good candidate for blood losses greater than 200 ml would be the levonorgestrel-releasing IUCD, which produces amenorrhoea and can be reversed, unlike hysterectomy and endometrial ablative techniques. Women, where treatment does not reduce blood loss, should be investigated for previously unsuspected uterine pathology.

In the past decade, endometrial ablative techniques have been introduced as alternatives to hysterectomy. It may be minimally invasive surgery but it is certainly not minor surgery and requires considerable skill and training. Patients need to be aware that the result may be light bleeding rather than amenorrhoea, that the procedure may fail, and of the rare hazards involved. Long-term studies are required to evaluate fully the role of endometrial ablative techniques.

Information packages need to be improved, and patient preferences need to be examined. Options must be discussed with the woman so that she can make an informed decision as to the best treatment for her as an individual.

Treatment of fibroids

Uterine fibroids are tumours which arise in the myometrium. They are the commonest form of pathology found in women, being present in about

30% of women over the age of 35. They are composed predominantly of smooth muscle with a variable amount of connective tissue. Three subtypes are recognized depending on their situation in relation to the uterine wall, namely submucous, subserous, and intramural. Submucous fibroids are often implicated in menorrhagia, while those in other sites may be innocent bystanders. The proportion associated with objective menorrhagia is not well-documented. They are commonly multiple and may result in considerable uterine enlargement. Fibroids are frequently asymptomatic, but may present with menorrhagia, pelvic pain, or pressure symptoms.

Fibroids are thought to be oestrogen-dependent since they do not occur prior to puberty and become smaller after the menopause. It is currently believed that oestrogen exerts an effect on fibroid growth by the stimulation of growth factors.

Uterine fibroids are usually diagnosed clinically but they may be difficult to differentiate from ovarian masses. Ultrasound is useful in this situation, but again there may be difficulty in distinguishing between pedunculated subserous fibroids and solid ovarian tumours. If any doubt remains patients need referral and laparoscopy or laparotomy may be considered.

The management of women with uterine fibroids depends on size, associated symptoms, as well as her age and reproductive wishes. Small asymptomatic fibroids rarely require treatment but need to be monitored regularly; say with annual ultrasound A concern is sarcomatous changes in fibroids, but this is now thought to be very low being less than 0.2%. Women with fibroids and menorrhagia are usually treated by hysterectomy. For those wishing to conserve their fertility, myomectomy may be offered. The advent of new endoscopic techniques means that it is possible to remove subserous and intramural fibroids by laparoscopy and submucous fibroids by hysteroscopy, and thus avoid laparotomy. Local destruction by laser or electrocoagulation are techniques currently being evaluated.

There is a considerable demand for an alternative to surgery in the management of fibroids. Prostaglandin synthetase inhibitors are probably of limited effect in reducing heavy menstrual bleeding. The 19-norsteroids danazol and gestrinone may be effective and may indeed shrink uterine volume. A therapeutic innovation is the use of GnRH analogues to induce a temporary and reversible menopausal state. These analogues produce amenorrhoea and fibroid shrinkage. Unfortunately, shrinkage is rarely complete and not sustained after cessation of therapy. Another concern is the bone mineral loss associated with a prolonged hypo-oestrogenic state, limiting the use of analogues to 6 months. GnRH analogues are especially useful prior to hysterectomy, making the operation technically easier and reducing operative blood loss. A combination of the GnRH analogue goserelin and endometrial resection is being evaluated as an alternative to hysterectomy for fibroids and the results look encouraging (Rees and Gillmer, in progress).

Dysmenorrhoea

Derived from the Greek meaning, difficult monthly flow, the word dysmenorrhoea has come to mean painful menstruation. Dysmenorrhoea can be classified as either primary or secondary. In the former type there is no pelvic pathology while the latter implies underlying pathology which leads to painful menstruation.

Primary dysmenorrhoea

In general, primary dysmenorrhoea appears 6–12 months after the menarche when ovulatory cycles have become established. The early cycles after the menarche are usually anovular and tend to be painless. The pain usually consists of lower abdominal cramps and backache and there may be associated gastrointestinal disturbances such as diarrhoea and vomiting. Symptoms occur predominantly during the first 2 days of menstruation. Primary dysmenorrhoea tends not to be associated with excessive menstrual bleeding: it is rare for women to have both dysmenorrhoea and menorrhagia.

It is only in the past two decades that intra-uterine pressure measurements were performed which demonstrated for the first time that women complaining of dysmenorrhoea were not neurotic. Primary dysmenorrhoea is associated with uterine hypercontractility, characterized by excessive amplitude and frequency of contractions and a high 'resting' tone between contractions. During contractions endometrial blood flow is reduced and there seems to be a good correlation between minimal blood flow and maximal colicky pain, favouring the concept that ischaemia due to hypercontractility causes primary dysmenorrhoea.

It is now generally agreed that the myometrial hypercontractility pattern found in primary dysmenorrhoea is associated with increased prostaglandin production. More recently, elevated levels of leukotriene C4, D4, and E4 (substances allied to prostaglandins) have been found in endometrium collected from dysmenorrhoeic women. Increased vasopressin levels have also been implicated.

Although excessive levels of prostaglandins, leukotrienes, and vasopressin have been found in primary dysmenorrhoea, the primary stimulus for their production remains unknown.

Secondary dysmenorrhoea

Secondary dysmenorrhoea is associated with pelvic pathology such as endometriosis, adenomyosis, pelvic inflammatory disease, submucous leiomyomas, and endometrial polyps. The use of an intrauterine contraceptive device may also lead to dysmenorrhoea. Secondary dysmenorrhoea tends to appear several years after the menarche and the patient may complain of a change in the intensity and timing of her pain. The pain may last for the whole of the menstrual period and may be associated with discomfort before the onset of menstruation. The mechanism by which various pathologies cause pain is uncertain and again prostaglandins may be involved though the evidence is less clear.

Assessment

A full gynaecological history is an essential part of investigation. The onset of dysmenorrhoea and its relation to menstruation usually differentiate between primary and secondary dysmenorrhoea. The presence of an intrauterine contraceptive device or a history of infertility should also be noted. In young girls one can usually assume a diagnosis of primary dysmenorrhoea and it is probably unnecessary to examine them. If the history is suggestive of secondary dysmenorrhoea, a bimanual pelvic and speculum examination should be performed. A particular search should be made for polyps protruding through the cervical os and for enlargement, tenderness, or fixity of the uterus or adnexae.

Referral to a gynaecologist may be necessary if pathology is suspected and the investigations may include ultrasound, MRI scans, hysteroscopy, and laparoscopy.

Treatment

The clear involvement of prostaglandins in primary dysmenorrhoea has led to the use of prostaglandin synthetase inhibitors such as mefenamic acid, naproxen, and ibuprofen to treat the disorder; and they are effective in reducing menstrual pain in 80–90% of patients. Commencing treatment before the onset of menstruation appears to have no demonstrable advantage over starting treatment when bleeding starts. This observation is compatible with the short plasma half-life of prostaglandin synthetase inhibitors. The advantage of starting treatment at the onset of menstruation is that it prevents the patient treating herself when she is unknowingly pregnant, which would only become apparent when a period is missed.

The presence of elevated leukotriene and vasopressin levels may explain why not all women respond to prostaglandin synthetase inhibitors. The role of the various agents which affect the leukotriene pathway has not yet been fully evaluated in the treatment of primary dysmenorrhoea. Vasopressin antagonists have been examined but are not available for routine use at present. It must not be forgotten that the combined oestrogen/progestogen oral contraceptive pill is a useful agent for the treatment of primary dysmenorrhoea, especially when contraception is required. The Pill is effective in 80–90% of women and probably acts by reducing the capacity of the endometrium to produce prostaglandins.

Concern remains about the 10–20% of patients with primary dysmenorrhoea who fail to respond either to prostaglandin synthetase inhibitors or to oral contraceptives. Some of these women may really be suffering from secondary dysmenorrhoea with pelvic pathology, requiring appropriate investigation, but the concern has led to the examination of new agents such as leukotriene and vasopressin antagonists.

Effective treatment of secondary dysmenorrhoea must be based on a correct diagnosis since different pathologies require different therapies. In addition the type of treatment offered must take into account the patient's age, her desire for conception, the severity of the symptoms, and the extent of the disease.

Amenorrhoea

Absence of periods disturbs women just as much as other disturbances of menstruation, especially since it has implications of loss of a normal bodily

Table 10.4 *Main causes of amenorrhoea*

Hypothalamic – pituitary disorders
  Prolactin hypersecretion ± prolactin-secreting pituitary adenoma
  Tumours
  Weight loss – anorexia nervosa
  Obesity
  Psychogenic
  Post-oral contraception
  Isolated gonadotrophin deficiency (Kallman's syndrome)

Ovarian, uterine, or vaginal disorders
  Polycystic ovarian disease
  Ovarian failure (premature menopause)
  Gonadal dysgenesis (e.g. Turner's syndrome)
  Absence of uterus (e.g. testicular feminization) or vagina
  Haematocolpos

Other diseases
  Thyroid hormone deficiency or excess
  Adrenal disorders (e.g. Cushing's disease, congenital adrenal hyperplasia)
  Severe general disease (e.g. leukaemia or Hodgkin's disease treated
  with chemotherapy)

---

function related to fertility. While some women may be concerned about loss of femininity, others will worry about an unwanted pregnancy. It seems relatively clear that women wish to menstruate regularly, not too much or too little, but not to be without altogether. There is also the connotation that amenorrhoea for 6 months or more, when associated with low oestrogen levels can increase the risk of osteoporosis, and bone density should be ascertained.

To menstruate women require a functioning, hypothalamic pituitary ovarian axis with a responding endometrium and genital outflow tract in the absence of endocrine or systemic disease or drug therapy, and in the presence of a normal chromosome complement. In the vast majority of women presenting in general practice the cause will be hormonal. There has been a preoccupation in the past in distinguishing between primary and secondary amenorrhoea, but this should be probably defused since there is so much overlap between the two. Instead, the differential diagnoses should be based on the pathological categories (Table 10.4).

Assessment

The initial step in the work up of the amenorrhoeic patient is exclusion of the possibility of pregnancy even in a woman with primary amenorrhoea. It is important that the GP should warn women with primary or secondary amenorrhoea of hormonal aetiology that they are not necessarily infertile and are at risk of pregnancy should a sporadic ovulation occur.

History-taking and examination should elicit the following information and physical characteristics in all cases of amenorrhoea:

(1) age at menarche;

(2) development of secondary sex characteristics – pubic and axillary hair, breasts, menstrual history before amenorrhoea;

(3) galactorrhoea

(4) recent change in body height and weight; and level of exercise;

(5) medication: oral contraception, chemotherapy;

(6) family history of genetic anomalies;

(7) recent emotional upsets;

(8) hirsutism, acne as markers of androgenization; voice changes, clitoromegaly as signs of virilization;

(9) hot flushes and sweats and dry vagina;

(10) previous surgery: curettage, oophorectomy, other endocrine organs;

(11) symptoms of endocrine disorders: thyroid, pituitary, adrenal;

(12) systemic, abdominal, and pelvic examination with special attention to reproductive tract and inguinal hernias, though in young girls pelvic examination is best replaced by ultrasound.

Laboratory tests to determine the cause of amenorrhoea involve measurement in serum in all cases of the anterior pituitary hormones FSH and LH, as well as prolactin and thyroid function tests. If FSH and LH are elevated they need repeating. Testosterone should be measured in women with hirsutism or where testicular feminization is suspected. Oestradiol levels are usually of limited value. The karyotype should be checked if there are suspicions of a chromosomal disorder such as testicular feminization and Turner's syndrome. It is important to remember that the presence of a Y-chromosome requires surgical removal of the gonadal areas because the presence of testicular components carry a 25% risk of malignant tumour formation. Even gonads of XY individuals (e.g mosaicism of XO/XY, etc.) who lack testicular tissue should have their gonads removed since there is up to a 50% chance of gonadoblastoma formation. About 30% of patients with a Y chromosome will not develop signs of virilization. Therefore this investigation should be undertaken also in women presenting with primary amenorrhoea and normal secondary sexual characteristics where gonadotrophin levels are high (Table 10.5).

If a patient is referred for specialist opinion the following investigations may be undertaken. In cases of hyperprolactinemia an MRI scan is used to evaluate the pituitary fossa. Vaginal ultrasound which may be followed by laparoscopy and examination under anaesthetic are used to evaluate pelvic organs. The endometrial cavity can be examined by hysteroscopy when a diagnosis of Ascherman's syndrome (endometrial adhesions) is suspected. Assessment of the renal tract may be instigated since abnormalities of this system are associated with developmental defects of the reproductive organs. Bone density will need assessment since bone mass is oestrogen-dependent in women.

Table 10.5 *Laboratory findings in major causes of amenorrhoea*

	FSH	LH	Prolactin	Testosterone	Karyotype
Hyperprolactinaemia	Normal	Normal	High	Normal	Normal
Premature menopause	Very high	High	Normal	Normal	Normal
Polycystic ovarian disease	Normal	Slightly raised	Normal or slightly raised	Slightly raised	Normal
'Hypothalamic'	Normal	Normal	Normal	Normal	Normal
Turner's syndrome	High	High	Normal	Normal	45XO or mosaics
Testicular feminization	High	High	Normal	High	46XY

Specific causes of amenorrhoea

Delayed menarche

1. *Age of menarche.* The menarche occurs between the ages of 10 and 16 in most girls in developed countries (Rees 1993). The first cycles tend to be anovular and there is wide variation in cycle length, and the menstruations are usually pain-free and occur without warning. By 6 years after the menarche 80% of cycles are ovulatory, and over 95% by 12 years.

There has been a secular trend to earlier menarche over the past century with a decrease of about 3–4 months per decade in industrialized countries (Europe, US, Japan). Thus the average age of menarche in 1840 was 16.5, and now averages 13. The reasons for the fall of menarcheal age are unclear but one interpretation is that it reflects improvement in health and environmental conditions. It now appears that this trend is levelling off in many countries such as the UK, Iceland, Italy, Poland, and Sweden. Indeed, there appears now to be a reversal of the fall with a gradual increase in the age of menarche in the UK since the birth cohort of 1945. However, in other countries such as Germany the fall in age is still continuing.

The age of menarche is determined by a combination of factors which include genetic influences, socio-economic conditions, general health and well-being, nutritional status, certain types of exercise, and family size.

The importance of genetic factors is illustrated by the similar age of menarche in members of an ethnic population and in mother/daughter pairs. Similarly, twin studies have shown a closer relationship in menarcheal age in identical (3 months) than in non-identical twins (12 months). Social class differences are disappearing in many countries. It is well-known that delayed menarche is a feature of chronic disease.

The role of body weight and proportion of body fat has received considerable attention. It is well-known that anorexia and malnutrition are associated with delayed menarche, and both conditions can induce secondary amenorrhoea. The mean weight at menarche is 47.8 ± 0.5 kg at the mean height of 158.5 ± 0.5 cm in the US. It has therefore been proposed that there is a threshold weight for height and critical proportion of body fat before the menarche can occur. Body composition changes in the adolescent growth spurt with the ratio of lean body weight to fat being 5:1 at the initiation of the spurt and 3:1 at the menarche, when about 22% of body weight is fat. Adipose tissue is a significant source of oestrogen, and its amount influences the direction of oestrogen metabolism to more potent or less potent forms. Very thin women have an increase in the 2-hydroxylated form of oestrogen which is relatively inactive. The reliability of methods to estimate fatness have been questioned, and it is currently generally agreed that body fat content, though a key player, is not the prime mover for the advent of menarche.

Intense exercise such as athletics, gymnastics, and ballet is associated with a delayed menarche, and it has been suggested that each year of pre-menarcheal training delays menarche by 5 months, but the mechanisms involved are not fully understood, though a more linear physique may be involved. The other alternative explanations are training and familial effects. The observation that athletes who begin training before the menarche tend to have later ages of menarche than their mothers and sisters and than those who begin training after menarche, has implicated training as a causative factor. The role of the amount of training has been examined in a recent study where three sports (gymnastics, swimming, and tennis) were examined. Analysis of covariance using maternal menarcheal age, socio-economic group, duration of training, and type of sport showed that maternal menarcheal age and type of sport were the best predictors of the athletes' age of menarche. In this study menarche was found to take place at a significantly later age (14.3 years) in gymnasts than in swimmers and tennis players (13.3 and 13.2 years respectively). The amount of training was estimated to be the same in the three sport groups, although the type differed. It was concluded that menarche was intrinsically late rather than delayed in gymnasts, and that some form of sport-specific selection may have occurred; other studies have come to similar conclusions. Thus it is thought that there is a combination of biological selection and social factors.

Family size and birth order influence age of menarche. There is a tendency to later menarche in girls from larger families and there is a tendency to precocity in girls born later in the family. Again the mechanisms are unclear.

As mentioned above, in some countries such as the UK, the age of menarche now seems to be increasing. The reasons for this are uncertain. It can be speculated that the secular trend in decrease in menarcheal age should end when the weight of children of successive cohorts remains the same because of attainment of maximal nutrition and child care. It is depressing to contemplate that deterioration of health and environmental conditions could be responsible for the increase. Popular fashion has favoured slim women and dieting to lose weight in industrialized countries, and this may be involved. However, it is likely that many factors such as biological selection could be involved and further research is required. A study is currently underway in Oxford to examine these.

2. *How and when should the GP investigate.* How long should a GP wait before investigating the girl who has never menstruated? Since most girls will have menstruated by the age of 16, it could be considered to be the upper age of the normal menarche. But referral is essential earlier if secondary sex characteristics have not developed, there appear to be anatomical disorders of the genital tract, or signs of a chromosome abnormality. Rarer possibilities are testicular feminization syndrome (maturation of breasts with absent axillary and pubic hair, absent uterus with normal or short vagina; 46XY with intraabdominal testes) or Turner's syndrome (many variants, but with typical short stature, sexual infantilism, webbing of the neck, cubitus valgus, 45XO with streak gonads). Absent development of the lower genital tract resulting in haematocolpos is another rare cause where secondary sexual development will be normal. There may be intermittent lower abdominal pain, a lower abdominal cystic swelling (confirmed on ultrasound), and a tense, blue-coloured membrane may be seen at the introitus. Referral is obviously necessary for incision and drainage.

If secondary sexual development is normal or appears to be progressing satisfactorily, and there is no anatomical problem, then the likely cause is hormonal which can be elucidated with an endocrine screen.

Hypothalamic amenorrhoea

This is the commonest cause of amenorrhoea seen in general practice. Hypothalamic problems are usually diagnosed by exclusion of pituitary lesions and are the most common category of hypogonadotrophic amenorrhoea. They usually present as secondary amenorrhoea. The condition normally should be investigated if the woman has been for 6 months or more without periods. Biochemically, it is found that gonadotrophins are normal or low with a normal prolactin.

The clinical picture is usually associated with weight changes, vigorous exercise, stress, and cessation of the combined oral contraceptive pill where the induced regular bleeds have masked an ongoing problem. Since weight loss and anorexia nervosa may lead to amenorrhoea it is important for the GP to enquire about recent weight changes and to check weight for height. Normal BMI is 20–25 kg/m2, with amenorrhoea occurring if BMI is less than 19 kg/m2. Where the problem is thought to be weight loss it is better to achieve a return of menstruation via weight gain than drug therapy; where there is no response to weight gain specialist referral should be considered. If weight gain is not being achieved then the doctor must consider whether the patient has anorexia nervosa and thus is in need of psychiatric help to prevent the serious consequences of that condition.

Those who take too much exercise have been observed since the first century AD by Soranus to have amenorrhoea. It is currently observed in athletes, some intensive joggers, and ballet dancers. A similar hypothalamic cause is found in association with stress, as in the student who always menstruated regularly until leaving school and home and coming to university or college; menstruation often returns once the final examinations are passed. Post-Pill amenorrhoea can also give the picture of normal FSH, LH, and prolactin, although there is no need to investigate this for 6 months after stopping the pill since spontaneous return to menstruation usually occurs during that time. Despite reassurance, many women find it difficult to accept amenorrhoea which is perceived as a loss of femininity. Some may want to know that their endocrine system can be switched on, and clomiphene may occasionally be used. But it should only be used for a limited amount of time and then reserved for achieving pregnancy. However, it must be remembered that in women with idiopathic or congenital (Kallman's syndrome) hypothalamic amenorrhoea, associated with absent puberty, there is no response to clomiphene but fertility may be achieved with pulsatile GnRH or HMG.

Recent concerns are the long-term consequences of the hypo-oestrogenic state on bone density and the cardiovascular system. Women with 6 months or more of amenorrhoea should have a bone density measurement. Cyclical oestrogen/progestogen HRT may be used but it must be stressed that this is not contraceptive. If contraception is needed the combined oral contraceptive pill is a better option.

Hyperprolactinaemia

The incidence of hyperprolactinaemia in amenorrhoeic populations varies with individual clinical practice but averages about one-third of women with no obvious cause for their amenorrhoea. Galactorrhoea is present in 30% of hyperprolactinaemic women but galactorrhoeic women who do not have menstrual disturbance only rarely have hyperprolactinaemia. High prolactin levels cause amenorrhoea by inhibiting the normal pulsatile secretion of GnRH by the hypothalamus.

There are many causes of hyperprolactinaemia, the most important which need to be diagnosed being prolactin-secreting tumours of the anterior pituitary and non-functional tumours such as craniopharyngiomas which impede the passage of dopamine to the pituitary and hence increase prolactin levels. Craniopharyngiomas need surgical removal. Prolactinomas less than 1 cm in diameter are referred to as microadenomas, and those greater than 1 cm as macroadenomas. The exact incidence of the clinical problem is uncertain; between 9–27% of pituitary glands in routine autopsy series have been found to contain adenomas. Women with hyperprolactinaemia (i.e. prolactin >1000 mu/l) should therefore have an MRI scan and visual field assessment.

It must be remembered that the commonest cause for a moderately-elevated serum prolactin level is stress (and also breast examination which is often done before a blood test!) and therefore it is important to take a repeat blood sample with the patient more relaxed, if that is possible. Drugs including metaclopromide, phenothiazines, reserpine, methyldopa, and cimetidine may also cause hyperprolactinaemia and therefore an accurate drug history is important.

Menstruation, ovulation, and fertility can be restored in patients with hyperprolactinaemia with drugs such as bromocriptine, cabergoline, and quinagolide which can be used for macro as well as microadenomas. If a patient wants her fertility restored then obviously she should be treated with bromocriptine and similar agents, which can be stopped during pregnancy. But there is controversy in patients with microadenomas who do not wish to become pregnant. If they are treated, they require contraception, preferably with a barrier method. Alternatively they could be given HRT to counteract the hypo-oestrogenic effects on their bones and cardiovascular system; these women need specialist referral since oestrogen can cause enlargement of a prolactinoma. Approaches over the years have become more conservative with documentation of a benign clinical course with spontaneous resolution in many patients. Surgical referral is required for women with macroadenomas, resistance to bromocriptine, or suprasellar enlargement prior to pregnancy.

Polycystic ovary syndrome (PCOS)
First described by two gynaecologists, Stein and Leventhal, in the early 1930s, this syndrome was originally ascribed to patients with amenorrhoea, hirsutism, obesity, and bilateral polycystic ovaries. It is clear, however, that any form of menstrual irregularity can occur – oligomenorrhoea, or menorrhagia with regular or irregular cycles – and the term polycystic ovary syndrome is now preferred. There is now a problem of definition and doctors may disagree as to whether a particular woman with less florid symptoms can be said to have the syndrome.

The condition involves:

(1) the presence of an excessive number of small follicles placed peripherally in the ovaries with a relative failure of follicular selection processes which should produce a dominant follicle

(2) a continuous background of oestrogen production by the small follicles;

(3) ovarian stromal hyperplasia associated with excessive androgen production;

(4) conversion of androgens in peripheral fat to oestrone, resulting in adequate oestrogenization;

(5) hypersecretion of insulin in obese and some slim women with PCOS; insulin secretion lowers SHBG and increases free androgen levels;

(6) disturbed ovarian pituitary feedback resulting in elevated secretion of LH. However the expression of excessive androgen production depends not simply on blood levels of testosterone and androstenedione but on the peripheral metabolism of testosterone to dihydrotestosterone in the specific androgen-sensitive end-organs (the hair follicles). This is the main difference between hirsute and non-hirsute women with PCOS.

In the UK, it is generally accepted that polycystic ovaries detected by ultrasound scan provide the unifying diagnostic criterion. On ultrasound, the classic picture is a string of small follicles, 2–8 mm in diameter, arranged like a necklace in the periphery of the ovary with a minimum of 10 follicles in each ovary. Several studies have tried to estimate the prevalence of polycystic ovaries in normal women and found it to be about 22%. However, the original description by Stein and Leventhal of amenorrhoea, obesity, and hirsutism does seem to be the extreme end of the spectrum. Indeed, many women with polycystic ovaries detected by ultrasound do not have any symptoms of polycystic ovary syndrome which may develop later, after weight gain for example. Thus not all women with polycystic ovaries have PCOS, but all women with PCOS have polycystic ovaries. The diagnosis should be reserved for when there are in addition to the ultrasound findings of polycystic ovaries, the associated symptoms (menstrual irregularity, hyperandrogenization, obesity) or endocrine abnormalities (raised serum LH and testosterone). A recent survey of 1741 women with PCOS referred to a specialist clinic showed that 39.8% and 29.8% respectively had raised serum LH and/or testosterone concentrations; while symptoms of obesity, hyperandrogenization, and menstrual cycle disturbance occurred in 38.4%, 70.3%, and 66.2% of patients respectively (Balen et al. 1995). Obesity was associated with hirsutism and an elevated serum testosterone concentration and was also correlated with increased rates of infertility and cycle disturbance. The rates of infertility and cycle disturbance also increased with serum LH concentrations (>10 iu/l). A rising serum concentration of testosterone was associated with an increased risk of hirsutism, infertility, and cycle disturbance. Furthermore, it is thought that obese women with PCOS hypersecrete insulin which stimulates ovarian secretion of androgens; the prevalence of diabetes in obese women with PCOS is 11%. It was therefore recommended that obese women (BMI >30 kg/m2) should be encouraged to lose weight; indeed weight loss may improve the symptoms and endocrine profile of PCOS.

Hypersecretion of LH is associated with menstrual disturbance, reduced conception rates, and increased miscarriages rates in both natural and assisted conception cycles. Suppression of LH levels with GnRH analogues or ovarian diathermy are two possible strategies which remain to be fully assessed. If the testosterone level is >4.8 nmol/l, the patient needs to be investigated to exclude androgen-secreting tumours, Cushing's syndrome, and congenital adrenal hyperplasia.

Treatment depends on the woman's desire for pregnancy. A first line is weight loss in overweight women. It must be remembered that the chronic anovulatory state in PCOS increases the risks of endometrial hyperplasia and cancer. If, on vaginal ultrasound, endometrial thickness is greater than 15 mm, a withdrawal bleed should be induced with progestogens, and if the endometrium fails to be shed, an endometrial biopsy performed. Cyclical progestogens can be given for 12 days each month, but this regime is not contraceptive. Alternatively, a combined oral contraceptive pill can be used. If hirsutism is a problem, one containing the anti-androgen drug cyproterone can be used; however, the role of waxing and electrolysis should not be forgotten. In the women who wish to become pregnant, ovulation induction with clomiphene may prove effective, but progression to gonadotrophin therapy, possibly with pituitary control using GnRH analogues to suppress LH production, is often required. In PCOS, women are at risk of an exuberant response to stimulation with gonadotrophins, with attendant risks of ovarian hyperstimulation syndrome and multiple pregnancy, and need close monitoring. Surgery in the form of laparoscopic laser or diathermy to the ovarian surface is now used instead of wedge resection. Its mode of action is uncertain, since unilateral diathermy can result in bilateral ovulation. This is believed to be less likely to cause the adhesions which were a problem after wedge resection.

1. Twenty per cent of women have polycystic ovaries, but not all have PCOS, a term reserved to women with additional symptoms or endocrine abnormalities.
2. Menstrual problems are varied and can be dealt with by progestogens or the combined contraceptive pill.
3. Fertility is reduced and the risk of miscarriage is increased, especially in women with increased LH levels.
4. Weight loss may improve the symptoms and hormonal profile of PCOS.
5. Contraceptive pills containing cyproterone or electrolysis can be used for acne/hirsutism.

Premature menopause

A menopause is considered to be premature if it occurs before the age of 45. It is characterized by high FSH and LH with normal prolactin levels. Other symptoms may be present such as hot flushes and night sweats, as well as atrophic vaginitis. Sadly, premature ovarian failure can occur at any age. While it may occur spontaneously, it may be due to previous chemotherapy or radiotherapy. Causes include autoimmune problems with ovarian antibodies and thus thyroid function should be checked for other endocrine compromise; viral oophoritis which may recover to some degree; and chromosomal abnormalities (patients with Turner's syndrome can menstruate for a while). Premature ovarian failure is difficult to distinguish from resistant ovary syndrome with fluctuating ovarian function and unpredictable ovulation.

If the woman is concerned about fertility, specialist referral is required. Treatment with cyclical oestrogen/progestogen therapy is indicated in women with premature ovarian failure, both to treat symptoms and to protect against premature heart disease and osteoporosis. The options are HRT or the contraceptive pill, depending on fertility goals. The combined oral contraceptive pill may be a more acceptable option in younger women. Bone density measurements are indicated in women who have 6 months or more of amenorrhoea. There is some controversy about the dose of oestrogen required to maintain bone mass, which will need monitoring in these women. Some may need the addition of bisphosphonates, but again this is controversial.

In the past these women were considered sterile and counselled that future pregnancy was impossible. However, in recent years it has become apparent that some may resume normal ovarian function either spontaneously or while taking HRT and may become pregnant. The picture has also changed with the possibility of fertilized ovum donation in some IVF programmes. Therefore it is important for women with premature ovarian failure to realize that there is a possibility of pregnancy. There are also new prospects being examined of freezing ovarian tissue before chemo or radiotherapy, with reimplantation after treatment.

Oligomenorrhoea

A woman with infrequent periods should be investigated in the same way as a woman with amenorrhoea, since the causes in general are the same. Scanty regular menstruation needs no investigation; blood losses as low as 2 ml per month have been found in normal parous women. It may herald the menopause or rarely have an endocrine basis but in general is not a worrying symptom.

Prolonged menstruation

On average, women menstruate for 5–6 days of each cycle and anything over this may be considered prolonged. As discussed earlier, the number of days of bleeding does not relate to menstrual blood loss since most of the loss is passed in the first 3 days of menstruation, whether the overall loss is light or heavy. Prolonged menstruation in itself does not require investigation but may go along with other complaints such as menorrhagia. The main menstrual flow can be prolonged by being preceded or succeeded by spotting in association with an IUCD or the progestogen-only pill: reassurance is usually all that is required. Several days of spotting before a period can be a sign of an endometrial or cervical polyp or even malignancy; and visualization of the cervix, a cervical smear, and pelvic examination should be carried out by the GP, with referral to the gynaecologist if there are suspicious findings.

Irregular menstruation and bleeding

Irregular periods

Women often worry if their previously regular periods become irregular, but as discussed earlier, this is most likely to be no more than a normal variation of hormonal changes. Irregular menstruation, both long and short cycles, is most common at the extremes of reproductive life, soon after the menarche or before the menopause. These cycles are usually anovulatory. In adolescent girls it does not need investigation and unless there are signs of obvious disease, hormonal therapy to regularize periods should be avoided. Rather, the GP should reassure the girl that it is part of the normal maturation process and her periods will become regular with time. If she requires contraception this may outweigh all other considerations and an oral contraceptive may then be used. In later life, nearer the menopause, irregularity of periods is extremely common. But if periods become heavy as well as irregular or there are problems such as intermenstrual or post-coital bleeding, referral to a gynaecologist is wise.

Intermenstrual and post-coital bleeding

Investigation and management mainly depend on the age of the patient. In peri-menopausal women these symptoms cannot be ignored. Speculum examination is essential to exclude a cervical lesion – malignancy, ectropion, or polyp – and pelvic examination will define any obvious uterine or ovarian problems. Referral to a gynaecologist should be made in older women (over 40) unless, for example, a cervical polyp is present. This can be easily avulsed by the GP, using long forceps to twist off the polyp and the resulting raw area cauterized with a silver nitrate stick. It is mandatory that the polyp should be sent for histology to exclude the rare malignancies. If the bleeding settles after removal of a polyp then referral is unnecessary. In young women, mid-cycle bleeding is often associated with ovulation and does not require investigation. Intermenstrual and post-coital bleeding in young women is rarely associated with malignancy but again it is important that the cervix be visualized, cervical smears taken, and a bimanual pelvic examination carried out to exclude pathology (see above). If the bleeding persists over several cycles referral should be considered.

Post-menopausal bleeding

This always requires examination and urgent referral because of the high incidence of malignancy. While the most common malignancy is endometrial, cancer of the cervix, vulva, or ovary may present in this way. It may, however, be due to non-malignant causes such as atrophic vaginitis or a polyp. Persistent heavy bleeding or breakthrough bleeding in women taking HRT also needs investigation to exclude endometrial pathology.

Variations in colour and smell of menstrual blood

Women may report to their doctor a change in the colour or smell of their menstrual blood which may worry them. There is no known association with pelvic pathology and these symptoms. If anything, these changes are associated with different rates of menstrual flow. Thus patients should be reassured.

Toxic shock syndrome

The only reason for including this section here is that there is the misconception that toxic shock syndrome (TSS), an extremely rare disease, is solely associated with tampon use. In fact it was first described in children in 1978 as a multi-system disease characterized by rapid onset of fever, hypotension, hyperaemia of the mucous membranes, and rash followed by desquamation and multi-system involvement. However, the descriptions of staphylococcal scarlet fever suggest that TSS was already noted in 1927. In 1980, an increase in TSS was noted in previously healthy young women with onset during menstruation. Initial studies of menstrual TSS suggested that tampon use was a risk factor for the disease, and a particular brand was implicated which was withdrawn in 1980. In the US, only half of the reported cases occur in menstruating women who use tampons. Non-menstrual cases in men, women, and children associated with hospital-acquired infections, surgery, boils, insect bites, burns, parturition, and contraceptive barriers have been increasingly recognized. Some women are subject to recurrences of menstrual TSS even when tampons have not been used.

The association between TSS and *Staphylococcal aureus* infection was firmly established when an exotoxin from isolates of TSS-associated *S. aureus* was isolated in 1981. The exotoxin has since been called toxic shock syndrome toxin-1 (TSS-1) and is generally considered to be the major cause of TSS. Other pathogens such as *Escherichia coli* have been more recently implicated as well.

The exact role of tampons in menstrual TSS is uncertain. Initially it was thought that high absorbency of tampons such as those containing carboxymethylcellulose or polyacrylate was an important factor. Indeed, these substances are no longer used. However, the role of absorbency is now being questioned since the original studies did not distinguish the effects of absorbency from the effects of chemical composition or other tampons' characteristics that are correlated with absorbency. One persistent problem in understanding the aetiology of TSS is that the vaginal environment is anaerobic but the production of TSS-1 requires the presence of oxygen. Therefore it has been suggested that the insertion of a tampon might provide the oxygen necessary for toxin production. Another theory is that highly-absorbent tampon material binds magnesium ions; in a magnesium-deficient environment, production of TSS-1 increases dramatically.

It is important to put the risk of developing TSS in perspective. It is a very rare disease with no justification for women to avoid using tampons. Tampon packets now carry warnings about TSS. On the other hand, if one suspects that a woman has TSS it is important to arrange hospital admission for appropriate antibiotic treatment since the disease has a high mortality.

Controversies

1. The management of menorrhagia is based on a subjective complaint which usually bears little correlation with objective blood loss.
2. Despite being an ineffective therapy for menorrhagia, low dose norethisterone is still a first line of treatment.
3. Prophylactic oophorectomy is undertaken at hysterectomy in women who are not at increased or high risk of developing ovarian cancer.
4. Premature ovarian failure can occur at any age and women should not be told 'they are too young'.
5. Women consult frequently for menstrual disorders and there is socioeconomic and educational variation in those having surgery.
6. Does lack of good information for consumers make menstrual disorders one of the commonest indications of use of NHS resources?

Acknowledgement

The author would like to thank Mr Adam Balen for his helpful comments and suggestions.

References and further reading

Anderson, A. B. M., Haynes, P. J., Guillebaud, J., and Turnbull, A. C. (1976). Reduction of menstrual blood loss by prostaglandin synthetase inhibitors. *Lancet*, 1, 774–6.

Balen, A., Conway, G. S., Kaltsas, G., Techatraisak, K., Manning, P. J., West, P. J., *et al.* (1995). Polycystic ovary syndrome: the spectrum of the disorder in 1741 patients. *Human Reproduction* 10, 2107–11.

Coulter, A., Peto, V., and Doll, H. (1994). Patients' preferences and general practitioners' decisions in the treatment of menstrual disorders. *Family Practice*, 11, 67–74.

Coulter, A., Kelland, J., Long, A., *et al.* (1995a) *The management of menorrhagia.* Effective Health Care Bulletin, no 9. Stott Bros., Halifax.

Coulter A., Kelland J., Peto, V., and Rees, M. (1995b). Treating menorrhagia in primary care: an overview of drug trials and a survey of prescribing practice. *International Journal of Technology Assessment in Health Care*, 11(3), 456–71.

Coulter, A., Peto, V., and Doll, H. (1995c). Gynaecology: the experience of patients referred to NHS and private clinics. *Health Trends*, 27, 57–61.

Kuh, D. and Stirling, S. (1995). Socio-economic variation in admission for diseases of the female genital system and breast in a national cohort aged 15–43. *British Medical Journal*, 311, 840–3.

Rees, M. (1991). Role of menstrual loss measurement in management of excessive menstrual bleeding. *British Journal of Obstetrics and Gynaecology*, **98**, 327–8.

Rees, M. (1993). Menarche when and why. *Lancet*, **342**, 1375–6.

Rees, M. (1997). Medical management of menorrhagia. (1996). In *Clinical disorders of the menstrual cycle* (ed. I. T. Cameron, I. S. Fraser, and S. K. Smith). Oxford University Press, Oxford. In press.

Rees, M. (1996). The menopause and the uterus. Baillière's (1996) *Clinical obstetrics and gynaecology*, 10: 419–32.

Vollman, R. F. (1977). *The menstrual cycle*. W. B. Saunders, Philadelphia.

CHAPTER ELEVEN

The menopause

Jean Coope

Natural history

The word menopause is derived from the Greek words '*men*' month and '*pausis*' halt. It means the end of menstruation and the last menstrual period marks the end of reproductive life.

The mean age at menopause is just over 50 and this is remarkably constant throughout the Western world. Moreover, a recent survey of Malaysian women showed a mean age at menopause of 50.7 years, and another of seven Asian countries found that most women reached menopause around 50. These findings relate to cross-sectional studies of large female populations. Longitudinal studies have been carried out in southern England, Norway, Canada, and Massachusetts, US (Holte 1990). These show similar results and confirm the only important factor to influence age at menopause: cigarette smoking advances it by about 2 years.

All the sociological studies confirmed the importance of cultural and social factors in determining a woman's attitude to menopause. For example, Rajput women of Northern India perceive the menopause as an end of taboos and social restrictions and do not suffer any symptoms. On the other hand, reports of North American women indicate that over 80% suffer from hot flushes and many suffer from a general decline in health status. In the US, and in Australia and Western Europe, the concept has emerged of the menopause as a deficiency disease which needs treatment by hormone replacement therapy.

The experience of British women at menopause has been investigated by sociologists (McKinlay and Jefferys 1974) and epidemiologists (Bungay *et al.* 1980). About 80% of women experience flushes but only 20% feel that their symptoms are severe enough to require medical help. Flushing and sweating are the only symptoms to show a sharp peak at or just after the menopause. Minor mental symptoms such as depression and loss of confidence show a smaller rise just before the last menstrual period. Other symptoms, such as headaches, urinary frequency, insomnia, back pain, and irritability are not specifically associated with menopause and major psychiatric illness

Fig 11.1 *Timing of problems related to menopause*

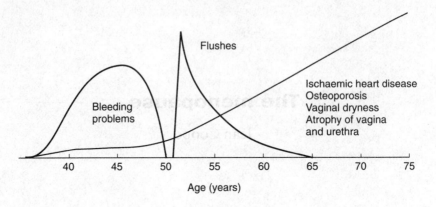

is not more common at this time. Sexual difficulties and loss of libido increase in frequency with advancing age in both sexes, and vaginal dryness and atrophy are common in post-menopausal women. Osteoporosis does not usually present with symptoms in mid-life but the imperceptible bone loss which begins at menopause may culminate in fractures or spinal pain 20 years later. Ischaemic heart disease is much commoner after menopause and is the most common cause of death in post-menopausal women. (See Fig 11.1.)

Longitudinal studies by McKinlay *et al.* in Massachusetts (1990) and Hunter in England (1990) have confirmed the importance of previous behaviour patterns and use of medical services in determining whether women actually experience symptoms and seek medical help at menopause. For individual women the experience of a worthwhile career and a satisfactory long-term sexual relationship protects against symptoms.

Recently, our knowledge of the events which accompany menopause has been helped by publication of four longitudinal studies of women who have been followed through the menopause by teams of research workers in different countries. Detailed and validated questionnaires were used and psychologists, gynaecologists, and sociologists participated in supervision and assessment. Table 11.1 shows their findings.

They concluded that psychological symptoms were not predominant and were usually temporary and related to negative beliefs and previous health problems. Major complaints were bleeding, insomnia, and vasomotor symptoms.

Definitions

Natural menopause. The permanent cessation of menstruation resulting from the loss of ovarian follicular activity. It is recognized to have occurred after 12 consecutive months of amenorrhoea, for which there is no other obvious cause, and can be known with certainty only in retrospect, a year after the final

Table 11.1 *Longitudinal studies of menopausal patients*

Authors	Country	Population and recruitment	Duration	Symptoms related to menopause and other findings
McKinlay S.M. Brambilla D.J. Posner J.G. (1992). The normal menopause transition, *American Journal of Human Biology,* **4**, 37–46	US	2 570 women aged 45–55 selected at random from Massachusetts census lists. Postal questionnaires and telephone interviews	5 years	Flushes in 50% women just after LMP; disturbed sleep due to flushes; irregular bleeding more troublesome than flushes; smoking accelerated menopause by mean of 1.5 years; Peri-menopause lasted nearly 4 years
Hunter, M. (1992). The South-East England longitudinal study of the climacteric. *Maturitas,* **14**, 117–26	UK	36 women from cross-sectional 3 years survey of 850 women aged 47 and over attending ovarian screen clinic, London. Postal questionnaire	3 years	Flushes +; insomnia +; depression + (related to psycho-social factors and negative beliefs)
Holte, A. (1992) Influences of natural menopause on health complaints. *Maturitas,* **14**, 127–41	Norway	200 pre-menopausal women randomly selected from 1 886 women aged 45–55 – Oslo Community Register. Yearly personal interview	5 years	Flushes and sweats +; vaginal dryness +; palpitations +; social dysfunction due to flushes; depression – no change
Kaufert, P.A., Gilbert, P. and Tate, R. (1992). The Manitoba Project a re-examination of the link between depression and menopause. *Maturitas,* **14**, 143–55	Canada	477 women aged 40–59, pre-menopausal or hysterectomized from mail screen of 2 500 women in Manitoba. Telephone interviews of subgroup of >45 year-olds	3 years	Depression in 25% but impermanent; not affected by natural menopause; hysterectomy, family stress, chronic illness associated with depression

menstrual period (FMP). An adequate **biological** marker for the event does not exist.

Induced menopause (often known as surgical menopause) is artificially-induced cessation of menstruation and ovarian activity. It includes either surgical removal of both ovaries (with or without hysterectomy) or other iatrogenic ablation of ovarian function, e.g. chemotherapy, radiation, etc.

Premature menopause. Menopause occurring before the age at which natural menopause is usually experienced. It is defined as occurring at an age less than 2 S.D. below the median for the referred population. Because of lack of data the age of 40 years is often used as an arbitrary cut-off point.

Post-menopause is the whole period of survival after the menopause. It is defined as dating from the final menstrual period, whether induced or spontaneous.

Peri-menopause is the period of a few years before and immediately after final menstruation. It includes the period just before menopause when endocrinological, biological, and clinical features of approaching menopause commence. The term menopausal transition is reserved for that period of time immediately before the FMP when menstrual cycle variability is usually increased.

Simple hysterectomy is removal of the uterus leaving at least one conserved ovary. It represents a distinct group in which ovarian function persists for a variable period after surgery. Objective assessment of ovarian function requires measurement of gonadotrophin and/or oestrogen concentrations.

The climacteric is waning of ovarian function which usually takes place over a number of years and has a powerful effect on bones, blood vessels, and collagen.

Hormonal changes

What happens at the menopause? Menstruation ceases and there is a sharp fall in the level of circulating oestrogen, although the ageing ovaries continue to secrete small amounts of oestradiol and testosterone. (Fig 11.2 shows the changing levels of hormones in women of different ages.)

Gonadotrophins

Positive and negative feedback systems operate between the ovaries and the pituitary gland and possibly also the hypothalamus. Ovarian secretion of oestradiol and the peptide inhibin acts on the pituitary gland to reduce production of the gonadotrophins: follicle stimulating hormone (FSH) and lutenising hormone (LH). High levels of FSH and LH occur in response to reduced ovarian function. FSH and LH estimations can be used to indicate whether a woman has reached the menopause (see Table 11.2). However, they are only reliable *after* the menopause. During the peri-menopause, patients' tests may revert to pre-menopausal levels temporarily, accompanied by further menstrual cycles.

Fig 11.2 *Plasma levels of oestradiol and testosterone in human females according to age*
(Source: (1988) The menopause and aging. In The menopause: comprehensive management (ed. B. A. Eskin)
MacMillan, New York.)

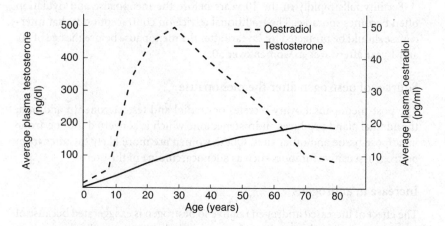

Laboratories vary in their estimation of the threshold of FSH concentration which is diagnostic of menopause. In our example taken from the Department of Clinical Endocrinology, Birmingham and Midland Hospital for Women, the threshold is defined as FSH 30 iu/l.

In ordinary circumstances it is not necessary to use a laboratory test to confirm menopause; the presence of flushes in a woman over 45 who has amenorrhoea for a year is sufficient. In hysterectomized patients, or those already taking the combined pill or HRT with regular bleeding, it may be useful to obtain FSH assay. A high level means that the patient is menopausal. A low level in a patient who is taking HRT or the combined pill does not necessarily exclude menopause as these preparations cause lowering of FSH and LH.

The ovarian follicles may become less sensitive to circulating gonadotrophins with time. The follicular phase shortens and shortening of the cycle to 18–24 days often occurs after the age of 40. After this the cycles

Table 11.2 *Reference ranges SI units*

Adult women	Oestradiol (pmol/l)	FSH (iu/l)	LH (iu/l)
Follicular	160–1310	1–9	1–12
Ovulatory	900–2290	6–26	16–104
Luteal	220–1480	1–9	1–12
Post-menopausal	<100	30–118	16–66

Note: Levels of FSH and LH decreases with age and are negatively correlated with the Body Mass Index
Source: Department of Clinical Endocrinology, Birmingham and Midland Hospital for Women

lengthen and there are often gaps of amenorrhoea before periods stop altogether. Women may need reassurance that short cycles are a normal pattern.

Fertility falls rapidly in the 10 years before the menopause and ovulation often becomes sporadic. The traditional advice on contraception is that intercourse should be protected for 2 years after the menopause before the age of 50, and 1 year afterwards in women over 50.

Sources of oestrogen after the menopause

The post-menopausal ovary secretes oestradiol and testosterone. In addition, the adrenal gland produces androstenedione which is converted into oestrone in adipose tissue and other sites. Obese women are more likely to suffer from oestrogen-sensitive tumours such as adenocarcinoma of the uterus.

Increase in androgens

The effect of increased androgen relative to oestrogen is exaggerated because of post-menopausal reduction in sex hormone-binding globulin. This has a greater affinity for testosterone than for oestradiol (Fig 11.2). Sex hormone-binding globulin exaggerates the clinical effect of oestrogen. It is only the unbound portions of the sex hormones that are clinically active and can be attached to receptors on the cells of target organs.

In young women and HRT-users, oestrogen stimulates the liver to produce sex hormone-binding globulin which binds selectively to circulating testosterone. Circulating free androgens are reduced thus raising the effect of oestrogen on the target organ. Older woman have lower oestrogen production, less sex hormone binding globulin is produced, and free circulating androgens rise. This probably explains the hirsutism and male pattern baldness which occurs in some elderly women.

Effects of HRT on thyroxine and cortisol levels

Increased thyroxine-binding globulin binds thyroxine, rendering it inactive, and patients who are taking thyroxine should be carefully assessed and warned that oestrogen therapy may reduce their levels of free thyroxine. The laboratory carrying out thyroid function tests should be informed that the patient is taking HRT. Cortisol-binding globulins are also increased and this may diminish the control of asthmatic symptoms in patients taking corticosteroids.

Interactions between HRT and anticonvulsant drugs

Oestrogens are conjugated in the liver and excreted via the kidneys and bowel. Care is needed with epileptic patients. Hormone actions on the liver may increase the clearance rates of anti-seizure medication and affect control of epilepsy (Herzog 1991). On the other hand, phenytoin and carbamazepine induce hepatic microsomal enzymes and increase elimination of oestrogen and progestogen. It may be appropriate to alter anticonvulsants to valproate or ethosuximide.

Smoking and HRT

A highly significant reduction in circulating oestrogen levels (about 50%) has been demonstrated in smokers taking HRT, when compared with non-smokers taking HRT (Jensen *et al.* 1985). This is probably caused by enhanced drug metabolism in smokers. It is important to take a smoking history as this sometimes accounts for non-resolution of menopausal symptoms on HRT. Also, bone mineral density is lower and fracture rate higher in heavy smokers (Daniell 1976).

Symptoms and signs of the menopause

Menses

Changes in menstrual pattern occur frequently in the last few years before the menopause. It is common for the cycle to shorten and after the age of 40 many women have cycles of 21 or even 18 days, which may lengthen to 2 or 3 months before ceasing altogether. Hot flushes often occur during the menstrual periods as this is the time when circulating oestrogen is at its lowest. Women who stop the contraceptive pill at this age often experience flushes which are triggered by falling oestrogen levels, rather than a constant low level of hormone.

Dysfunctional bleeding

Irregular and falling production of progesterone means that the endometrium may be exposed to unopposed oestrogen stimulation for many weeks. This causes prolongation of the proliferative phase and perhaps hyperplasia, which may progress to cystic or atypical hyperplasia, a precancerous condition.

Heavy bleeding occurs when oestrogen levels fall and the thick endometrium separates. Very heavy, painful, or irregular bleeding needs investigation to exclude uterine pathology and women need to be educated that this is not simply 'part of the menopause'. Post-menopausal bleeding needs investigation and so does very late menstruation past the age of 54 as there is a higher incidence of malignancy in these patients.

Flushes and sweats

Vasomotor symptoms consist of hot flushes, sweats, and possibly palpitations. Ginsburg (1981) investigated women who flush compared with a group who do not, and found that flushes are accompanied by an immediate rise in blood flow to the hand and increased pulse rate. There is no change in blood pressure. The rise in skin temperature in the hand occurs simultaneously with a fall in core body temperature measured on the tympanum or in the bladder.

No one hormone has been found to be responsible for flushes and it has been suggested that a change in the body thermostat which reduces core temperature creates a response in the hypothalamic thermoregulatory centre and sets off mechanisms to promote heat loss (flushes and sweats). The administration of a GnRH agonist may promote flushes. Animal studies have identified three different substances – dopamine, noradrenaline, or endogenous opiod peptides – as transmitters but these findings are not confirmed in human subjects. It is possible that a similar mechanism is the reason that men also experience flushes after removal of the testes. Some women never flush but others experience reduced quality of life due to loss of sleep caused by nocturnal sweats. However, oestrogen in sufficient dosages abolishes menopausal flushes in nearly all women. Insomnia due to vasomotor symptoms improves on oestrogen.

Psychological symptoms

It is common for middle-aged women who are tired, depressed, or unhappily married to complain of 'the menopause' and expect alleviation and quality of life from a prescription for HRT.

A survey of a population of women in Dundee (Ballinger 1975) found that there was a peak of mild depressive illness and anxiety just before the menopause. However, Jenkins and Clare (1985) in a review of the literature concluded that true depressive illness is not commoner at this time; and depression was not observed more commonly at the natural menopause in a large longitudinal study of Canadian women (Kaufert 1992 – see Table 11.1).

There is no doubt that depression is commoner in women than in men but this may be largely due to social factors such as the psychological pressures of childbearing, shortage of money, and lack of interesting, well-paid work. Careful research on a population of 408 menopausal women in Glasgow (Cooke and Greene 1981) found that psychological stress was directly related to adverse life events, particularly bereavement.

On the other hand, some workers have treated depression successfully with large doses of oestrogen (Klaiber et al. 1979) although the safety of very high dosage must remain in doubt. Women who experience depression and loss of libido after surgical castration are enormously helped by oestrogen/androgen implants but they often become dependent on this treatment and much of the effect may be due to testosterone.

Montgomery et al. (1987) have attempted to reduce scores of depression measured on Kellner and Sheffield scales, using oestradiol/testosterone implants or placebo. They found that after the menopause women responded better to placebo but peri-menopausal patients were significantly improved on oestrogen. This group has also demonstrated the efficacy of anovulatory doses of oestrogen in treating premenstrual depression. My own double-blind study of 55 women in general practice (1981) did not show a significant difference between oestrogen and placebo in the treatment of depressed patients over a period of 6 months. However, the oestrogen used (piperazine oestrone sulphate) was not as potent as the oestradiol implants.

The conclusion must be that depression at the menopause is caused by many factors and careful assessment of the social and cultural environment is needed.

Assessment of psychological symptoms

Accurate diagnosis is essential and must exclude major or chronic diseases. Anaemia due to causes ranging from leukaemia to fibroids and menorrhagia, familial endogenous depression, myxoedema, and polymyalgia have all presented as 'the menopause' at our practice. Assessment indices such as the Kuppermann Blatt Index which includes many symptoms of anxiety should be avoided in favour of questionnaires specially validated for use at the menopause. Hunter (1992) has devised the Women's Health Questionnaire which measures women's perceptions of their own emotional and physical health, after studying over 680 women attending a London hospital clinic. Test – retest reliability using the questionnaire was high and was confirmed by comparison with the General Health Questionnaire.

The effect of menopausal symptoms on quality of life has been measured at the Department of Public Health and Primary Care, University of Oxford (Daly *et al.* 1993). Two methods of assessment were used. In the first, a visual analogue scale from 0–10 was completed by the patients, to show how they rated their quality of life (0=death, 10=normal health). The second method used 'time trade-off' in which the patients were asked to choose between having menopausal symptoms for a certain period and normal health for a shorter period (trade-off between the length of life and quality of life). The two methods produced disparate results. Although many women measured 'severe symptoms' on the numerical scale, most were not inclined to sacrifice length of life for quality. However, this may reflect their altruistic role of caring for the family.

If you suspect depressive illness the Beck Inventory is useful as a screening method to assess suicidal intent and severity of illness (Beck *et al.* 1961).

Sexuality and the menopause

If sex is satisfactory before the menopause it is usually satisfactory afterwards. The most significant factor affecting the sex life of older women is the loss of a partner. Many older men suffer from impotence which may be due to the effects of treatment of hypertension or depression, or to diabetes or heavy drinking. The menopause causes vaginal atrophy in some women but this is very variable and cytological studies show high oestrogen status and 'young' smears in a percentage of older women. If a woman restarts a sexual relationship after a gap, perhaps due to divorce, remarriage, or bereavement, she may have problems with a tight, dry vagina. This can be treated by taking oestrogen in any form and a lubricating jelly also helps. Castrated women suffer from severe loss of libido. Controlled studies have shown that androgens are often effective, either as implants combined with oestrogen or depot injections plus HRT. They should be given for as short a time as possible, until libido is re-established, as unwanted androgenic side-effects may occur.

Urinary problems

Urinary problems are common in post-menopausal women. Incontinence, nocturia, and urgency occurred in 25% of large populations in the Netherlands, UK, and the US.

Stress incontinence does not respond to HRT according to carefully controlled trials. It needs skilled investigation and surgery. However, local oestrogen treatment to the vagina improves the condition of the tissues pre-operatively and may contribute to the success of the operation.

Recurrent urinary infections in older women have been shown to be reduced in patients using local oestrogen. An oestrogen-releasing vaginal ring has a significant effect on urinary urgency, dryness, and pruritis vulvae.

Oestrogen and ischaemic heart disease

An early study of Scottish women whose ovaries were removed showed that they were more likely to develop atherosclerosis and anginal symptoms than other women of their age. The menopause approximately doubles the risk of developing ischaemic heart disease. A woman of 40 who is pre-menopausal has a lower risk of ischaemic heart disease than a woman of 38 who is post-menopausal. Why is this?

Rigidity of the arteries, measured by the pulsatility index, increases rapidly after the menopause. Clotting factors change and accelerate blood coagulation. Lipid patterns alter with age and menopause, increasing cholesterol, reducing high-density lipoprotein (HDL) and increasing low-density lipoprotein (LDL) levels. All these changes, except for coagulation factors, are reversed by oestrogen.

Clinical experiments show that sublingual oestradiol increases blood flow and reduces peripheral vascular resistance in the forearm. Pulsatility index is reduced in the carotid arterial bed in response to oestrogen. Long-term administration of oestrogen reduces LDL and total cholesterol levels and increases HDL, especially HDL 2. Experiments on monkeys have shown that castrated animals build up plaques of atherosclerosis in the coronary arteries but animals treated with oestrogen show a much smaller plaque size.

Observational studies from the US, Sweden, and the UK demonstrate an enormous reduction in the incidence of deaths from ischaemic heart disease in post-menopausal women currently taking oestrogen. The addition of progestogen does not seem to remove the protective effect, which is approximately 50%. The Nurses' Health Study found that current users of HRT had the risk of illness from ischaemic heart disease reduced by 50% (Stampfer 1991). Probably *current* users are protected as the effect of oestrogen on vessel walls is immediate and transient (see experimental work by Gangar *et al.* 1993). But past use prevents build up of atherosclerotic plaque in monkeys. We do not know how long women need to take HRT to obtain the full benefit of cardiovascular protection.

Women who already suffer from heart disease have improved survival if they take oestrogen. Ten years observation of patients with left main coronary

Fig 11.3 *Ten-year survival of group 2 patients with left main coronary stenosis of 50% or greater or other stenosis of 70% or greater*

(From: Sullivan et al. (1990). Archives of Internal Medicine, 150)

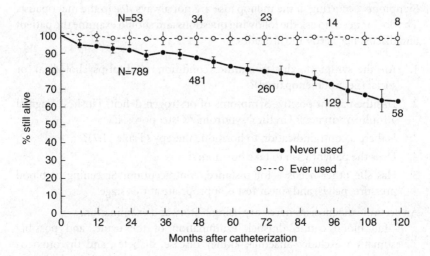

stenosis of 50% or greater, showed that those taking HRT survived significantly longer than the control group (Fig 11.3).

The OPCS provides data on mortality in Great Britain which show that nearly 30 000 women die of ischaemic heart disease each year before the age of 74. As the average age at death of British women is over 80 years, these deaths can be regarded as premature. Heart disease is underdiagnosed in women. Exercise ECGs are more likely to give misleading results and women have higher mortality than men after cardiac surgery.

Oestrogen protects women against ischaemic heart disease although the true level of protection is probably lower than the 50% reduction seen in observational studies owing to the self-selection of low-risk women taking HRT (see Controversies, p. 371). It is useful to regard oestrogen as a cardioprotective drug which can be added to the armamentaria of stopping smoking, healthy diet and exercise, and control of blood pressure. Some centres already use HRT as a lipid-lowering drug in high-risk women. HRT is relatively safe and is much cheaper than cardiac surgery. The advent of continuous oestrogen/progestogen packs has removed the objection of older women (who are at higher risk of ischaemic heart disease) to 'periods' after the menopause.

Oestrogen and cerebrovascular disease

At present there is still too little data to clarify the effect of hormones on the risk of stroke. The results from studies continue to be conflicting with some showing a decrease and others showing no effect or even an increased risk with high doses of oestrogen (Grodstein *et al.* 1996).

General management of the menopause

Diagnosis

Symptoms occurring *at* the menopause are not always *due* to the menopause. The doctor needs to ask the following questions and should examine the patient and discuss her needs and attitudes.

1. Are the symptoms due to another condition, medical psychological, or social (i.e. not menopausal)?
2. Has the patient positive symptoms of oestrogen deficit? Flushes? Vaginal atrophy or dryness? Urethral syndrome? Osteoporosis?
3. Is there a contraindication to hormone therapy (Table 11.7)?
4. Does the patient wish to take hormones?
5. Has she other needs – for instance, contraception? Screening of blood pressure, pelvis, and smear test is appropriate at this stage.

An accurate diagnosis is necessary using history and examination.

A full blood count, dipstick examination of the urine, and possibly T_4 estimation excludes anaemia, kidney disease, diabetes, and thyrotoxicosis which may mimic menopausal symptoms or contraindicate hormone therapy. Abnormal vaginal bleeding such as intermenstrual, post-coital, or post-menopausal must be investigated and hospital referral is essential.

Health promotion

The opportunity should be taken to promote a healthy lifestyle, discussing in particular smoking, alcohol intake, diet, and exercise (see Chapter 2). Any family history of breast cancer, ischaemic heart disease, and stroke should be recorded, including age of onset, and cholesterol measured in the case of premature heart disease. Weight, Body Mass Index, and blood pressure should be checked. Current medical conditions and medication which predispose to ischaemic heart disease or osteoporosis should be discussed with the patient, as these are relevant to her decision concerning long-term HRT. Non-hormonal measures to promote bone density should be explained, especially smoking cessation, regular exercise, and recommended dietary calcium intake (see Table 11.4, p. 358). The importance of regular cervical and breast screening should be stressed, and the patient reminded that she will be called for regular mammograms from the age of 50.

Non-HRT treatment of flushes

Exercise has been used in a controlled study of 1600 women in Sweden. Flushes were reduced by 50% in the actively-exercising group.

Cognitive behavioural therapy is used by psychologists to cope with flushes, and paced respiration (deep breathing) is effective.

A cool ambient temperature is important and controlled studies have shown

Fig 11.4 *Relationship between number of flushes and daily temperature*
(Coope et al., 1978)

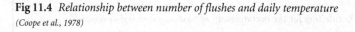

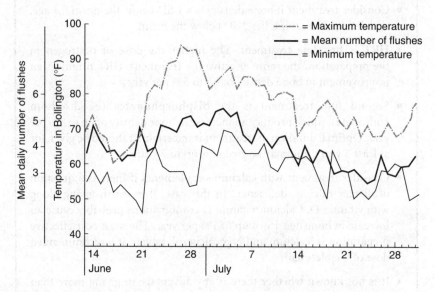

that the number of flushes experienced by a group of untreated women varies significantly with the temperature of the environment (Fig 11.4).

Other treatments such as clonidine, evening primrose oil, and tranquillisers have not proved to be more effective than placebo. There is particular interest at present in the use of natural progesterone (either topically as skin cream or orally) for the treatment of menopausal symptoms, but this has not been formally evaluated (see Chapter 20). A summary of menopausal symptoms and non-hormonal treatments is available. (Coope 1996).

Osteoporosis

There are no symptoms due to low bone density although it is the most important risk factor for fractures in people below the age of 75. After this age other factors such as poor nutrition, dangerous environment, and lack of sunlight become prominent, although loss of bone is still an important cause. The architecture of bone is lost in severe cases, so that rebuilding of the structure becomes impossible.

In the UK there are 50 000 wrist fractures and 60 000 hip fractures each year. Spinal fractures are thought to reach 40 000 annually, but this is probably a low estimate. A 50-year-old white woman has a 15% lifetime risk of hip fracture, 30% vertebral, and 15% Colles fracture. Chinese and Indian women are also at high risk but negroes do not generally develop osteoporosis.

Throughout life there is constant removal of defective bone cells and replacement by new bone. Peak bone mass is achieved in young adult life. It is influenced by the date of menarche, whether a girl has amenorrhoea, lack

---

Box 11.1 *Guidelines for the management of post-menopausal osteoporosis*

- Consider treatment if bone density lies 1 SD below the norm for age, and definitely treat if it lies 2 SD below the norm

- **HRT** is first line treatment. The higher the dose of oestrogen in the preparation, the more effective the treatment. HRT produces an improvement in bone density of up to 5% per year

- Second line treatment is the **bisphosphonates** (eg disodium etidronate), which produce an increase in bone density of up to 4% per year. Optimal duration of treatment is uncertain: it should be given for at least 3 years, and may be given for up to 7 years

- Consider treatment with **calcium supplements** if there is a question of dietary calcium deficiency. In this case, it is worth giving along with vitamin D. Calcium/vitamin D combinations probably cause an increase in bone density of up to 1% per year. The most cost-effective preparation is 'calcium and ergocalciferol' tablets at a recommended dose of 2 tablets daily

- It is not known whether there is any advantage in giving more than one treatment for osteoporosis concurrently. Studies are currently in progress to determine this

Source: J. A. H. Wass (1966). Personal communication

---

of exercise, smoking habit, and intake of dietary calcium. Genetic factors are also important. At the menopause, bone resorption exceeds the formation of new bone and bone density is reduced at the rate of 1–3% per year. Sufficient dosage of oestrogen for a long period, perhaps 7–10 years post-menopause, can prevent this loss of bone density, but even this may have little effect after the age of 75 when fracture risk is increased.

The diagnosis of osteoporosis may be suspected if women show rapid loss of height or kyphosis but can only be confirmed by densitometry. X-ray of the spine discloses fractures but is too insensitive to detect loss of bone density under 30% reduction.

Measurement of bone density

There are now two methods of bone density estimation in common use. (WHO 1994). The first, DEXA (dual energy X-ray absorptiometry), uses a pair of X-ray generators and produces a rapid scan (less than 5 minutes for the lumbar spine). The patient does not need to undress. The sites measured are generally the lumbar spine, hip, forearm, or whole body. Error in reproductibility is 0.4%. The radiation dose is very low.

QCT (quantitative computed tomography) images a series of thin transverse slices through the body and these can be quantified to give a measure of

Table 11.3 *Minimum bone-sparing doses of HRT*

These achieve plasma concentrations of approximately oestradiol >200 pmol/l or the equivalent and are usually successful in preventing reduction of bone density

Bone-conserving steroids	Minimum daily doses in common use	
Conjugated equine oestrogens	0.625 mg*	Equally effective with progestogen
Piperazine oestrone sulphate	1.5 mg	
Oestradiol 17 beta (oral)	2.0 mg	
Oestradiol 17 beta (gel)	5 G (=2 mgE₂)	
Oestradiol 17 beta (implant)	50 mg (6 monthly)	
Norethisterone	5–15 mg daily	
Livial (Tibolone)	2.5 mg (awaits formal produce licence for prevention of osteoporosis)	

These doses are used for at least 5 years in post-menopausal, healthy women. Lower doses may suffice for older women; younger women with premature menopause may require higher doses

volumetric bone density. QCT of the spine takes about 20 minutes during which the patient is positioned over a calibration standard (the phantom) of known density. Radiation dose is higher than in DEXA but is still no higher than that of an AP chest X-ray. Very debilitated patients may not be able to complete the test.

Bone density measurement may be compared with the average reading for the patient's sex and age (Z score) or with the reading obtained in a young adult (T score). There is considerable variation between the reference ranges provided by various manufacturers and also those in use in different areas of the country. Your local radiology department which carries out the test will report on the result and advise as to whether the patient is at increased risk of fracture. A reduction of 1 SD in bone density is associated with approximately double the risk of future fracture. Bone density estimation is the most reliable indicator of fracture risk and should be widely available to GPs.

Patients who are especially vulnerable to osteoporosis include women with early fracture; long-term corticosteroid-users; and those with a positive family history of osteoporosis, premature menopause, or a period of early amenorrhoea. There is disagreement over the effect of hysterectomy with conservation of the ovaries. Two British surveys of patients attending gynaecological clinics detected early ovarian failure in hysterectomized patients. However, a Danish study of women in the community aged 50–59 years found similar bone density in patients who had undergone pre-menopausal hysterectomy and matched controls (Ravn 1995).

Bone density should only be measured if it will affect the management of

Table 11.4 *Typical calcium content of food*

⅓ pint (195 ml) silver top milk	230 mg
⅓ pint (195 ml) semi-skimmed milk	240 mg
⅓ pint (195 ml) skimmed milk	250 mg
1 oz (28g) Cheddar or other hard cheese	220 mg
5 oz (140g) pot of yogurt	270 mg
4 oz (112g) cottage cheese	60 mg
4 oz (112g) ice-cream	157 mg
2 oz (56g) sardines (including bones)	220 mg
2 large (60g) slices white bread	60 mg
2 large (60g) slices wholemeal bread	14 mg
4 oz (112g) broccoli	76 mg
4 oz (112g) baked beans	45 mg
2 oz (56g) peanuts	34 mg
2 oz (56g.) dried apricots	52 mg

the patient. A woman who says 'under no circumstances will I take HRT' is not a candidate for densitometry unless she is willing to take alternative treatment such as bisphosphonates (Etridonate, Alendronate, etc.).

Treatment of low bone density

HRT is extremely effective in the treatment of low bone density. Women at high risk, (e.g. corticosteroid users and/or family history) should be advised to continue with HRT throughout life if possible. (Table 11.3) A woman who sustained an osteoporotic fracture could be prescribed HRT at a later age as it is effective after 70 years. Oestrogen therapy is the most effective treatment in women just past the menopause and later in life. Livial (Tibolone) is not yet approved for this purpose but it is popular, particularly with older women as it does not cause 'periods'.

Calcium supplements are partly effective in older women. Calcium 1000 mg daily should be the aim, preferably through dietary sources such as dairy products (Table 11.4). Sunlight is essential because of its action on the skin to synthesize Vitamin D. Housebound elderly patients would benefit from Vitamin D supplements which have been shown to reduce the incidence of fracture in French nursing home patients (Chapuy *et al.* 1992). Exercise, particularly walking, increases bone mass. Loss of weight-bearing activity in astronauts, hemiplegic patients, and rheumatoid arthritis sufferers has been associated with rapid reduction in bone density.

Patients (male and female) who do not wish to take hormones can be prescribed etidronate (Watts *et al.* 1990; Compston 1994) which is useful both for prevention and those who have already sustained a fracture. Alendronate now has a product licence and does not cause the mineralization defect as seen in etidronate if used for long periods. Other products such as tilodronate, pamidronate, clodronate, and risedronate may be on the market in the next

Table 11.5 *Safe doses of progestogen*

Safe doses of progestogen

Continuous	Norethisterone	1 mg daily
	Medroxyprogesterone acetate (MPA)	5 mg daily
	Dydrogesterone	10 – 20 mg daily
Cyclic	Norethisterone	1 mg 10–12/28 days
	Levonorgesterel	75–250 μg 12/28
	MPA	10 mg 14/28
	MPA	20 mg 14/91
	Dydrogesterone	10–20 mg 14/28

few years. Anabolic steroids which cause weight gain and fluid retention are not widely used in the UK.

Hormone replacement therapy

Oestrogen levels fall at the menopause, putting the woman at risk of temporary symptoms such as flushes and insomnia and long-term effects such as osteoporosis, increased risk of heart disease, and urethro/vaginal problems. Replacement therapy is an attempt to provide enough exogenous oestrogen to reverse these processes. There are many different routes and preparations and the reader is advised to consult the British National Formulary for an up-to-date list.

Each general practice needs to agree on a prescribing policy which takes into account both the short-term relief of symptoms and long-term prevention of serious disease. In addition, time needs to be allocated for counselling and education of patients, initial assessment and screening, and regular supervision. A study in Lancashire (Roberts 1994) found that a dedicated menopause clinic run by a doctor and nurse was preferred by patients.

Principles of prescribing

Women with a uterus need progestogen supplements to eliminate the otherwise increased risk of endometrial cancer (Table 11.5). Peri-menopausal patients are treated with continuous oestrogen and sequential progestogen 10–14 days each month. Withdrawal of progestogen is usually followed by a monthly bleed, although 10% of users have endometrial atrophy and do not bleed. Amenorrhoea is not dangerous provided the full course of progestogen has been taken. The bleeding pattern is not a sensitive guide to the state of the endometrium and unfortunately hyperplastic patterns have been diagnosed in biopsy in patients who bleed regularly.

It has to be remembered that the endometrium may not have been normal *before* treatment. Patients with undiagnosed endometrial polyps or hyperplasia may start treatment and it is usually the occurrence of heavy or irregular bleeding which alerts the physician to the need for investigation.

Initial screening should include enquiry into bleeding pattern, previous hormonal therapy (? unopposed oestrogen or implants), and pelvic examination to exclude fibroids. If there is abnormal bleeding or uterine enlargement or ovarian pathology is suspected, vaginal ultrasound should be arranged and biopsy may be necessary (endometrial thickness ≤4 mm=normal; endometrial thickness ≥8 mm needs further investigation).

Women who are over 1 year post-menopausal can use continuous combined oestrogen/progestogen as in Kliofem, or Tibolone which has weak oestrogenic, progestogenic, and androgenic properties. Younger women who use continuous preparations often suffer from unacceptable irregular bleeding.

Recent advances in HRT

Continuous oral preparations

Continuous oestrogen/progestogen packs for older women who do not wish to bleed are more acceptable than the 'do-it-yourself' arrangements previously available (the physician prescribed separately continuous oestrogen, and progestogen as Micronor HRT or other preparation).

Kliofem is continuous oestradiol 2 mg and norethisterone 1 mg in a single tablet. There is only one prescription charge. After a year nearly all users experience amenorrhoea although there may be unacceptable spotting in the early months. Premique is a combination of conjugated oestrogen 0.625 mg and medroxyprogesterone acetate (MPA) 5 mg in a single tablet. A controlled study of 1724 women showed that 50% developed amenorrhoea after 6 months.

These and similar preparations should aid compliance in older women, many of whom are at high risk of fracture and heart disease. HRT is effective over the age of 70.

Periods which occur every 3 months instead of monthly are now possible with the availability of Tridestra. This contains oestradiol 2 mg daily for 70 days, followed by oestradiol 2 mg plus MPA 20 mg for 14 days, then placebo for 7 days during which the patient bleeds. This preparation represents an advance over previous 'do-it-yourself' arrangements when women who were going on holiday would manipulate their dosage of progestogen to postpone a period. This practice is sometimes dangerous and may lead to catastrophic bleeding.

Patches and gel

Several new types of transdermal oestrogen patch are available. Some women whose skin reacts to the older type of reservoir patch which contains alcohol may prefer the newer matrix patch. In these the oestrogen is contained in the adhesive film. Doses vary from 25 μg, 50 μg, 80 μg to 100 μg daily, so it is possible to accommodate young castrated patients who may need as much as 200 μg daily, and also women who develop side-effects and can only tolerate small doses. Oestrogen gel has a similar action and is often useful for 'difficult'

Table 11.6 *Progestogens*

Androgenic	*Less androgenic*
Norethisterone	Dydrogesterone
Norgestrel	Medroxyprogesterone
Levonorgestrel	
Side effects	Side effects
Weight gain	Minimal
Adverse changes in lipids	
Acne, 'premenstrual' symptoms	
Highly effective in protecting	
endometrium against hyperplasia	

cases and those who are being weaned off implants. It is marketed as Oestrogel in a pressurized dispenser. Two measures (2.5 g) daily are applied to arms, shoulders, or thighs and the dose can be increased to four measures daily after a month if symptoms are not controlled. The plasma levels of oestradiol which are achieved are similar to those using a Estraderm 50 µg patch and are sufficient to prevent osteoporosis. However, the product licence only includes its use for flushes, sweating, atrophic vaginitis, and urethritis.

Local oestrogen

A silicone ring impregnated with oestradiol has become available. It is small (55 mm diameter) and is easily inserted and removed by the patient. Delivering 7.5 µg of oestradiol per 24 hours it does not raise plasma oestrogen and can be safely used by women who have contraindications to HRT. It is less messy than creams or pessaries and a controlled trial has shown that urinary symptoms are improved in users. It has no effect on bone density or cardiac risk as very little oestrogen is absorbed. Progestogen supplements are unnecessary.

Problems with progestogens

Side-effects such as headache, weight gain, bloating, and depression are common during the days when women are taking the progestogen supplement. These are sometimes reduced by using a less androgenic progestogen such as medroxyprogesterone or dydrogesterone (Table 11.6). The latter is available in Femoston which combines continuous oestradiol 2 mg with 14 days dydrogesterone, which may be prescribed at different strengths. Women who take high-dose androgenic progestogens such as norethisterone 5 mg for cycle control, or HRT when oestrogen is contraindicated, may experience weight gain and blood pressure should be monitored. Serum lipid pattern is altered with a fall in HDL and rise in LDL cholesterol. The levonorgestrel IUCD (Mirena) is effective, although not yet marketed for this purpose, in preventing endometrial hyperplasia in women taking conjugated oestrogens. It should prove particularly useful for women using gel or patches (Shoupe *et al.* 1991). It also provides effective contraception and prevents menorrhagia.

Benefits, risks, and costs of HRT

It has been suggested that prevention of fractures and heart disease in the population by use of long-term HRT may be cost-effective because the savings in costs of treatment and hospitalization could possibly outweigh the cost of therapy.

A computer model has been established by a team working at the Department of Public Health and Primary Care at the University of Oxford (Daly *et al.* 1994) to examine this hypothesis, assuming a hypothetical population of women aged 50, taking oestrogen or oestrogen plus progestogen for 10 years with full compliance. They investigated:

(1) mortality induced or prevented by HRT;

(2) morbidity induced or prevented by HRT;

(3) quality of life following relief of menopausal symptoms;

(4) Cost of treatment.

Hospital admission rates were taken from the most recent Hospital In-patient Enquiry. Mortality rates were national mortality figures for 1990. It was assumed that breast cancer risk increased by 30% after 10 years use of HRT and 50% after 15 years. Osteoporotic fractures were assumed to be reduced by 20% after 5 years use and 60% after this, the reduction continuing for a period equal to the length of treatment. Ischaemic heart disease was assumed to decrease by 25% after 5 years and 50% after 10 years' use of oestrogen alone, with halving of protective effect in women using progestogen supplements. Stroke

Fig 11.5 *Hospital admissions induced/prevented by cause to age 69 following 10 years' treatment with oestrogen only (ORT) or oestrogen plus progestogen (CRT) replacement therapy. IHD, ischaemic heart disease; CVD, cerebrovascular disease*
(*Daly et al., 1994*)

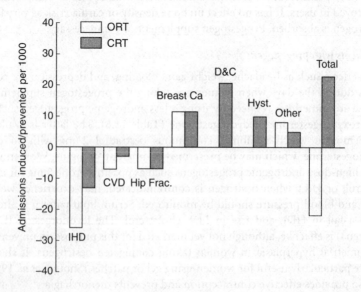

Box 11.2 *Reasons for positively recommending HRT if there are no contraindications*

1. Removal or irradiation of both ovaries before menopause, or natural menopause before 45 years. Bone loss occurs rapidly in these women and oestrogen prevents this for the duration of therapy. Give HRT until 55–60 years-old or longer. Oophorectomized patients may need HRT for 20–30 years. Periodic mammography is important as there is increased breast cancer risk after 9 years' treatment

2. Hysterectomy before the menopause, even if ovaries are conserved. 25% of these women have early ovarian failure. The appearance of hot flushes and FSH >20 μ/l is confirmation of menopause. Oestrogen can be given without progestogen and is protective against ischaemic heart disease for the duration of therapy. If given for 5 years, it halves the risk of future fractures

3. Sexual difficulty due to tight atrophic vagina, which usually occurs in women over 55 but may occur earlier in hysterectomized patients. This responds dramatically to oestrogen

4. Fractures, particularly if occurring before the menopause and with minimal trauma. The appearance of a second fracture or compression fracture of vertebra indicates the need for immediate treatment with oestrogen to prevent further fractures. HRT is the safest and cheapest form of treatment. If the patient cannot take this, refer her for bone density measurement and if low ask advice of specialist unit. Etidronate is effective. Calcitonin is useful but expensive. Stanozolol is useful in older women

5. High risk of ischaemic heart disease, e.g. diabetic, patient already suffering from angina, or high cholesterol >6.8 not responding to diet. Severe family history of cardiac or stroke death <60. Oestrogen is the cheapest and most effective lipid-lowering drug for women

6. Flushes and sweats interfering with sleep or work

7. Increased risk of osteoporosis. Thinness, lack of exercise, rheumatoid arthritis, use of corticosteroids, heavy smoking at peri-menopause, low calcium diet, family history of osteoporosis

8. Depression associated with labile mood at the peri-menopause. Careful assessment of psycho-social background is needed. Also assess depth of depression and suicide risk (Beck Inventory is useful). Psychotherapy or antidepressant drugs may be first-line treatment. Refer if suicidal

Fig 11.6 *Management of the climacteric.*
(Source: Mellor (1996)

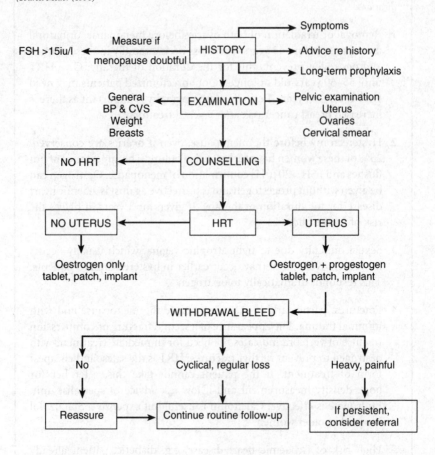

reduction of 25% or 12.5% was assumed, using oestrogen or supplemented HRT respectively. Increased gynaecological intervention of 25% was assumed in women with a uterus.

The cost of treatment was calculated assuming that all prescriptions were for Premarin 0.625 mg at £24 p.a. or Prempak C at £53 p.a. Also, two extra GP consultations at £9.10 each were included. Out-patient hospital appointments at £42.75 and in-patient stays at £157 per day were derived from 1992–93 average prices (e.g. breast cancer was estimated at £1950–6910 and wrist fracture at £170). Estimated savings due to use of HRT over 10 years were: deaths, 16 out of 710; hospital admissions, none (Fig 11.5).

Quality of life also needs to be taken into account and there is no doubt that HRT improves this for women with severe menopausal symptoms (Box 11.2). The study concludes that there is an average overall cost (and not a saving) to the health service of £316–£547 per woman treated for 10 years. However, the cost of HRT compares favourably with other health interventions such as

GPs' advice to stop smoking and very favourably with long-term treatment for hypertension or coronary artery bypass grafting.

From the point of view of the individual woman, selection of patients for therapy is very important. The high-risk patient, suffering from angina, osteoporotic fracture, or early menopause should be strongly advised to consider using HRT. For the general population it is not necessarily true that prevention is better than cure as we have to consider the costs of prevention and the possibility that resources could be better used elsewhere (Cairns 1995).

HRT protocols

HRT spans a wide variety of specialties although the work of initial screening, decision on therapy, and supervision usually falls on general practice. Gynaecologists, physicians with special interest in bone disease, cardiologists, rheumatologists, radiologists, hospital pharmacists, and orthopaedic surgeons should have an interest in HRT as preventive therapy and work with general practitioners (GPs) to devise joint protocols for management.

Individual practice protocols are useful (Fig 11.6) and the menopause clinic is often shared between nurse and doctor, possibly working in parallel rooms, with separately-booked patient appointments. The nurse should always have full access to discuss patients with the doctor.

Protocol for doctor/nurse HRT clinic

Aims:

To offer screening, prescription, advice, and supervision for women considering HRT. HRT is regarded as a preventive strategy against heart disease and osteoporosis.

Personnel:

Doctor
Nurse
Receptionist/clerk.

Method:

Weekly 2-hour session at surgery, using two consultation rooms and a reception desk.

Appointments 15 minutes or more (depending on problem).

Equipment Examination couch, hand basin, light, etc. Clinical records, and computer if in practice use.

Initial assessment:

Indications for HRT:

1. **Patients should be menopausal**.
   - Accurate diagnosis is essential if patient complains of symptoms such as flushes or mood swings. Exclude physical illness (e.g. thyroid disease), side-effects of medication, social problems, or psychiatric illness.
   - FSH level can be used to establish menopause status in hysterectomized or doubtful cases.
   - Detection of menopause in COC users can be difficult. There are two methods. Either change to barrier method for 6 months and await menses. Flushes + amenorrhoea=menopause. Or carry out serial FSH estimation, at least 6 weeks apart. FSH >20=menopause (see Chapter 6).
2. **Peri-menopausal women** can safely take cyclical oestrogen/progestogen for cycle control, but some may prefer to wait because of increased risk of breast cancer with prolonged use.
   - Contraceptive advice should be offered to this group. For non-smokers the COC provides adequate HRT.
3. **Post-menopausal women** – oestrogen is effective for older women, though the maximum benefit in osteoporosis prevention is gained at the menopause when bone loss is most rapid.

Table 11.7 *Contraindications to oestrogen treatment*

Absolute contraindications
- Cancer of breast or endometrium
- Major thromboembolic disease (including atrial fibrillation)
- Severe liver or kidney disease

Relative contraindications
- Lump in breast (needs investigation and possibly removal)
- Lump in pelvis (needs investigation and possibly removal)
- Intermenstrual, post-menopausal, or heavy bleeding (needs investigation and possibly removal of uterus)
- Gall-bladder disease
- Previous adverse reaction to hormone replacement or the Pill

4. **Medical problems** that increase the risk of osteoporosis (e.g. rheumatoid arthritis, thyroxine or corticosteroid therapy, past history of anorexia nervosa) and/or current ishcaemic heart disease are positive indications for HRT. Bone density estimation will sometimes help her make a decision.

Contraindications for HRT:
See Table 11.7. The relative pros and cons of HRT need to be discussed with each women in the light of her personal risk profile and a shared decision reached. If HRT is not appropriate, other non-hormonal methods of keeping well can be discussed.

History and examination of patient:
1. Enquire about bleeding pattern – post-menopausal, heavy or irregular bleeding should be investigated.
2. Vaginal examination should be conducted before commencing therapy to exclude pelvic masses. Any masses found should be investigated. Endometrial biopsy, hysteroscopy, pelvic ultrasound, or laparoscopy may be indicated.
3. Breast examination prior to HRT is mandatory with referral if a lump or nipple discharge is found. Whether mammography is desirable before embarking on long-term therapy in women under 50 is controversial (Chapter 5). All women over 50 should be encouraged to attend for 3-yearly mammography screening. Ideally, women over the age of 65 on HRT should continue to have regular mammograms.
4. Weight should be recorded. Weight gain on HRT is a common complaint. However, in research studies of large groups of patients the mean weight did not increase on HRT. Some women gain weight due to fluid retention and may improve on diuretics. It is worth experimenting with different

HRT preparations as the progestogenic component may differ in dosage and anabolic effect.

5. Blood pressure is measured routinely. In a few patients BP rises on HRT and can usually be controlled with hypotensive medication. However in a few idiosyncratic cases HRT may need to be stopped.

6. Smoking and alcohol status, exercise, diet, and any family history of ischaemic heart disease and breast cancer should be discussed and recorded.

Prescribing HRT:

The lowest effective maintenance dose to control symptoms should be found for each patient.

Choice of preparation:

(1) oestrogen patches or tablets (continuous) for hysterectomized women;

(2) oestrogen patches/gel and progestogen or oestrogen tablets and progestogen (cyclical or continuous) for women with a uterus;

(3) tibolone (in post-menopausal women);

(4) local oestrogen ring, cream or pessaries for vaginal/urethral problems (only small doses administered or progestogen is required).

The prescription must be given by a doctor, initially for 3 months, then reviewed. If she is taking combined, cyclical HRT, the bleeding pattern may be irregular for the first 2 months, but should appear after progestogen supplement in subsequent months. Continuous oestrogen/progestogen regimes may cause spotting for several months (can be up to 12 months) but should lead to amenorrhoea. This should only be given to post-menopausal women.

Follow-up:

1. **Annual follow up** is recommended with more frequent assessment if problems arise. Assessment includes blood pressure and weight measurements and breast examination. Computerized prescription records can be programmed to ensure that patients on long-term therapy are called for review before a further script is issued.

2. **Common side-effects of HRT include:**

   (a) oestrogen – fluid retention, breast enlargement and tenderness, nausea, headaches;

   (b) progestogen – premenstrual syndrome, depression and mood swings, bloating, headache. It is worth trying a different preparation if side-effects are a problem.

3. **Coming off therapy** may be difficult. Slow withdrawal by halving dosage is helpful and therapy is better withdrawn in cold weather. Withdrawal flushes can be severe and distressing to the patient and she needs reassurance that they are harmless and will eventually cease.

Controversies

Many aspects of hormone therapy are controversial and further research is necessary to throw light on these areas.

Is there an increased risk of breast cancer in women taking HRT?

Breast cancer affects one in 12 women in Britain and the question of whether the risk is increased by hormone therapy is enormously important.

A recent editorial by McPherson in the *British Medical Journal* (1995) points out that a 50-year-old woman faces a lifetime risk of coronary heart disease of 45%, hip fracture 15%, and breast cancer 8%. Most of the meta-analyses to date measure the effect of oestrogen alone and show that long-term use of oestrogen (over 10 years) increases the risk of breast cancer, possibly by up to 50%, but shorter use does not affect risk.

It was hoped that added progestogen would protect oestrogen-users against breast cancer but this has not proved to be the case, either in the Swedish study of 23 000 users (Bergkvist *et al.* 1989), or the recent updated analysis of the ongoing American study of the health of over 48 000 nurses (Colditz *et al.* 1995). In the Nurses Health Study there was a 50% increase in the risk of breast cancer in women currently using HRT for over 5 years. A 70% increase occurred in older women aged 60–64 years. Reliable information is lacking on how long the increased risks continue after stopping treatment.

However, the results of the Nurses Health Study are regarded as an 'outlier' by other experts in this field, including Howell and his team at the Christie Hospital, Manchester, who have recently published an overview of the analyses dealing with this subject (1995). They conclude that 10 or more years use of oestrogen in the general population results in 30% increased risk. Shorter use does not increase risk. There is no evidence of increased mortality from breast cancer in long-term HRT users.

This is an important point as modern treatments such as tamoxifen have improved the outlook for survival and quality of life for breast cancer sufferers. Early diagnosis is extremely important and lumps which are found in the course of HRT surveillance may be spotted earlier in the course of the disease (our practice protocol suggests yearly breast examination by the doctor or nurse in HRT users). A woman who is at high risk of dying from ischaemic heart disease may think the odds worthwhile in taking HRT to prevent myocardial infarction and accepting an increased risk of breast cancer.

Women with a family history of breast cancer before the menopause in one or two first-degree relatives have double the risk of breast cancer until they reach the age of 60. They may well be reluctant to take HRT. Overviews of the various epidemiological studies do not show that taking HRT increases their risk beyond the increase in the general population. However their **absolute** risk remains high and it is often helpful to refer them to a genetic counsellor. If HRT is considered it should be given as part of a national trial such as that taking place under the auspices of the Royal Marsden Hospital. The same advice would apply to women with treated breast cancer who wish to take

HRT: they should be referred to a specialist unit and offered entry into a randomized trial.

Only one small, randomized controlled study of 84 women on continuous HRT and 84 on placebo has been published and after 22 years of follow-up no cancer occurred in HRT users, whereas 7 controls developed breast cancer. It is hoped that large randomized studies being launched by the MRC and the NIH will provide answers to these questions.

What is the optimum length of time for women to take HRT?

Women and their doctors are faced with a difficult equation in balancing risks and benefits of HRT. The Framingham Study of 670 elderly women (Felson 1993) has shown that at least 7 years oestrogen therapy after the menopause is needed to provide protection against osteoporosis. Yet over 10 years use increases the risk of developing breast cancer. Long-term therapy should therefore last from 7–10 years unless the patient has lost both ovaries before the menopause. In this case the risk of breast cancer is lower, and therapy should continue for 20 years or at least until the expected date of natural menopause (50 years). It is the author's practice to postpone HRT until after the menopause so that the envisaged 7–10 years of oestrogen therapy may protect against the rapid bone loss expected at this age.

Bone density screening: is it worthwhile?

Bone densitometry is the most effective method of ascertaining the risk of fracture in an individual woman. Below the age of 75 bone density is the most sensitive predictor of fractures; after this age other factors become more important, such as likelihood of falling due to the use of sedatives, badly-lit environment, or poor nutrition. The most important question to put before ordering measurement of bone density is whether the result will alter the management of the patient. Many women are willing to take long-term preventive HRT only if it is demonstrated that their bone mass is reduced. A patient who is unwilling to take treatment whatever the result will not benefit from measurement of bone density. However, there is now a range of non-hormonal treatments available, such as etidronate and alendronate, and calcium and Vitamin D for housebound patients. Densitometry is also useful to monitor patients on corticosteroids as modification of therapy is indicated where possible, e.g. reduction in dose of corticosteroids or alteration of route (inhaled for asthmatics).

Should bone density screening be offered to the whole population?

Bone density measurements are poor at identifying those patients who develop fractures later in life. Over 60% of fractures occur in those with 'normal' bone densities. Although HRT preserves bone density in most women it is not known how long the effect lasts after treatment stops. Because of increased risk of breast cancer, patients are advised to stop HRT well before the age of 70, after

Fig 11.7 *Social class distribution of attenders and non-attenders at the clinic*
(Coope and Roberts, 1990)

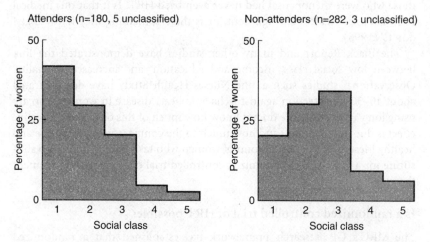

Attenders (n=180, 5 unclassified)   Non-attenders (n=282, 3 unclassified)

which most fractures occur. Compliance with long-term treatment is poor, probably less than 30%. It is likely that a population bone density screening programme followed by HRT for the lowest bone density groups would prevent no more than 5% of fractures in elderly women. On current evidence it would be inadvisable to establish a population bone screening programme with the aim of preventing fractures (Effective Health Care 1992).

Is the woman who uses HRT a special kind of person?

Most GPs are familiar with the healthy, non-smoking, comfortably-off, middle-aged woman who asks for HRT perhaps because her friends are taking it or she has read about it. Behind her is an army of poorly-paid, unhealthy, smoking, and badly-fed female workers who do not demand HRT but probably need it. The inverse care law which states that those most in need of medical care are least likely to receive it applies to the menopause as in most other areas of medicine. The analysis of attendances at our women's health clinic, which aimed at contacting and educating all women in the practice aged 40–60, found a highly significant social class gradient between attenders and non-attenders (Fig 11.7). In the audit carried out after 12 months the women who attended were twice as likely to use HRT and half as likely to smoke as the non-attenders.

A postal survey of over 1000 women doctors showed current use of HRT was 41% for menopausal women in the 45–64 age group and ever use was 55%. Over half of the women doctors starting HRT were expected to continue treatment for 10 years of more (Isaacs *et al.* 1995). Other surveys on use of HRT by menopausal women in the general population in the UK have found a prevalence between 7–9% for current use and 10–16% for ever use. Isaacs *et al.* suggest that the high rates of personal use of HRT by women doctors are likely to predict increased use in the general female population as the benefits of HRT become more widely understood. It is as well to consider why more menopausal women doctors have not tried HRT. In his paper on controversies in management, Jacobs remarks that the authors 'found 40% of those who were menopausal had never even tried HRT. Is it that our medical colleagues are feckless and ignorant, or is there something they know that I don't?' (1996).

The Black Report and many other studies have demonstrated the link between low social class, income and education, and increased mortality. Observational studies such as the Nurses Health Study have demonstrated about 40–50% protection against ischaemic heart disease in women who are using long-term HRT. We do not know how much of this observed protective effect is due to hormones, and how much to the comparatively stress-free and healthy lifestyle of the select group of women who take HRT. There is no sub-stitute for a large-scale, randomized controlled trial of hormone replacement therapy.

Is a randomized controlled trial of HRT possible?

The MRC's GP Research Framework has established that a randomized controlled trial of HRT would take at least 30 years. Cardiovascular disease and vertebral fractures could be evaluated at 10 years, hip fractures and breast cancer at 15–20 years. Depending on the assumptions made (e.g. the number of fatal to non-fatal coronary events) and the power of the study, between 34 000 and 43 000 women would be required. The UK alone would be unable to contribute this many women to the study, so recruitment would need to be from more than one country. A recent, randomized double-blind study comparing compliance of oestrogen therapy alone versus a combined preparation of oestrogen/cyclical progestogen in 321 hysterectomized women (MRC GP Research Framework 1996) found that after 2 years over 30% of women had stopped therapy; there was no difference in compliance between the two groups. The research team suggests that compliance with HRT over a longer trial period of 5–10 years would be likely to be even lower, less than 60%.

In the US, a multi-centre, randomized controlled trial of HRT is currently taking place, involving 57 000 women, with follow-up planned over 9 years. Perhaps this will go some way to answering our questions, but whether it will prove possible to retain sufficient numbers for the duration of the study awaits to be seen.

Is oestrogen an addictive drug?

Most women who stop oestrogen therapy suffer from withdrawal symptoms such as flushes, poor sleep, and irritability which may continue for several months, and always improve on restarting therapy. In our double-blind, ran-domized placebo/oestrogen trial in 30 women in general practice we found that even those women who had not experienced flushes before the trial suffered symptoms when oestrogen was replaced by placebo. It is falling oestrogen levels, not the absolute level, which precipitates flushing and other symptoms.

Women who wish to stop therapy need reassurance that flushes are unpleasant but not permanently damaging and eventually they will cease. The decision to stop therapy needs to be taken on other grounds, i.e. the risk/benefit equation regarding their individual risks of osteoporosis, heart disease, and breast cancer.

Oestrogen implants can raise the serum oestradiol dramatically to supra-physiological levels. These gradually fall and women may experience flushes and demand a replacement implant before the end of the life of the existing implant. This phenomenon is known as tachyphylaxis and is managed by arranging serial oestradiol estimations and avoiding a further implant before it is due. If oestradiol is above the optimum level of 200–400 pmol/l, oestrogen patches of various strengths or oestrogen gel can be useful in these patients.

Does HRT protect against Alzheimer's disease?

A New York-based study suggests that oestrogen therapy may significantly delay the onset and reduce the risk of Alzheimer's disease in post-menopausal women (Tang *et al.* 1996). A total of 1124 non-demented women (mean age 74 years) were entered into the study after neuropsychological testing and examination. After 1–5 year follow-up, 167 (15%) developed Alzheimer's disease (as assessed by an independent group of doctors using standardized tests). Of the 968 women who had never used HRT, 158 (16.3%) developed the disorder, compared with 9 of the 156 women (5.8%) who had taken oestrogen after the menopause. (Relative risk of developing Alzheimer's disease in oestrogen users=0.4, 95% Cl 0.22–0.85, p<0.01.) Women who had taken oestrogen for longer than 1 year showed the greatest reduction in risk, and none of the 23 women who were taking oestrogen when the study started developed dementia. The significant differences between women who had taken oestrogen and those who had not were still apparent even after adjustment for differences in education, ethnic origin, and apolipoprotein E genotype in the two groups of women.

Why might oestrogens be protective? Oestrogens have a wide range of benefits for the human brain. They are known to modify development and ageing of the hippocampus and associated neocortex, the regions affected by Alzheimer's disease. They may also affect neurotransmitters which are compromised in Alzheimer's disease: oestrogens stimulate cholinergic markers, known to be deficient in the disease. Oestrogens are an important co-factor in the actions of nerve growth factors. They also improve cerebral blood flow. The protective effect reported in this study is likely to be multifactorial. Although these results are promising, an unexplained bias could still account for the differences. HRT cannot be recommended universally on the basis of this one study, but if an individual has a strong family history of Alzheimer's disease or is showing early clinical signs of the disease it might be worth considering as a potential means of slowing down disease progression. Prospective studies are clearly needed to consolidate these findings and establish the dose and duration of oestrogen required.

Case histories of patients attending the menopause clinic

We have over 300 long-term users of HRT in our practice who are well and happy on treatment. They attend yearly for routine surveillance and their main concern is to discuss the length of time they should stay on therapy. The following case histories have been chosen to illustrate 'problems' and the practical aspects of clinical management. Doctors' questions have been omitted, and the individual voices of the women can be heard, followed by the doctors' comments on the management of each case.

Gillian: aged 50

I have been worried about breast cancer. I would like you to have a look at my breasts. My mother was treated for breast cancer when she was 44; that was before the menopause and she had an operation. Yes, she is still alive now. My grandmother developed breast cancer when she was 60 and she died of it. I have a tingling feeling in my right breast. Yes, I have had a mammogram this year (1995) and it was normal, but I feel very anxious.

Doctor. This patient's breasts were examined and they were normal. She had a hysterectomy in 1986 so we arranged blood tests to find out if she had reached the menopause. Result: FSH 4.1 u/l, LH 9.5 u/l (not menopausal). In view of her extreme anxiety and the family history of breast cancer she has been referred to a family history breast clinic for further advice and counselling. HRT is not appropriate medication as she has not yet reached the menopause; also we felt unsure about a possible increased risk due to the combination of positive family history and HRT. She will probably return in a couple of years for further blood tests and, possibly, estimation of bone density. One of the advantages of working in general practice is the possibility of seeing your patient again at a later date and deferring the decision on long-term treatment. She may be asked to enter one of the randomized multi-centre trials which are being arranged for patients with a family history of breast cancer.

Frances: aged 45

I had a hysterectomy and one ovary removed for a cyst 3 years ago and got very depressed, perhaps the other ovary wasn't working very well; anyway, I felt awful and the doctor started me on HRT – Premarin. Since then I have felt a lot better and my sex life has been fine, but I have gone on gaining weight. I have gained 2 stone and dieting doesn't make any difference. Will it make any difference if I go on to a different kind of HRT?

Doctor. Although scientific studies of large groups of women have not found that there was an average gain in weight on HRT, individual women often put on weight in a startling fashion. This is a serious matter and many would rather stop treatment than become obese. Diuretics such as bendrofluazide may be helpful as some of the weight gain is due to sodium and water retention. The only sure way to reduce weight is to stop HRT temporarily. This patient was advised to do this when the weather becomes colder as she could expect to suffer severe withdrawal flushes. After losing weight she could then restart therapy. Small doses of bendrofluazide were also prescribed. It is interesting that oestrogen therapy greatly improved her post-operative depression which followed hysterectomy and the removal of what was probably the only effectively-functioning ovary.

Elizabeth: aged 66

The doctor suggested I take HRT as my father and brother both died of a heart attack and he thought it might help protect my heart. I have had angina for 10 years and my cholesterol is high. I have taken HRT for a year and I feel a lot better. I don't get as much chest pain and I feel younger than my age.

Doctor: This patient is at high risk of myocardial infarction and is a suitable case for preventive HRT. Her cholesterol has dropped from 9.1 mmol/l to 5.8 mmol/l and fasting LDL cholesterol from 5.5 mmol/l to 3.9 mmol/l while she was taking HRT. This effect on lipids is beneficial and is typical of the effect of long-term oestrogen therapy, even if, as in this case, progestogen is added. She takes Premarin 0.625 mg plus Micronor two tablets daily, continuously. She is well and does not experience any bleeding. However, despite the adverse effect of androgenic progestogens on the lipid pattern, making it advisable to keep the dose as low as possible, compatible with endometrial safety this patient's medication has not been changed to a continuous combined pack as she does not want to change and is anxious that another treatment may not suit her.

Ellen: aged 56

Some years ago I went to the health clinic to get advice about my moods which got very bad before my periods. Often I could not cope with my job as a teacher and I was lucky that the headmaster was really understanding. You gave me HRT and as they say, the rest is history! I began to feel much better, although I found I needed the higher dose of oestrogen. Last year I had a stroke and as you see I am now in a wheelchair. I have just had surgery to the carotid artery in my neck and the surgeon has told me to stay on hormones as they are good for the arteries. I am a bit worried about periods as my husband has to help me get to the toilet. I have heard about a kind of hormone treatment that does not cause periods.

Doctor: Ellen was hypertensive on HRT 2 years ago and was treated with bendrofluazide. Her father died of a stroke at 56. She is a non-smoker. There is no evidence that HRT increases the risk of stroke and some evidence that it may help to prevent it. Experimental evidence supports the suggestion that oestrogen protects against atherosclerosis. Ellen was taking Prempak C which causes cyclical bleeding, a nuisance in a wheelchair-bound patient. We have now prescribed Kliofem which does not cause bleeding and is appropriate in a post-menopausal patient (at the age of 56 she is presumed to be past the menopause). She also takes low-dose aspirin, diuretics, and attends physiotherapy.

Sandra: aged 49

My periods are very frequent. I have brought you a list of the dates; they are all over the place, the shortest time between is 14 days, the longest 23 days. I have been wondering if HRT would help. The bleeding is heavy and the periods are very painful; tablets don't seem to help.

Doctor. On examination, this patient had an IUD *in situ* which may be causing the heavy and painful bleeds. She does not smoke. She needs contraception and has been given a prescription for the COC (Ovranette) for 3 months and asked to re-attend for removal of IUD after a month on the Pill. Her Body Mass Index is only 20. Research shows reduced bone density in women of low body weight, presumably due to reduced oestrogen levels. (There is significant correlation between Body Mass Index and circulating oestrogen levels.) The contraceptive pill will provide sufficient oestrogen to protect bone density. Eventually she may change to HRT but at the moment the Pill is the best option as it provides control of menorrhagia and contraception. Another useful alternative would be the progestogen-releasing IUD, Mirena.

Doreen: aged 50

Just after my 50th birthday I began to experience several mild flushes every day. My GP carried out some blood tests as I had not had a period for 8 months and found that I was menopausal. There was a delay of some weeks while I had another medical investigation. The doctor then repeated the menopausal blood tests and in the same week I had a period! Apparently the tests showed I was not yet truly menopausal but I decided anyway to start HRT to prevent osteoporosis. I have now been taking HRT for 3 months and I cannot say that it has made a great deal of difference to my life. I do not feel 10 years younger but neither have I experienced any unpleasant side-effects. During the first course I did experience a bad headache and very heavy bleeding but this usually occurred during periods when I was a younger woman. Obviously my body will need time to adjust to HRT but I have every confidence that it is the correct way forward.

Doctor. This patient had typical menopausal symptoms and blood tests showed FSH 100 iu/l, oestradiol30 pmo/l (post-menopausal level). However after a delay of some weeks she regressed to a pre-menopausal state: FSH 16 iu/l, oestradiol 410 pmol/l. Some women can go in and out of the menopause and therefore need a check on contraception: luckily her husband had had a vasectomy.

References and further reading

Ballinger, C. B. (1975). Psychiatric morbidity and the menopause: screening of general population sample. *British Medical Journal*, **3**, 344–6.

Beck, A. T., Ward, C. H., Mendelson, M., *et al.* (1961). An inventory for measuring depression. *Archives of General Psychiatry*, **41**, 561–71.

Bergkvist, I., Adami, H-O., Persson, I., *et al.* (1989). The risk of breast cancer after estrogen and estrogen-progestin replacement. *New England Journal of Medicine*, **321**, 293–7.

Bungay, G. T., Vessey, M. P., and McPherson, C. K. (1980). Study of symptoms in middle life with special reference to the menopause. *British Medical Journal*, **281**, 181–3.

Cairns, J. (1995). The costs of prevention. *British Medical Journal*, **311**, 1510.

Chapuy, M. C., Arlot, M. E., Duboeuf, F. *et al.* (1992). Vitamin D and calcium to prevent hip fractures in elderly women. *New England Journal of Medicine*, 327, 1637–42.

Colditz, G. A., Hankinson, S. E., and Hunter, D. J. (1995). The use of estrogens and progestins and the risk of breast cancer in postmenopausal women. *New England Journal of Medicine*, **332**, 1589–93.

Compston, J. E. (1994). The therapeutic use of biphosphonates. *British Medical Journal*, **309**, 711–15.

Cooke, D. J. and Greene, J. G. (1981). Types of life events in relation to symptoms at the climacterium. *Journal of Psychological Research*, **25**, 5–11.

Coope, J. (1981). Is oestrogen therapy effective in the treatment of menopausal depression? *Journal of the Royal College of General Practitioners*, **3**, 134–40.

Coope, J. (1996). Hormonal and non-hormonal interventions for menopausal symptoms. *Maturitas*, **23**, 159–68.

Coope, J., Williams, S., and Patterson, J. S. (1978). A study of the effectiveness of propanolol in menopausal hot flushes. *British Journal of Obstetrics and Gynaecology*, **85**, 472–5.

Coope, J. and Roberts, D. (1990). A clinic for the prevention of osteoporosis in general practice. *British Journal of General Practice*, **40**, 295–9.

Daly, E., Gray, A., Barlow, D., *et al.* (1993). Measuring the impact of menopausal symptoms on quality of life. *British Medical Journal*, **307**, 836–40.

Daly, E., Vessey, M. P., Barlow, D., Gray, A., McPherson, K., and Roche, M. (1994). Hormone replacement therapy in a risk-benefit perspective. In *The modern management of the menopause. A perspective for the 21st century* (ed. G. Berg and M. Hammar), pp. 473–97. Parthenon Publishing Group.

Daniell, H. W. (1976). Osteoporosis of the slender smoker: vertebral compression fractures and loss of metacarpal cortex in relation to postmenopausal cigarette smoking and lack of obesity. *Archives of Internal Medicine*, **136**, 298–304.

Effective Health Care (1992). *Screening for osteoporosis to prevent fractures.* University of Leeds, University of York, Royal College of General Practitioners.

Felson, D. T., Zhang, Y., Hannan, M. T., Kiel, D. P., Wilson, P. W. F., and Anderson, J. J. (1993). The effect of postmenopausal estrogen therapy on bone density in elderly women. *New England Journal of Medicine*, **329** (16), 1141–6.

Gangar, K. V., Reid, B. A., Crook, D., *et al.* (1993). Oestrogens and atherosclerotic disease – local vascular factors. In *Ballière's clinical endocrinology and metabolism*, Vol. 7, No. 1, pp. 47–59. Ballière Tindall, London.

Ginsburg, J., Swinhoe, J., and O'Reilly, B. (1981). Cardiovascular responses during the menopausal hot flush. *British Journal of Obstetrics and Gynaecology*, **88**, 925–30.

Grodstein, F. *et al.* (1996). Postmenopausal estrogen and progestin use and the risk of cardiovascular disease. *New England Journal of Medicine*, **335**, 453–61.

Herzog, A. G. (1991). Reproductive endocrine considerations and hormonal therapy for women with epilepsy. *Epilepsy*, **62** (6), 527–33.

Holte, A. (1990). The *Norwegian menopause project (NMP)*. Abstract of Sixth International Congress on the Menopause, Bangkok, p. 227. Parthenon Publishing Group, Carnforth.

Howell, A., Baildam, A., Bundred, N., *et al.* (1995). Should I take HRT doctor? Hormone replacement therapy in women at increased risk of breast cancer and in survivors of the disease. *Journal of the British Menopause Society*, **1** (2), 294–7.

Hunter, M. (1990). *Longitudinal studies of the climacteric – the South-East England study*. Abstract of Sixth International Congress of the Menopause, Bangkok, p. 228. Parthenon Publishing Group, Carnforth.

Hunter, M. (1992). The Women's Health Questionnaire: a measure of mid-aged women's perceptions of their emotional and physical health. *Psychology and Health*, **7**, 45–54.

Isaacs, A. J., Britton, A. R., and McPherson, K. (1995). Utilisation of hormone replacement therapy by women doctors. *British Medical Journal*, **311**, 1399–1401.

Jacobs, H. (1996). Controversies in management. Not for everybody. *British Medical Journal*, **313**, 351–2.

Jenkins, R. and Clare, A. W. (1985). Women and mental illness. *British Medical Journal*, **291**, 1521–2.

Jensen, J., Christiansen, C., Rodbrø, P. (1985). Cigarette smoking, serum oestrogens, and bone loss during hormone replacement therapy early after menopause. *New England Journal of Medicine*, **313**(16), 973–5.

Klaiber, E. L., Broverman, D. M., Vogel, W., *et al.* (1979). Estrogen therapy for severe persistent depression in women. *Archives of General Psychiatry*, **36**, 550–4.

Lee, S. (1992). *The Sheffield protocol for the management of the menopause and prevention of osteoporosis* (2nd edn).

Lindsay, R., Hart, D. M., Purdie, D., *et al.* (1978). Comparative effects of oestrogen and a progestogen on bone loss in postmenopausal women. *Clinical Science and Molecular Medicine*, **54**, 193–5.

McKinlay, S. M. and Jefferys, M. (1974). The menopausal syndrome. *British Journal of Preventative and Social Medicine*, **28**, 108–15.

McKinlay, S. M., *et al.* (1990). *The Massachusetts women's health study: a prospective study of menopause*. Abstract of Sixth International Congress on the Menopause, Bangkok, p229. Parthenon Publishing Group, Carnforth.

McPherson, K., (1995). Breast cancer and hormonal supplements in post-menopausal women. *British Medical Journal*, **311**, 699–700.

Mellor, S., Stirling, A., and Ramsden, V. (1994) *Guidelines for the use of hormone replacement therapy: management of the climacteric.* East Cheshire Trust Working Party, Macclesfield District General Hospital.

Medical Research Council's General Practice Research Framework (1996). Randomised comparison of oestrogen versus oestrogen plus progestogen hormone replacement therapy in women with hysterectomy. *British Medical Journal,* **312,** 473–8.

Montgomery, J. C., Brincat, M., Tapp, A., *et al.* (1987). Effect of oestrogen and testosterone implants on psychological disorders in the climacteric. *Lancet,* **i,** 297–9.

Ravn, P. (1995). Lack of influence of simple premenopausal hysterectomy on bone mass and bone metabolism. *American Journal of Obstetrics and Gynecology,* **172,** 891–5.

Roberts, P-J. (1994). Reported satisfaction among women receiving hormone replacement therapy in a dedicated general practice clinic and in a normal consultation. *British Journal of General Practice,* **45,** 79-81.

Shoupe, D., *et al.* (1991). Prevention of endometrial hyperplasia in postmenopausal women with intrauterine progesterone. *New England Journal of Medicine,* **325** (25), 1811–12.

Stampfer, M. K., Colditz, G. A., Willett, W. C., *et al.* (1991). Postmenopausal estrogen therapy and coronary heart disease: ten year follow-up from the Nurses Health Study. *New England Journal of Medicine,* **325,** 756–62.

Sullivan, J. M., *et al.* (1990). *Archives of Internal Medicine,* **150,** 2557–62.

Tang, M-X., Jacobs, D., *et al.* (1996). Effect of oestrogen during menopause on risk and age at onset of Alzheimer's disease. *Lancet,* **348,** 429–32.

Toozs-Hobson, P. and Cardozo, L. (1996). Controversies in management: HRT for all? Universal prescription is desirable? *British Medical Journal,* **313,** 350–2.

Watts, N. B., Harris, S. T., Genant, H. K., *et al.* (1990). Intermittent cyclical etidronate treatment of postmenopausal osteoporosis. *New England Journal of Medicine,* **323,** 73–9.

World Health Organization (1994). *Assessment of fracture risk and its application to screening for postmenopausal osteoporosis.* Report of WHO Study Group, Geneva.

Further reading for patients

Coope, J. (1997). *The menopause: coping with the change.* Vermilion (Ebury Press), London.

Furman, C.S. (1995). *Turning point: the myths and realities of menopause.* Oxford University Press, Inc., New York.

Greer, G. (1993). *The change: women, ageing and the menopause.* Penguin Books, London.

Ojeda, L. (1993). *Menopause without medicine: feel healthy, look younger, live longer.* Thorsons, UK.

Sand, G. (1994). *Is it hot in here or is it me?: facts, fallacies and feelings about menopause.* Bloomsbury, London.

Stoppard, M. (1994). *Dr Miriam Stoppard's practical guide to the menopause.* Dorling Kindersley, London.

CHAPTER TWELVE

Cervical cytology

Ann McPherson and Joan Austoker

Introduction

There has been a screening programme for cervical cancer in the UK since 1964. However, it was not until 1988 that a systematic call and recall system was introduced with coordination by an NHS cervical screening programme national coordinating network. This has resulted in an increase in the number of women having cervical smears, with better coverage of those most at risk, i.e. older women and those from lower social class. At last we are beginning to see an overall fall in the number of deaths from squamous cell cervical cancer, most strikingly in older women, as has happened in other countries with a well coordinated screening programme. This chapter will look at the facts and figures, the natural history, risk factors, and the organization of the service within general practice. Classification of what is meant by an abnormal smear has changed over the years and there will be a review of the new consensus management and treatment of abnormal smears, and a discussion of the current controversies relating to cervical screening.

Facts and figures

Incidence

During 1989 in England and Wales there were over 4000 new cases of invasive carcinoma of the cervix registered, making it the eighth most common cancer in women with an incidence rate of 68.8 new cases per 100 000 population and an incidence to mortality ratio of 2.29 (OPCS 1994). It is the most common cancer in women under 35 although only 15% of cases occur in this age group. There has been a significant increase in the incidence of carcinoma *in situ* as well as invasive carcinoma in young women, but this may partly reflect detection by screening and changes in classification. Carcinoma *in situ* (CIS) now includes grade 111 cervical intraepithelial neoplasia. There were 17 818 women in England and Wales registered as having CIS in 1989 and 85% of these were in women under the age of 45 (see Table 12.1). There are also regional and socio-

Table 12.1 *Age distribution for screening, abnormal/positive results on smear testing, new cases of carcinoma in situ and invasive carcinoma, and death from carcinoma of the cervix. Values are percentages*

Age (years)	Women screened*, 1994–95	Abnormal/positive smear, 1994–95	New cases† of carcinoma in situ or CIN III, 1989	New cases of invasive carcinoma, 1989	Death from carcinoma of the cervix, 1992–93
≤24	11.7	24.5	13.9	1.1	0
25–34	31.9	35.0	43.4	14.1	5.3
35–44	27.5	20.7	27.6	21.2	14.1
≥45	28.9	19.8	15.1	63.6	80.6

* Call and routine recall

† Not true incidences as cases can be detected only by screening. Reflects a mixture of prevalence rates for women screened for the first time and cumulative incidence rates from the date of the last screening for women screened previously

CIN III = cervical intraepithelial neoplasia grade III

Sources: OPCS (1994); (1995); DoH statistical bulletin (1996)

Table 12.2 *Cervical cancer deaths per year (England and Wales)*

Year	No. of deaths
1970s – late 1980s	>2 000
1989	1 816
1990	1 781
1993	1 485
1994	1 369

Source: OPCS (1996)

economic variations for cervical cancer incidence with Wales and the north having higher rates and women in social class V being five times more likely to develop cancer of the cervix than those in social class I (Cancer Research Campaign, 1990).

Mortality

Although age-standardized mortality rates for cervical cancer in England and Wales have been falling by about 1–2% per year from 1970 to 1988, it is only latterly that we seen this fall increase to 7% annually in 1993 and 1994.

In 1994 there were 1369 deaths from cervical cancer in England and Wales (Table 12.2); 95% of these were in women aged 35 and over. Over the last 20–30 years there has been a marked decrease in the mortality of women aged 55 and over. Detailed analysis in younger age groups where there had been a doubling of deaths in the 1970s and 1980s has also slowed in the 1990s. It is probable that the screening programme has had an important role to play in this, though there are other possible contributing factors, including a cohort effect (Sasieni *et al.* 1995) (Fig 12.1). The fall in death rate is due to a fall in deaths from squamous cell carcinoma as there has been no observed effect on the incidence or mortality from adenocarcinoma. These latter cancers now make up 20% of cervical cancer, and as high as 30% in the younger age group, whereas in the 1950s the proportion with a glandular component was only 5%.

There is also a considerable regional variation in cervical cancer mortality in the UK, showing a marked north–south divide. Analysis of the figures for district health authorities (DHAs) show that the 20 DHAs with the highest standardized mortality ratios are all in the northern half of the country.

Natural history

The natural history of invasive cervical cancer and carcinoma *in situ* remains uncertain, a factor which obviously has a profound influence on trying to formulate a screening policy. The natural history is complicated by the fact that the investigative procedure of performing a biopsy on the cervix may itself in

Fig 12.1 *Age-specific mortality rates by birth cohort, England and Wales, 1950–94.*
(From: Sasieni et al., (1995). Lancet, 346, 1566–7)

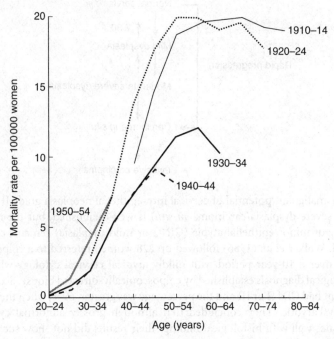

some cases be curative. The questions to which one would theoretically like definite answers *are*:

(1) what number of abnormal/positive smears progress to invasive carcinoma?
(2) what numbers regress to normal?
(3) how long do these changes take to occur?
(4) what factors influence these changes?

The studies dealing with the first question are conflicting and not made easy to compare by the variation in what has been identified as the different stages of dysplasia as against carcinoma *in situ*. The popular theory is that there is a progression to invasive carcinoma of the cervix through various different phases, as illustrated in Fig 12.2, although histologically all stages may be present at the same time – a fact that neither refutes nor confirms this hypothesis. Evidence to support this theory comes from several studies.

There is much confusion over the terms dyskaryosis, dysplasia, and cervical intrapithelial neoplasia (CIN). Cytological surveillance is different from histological diagnosis. Dyskaryosis is used to describe cytological appearances of smears. Dysplasia is used to describe histological appearances. In practice, mild and moderate dyskaryotic smear results do not correlate well with the histological diagnosis of mild and moderate dysplasia, that is grade I and grade II CIN. The difference is more in quantity of CIN rather than quality. Severe dyskaryosis is more likely to mean that there will be a high proportion of grade III CIN in the biopsy specimens.

Fig 12.2 *Possible phases of progression to invasive carcinoma of the cervix*

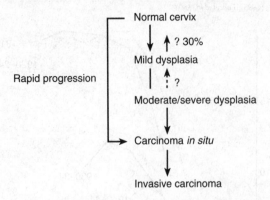

The malignant potential of cervical intraepithelial neoplasia grade III (CIN III or severe dysplasia/carcinoma *in situ*) is well-established, but the natural history of minor epithelial atypia (CIN I or mild dysplasia) remains controversial. Walker *et al.* (1986) followed up 228 women referred to a colposcopy clinic over a 10-year period with mildly atypical cervical cytology who had histological diagnosis established by colposcopically-directed biopsy. Sixty-two per cent had CIN II or III and the percentage was greater, 69%, when the smear was dyskaryotic. They concluded that although grossly abnormal cytology correlates well with histological findings their results did not show such good correlation with lesser grades of cytological abnormality.

The older literature based on cytological and epidemiological evidence suggests that progression from cervical dysplasia to carcinoma *in situ* normally takes over 10 years. Most invasive carcinomas occur in women over 40, most dysplasia in the younger age group (see Table 12.1). However, reports have appeared that in a small number of cases progression may be more rapid and invasive cancer may develop within 5 years of a normal test (Roberts *et al.* 1985). It is not known what percentage progresses rapidly nor which patients they will be. Obviously an increase in the overall number of rapidly-growing cancers could result simply from an overall increase in the incidence of cervical cancer. Some patients with apparently rapidly-progressive lesions have had only one previous smear, because of the probability of false negative results two consecutive satisfactory smears are better evidence that no abnormality is present. It should be stated that prior to 1988 in Aberdeen where a large percentage of the population have had a smear, only 2% of women found to have invasive cervical carcinoma had had a negative smear within the preceding 5 years while 90% had never had a smear (MacGregor *et al.* 1985). In a recent audit of the smear histories of women with and without cervical cancer it was estimated that in women under the age of 70, the number of cases of cervical cancer would have been approximately 75% greater if there had been no previous screening (Sasieni *et al.* 1996). Extrapolation of the results from this pilot study suggests that screening prevented between 1100 and 3900 cases of invasive cervical cancer in the UK in 1992.

Table 12.3 *Stage and prognosis of cancer of the cervix*

Stage	Description	5-year survival rate %
	Precancerous lesions	99–100
I	Cancer confined to cervix	7
II	Cancer has spread beyond the cervix but not on the pelvic wall	47
III	Cancer has spread on to the pelvic wall	22
IV	Cancer has spread more widely	7
All stages		57

Source: Cancer Research Campaign (Factsheet 12)

Further light on the subject comes from the Green experiment in New Zealand. This experiment or trial was set up in 1966 and followed women with minor abnormalities by repeated smears and colposcopy (Coney 1988). Green did not believe that minor abnormalities developed into invasive cancer and therefore watched the progress of these lesions without giving treatment. Those that did progress were excluded from the trial. The conduct of the trial was seen as a scandal. Unfortunately, because of political sensitivities a full analysis of the data which could give good information on natural history has not been carried out.

Prognosis

Although this chapter deals primarily with precancerous lesions of the cervix, it is important to know the prognosis once the diagnosis of invasive cancer has been made. It is staged, which is a way of describing how far it has spread, and the stages are:

Stage I   : Cancer confined to the cervix
Stage II : Cancer has spread beyond the cervix but not on to the pelvic wall
Stage III : Cancer has spread on to the pelvic wall
Stage IV : Cancer has spread more widely.

The percentages of women who will survive 5 years after treatment for the different stages are given in Table 12.3.

Risk factors

In order to develop a screening programme it helps to know the risk factors involved in developing carcinoma of the cervix. Factors related to risk either

Table 12.4 *Risk factors in developing carcinoma of the cervix*

Risk factor	Low risk	High risk	Relative risk <2	2–4	4+
Sexual partners	Few	Many			X
Age at first intercourse	Old	Young			X
Social class	Non-manual	Manual	X		
Smoking	No	Yes		X	
STD	Never	Ever			X
OC use	<5 yrs	5 yrs+	X		
Cervical smear	Ever	Never			X
Age	Young	Old			X

directly or indirectly include:

(1) sexual behaviour;
(2) sexually-transmitted factors;
(3) parity and age at first pregnancy;
(4) method of contraception;
(5) occupation anal social class;
(6) smoking;
(7) history of dyskaryosis.

One could make up a scoring system as indicated in Table 12.4 to try and develop a risk table and thus work out a screening policy for each woman.

Sexual behaviour

Epidemiological studies of risk factors for carcinoma of the cervix initially paid more attention to the sexual behaviour of women than to that of men. It was not realized that not only age at first intercourse, number of sexual partners, and frequency of intercourse of the women may be important but also the sexual habits of their partners or husbands. Evidence for this came from a study of two groups of women with and without cervical pathology, all of whom had had only one sexual partner. When these partners were interviewed the number of their sexual contacts was found to be a significant risk factor in the development of cervical pathology (Buckley *et al.* 1981).

Age at first intercourse was always thought to be an important risk factor but more recently it has been shown that when adjustment is made for the number of sexual partners there appears to be no clear relationship with age. However, in trying to identify at-risk categories young age at first intercourse can be included as this group of women are likely to have more partners during their lives than those starting sexual activity later, and will thus be at increased risk. The number of sexual partners is a definite risk factor and there is a linear relationship between the number of partners that a woman has had a and the likelihood of her developing cervical changes. Compared to having one partner, two partners increase the age-standardized incidence rate by 3, and three or more partners by 5. What evidence there is does not link increased frequency of intercourse *per se* with increased cervical changes.

Sexually transmitted factors

The most popular theory of the causation of cervical cancer is an infection passed venereally. There is an increasing mass of evidence to implicate certain strains of papilloma or wart virus. In 1976 and 1977 two laboratories working independently reported an association between wart virus infection and cervical cancer. Since then there have been great advances in our knowledge of human papilloma viruses (HPV) and their relationship with cervical neoplasia. Different strains of HPV have been identified. Correlation of virus type with the morphology of the cervical lesion shows that HPV types 16 and 18 are present in over 28% of invasive squamous cancers of the cervix, vulva, and penis, and in the higher grades of intraepithelial neoplasia of the cervix and vulva (CIN III and VIN III). In contrast, HPV 6 and 11 are more often associated with benign warts or mild dysplasia (CIN I or II). It is therefore thought that different HPV strains vary in their oncogenic potential.

A prospective study of 100 women under 30 years-old with cytological and colposcopic evidence of mild cervical atypia consistent with CIN I showed that 26% progressed to CIN III; spontaneous regression occurred in only 11 cases, and in four of these CIN recurred. The prevalence of HPV 16 in this group was 39%, but in the cases with progressive disease 85% were positive for HPV 16 (Campion *et al.* 1986). More recent studies (Woodman 1996) have further strengthened this association as well as with HPV 18, though we still await the outcome of cohort studies in which longitudinal observations are made on subjects whose exposure status has been defined before the onset of the disease.

Other theories put forward have included an association with herpes virus type II, a carcinogenic effect of smegma, and that products from sperm may induce malignant change in cervical cells at a particular stage of cell division.

Parity and age of first pregnancy

There appears to be no association between risk and age at menarche. Virgin women have the lowest risk of severe dysplasia and carcinoma *in situ*, and women having a late pregnancy have relative risks lower than those with an early pregnancy. An increased number of pregnancies increases the risk of cervical abnormalities but there appears to be no clear relationship once other confounding factors such as number of sexual partners is allowed for, and it is likely to be an associative rather than a causative factor. Pregnancy outside marriage, termination, and divorce have at some time all been shown to be associated with increased risk, but it is unlikely that these will all hold up to closer scrutiny once other variables are allowed for.

Method of contraception

Certain methods of contraception may have a direct adverse effect, such as the hormonal influence of the Pill, while others, such as the barrier methods, may actually have a protective effect. Long-term use of oral contraceptives has been shown in several studies to be associated with cervical abnormalities. Some of these findings have been questioned because of inadequate control of confounding factors such as age at first intercourse, number of sexual partners (both men and women) and inclusion of diaphragm-users in the control groups. In several studies (Wright *et al.* 1978; Vessey *et al.* 1983; WHO Collaborative Study 1985) in which many of these factors were taken into account, there was still a higher relative risk for people on the contraceptive pill. Another difficulty in trying to evaluate the effect of the Pill is that oral contraceptives may cause eversion of the endocervix, making abnormalities easier to detect. Thus, the direct importance of the oral contraceptive (OC) in the pathogenesis of cervical dysplasia and invasive carcinoma is still controversial and the issue is unlikely to be resolved until more prospective long-term studies are reported. Several recent studies support earlier findings that the risk of cervical neoplasia increases with longer duration of OC use and that increased risk is confined to women who have used OCs for 5 or more years, with risk estimated at nearly twice that of non-users in studies that controlled for the differences in sexual and cytological screening behaviours between OC-users and non-users (Irwin 1996).

However, recent studies of the effects of age at first OC use remain conflicting: some indicate that women who first used the Pill before age 18 are approximately twice as likely as those who never used it to develop invasive cancer, while other studies have observed no increased risk in this subgroup. Thus, it remains uncertain if OC exposure at a critical period in the development of a woman's cervix influences the risk of neoplasia. Most studies that examined risk by recency of use found that the risk of high-grade intraepithelial neoplasia and *in situ* carcinoma was greater among current and recent users than among past users. Enhanced cytological screening of OC users, i.e. detection bias, may explain this observation because CIN is usually diagnosed with routine cytology. However, late-stage carcinogenic effects of OCs cannot be ruled out.

On the other hand, diaphragm-users and users of other barrier methods have a decreased risk of cervical abnormalities, as shown in several studies. However, diaphragm-users are less likely to have had coitus at an early age and have usually had fewer sexual partners. Even when these factors and the frequency of intercourse are allowed for, they have a much lower risk; though when looking at barrier methods the possible effect of spermicides should also be considered. But again the difficulties of interpretation are many, for although spermicides may have a direct effect, protective or otherwise, they are not applied by all users of barrier methods.

Social class

Mortality statistics for cervical cancer show a steep social class gradient. Women in social class V are three times more likely to die of cervical cancer than those in social class I which may in part explain the regional variation within England; and it is more common in urban than rural areas. Social class variation may also reflect women's different usage of preventive medical services. It may, of course, not be a direct effect of social class. In one study (Harris *et al.* 1980) that looked at the characteristics of women with dysplasia or carcinoma *in situ*, no social class influence was found once the other risk factors had been taken into account, such as earlier marriage, more pregnancies, more partners, etc.

Smoking

The emergence in several studies of cigarette smoking as a major risk factor for cervical neoplasia is difficult to understand as at first sight it seems unlikely that the use of tobacco has any direct effect on the cervix. It may be that smoking reflects some important aspect of sexual behaviour or is indirectly linked via other social-class factors. There are no published laboratory findings establishing a direct effect of smoking on cervical cells, although it has been suggested that this is possible as (1) it is known that the carcinogenic products of cigarette smoke are absorbed from the respiratory tract and excreted at distant sites, e.g. breast ducts and in the urine; (2) nicotine and cotinine have been detected in the cervical fluid of smokers; and (3) chemical carcinogens can enhance the *in vitro* carcinogenicity of certain viruses. In many of these studies the sexual habits of the male partner and his occupation have not been allowed for, but where they have, smoking still comes out as a strong independent risk factor (Barton *et al.*, 1988).

Primary prevention

Cervical screening is secondary prevention. At present, the ***exact*** cause of cervical cancer is not known but it seems that it is sexually transmitted with HPV heavily implicated. From the risk factors already mentioned information can and should be given to women (and men) to allow decisions to be made which may help in primary prevention. Thus available information on primary prevention would include:

(1) fewer partners (for both men and women);
(2) barrier methods of contraception and avoidance of long-term use of the Pill;
(3) avoidance of intercourse with partners with genital or rectal warts, and hence avoidance of the spread of papilloma virus;
(4) advice to heavy smokers to stop or reduce smoking.

Guidelines for screening

The present guidelines in the UK are that all women aged 20–64 who are or ever have been sexually active should be screened. It is suggested that screening should stop at age 65 if a woman has had regular negative smears, but that there is no upper age limit for having a first smear. It is also suggested that a smear should be taken at least every 5 years. Women who have never been sexually active do not need to be screened. Different countries and individual doctors operate under different guidelines. Trying to establish consensus has been extremely difficult.

Organization

The aim of the cervical screening programme is to reduce the deaths from cervical cancer. The *Health of the Nation* has set targets to reduce the incidence of invasive cervical cancer by at least 20% by the year 2000 from 15 per 100 000 population to no more than 12 per 100 000. For the screening programme to be effective there must be:

(1) a high uptake of smears across all age groups and social classes;
(2) repeat tests at regular intervals of not more than 5 years;
(3) a service which women find acceptable;
(4) adequate smear-taking with training of smear-takers;
(5) quality control for interpreting smears;
(6) a reliable fail-safe mechanism;
(7) efficient and good treatment facilities;
(8) systematic evaluation and monitoring.

The organization of the national screening programme depends on cooperation between the health authorities and general practice. Two major changes have taken place since 1988; the introduction of a national call and recall system and a change in the method of payment to general practitioners (GPs).

Since 1988 there has been a national call and recall system. However, there are still local variations; for example, the screening interval is different in different areas. The current national guidelines recommend women aged 20–64 years be offered a smear at least every 5 years but many screening programmes adopt a 3-year recall policy, whilst in other areas it varies according to age. Practices get sent regular lists of women within that age group who need smears at intervals dependent on local policy and individual patient needs according to previous smear results.

Since the 1990 contract, GPs have been set targets on which payment for cervical screening depends. Payment is dependent on reaching quarterly targets of 80% or 50% coverage of the eligible population within the preceding 5.5 years with a differential of 3:1 in favour of the former. There was considerable doubt as to how effective these target payments would be, but in the event, they appear to have been very effective in increasing screening activity. Between April 1990 and October 1993, the percentage of GPs reaching the higher target increased from 53% to 83% with only 3% reaching neither target in 1993 compared with 15% in 1990. From 1989/90 to 1994/95 coverage of the target population increased from 61% to 85% (in future statistics will be presented based on a 5-year period). Coverage particularly improved in the older age group. Between 1988/89 and 1994/95 coverage of women aged 55–59 increased from 37% to 81% and that for women aged 60–64 increased from 25% to 87%. A survey in 1992 showed that there was also a decline in the social class differential that had previously been observed. However, there are still problems in some areas. The metropolitan areas, especially the Thames regions, have been slower to raise their coverage partly because of a more mobile population and difficulties with inaccurate registers such that many invitations are sent to the wrong address.

Practice organization

Over 4.5 million smears are taken in England annually from 3.9 million women, with over 80% taken in primary care (DoH 1996). Organization of cervical screening varies from one practice to another and there is no right way. Regular lists of women needing a smear are sent to the practice. These need to be checked before letters of invitation are issued either from the practice itself or via the health authority. Smears can be taken in smear clinics, women's health clinics, family planning clinics, or during normal surgery appointments. The best rates of coverage will be reached by combining a mixture of a call and recall system with opportunistic screening of those who fall through the call/recall net. However it is arranged, it is necessary to have a system and to have someone responsible for running it. Whoever takes the smear needs to be adequately trained. The sex of the smear-taker is important for some women. One study showed that 41% of women would prefer a female doctor and this proportion was higher among older women and those from lower socio-economic classes (Nichols 1987).

Invitation letters

The invitation letter that a woman receives asking her to attend for a smear will affect her response. The style, presentation, tone, and contents are all important. The purpose and applicability of the test to the individual women should be clearly stated, and an explanatory leaflet enclosed. The inclusion of a fixed appointment time results in better uptake, rather than asking a women to make her own appointment, and a reply slip helps the practice. It also helps if the letter is signed by the patient's usual doctor and it should state who will take the smear, giving the option of a woman doctor or nurse if this is possible. A study in Australia showed that a personal letter from a GP combined with a television campaign to increase awareness was the most effective way of improving uptake of cervical smears (Byles *et al.* 1994).

New patients

For *new* patients the registration medical is the ideal time to check on their cervical screening status, and if they have fallen through the net or are due for a smear they can be put on the appropriate call/recall system immediately. It is important to do this as there is a time-lag before old notes come through.

Special groups

Temporary and emergency patients are a group who may never get asked about a cervical smear. This does not mean the temporary patient visiting her mother for a few days at Christmas who comes to see the GP because she has a cough. The temporary patients at risk are those who never register permanently, who are frequently on the move, who never get on to an operative call/recall list, and whose lifestyle may put them at increased risk. They are not included in practice targets but even in this money-oriented age they should not be neglected! Other groups that may require special inputs to encourage them to have smears taken are Asian women and travellers. Personal visits and videos have proved effective in increasing the uptake of cervical smear testing among Asian women in Leicester who have never been tested previously (McAvoy and Raza 1991).

Fail-safe

The GP has certain clearly laid-down responsibilities in the fail-safe mechanism:

(1) checking that all smear reports have been received;
(2) informing the woman of the result;
(3) initiating further investigation;
(4) contacting women who do not attend for further investigation;
(5) informing the health authority if a woman requiring investigation has moved away;
(6) monitoring the 'suspend' and 'repeat advised' lists sent by the FHSA.

Where smears are taken by GP trainees or practice nurses, responsibility lies with the GP principal recorded on the request form.

Where smears are taken outside the primary care setting and the result is sent to the GP, it is important to check who is looking after the follow-up and referral as necessary. Some cervical smears continue to be taken in, for example, genitourinary clinics, often outside the screening guidelines. However, this practice may decrease as a recent paper (Stedman *et al.* 1995) concluded that a policy of cervical screening of all genitourinary medicine patients could no longer be sustained, and that smears should be offered to those women who had not been screened in the previous 3–5 years.

Non-attenders and attitudes of women

There are two groups to be considered among non-attenders for cervical smears, those who have received an appropriate invitation and non-attendance due to administrative failure. For many years the main reason women failed to have a smear was that they had never been asked. With the more efficient working of a call/recall system this is much less true, though studies in some inner cities have shown invitations were sent to wrong addresses in 30% or more cases. Although the percentage of women who do not attend for a smear has fallen, some women even if invited will not come forward. There may be many reasons why women will not have a smear and myths need to be dispelled. The reasons for their non-attendance include high level of anxiety about the test, fear about cancer, erroneous beliefs about the relevance of the test, concurrent family difficulties, and seeing it as a low priority. A survey in east London showed that 71% of women thought a cervical smear was a test to pick up cancer, and only 12% realized it was to detect disease at the pre-cancerous stage (Savage and Schwartz 1985).

A recent study looking at women's views on the screening programme since 1990 (Summers and Fullard 1995) found that three-quarters of the women who had had a smear made positive comments on the experience, but when asked specifically about the information they had received felt it was inadequate. Improvements in health education, be it by mass media or health professionals, may have the most impact on improving coverage and quality of cervical screening from the viewpoint of women.

The Women's Institute carried out a survey of members in their groups. Common worries expressed by patients include:

'I thought it would hurt'
'I felt embarrassed about being examined'
'I didn't want to see a male doctor'
'I didn't want to bother the doctor'
'I no longer have sex, so I didn't think I needed one'
'I'm too old to need one'
'You can't do anything about it anyway'
'It's only promiscuous women who get it'
'I wouldn't want to know if I had cancer anyhow'

Women who do not attend should have their notes tagged so that the opportunistic approach can be used when they next attend the surgery. This is useful backup as 75% of women consult their GP in any 1 year and 90% over a 5-year period. Reminders by telephone are more effective than standard letters in getting women to attend for a smear but care must be taken not to make women feel they are being coerced into having a smear. They need to be given the relevant information and left to make their own choice.

Taking a cervical smear

The objective of taking the smear is to identify women whose cytological pattern is suggestive of CIN. One of the key factors determining the effectiveness of a cervical screening programme is the quality of smear-taking. Poor smear-taking can miss 20% or more of pre-cancerous abnormalities of the cervix (BSCC 1989).

The practicalities of exactly how to take a smear can be found in the second edition of *Cervical screening* (Austoker and McPherson 1992) and BSCC booklets. Whoever takes the smear should be adequately and appropriately trained, whether a doctor or a nurse, and should make sure that the environment and equipment is prepared; the patient is properly interviewed, a history taken, and the form accurately completed; the right-sized speculum – adequately sterilized or single-use disposable – is used; the spatula is appropriate to the size and shape of the cervix; and the cervix is properly visualized before the smear is taken.

Courses are available for training in cervical smear-taking with quality assurance guidelines laid down and a suggestion that there should be formal updating of skills every 3 years (RCN 1994; NHSCSP 1996). In practice this

Table 12.5 *Adequate smears results 1994–95*

	%	Number
Negative	94.4	3 544 575
Borderline changes Mild dyskaryosis	4.4	165 706
Moderate dyskaryosis	0.7	25 005
Severe dyskaryosis ?Invasive carcinoma ?Glandular neoplasia	0.6	20 842

Source: DoH statistical bulletin (1996)

does not happen but if GPs are delegating smear-taking to nurses it is essential that the nurses are properly trained and updated as should the GPs be themselves!

Results

There is no point in taking cervical smears unless the results are transmitted to the women. The most commonly-used system until recently has been 'no news is good news' or 'the test is normal unless you hear from us'. Unfortunately, this has in some cases resulted in poor follow-up of patients who have had abnormal smears. It is now a necessary standard to send out results to all women who have had a smear, informing them of the result and when the next smear is due (NHSCSP 1996).

Before women have a cervical smear, or at least sometime during the consultation, it is good practice to tell them:

(1) that the condition being looked for is precancerous;
(2) how and when the results will be obtained, e.g. the result will be sent in 4 weeks time and if you do not hear please contact the practice;
(3) what percentage of smears are negative or abnormal (see Table 12.5) and what that means (see Table 12.6)
(4) that approximately 8% of smears are inadequate or unsatisfactory;
(5) what an inadequate or unsatisfactory smear means;
(6) the significance of being recalled;
(7) what the options are if the result is abnormal.

Women are less likely to be worried when they are recalled if they have been prepared at the time the smear is taken. However, there is considerable evidence to suggest no matter how they are told, women with abnormal results on smear testing do feel very anxious because of fears of cancer and the investigative procedures such as colposcopy. In one study 27% felt shocked, stunned, or

Table 12.6 *Interpretation of smear results result codes and action*

Result	Explanation	Action
Inadequate	Insufficient cellular material Inadequate fixation Smear consisting mainly of blood or inflammatory cell exudate Little or no material to suggest that the transformation zone has been sampled	Repeat smear
Negative	Normal. Includes simple inflammatory changes including a mild polymorph exudate	Routine recall
Borderline changes, with or without HPV change	Cellular appearance that cannot be described as normal. Smears in which there is doubt as to whether the nuclear changes are inflammatory or dyskaryosis	Repeat smear at 6 months. Consider for colposcopy if changes persist
Mild dyskaryosis with or without HPV change	Cellular appearances consistent with origin from CIN I (mild dysplasia)	Repeat smear at 6 months. Consider for colposcopy if changes persist
Moderate dyskaryosis with or without HPV change	Cellular appearances consistent with origin from CIN II (moderate dysplasia)	Refer for colposcopy
Severe dyskaryosis with or without HPV change	Cellular appearances consistent with origin from CIN III (severe dysplasia/carcinoma *in situ*)	Refer for colposcopy
Severe dyskaryosis/? invasive carcinoma	Cellular appearances consistent with origin from CIN III, but with additional features which suggest the possibility of invasive cancer	Refer for colposcopy
Glandular neoplasia for suspicion of glandular neoplasia	Cellular appearances suggesting pre-cancer or cancer in the cervical canal or the endometrium	Refer for colposcopy

Note: The use of the term atypical cells is no longer recommended in the result Codes and its use should be discontinued. The preferred term is Borderline changes (atypia may still be used in the free-text comment, but the degree of atypia should be clarified in the Result Code)

Sources: BSCC (1989); I. Duncan (1991); Austoker and McPherson (1992); Austoker and Davey (In press)

devastated whilst 65% were worried or alarmed (Posner and Vessey 1988). A randomized study showed that inclusion of an information leaflet with the postal notification of the results decreased the levels of anxiety significantly (Wilkinson *et al.* 1990). Studies have also shown that the written information does have to be understandable and not too alarmist if it is to be useful and help women cope with any treatment or future follow-up.

Interpretation of smear results

Smear results can sometimes be difficult to interpret and over the years there has been much confusion in reporting. Recently, a working party (Herbert *et al.* 1995) has developed national criteria for evaluating cervical cytopathology. The smear may be normal in that there is no nuclear abnormality, but other comments may be made (Table 12.7). When a smear is reported with some abnormal cells the action required will depend on many factors, including the appearance of any previous smears. If you do not understand a smear result, contact your local cytopathologist for clarification.

It must be borne in mind that there is a whole spectrum of abnormality, from completely normal to definitely malignant, and cytological grading is an inexact science. The exact risk consequent on each grade is not clear either.

It also needs to be remembered, when recommending further action, that referral of *all* grades of abnormality would lead to considerable over-diagnosis and over-investigation. A careful balance thus has to be reached, taking into account both the benefits that are likely to ensue and the costs – to women and to the health service in terms of resource implications. Inevitably, opinions will differ on how such a balance is arrived at. Tables 12.6 and 12.7 summarize the more commonly-used terms in the reporting of cervical smears, with guidelines for action.

Management of women with abnormal cervical smears

The management of patients with abnormal smears is based on the limited available information about the behaviour of CIN. It is known that patients with severe dyskaryosis (suggesting a large proportion of CIN III) have a risk of progression to invasive cancer sufficiently high and immediate to merit early biopsy for histological confirmation followed by treatment. This action is also to exclude reliably the presence of an invasive carcinoma in such cases. The behaviour of mild and moderate dyskaryosis is less certain, but there is no doubt that a number of these abnormalities will progress to invasive cancer if untreated. It is not possible at present to predict behaviour from morphological appearances, and there is disagreement as to whether all patients with mild dyskaryosis should be referred for further investigation.

Colposcopy

The colposcope is a low-powered microscope for viewing the cervix. During the investigation the patient lies on her back with her legs up in stirrups.

Table 12.7 Interpretation of specific incidental observations on negative cervical smear reports

Result code	Explanation	Action
Specific infections	*Trichomonas*, *Candida*, and cell changes associated with herpes simplex can be identified	*Trichomonas* – treat *Candida* – treat if symptoms *Herpes* – no treatment – to discuss with patient
Actinomyces	Organisms associated with IUD	No consensus. Alternatives (1) do nothing unless other symptoms, e.g. pain or discharge; (2) change coil and the *Actinomyces* organisms will disappear
Endocervical cells	Cells from the glandular epithelium of the cervical canal. During its formation the transformation zone will include similar epithelium	No action needed
Metaplastic cells (metaplasia/squamous metaplasia)	Normal cells from the transformation zone that are ideally contained in a smear	No action needed
Cytolysis	Normal process of cell disintegration	No action needed
Endometrial cells	Cells derived from the endometrial lining of the uterine cavity. Shed during menstruation and in some other circumstances	If IUD present – probably normal finding. If 1–12 day of 28-day cycle – normal finding. Otherwise discuss with laboratory or local gynaecologist
Inflammatory changes	Cellular appearance present in some degree in many smears and not evidence of CIN	No consensus. Alternatives (1) do nothing; (2) take high vaginal swabs for culture and sensitivity and take chlamydial swabs. Then treat as necessary
Atrophic smear	Common in post-menopausal smears, i.e. when oestrogen and progesterone levels are low. Similar changes are seen in postnatal smears	No action needed

A speculum is passed into the vagina to visualize the cervix before using the colposcope, which is mainly used for the investigation and management of cervical intraepithelial neoplasia (CIN) and to assess more thoroughly a clinically-suspicious cervix even when the smear test is normal.

Colposcopy takes about 15 minutes to carry out, and should not be painful, although it is uncomfortable. It allows the clinicians to view the cervix very carefully in order to assess the extent and severity of any lesion properly and to provide appropriate treatment. A biopsy is usually taken and this can be acutely painful. Approximately 2–4% of all smears will need referral of the woman for colposcopy, depending on what guidelines for referral are used. Women having colposcopy may have very high levels of anxiety about both the procedure and the outcome. A randomized study showed that this anxiety was reduced by providing a simple booklet about colposcopy with the appointment letter (Marteau *et al.* 1996). More detailed information, though adding to knowledge, did not reduce anxiety levels. Many patients also complain of profuse vaginal discharge which may last up to a month after cryocautery. Fifty-two per cent also had disturbed feelings about sexual relationships after colposcopy (Posner and Vessey 1988).

If the smear is reported as having malignant cells or carcinoma *in situ*, confirmation of the cytology report requires cervical biopsy. By arranging this quickly, the doctor can relieve the patient's anxiety about the extent of the disease as soon as possible. If the cervix looks malignant clinically, then it is best to prepare the woman for hearing this in hospital, possibly suggesting that she is accompanied there by her partner or a friend. If the cervix is clinically normal on examination by the naked eye, then the question of frank malignancy need not be raised and one should prepare the woman for colposcopy and/or biopsy.

Treatment of the cervix

Before the advent of colposcopy, cone biopsy or hysterectomy were the standard treatments for the most severe grades of CIN. These can be avoided in 80–90% of patients by the use of colposcopically-directed biopsies. In order to know when to treat the cervix it is important to have some idea of the rate of progression of abnormalities. Those at high risk of progression must be treated. There is currently inadequate information about the natural history of the lower grades of abnormality. The majority may not progress, but some would lead eventually to invasive disease if not treated at any stage. A balance must thus be reached between potential over-diagnosis and over-treatment and the need to ensure that progression to invasive cancer does not occur. It is therefore not possible to define a treatment policy with any degree of certainty. Although grade I cervical intraepithelial neoplasia carries low risk and grade III carries high risk, grade II cervical intraepithelial neoplasia is more difficult to categorize. On balance, it is currently believed that grades II and III cervical intraepithelial neoplasia should be treated once diagnosed. Grade I cervical intraepithelial neoplasia may be treated or kept under close surveillance.

Treatment aims at destroying cells in the transformation zone of the cervix. Extremes of heat or cold are equally effective. Some methods of treatment require two visits, while others deal with diagnosis and treatment in one visit, which has obvious advantages for the women. CIN can be effectively destroyed by electrodiathermy, cryosurgery, laser evaporation, or cold coagulation. Alternatively, the transformation zone may be excised using a large cutting electrosurgical loop (laser loop excision). The benefit of the latter is that it combines diagnosis and treatment in one visit which is advantageous to the patient. These procedures are usually associated with uterine pain. Local anaesthetic is of limited value and general anaesthesia is rarely required. These locally destructive methods have the advantage of preserving cervical function and have thus become acceptable in treating more minor degrees of CIN.

Follow-up after treatment

Follow-up is necessary to identify any residual disease, to identify new CIN or invasive disease, and, perhaps most important, to reassure the patient (and the doctor). Duncan (1991) has recommended the following guidelines:

1. Cytological follow-up is essential following treatment for CIN. Colposcopy is not essential but may enhance detection of persistent disease at 6 months.
2. Following treatment, the first smear should be taken at 6 months and, if normal, repeated at 12 months.
3. More frequent surveillance need not be continued beyond 5 years of normal findings after conservative treatment for CIN III.
4. Women undergoing hysterectomy with a past or current history of CIN III need have no further smears if the vault cytology is normal 6 and 12 months after surgery; but if there is suspicion that the pre-malignant condition is not completely removed, continue with 3-yearly screening.

The negative aspects of screening

In evaluating any screening programme the negative aspects are sometimes forgotten and are rarely quantified. Campion *et al.* (1988) looked at women under investigation for CIN compared to women investigated as partners of men with sexually-transmitted diseases, and found that CIN had a strong negative effect on sexual feelings and behaviour 6 months later, whereas the psychosexuality of those who had not had CIN treatment did not change.

There are many anecdotal stories and books now written of how women feel about having an abnormal smear (e.g. Quilliam 1992), and the doctor should always be humble enough to listen to patients' opinions:

I felt dirty inside, as if I was rotten to the core. My imagination ran riot – I felt as if I was 'had' in the most intimate and feminine part of my body. I was like an apple that looks crisp and juicy from the outside but inside is crawling with maggots. As you can imagine, this had a devastating effect on my sex life. Why wasn't I able to go to my doctors and tell them honestly how I felt?

Controversies

Over the last few years there has been an attempt to get consensus in areas of screening policy. However, there are still many areas of uncertainty and further research and information are necessary to resolve these areas of controversy. Some of these issues are discussed below.

Is screening cost-effective?

It has been argued by Skrabenek, McCormick, and others that the screening programme in the UK was not cost-effective and should be stopped (McCormick 1989). This of course begs the question of who judges the cost-effectiveness – the women, the doctors, or the politicians. It was true until recently that the overall mortality from cervical cancer had not been significantly reduced in the UK compared to other countries. But since the introduction of a proper call and recall system and the attainment of good population coverage, this is no longer true. The reduction in mortality, however, cannot all be attributed to screening, in that a cohort effect, increased use of condoms, etc. may also play a part. The sensitivity and specificity of the test available is wanting. Raffle *et al.* (1995) reviewed cervical screening in the Bristol area during the 1988–93 screening round. 225 974 women were tested, new smear abnormalities were found in 15 551, and approximately 6000 were referred to colposcopy. They felt the numbers investigated were high in comparison to the number of potential malignancies and the effect of screening on death rates in Bristol were too small to detect, with much effort being put into limiting harm done to healthy women and protecting staff from litigation. There are limitations to screening as women who have been screened do still die of cervical cancer. One lesson that can be learnt is never again to introduce an unevaluated screening programme, but we have passed the point where its effectiveness can be tested by a randomized trial.

How often should smears be taken?

The Department of Health has recommended that a smear should be taken 'at least every 5 years'. There is considerable local variation – some health authorities do 5-yearly screening, some 3-yearly, and some a mixture of both. This is further complicated by the fact that GP target payments relate to smears taken over a 5.5-year period (although this is now changing to a 5-year period). Because the natural history of the disease is not well-understood, the optimum interval remains a subject of debate and an important research issue. Attempts have been made to show the effects on cervical cancer incidence of different screening policies. As can be seen from Table 12.8, the advantage of 1-year over 3-year screening intervals is very small (2%), whereas there is a 7% difference between 3 and 5-yearly screening. This is the rationale for 3-yearly screening.

Should younger women be screened more frequently?

For younger women, particularly those aged 25–34, there has been a significant increase in cervical cancer incidence and mortality rates over the past 10–15 years, though the mortality rates are now starting to decline. Some health authorities screen women under 35 at 3-year intervals, and women over 35 at

Table 12.8 *Effects on cervical cancer incidence of different screening policies, starting at age 20*

Screening schedule	Reduction rate (%)	No. of tests
Every 10 years, 25–64	61	4
Every 10 years, 35–64	55	3
Every 10 years, 45–64	43	2
Every 5 years, 20–64	84	9
Every 5 years, 30–64	81	7
Every 3 years, 20–64	91	15
Every year, 20–64	93	45

Source: Day (1986); assuming incidence rates from Cali Colombia. The first screening test is assumed to be 70% sensitive

5-year intervals. There is no good evidence to support this decision one way or another. Further research on the natural history of the disease is necessary, for example, to clarify whether the disease is more aggressive in younger women or not.

Should high-risk women be screened more frequently?

Although there are several risk factors associated with an increased risk of invasive cervical cancer, it is not possible to use these factors reliably to predict which women will develop CIN. Moreover, there is no evidence that these risk factors affect the rate of progression of CIN. Thus it has been argued that there is little value in targeting these women for screening or selecting them for more frequent screening.

Is screening teenagers worthwhile?

The prevalence of invasive carcinoma of the cervix does not justify including women under the age of 20 in the routine screening programme, provided that there is good uptake in women aged 20–25. While CIN does exist in teenagers, invasive cancer is extremely rare. There is no rational basis for routinely screening teenagers, regardless of whether they are 'promiscuous' or not; a smear is not needed for at least 2–3 years after becoming sexually active. In particular cases an approach could be to take a smear where a teenage girl has had multiple sexual partners for over 3 years. This is *not* screening, but a matter of responding to individual cases on merit.

Is screening 65-year-olds and over worthwhile?

Although a substantial number of cases of cervical cancer occur in women aged 65 and over, an effective screening programme should detect pre-cancerous lesions in those under 65, and thus reduce the incidence of invasive disease in older women. Women aged 65 and over should be encouraged to have a smear if they have not previously been screened; but there is, of course, the added complication that the smear is more difficult to take for the smear-taker and the woman for physiological reasons.

Which spatula?

There are many different spatulae on the market. The Aylesbury spatula is most widely-used and is a wooden spatula which has a tip larger than the old Ayres spatula and has been shown to be more likely to sample cervical cells as well as transformation zone squamous cells. The flatter reverse end may be used for a patulous cervix or a vault smear.

A study in general practice showed that the plastic Cervex sampler gave a better pick-up of endocervical cells (78.2% compared to 62.8%) and fewer inadequate smears, although the percentage of abnormals was the same (Cumbrian Practice Research Group 1991). Other studies have shown an increased number of bloodstained smears with the Cervex or other plastic samplers. A recent large study found that the Cervex brush offers no advantage over the Aylesbury spatula in reducing inadequate smear rates in the primary care setting with 5.4% and 5.5% respectively of smears taken reported as inadequate (Dey et al. 1996). The Cervex sampler costs about five times as much as the Aylesbury type (15.5p compared to 3p). These results do not support the routine use of the more expensive Cervex brush to reduce inadequate smear rates.

Another alternative is the cytobrush, which can also be used to sample the endocervix, and is mainly used in colposcopy clinics or when the cervix is distorted by surgery or local ablation. It may be used in addition to a spatula in some instances, for example, when the woman has had two previous smears showing insufficient cells. Beware, as one is likely to get more bleeding; so get the spatula sample first. The cytobrush is *not* the method of choice in primary screening, because it does not always sample the transformation zone, and provides smears of sparse cellularity which dry quickly and need very rapid fixation. It is also more expensive than the Aylesbury spatula.

What is the best way to sterilize the equipment?

It is important that the practice has adequate facilities for sterilizing the equipment used: soaking in Savlon and/or reusing a plastic speculum does *not* destroy the papilloma virus (Skegg and Paul 1986). Papilloma viruses are stable viruses and it is recommended that all instruments are autoclaved between patients. If this is not possible the instruments should be washed and put in boiling water for 10 minutes. The HIV virus will also be destroyed by these procedures.

When in the menstrual cycle to take the smear?

There are changes in the cervical epithelium during the menstrual cycle, although these do not reflect the hormonal changes as accurately as do the changes in the vaginal epithelium. Taking smears during menstruation is not a practice welcomed by most cytologists as erythrocytes, leukocytes, endometrial cells, and blood pigments obscure the field. However, in high-risk women any chance should be seized as they may not present again, and a note should be made about menstruation on the request form. Following menstruation and after ovulation, i.e. days 10–20 of the 28-day cycle, is probably the best time to take a smear as there are few polymorphs and the cells are mature. Histiocytes may be seen up to the twelfth day of the cycle, which gives a dirty background to the smear. However, while in planning screening mid-cycle smears are ideal, rarely should a woman needing a smear (especially if high-risk) be asked to return at another time.

Do you need endocervical cells present on the smear for it to be adequate?

A cervical smear if properly taken should contain cells from the whole of the transformation zone, which should therefore be adequately sampled (BSCC 1989; Herbert 1995). Squamous epithelial cells will normally be the most numerous cell type. The main evidence of an adequate smear is that it should contain a sufficient quantity of epithelial cells, taking into account a woman's age and her hormonal status.

An indication that the transformation zone has been properly sampled is the additional presence of endocervical columnar cells and recognizable metaplastic cells, but these can sometimes be difficult to identify as they become more mature. Owing to the variable nature of the transformation zone, *only one* of these cell types may be present on the smear. Endocervical cells may not always be seen in smears from post-menopausal women or those with atrophic smears. If the smear-taker is sure that the cervix was well-sampled and the appropriate area was fully sampled, the absence of endocervical cells is not necessarily an indication to repeat the smear. But if the smear-taker feels there was a problem in sampling and there is no good evidence of transformation zone materials in the smear, then an early repeat is necessary. Best to make a note at the time!

How should HPV be managed?

The exact role of HPV in cervical cancer is still uncertain but strong evidence is now accruing to implicate certain strains. Different strains of HPV have been identified which vary in their oncogenic potential. Correlation of virus type with the morphology of the cervical lesion shows that HPV types 16 and 18 are present in over 80% of invasive squamous cancers of the cervix and grade III cervical intraepthelial neoplasia. No cell with evidence of HPV is normal. No smear in which there is evidence of HPV should be reported as normal whether or not there is substantial nuclear abnormality, though the majority of smears showing evidence of HPV will also have nuclear abnormalities (Joint Working Party 1994, Herbert 1995). Cells in which there is dyskaryosis in addition to cytoplasmic features of HPV should be reported according to the grade

---

Box 12.1 *What women will need to know if the presence of HPV is reported*

- The wart virus in its subclinical state requires no specific treatment such as antibiotics. Referral to an STD/GUM clinic is not necessary
- The changes are evidence of contact with the virus at some stage in the woman's life, and may not indicate an active infection
- There are parallels with skin wart, and many other viral conditions, where only very few contacts develop the clinical infection
- The virus is usually transmitted sexually; but this is not the only way, as it has been isolated from other sites in the body and has also been found in children
- The natural history of wart virus changes is to regress over a period of several years. Two particular strains of the virus, HPV 16 and HPV 18, may be important prognostic markers for identifying patients who are at risk of developing severe cervical disease. Other factors such as smoking or lowered immunity may also come into play
- In a steady relationship there is no need to change contraception; but if a woman is likely to have any sexual contact outside an established relationship, barrier methods might be used
- Subclinical warts are not known to affect pregnancy, fertility, or the baby. Clinical warts should be treated prior to delivery
- Visible cervical warts are thought to be more easily transmitted than subclinical HPV
- Colposcopic treatment does not eradicate the presence of wart virus

Source: Oxfordshire DHA (1991)

---

of dyskaryosis and the management based on this, regardless of cytoplasmic changes. The presence of HPV is the main reason for reporting borderline nuclear changes (Joint Working Party 1994). Smears with HPV or borderline nuclear changes should be repeated at 6–12 monthly intervals at least once before considering colposcopy. At some time in the future, routine viral typing may be a second discriminator in the process of deciding which lesions to treat, but this is not the case at present.

Included in Box 12.1 is information that women will need to know if HPV is reported on a smear as it often causes considerable anxiety.

What is the appropriate management of mild dyskaryosis?

Mild dyskaryosis reflects the cytological appearance of a cervical smear. While the consensus view is that a single mildly-dyskaryotic smear should be managed by a repeat smear at 6 months and only referred for colposcopy if the abnormality persists, there are those who believe that such smears should be referred immediately for colposcopy. This is because, although the majority of such smears revert to normal or persist as mildly dyskaryotic, a small proportion do progress to severe dyskaryosis. One is therefore faced with achieving a balance between ensuring appropriate management and not over-investigating too many women. A recent study from Aberdeen (Flannelly *et al.* 1994) concluded that cytological surveillance, although safe, is not an efficient strategy for managing women with mildly-abnormal smears as three-quarters of the women eventually needed colposcopy and there was a high default rate in those put on surveillance. However, others have argued that referring all women with one mildly-dyskaryotic smear for colposcopy would result in over-investigation of very many more women than would ever go on to develop invasive disease (Raffle *et al.* 1995). Until we have better ways of differentiating which women are going to develop invasive disease, possibly by testing for high-risk human papilloma virus types, it is unlikely that a real consensus will be reached. Further research is also needed into the impact of the psychological well-being of the women having surveillance or colposcopy.

When should the cervix be treated?

Treatment of the cervix depends on the histological diagnosis of CIN from a biopsy specimen. There is a whole spectrum of abnormality from completely normal to definitely malignant. Ideally, it is important to have some idea of the rate of progression of abnormalities. Currently, however, there is inadequate information available about the natural history of the lower grades of abnormality. A balance must thus be reached between potential over-diagnosis and over-treatment and the need to ensure that invasive cancer does not occur. A treatment policy cannot be defined with any degree of certainty. On balance, the present belief is that CIN II and CIN III should be treated once diagnosed, while women with CIN I may be treated or kept under close surveillance.

What is the role for bimanual pelvic examination in cervical screening?

It has been suggested that routine pelvic examination could be performed as a screening test for ovarian cancer on asymptomatic women who attend for cervical smears. This would have implications for training as most cervical smears are taken by nurses who have not been trained in conducting this procedure. At present, the evidence does not support its use as a screening test (Austoker 1996). Bimanual pelvic examination has a low specificity and sensitivity. It is not able to distinguish between benign and malignant ovarian cysts and the false positive rate is accordingly high because of benign disease, particularly in pre-menopausal women. Moreover, pelvic examination does not seem to be effective in detecting early stage ovarian cancer. On the basis of the current evidence, bimanual pelvic examination should not be undertaken as a routine screening procedure performed on asymptomatic women (RCN 1995). If a woman is symptomatic (e.g. with troublesome fibroids) or is about to start on HRT, this represents a clinical indication for performing a bimanual examination and does not constitute screening. When women do present for a cervical smear it is very important to have a checklist of questions to exclude any

underlying possible pathology, for example, the detection of pelvic inflammatory disease (PID). Women are not always aware of the symptoms they should
be looking out for and therefore the positive effects of reminding them by direct
questions is extremely important. These questions should include:

- abdominal swelling?
- intermenstrual bleeding?
- very painful and/or heavy periods?
- lower abdominal pain or discomfort?
- post-coital bleeding?
- pain on intercourse?
- urinary symptoms?

Women who have any of these symptoms or signs should have a bimanual
pelvic examination by a doctor or nurse who has been appropriately trained.

Conclusion

In summary, what we perform in the way of cervical screening is the best we
have at the moment, but we should not pretend that it is ideal as the test
itself and our knowledge of the disease are both limited. Recent decreases in
mortality from the disease have occurred and are encouraging, and can at least
in part be attributed to the screening programme which is now well-run, with
most practices providing a good and efficient service.

References and further reading

Austoker, J. (1994). Screening for cervical cancer. *British Medical Journal*, **309**, 241–8.

Austoker, J. (1996). Screening for ovarian cancer. In *Evidence-guided prescribing of the Pill* (ed. P. C. Hannaford), pp.167–73. Parthenon Publishing Group, Camforth.

Austoker, J. and McPherson, A. (1992). *Cervical screening. Practical Guides for General Practice*, No. 14. Oxford Medical Publications, Oxford.

Austoker, J. and Davey, C. (1997). *Cervical smear results explained – a guide for primary care*. NHS Cervical Screening Programme Publications, Sheffield. (In press.)

Barton, S. E., et al. (1988). Effect of cigarette smoking on cervical epithelial immunity: a mechanism for neoplastic change. *Lancet*, **ii**, 652–4.

BSCC Booklet and Video (1989). *Taking cervical smears*. British Society for Clinical Colposcopy. (For further information contact Dr Keith Randall, Red Tree House, Pine Glade, Keston Park, Orpington, Kent BR6 8NT.)

Buckley, J. D., Harris, R. W. C., Doll, R., et al. (1981). Case control study of husbands of women with dysplasia or carcinoma of the cervix uteri. *Lancet*, **ii**, 1010–14.

Byles, J. E., et al. (1994). Effectiveness of three community-based strategies to promote screening for cervical cancer. *Journal of Medical Screening*, **1**, 150–8.

Campion, M. J., Cuzick, J., McCance, D. J., *et al.* (1986). Progressive potential of mild cervical atypia: prospective cytological, colposcopic, and virological study. *Lancet*, **ii,** 237–40.

Campion, M. J., *et al.* (1988). Psychosexual trauma of an abnormal cervical smear. *British Journal of Obstetrics and Gynaecology*, **95,** 175–81.

Cancer Research Campaign factsheets (1990). *Cervical cancer* (Factsheet 12). *Cervical cancer screening* (Factsheet 13).

Coney, S. (1988). *The unfortunate experiment.* Penguin, New Zealand.

Cumbrian Practice Research Group (1991). Sampling endocervical cells on cervical smears: a comparison of two instruments used in general practice. *British Journal of General Practice*, **41,** 192–3.

Cuzick, J. (1991). Organization of cervical screening in England and Wales. In *Cancer screening* (ed. A. B. Miller, J. Chamberlain, N. E. Day, *et al.*). Cambridge University Press, Cambridge.

Day, N. E. (1986). The epidemiological basis for evaluating different screening programmes. In *Screening for cancer of the uterine cervix* (ed. Hakeama, M., *et al.* IARC Scientific Publications No. 76, Lyon.

Dey, P. *et al.* (1996). Adequacy of cervical cytology sampling with the Cervex brush and the Aylesbury spatula: a population-based randomized controlled trial. *British Medical Journal*, **313,** 721–3.

DHSS (Department of Health and Social Security) (1988). *Cervical cancer screening.* Health circular HC(88)1.

DoH (Department of Health) (1988). *Cervical cytology and cervical cancer statistics 1976–1986, England and Wales.* Department of Health, London.

DoH (Department of Health) (1989). *Cervical cytology 1987/88.* Department of Health, London.

DoH (Department of Health) (1990). *Cervical cytology 1988/89.* Department of Health, London.

DoH (Department of Health) *Cervical cytology, England, 1988/89–1993/94.* (Form KC 53.)

DoH statistical bulletin. (1996) *Cervical screening programme, England 1994–95.* (February 1996.)

Duncan, I. (ed.). (1991). *Guidelines for clinical practice and programme management.* NHS Cervical Screening Programme, Oxford.

Flannelly, G., *et al.* (1994). Management of women with mild and moderate dyskaryosis. *British Medical Journal*, **408,** 1399–1403.

Harris, R. W. C., Brinton, L. A., Cowdell, R. H., *et al.* (1980). Characteristics of women with dysplasia or cancer *in situ* of the cervix uteri. *British Journal of Cancer*, **42,** 359–69.

Herbert, A., *et al.* (1995) Achievable standards, benchmarks for reporting and criteria for evaluating cervical cytopathology. *Cytopathology*, **6(2)**, 1–32.

Irwin, K. L. (1996). The association between oral contraceptive use and neoplasia of the cervix, vagina and vulva. In *Evidence-guided prescribing of the Pill* (ed. P. C. Hannaford), pp.145–56. Parthenon Publishing Group, Carnforth.

Joint National Co-ordinating Network (National Cervical Screening Programme), British Society for Clinical Cytology, and Royal College of Pathologists' Working Party (1994). Borderline nuclear changes in cervical smears: guidelines on their recognition and management. *Journal of Clinical Pathology*, **47**, 481–92.

McAvoy, B. R. and Raza, R. (1991). Can health education increase uptake of cervical smear testing among Asian women? *British Medical Journal*, **302**, 833–6.

McCormick, J. (1989). Cervical smears: a questionable practice? *Lancet*, **ii**, 207–9.

MacGregor, J. E., Moss, S. M., Parkin D. M., *et al.* (1985). A case-control study of cervical cancer screening in north east Scotland. *British Medical Journal*, **290**, 1543.

Marteau, T. M., Holland, A., Kidd, J., Cuddeford, L. and Walker, P. (1996). Reducing anxiety in women referred for colposcopy using an information booklet. *British Journal of Clinical Psychology*. (In press.)

NHSCSP (1996). *Quality Assurance Guidelines for the Cervical Screening Programme.* NHSCSP Publications No. 3, January 1996.

Nichols, S. (1987). Women's preferences for sex of doctor: a postal survey. *Journal of the Royal College of General Practitioners*, **37**, 540–3.

OPCS (1994). *Cancer statistics: registrations, 1989 (England and Wales).* HMSO, London.

OPCS (1995). *Mortality statistics: cause, 1993 (England and Wales).* HMSO, London.

OPCS (1996). *Mortality statistics: cause (England and Wales 1970–1994).* HMSO, London.

Oxfordshire DHA (1991). Cervical screening information factsheet No.9. *Genital wart (human papilloma) virus infection.* Cytology Department, John Radcliffe Hospital, Oxford.

Posner, T. and Vessey, M. (1988). *Prevention of cervical cancer: the patient's view.* King Edward's Hospital Fund for London.

Quilliam, S. (1992). *Positive smear* (2nd edn). Charles Letts & Co. Ltd., xxx

Raffle, A. E., Alden, B., and Mackenzie, E. F. D. (1995). Detection rates for abnormal cervical smears: what are we screening for? *Lancet*, **345**, 1469–73.

Roberts, A. W., Lane, D. A., Buntine, D., *et al.* (1985). Invasive carcinoma of the cervix in young women. *Medical Journal of Australia*, **143**, 333–5.

Royal College of Nursing (1994). *Cervical screening: guidelines for good practice. Issues in nursing and health*, April 1994.

Royal College of Nursing (1995). *Bimanual pelvic examination guidance for nurses. Issues in nursing and health*, November 1995.

Sasieni, P., Cuzick, J., Farmery, E. (1995). Accelerated decline in cervical cancer mortality in England and Wales. *Lancet*, **346**, 1566–7.

Sasieni, P. D., Cuzick, J., Lynch-Farmery, E., and the National Co-ordinating Network for Cervical Screening Working Group (1996). Estimating the efficacy of screening by auditing smear histories of women with and without cervical cancer. *British Journal of Cancer*, **73**, 1001–5.

Savage, W. and Schwartz. M. (1985). [Letter]. *Lancet*, **ii**, 1305.

Skegg, D. C. G. and Paul. C. (1986). Viruses, speculae and cervical cancer. *Lancet*, **i**, 747.

Stedman, Y., Woodman, C. B. J., and Donnelly, B. (1995). Is a policy of cervical screening for all women attending a genitourinary medicine clinic justified? *Journal of Public Health Medicine*, **17**, 90–2.

Summers, A. and Fullard, B. (1995). Improving the coverage and quality of cervical screening: women's views. *Journal of Public Health Medicine*, **17**, 277–81.

Vessey, M. P., McPherson, K., Lawless, M., *et al.* (1983). Neoplasis of the cervix uteri and contraception: a possible adverse effect of the pill. *Lancet*, **ii**, 930–4.

Walker, E. M., Dodgson, J., and Duncan, I. D. (1986). Does mild atypia of cervical smears warrant further investigation? *Lancet*, **2**, 672–3.

WHO Collaborative Study (1985). Invasive cervical cancer and combined oral contraceptives. *British Medical Journal*, **290**, 961–5.

Wilkinson, C. (1992). Abnormal cervical smear test results: old dilemmas and new directions. *British Journal of General Practice*, **42**, 336–9.

Wilkinson, C., Jones, J. M., and McBridge. J. (1990). Anxiety caused by abnormal result of cervical smear test: a controlled trial. *British Medical Journal*, **300**, 440.

Wolfendale, M., Howe-Guest, R., Usherwood, M., *et al.* (1987). Controlled trial of a new cervical spatula. *British Medical Journal*, **i**, 33–6.

Woodman, C. B. J., Rollason, T., Ellis, J., Tierney, R., Wilson, S., and Young, L. (1996). Human papilloma virus infection and risk of progression of epithelial abnormalities of the cervix. *British Journal of Cancer*, **73**, 553–6.

Wright, N. H., Vessey, M. P., Kenward, K., *et al.* (1978). Neoplasis and dysplasis of the cervix uteri and contraception: a possible protective effect of the diaphragm. *British Journal of Cancer*, **38**, 273–9.

CHAPTER THIRTEEN

Vaginal discharge and sexually transmitted diseases

Pippa Oakeshott

Good general practice management of women with vaginal discharge and sexually transmitted infections can make an important difference to their health. It may prevent the potentially devastating consequences of undiagnosed or inadequately treated cervical chlamydia infection. It can also help to reduce the discomfort, embarrassment, and anxiety often associated with genitourinary problems.

Not every woman needs investigation. If a woman in a long-term stable relationship develops symptoms of thrush after a course of antibiotics, blind treatment is perfectly reasonable. But in young women with abnormal vaginal discharge or suspected sexually transmitted infection, microbiological tests are essential for accurate diagnosis and management. Specimens obtained should always include appropriate swabs for chlamydia or gonorrhoea. It is totally unacceptable to reassure a woman that she has no serious infection merely on the basis of a normal high vaginal swab, or to treat for pelvic inflammatory disease without reference to sexual partners (Hopwood and Mallinson 1995).

General practitioners (GPs) and practice nurses performing pelvic examinations should therefore ensure they have suitable diagnostic swabs available. Since women with sexually transmitted infections often have few or no symptoms, opportunistic testing should be considered for those thought to be at risk. Women found to have a sexually transmitted infection should be given appropriate antibiotics and advised that it is essential that their partners receive treatment. In addition, referral to a department of genitourinary medicine for further tests and follow-up is usually recommended. However, effective management in general practice should be available for women who insist on seeing their GP or who do not have easy access to a genitourinary clinic (Owen *et al.* 1991). GPs should only undertake this work if they can do it properly and know their limitations.

Prevalence

Vaginal discharge is a common problem in general practice. O'Dowd estimated

Fig 13.1 *New cases of sexually transmitted diseases in women aged 15–59 in England, 1988–94*

(Source: GUM clinic returns)

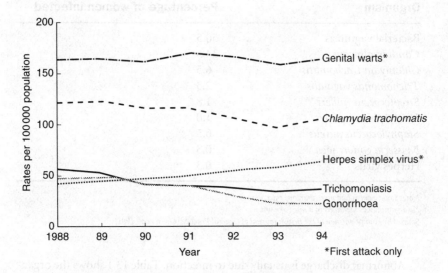

that one in 10 women presenting to her GP complains of vaginal symptoms (O'Dowd and Bourne 1994). The 1991–92 National Morbidity Survey found there were 421 general practice consultations annually for inflammatory disease of the cervix, vagina, or vulva per 10 000 women aged 16–44 (OPCS 1995).

Fig 13.1 shows the prevalence of sexually transmitted diseases in women attending English genitourinary clinics. Although the prevalence of gonorrhoea and trichomoniasis has fallen since 1988, there has been little change in the prevalence of chlamydia infection and genital warts, and the prevalence of a first attack of genital herpes has increased. In Denmark, a study of women attending a genitourinary clinic found that although 'safer sex' campaigns increased condom use, there were no significant reductions in the number of sexual partners or unplanned pregnancies, and the number of women with genital warts increased (Olivarius *et al.* 1992). Thus sexually transmitted infections in women remain an important problem. This chapter will cover the common infections seen in general practice, excluding HIV infection.

Causes of vaginal discharge

Vaginal discharge may be physiological or pathological. Physiological vaginal discharge is white, becoming yellow on contact with air due to oxidation. The amount of discharge produced varies considerably between women. It may increase at ovulation, premenstrually, or when using oral contraception or an IUCD. What matters is that a woman is complaining of a change in her normal discharge.

Table 13.1 *Organisms identified in 386 women aged 15–65 years presenting with lower genital tract symptoms*

Organism	Percentage of women infected
Bacterial vaginosis	56.5
Candida albicans	34.5
Chlamydia trachomatis	6.5
Trichomonas vaginalis	2.3
Streptococcus milleri	1.8
Haemophilus species	1.0
Staphylococcus aureus	0.5
Neisseria gonorrhoea	0.3
Herpes virus	0.3

Note: Some women had more than one infection
No organism was identified in a third of women
Source: By kind permission of the British Journal of General Practice (Owen et al. 1991)

Abnormal discharge is usually due to infection. Table 13.1 shows the organisms isolated from 386 consecutive women (mainly social classes III and IV) who presented with vaginal discharge, soreness, or vulval irritation in Owen's suburban general practice in Cardiff (Owen *et al.* 1991). Bacterial vaginosis and *Candida albicans* are the commonest infections. They are relatively harmless and not generally regarded as sexually transmitted. *Trichomonas vaginalis* is also a vaginal pathogen. Its main significance is that it is sexually transmitted and a marker for other sexually transmitted diseases. However, the most important sexually transmitted causes of vaginal discharge are *Chlamydia trachomatis* and *Neisseria gonorrhoea* since they can cause pelvic inflammatory disease leading to tubal infertility, ectopic pregnancy, or chronic pelvic pain. Effective management in general practice should prevent many such sequelae.

Herpes and genital warts are sexually transmitted viral infections which can be distressing for the patient. Unfortunately, treatment for these infections is only suppressive and not curative. *Streptococcus, Staphylococcus aureus,* and *Haemophilus* species may be commensals in the vagina but should be treated if causing symptoms. *Streptococci* should always be treated in pregnant women near term or after delivery because of the risks of neonatal infection or post-partum endometritis.

Non-infective causes of vaginal discharge are usually diagnosed on clinical examination. They include cervical ectropion, polyp or carcinoma, retained products, and foreign bodies in the vagina, notably 'lost' tampon. The latter should be disposed of in a self-sealing plastic bag before the smell in the surgery becomes intolerable. Fortunately, toxic shock syndrome is rare (see Chapter 10). Vulvovaginitis may also be due to dermatological problems such as eczema, or associated with irritants.

Diagnosis of vaginal discharge

History

Most causes of vaginal discharge will be elucidated by clinical examination and tests. Thus during a busy surgery it is tempting to move straight to the examination without taking a relevant history. However, it is important at some stage to ask the patient why she is worried about the discharge; how is it different from normal; is she worried about sexually transmitted infections; and is there associated soreness, dysuria, intermenstrual bleeding, or pelvic discomfort? A sexually transmitted infection is more likely if the discharge is associated with recent change of sexual partner, multiple partners, or a partner with urethritis. Finally, has she already treated herself unsuccessfully with an over-the-counter preparation such as clotrimazole cream or oral fluconazole?

If clinical history and prior knowledge of the patient suggest a sexually transmitted infection is highly likely, and the local genitourinary clinic is easily accessible, it may be simpler to give the patient a letter and clinic leaflet and send her straight there. However, a study from Liverpool family planning clinics found that only 40% of women with untreated chlamydia infection who were referred to a genitourinary clinic attended within 4 weeks (Hopwood and Mallinson 1995). For many patients therefore it will be better to arrange screening in the practice, either by the GP or by an appropriately trained practice nurse. Both need to have the right equipment available and know how to take suitable specimens, especially endocervical swabs.

Examination

The vulva should be examined for genital warts or herpetic ulcers. A bimanual examination may reveal adnexal tenderness or cervical motion pain suggestive of pelvic inflammatory disease. It is preferable to use warm water as a lubricant as other substances may interfere with cultures. A speculum should be passed and the appearance of the cervix and any discharge should be noted. However, as with symptoms, physical signs are not reliable in making a diagnosis.

Tests

If these are to be done at all they should be done properly. Although specimens taken will depend on arrangements with the local laboratory, minimum tests should include:

1. *Cervical swab for culture* in Stuart's transport medium. The swab should be inserted in the endocervix to sample pus and discharge for gonorrhoea. This will also usually pick up vaginal infections such as bacterial vaginosis, candidiasis, and trichomoniasis.

2. *Opportunistic cervical smear* if the patient has not had a normal routine smear, or there is some clinical indication.

3. *Endocervical swab for chlamydia.* Chlamydia are intracellular bacteria so specimens for chlamydia should contain cells from the endocervix or an ectropion if present, not pus or discharge. Sampling should be done *at the end* of a speculum examination after cleaning the cervix. (In practice, if a cervical smear or other swabs have been taken first, cleaning may not be necessary.) A cotton-tipped swab is rotated gently in the endocervix for at least 10 seconds to collect as much material as possible. Then it may be placed in transport medium for enzyme immunoassay or smeared on to two wells on a teflon-coated slide for the direct fluorescent antibody test. Exact details will depend on the local laboratory.

Box 13.1 *Basic investigations of a sexually active young woman complaining of abnormal vaginal discharge*

- Endocervical swab for *Neisseria gonorrhoea* in Stuart's medium. May also diagnose *Candida albicans*, bacterial vaginosis, or *Trichomonas vaginalis*
- Cervical smear if not recently done
- Endocervical swab for *Chlamydia trachomatis* after cleaning the cervix

---

The common practice of investigating vaginal discharge with a high vaginal swab is totally inadequate since it will miss the most important bacterial pathogens *C. trachomatis* and *N. gonorrhoea* (see Box 13.1). In fact, a high vaginal swab can probably be omitted since most vaginal infections will be picked up on the first endocervical swab. However, some laboratories prefer a separate high vaginal swab for *T. vaginalis*.

If vulval or cervical ulcers are seen a special viral swab should be taken for herpes simplex culture (see p. 424). Practices without access to viral swabs should normally refer women with a first attack of genital ulcers to the local genitourinary clinic so a definitive diagnosis can be made, contacts traced, and full screening performed.

Management

Ideally the patient should be asked to come back in a week when all the swab results will be available and appropriate treatment can be given. However, if she requests treatment for symptoms of possible thrush or bacterial vaginosis, it is not unreasonable to treat blind provided she returns for follow-up. Similarly, if pelvic inflammatory disease is suspected clinically, she should be given a 2 week course of doxycycline and metronidazole on the understanding that it is essential she returns for the swab results in case additional treatment or contact tracing is required. Detailed management will be discussed under the section for each infection and is summarised in Table 13.3, p. 421.

Infective causes of vaginal discharge

Candidiasis

Candida albicans or thrush is an ubiquitous yeast-like fungus which is commonly carried as a commensal. It is present in the vaginas of 20% of women with no symptoms. Predisposing factors include diabetes (therefore exclude glycosuria), pregnancy, broad-spectrum antibiotic treatment, steroid treatment, and immunodeficiency as in AIDS. Contrary to popular opinion, the low-dose oral contraceptive pill is not a cause of thrush (Adler 1995) and the pill should not be discontinued for this reason alone. Although vaginal candidiasis in healthy women does not result in serious complications, it can cause considerable distress. In addition, in the lay press thrush has been blamed (with little scientific evidence) for a multitude of symptoms, including those often attributed to irritable bowel syndrome.

Symptoms and signs

Candida may cause itching and soreness of vulva and vagina leading to dysuria and dyspareunia. However, it can improve spontaneously, and often causes no symptoms. On examination, the vagina and vulva may be inflamed and oedematous, and fissures can occur. The typical discharge is white or yellow, like cottage cheese. But clinical examination is notoriously unreliable for diagnosis.

Diagnosis

This is by culture and microscopy of a high vaginal or cervical swab. Candida may occasionally be diagnosed on cervical cytology. However, most women in stable partnerships who have had microbiologically diagnosed thrush previously will not need swabs unless their symptoms fail to improve on treatment.

Treatment

This is only required for symptomatic candida. Topical or oral treatments are both 80–90% effective in uncomplicated candida, but topical treatment is cheaper and less toxic. Common regimes are:

(1) clotrimazole pessaries 200 mg *per vaginam nocte* for 3 nights or 500 mg for 1 night; or

(2) fluconazole 150 mg orally as a single dose. This is contraindicated in pregnancy or lactation;

Additional cream containing steroid, e.g. clotrimazole with hydrocortisone is useful for local irritation. All these treatments are available over the counter.

Recurrent candida

Ideally, 'thrush' should only be treated blind on one occasion before being investigated, and then only in low-risk women who will return if symptoms persist. Many women with so-called 'recurrent candida' do not have candida at all. Therefore clinical examination and full microbiological tests are essential. The patient may have bacterial vaginosis, herpes, or dermatological conditions such as eczema, lichen planus, or lichen sclerosis. There may be psychosexual problems and some women may use their symptoms as an excuse to avoid sexual intercourse (see Chapter 19).

Management of women with proven recurrent vaginal candidiasis can be difficult. They should be advised to use emollients, not to wash excessively, and to avoid vaginal deodorants, bubble baths, and other additives such as Dettol and TCP. KY jelly can be used to reduce trauma during sexual intercourse. Loose clothing is recommended. Two-week courses of clotrimazole pessaries 100 mg *nocte* or oral fluconazole 50 mg daily may be effective. Unfortunately, oral treatment is no more likely than topical treatment to prevent relapse. If thrush occurs premenstrually, pessaries can be used prophylactically. Partners should be treated if symptomatic.

The scientific basis for the benefits of yoghurt in the prevention of recurrent candidiasis is sketchy. In a small crossover study of 33 women, daily ingestion of 8 oz of yoghurt containing *Lactobacillus acidophilus* reduced attacks of candidiasis from 2.5 to 0.4 over 6 months; but only 13 women completed the protocol (Hilton *et al.* 1992). Further prospective controlled trials are needed; but meanwhile eating yoghurt is unlikely to be harmful! There is no clear evidence that local application of yoghurt is effective, but some women find it soothing. Self-help books (p. 429) and complementary therapies may be useful.

Bacterial vaginosis

Bacterial vaginosis is due to an overgrowth of *Gardnerella vaginalis* and mixed anaerobes. It is the commonest cause of abnormal vaginal discharge in women of childbearing age. Once regarded simply as a nuisance which could be ignored if the patient was asymptomatic, bacterial vaginosis is being suggested as a preventable cause of pre-term labour and premature rupture of the membranes (Hay *et al.* 1994; Macdermott 1995; McGregor *et al.* 1995). It is not generally regarded as a sexually transmitted infection although its prevalence increases with increasing sexual activity.

Symptoms and signs

Bacterial vaginosis has a characteristic fishy smell because of the production of diamines. The smell is worse after sexual intercourse and may be associated with a watery, grey, offensive discharge. It causes little irritation and up to 50% of women with bacterial vaginosis have no symptoms.

Diagnosis

In general practice this is usually by culture and microscopy of a high vaginal or cervical swab. Clue cells – vaginal epitheliel cells covered with adherent bacteria – may be seen on a wet mount of vaginal fluid. In the amine test a sample of vaginal discharge is mixed with a drop of 10% potassium hydroxide on a glass slide. A pungent fishy odour is produced if the woman has bacterial vaginosis.

A visual diagnostic desk-top test for bacterial vaginosis may become available in future (O'Dowd and Bourne 1994).

Treatment

There is no absolute indication to treat healthy asymptomatic women with bacterial vaginosis. For those complaining of smelly vaginal discharge, a 90% cure rate is produced by metronidazole orally 400 mg twice a day for 5 days or a single dose of 2 g orally. (Metronidazole is contraindicated in the first trimester of pregnancy, and patients should be advised to avoid alcohol because of the antabuse-like effect.) Alternatively, clindamycin 2% cream, one 5 g application may be inserted *per vaginam nocte* for 7 nights.

If initial treatment is unsuccessful the alternative treatment may be tried. In resistant cases oral clindamycin 300 mg twice daily for one week is occasionally used. Treatment of the male partner has not been shown to increase cure rate or reduce recurrence, but is probably worthwhile in women with recurrent bacterial vaginosis.

Bacterial vaginosis and adverse pregnancy outcome

Cohort studies show that women with bacterial vaginosis antenatally have a two to three times increased rate of pre-term labour (Hay *et al.* 1994; Macdermott 1995). A recent prospective controlled trial found orally administered clindamycin treatment was associated with a 50% reduction of bacterial vaginosis-linked pre-term birth and pre-term premature rupture of the membranes (McGregor *et al.* 1995). However, treatment in pregnancy may be teratogenic, and it is not clear whether all pregnant women should be screened or only those with a past history of recurrent pre-term labour.

Trichomoniasis

Trichomonas vaginalis is a protozoan which is a relatively harmless, sexually transmitted vaginal pathogen. It can cause severe vaginal inflammation, but may also be asymptomatic and diagnosed on a routine cervical smear. Although it may occasionally be linked to adverse pregnancy outcome or possibly pelvic inflammatory disease, its main importance is that it can be a marker for other sexually transmitted diseases and indicates the need for screening.

Symptoms and signs

Women with trichomoniasis may complain of an intensely irritating, bubbly, purulent discharge and vaginal soreness (more than irritation). There may be a fishy smell due to associated bacterial vaginosis.

Diagnosis

This is by culture and microscopy of a high vaginal or cervical swab, either in Stuart's medium or special *T. vaginalis* transport medium. *T. vaginalis* may also be seen on a cervical smear and associated with inflammatory changes. In one study the sensitivity of cervical cytology for diagnosis of trichomoniasis was 90% compared with culture (Dimian *et al.* 1992).

Treatment

Metronidazole 2 g stat or 400 mg twice a day for 5 days will cure 90% of women with trichomoniasis. Intravaginal 2% clindamycin cream may sometimes be used during pregnancy (Corcoran and Ridgway 1994). Sexual partners should be treated. Ideally, both the woman and her partner should be screened for other sexually transmitted infections.

Chlamydia

Cervical *Chlamydia trachomatis* infection is the commonest bacterial sexually transmitted disease in women, with prevalences in general practice populations of 2–12% (Table 13.2). Untreated chlamydia can cause pelvic inflammatory disease leading to tubal infertility, ectopic pregnancy, or chronic pelvic pain. Since many women with chlamydia infection are asymptomatic, the first sign that a woman has had chlamydia infection may be when she presents with infertility. Forty per cent of women thought to have uncomplicated chlamydial cervicitis have histological evidence of endometritis. Although the exact risk of infertility following cervical chlamydia infection is unknown, estimates suggest it may be 2–4% (Oakeshott and Hay 1995).

Symptoms and signs

Up to 70% of women with cervical chlamydia infection have no symptoms; the remainder may have mild symptoms of vaginal discharge, intermenstrual bleeding, lower abdominal pain, or dysuria. Occasionally the first indication of infection in a mother may be chlamydial conjunctivitis in a neonate. Pelvic examination may be normal or show mucopurulent cervicitis or a friable cervix. Signs of pelvic inflammatory disease indicate the need to take endocervical swabs for *N. gonorrhoea* as well as *C. trachomatis*. Since clinical findings in chlamydia infection are often variable, screening should probably be performed on the basis of risk factors (see Box 13.2 and p. 427).

Box 13.2 *Indications for chlamydia testing in sexually active young women*

- Mucopurulent vaginal discharge
- Suspected pelvic inflammatory disease
- Suspected sexually transmitted infection
- Before termination of pregnancy or IUCD insertion
- Sexually active teenagers

Diagnosis

The test used will depend on arrangements with the local laboratory. At present, antigen detections tests – enzyme immunoassay or direct fluorescent antibody test – are the most suitable tests for general practice. Culture involves complicated storage and transport, while near-patient tests are currently limited by their low sensitivity, time-consuming nature, and difficulties with quality

Table 13.2 *Prevalence of cervical chlamydia infection in UK general practices*

First author, year of publication	Location	No. of practices	Study populations	Age range (years)	Test used	No. infected/ no. studied	Prevalence (%)
Southgate 1983	East London	3	Women having speculum examination	15–45	Culture	19/248	8
Longhurst 1987	Central London	1	Women having speculum examination	Pre-menopausal	DFA	18/169	11
Southgate 1989	East London	4	Women requesting termination of pregnancy	16–44	DFA	12/103	12
Owen 1991	Cardiff	1	Women with lower genital tract symptoms. Mainly social classes III and IV	15–65	DFA	25/386	6
Smith 1991	Glasgow	1	Women attending for cervical smear. Mainly social class III	19–58	Culture	24/197	12
Oakeshott 1992	South-east London	2	Women having speculum examination. Mainly social classes IV and V	17–45	DFA	36/409	9
Thomson 1994	Fife	10	Women attending for cervical smear	15–40	DFA	5/287	2
Oakeshott 1995	South London	28	Women attending for cervical smear	17–35	EIA	39/1255	3

DFA = direct fluorescent antibody test. EIA = enzyme immunoassay
Source: By kind permission of the British Journal of General Practice (Oakeshott and Hay 1995)

control. In future, DNA detection tests on first pass urine specimens may become available.

The method of taking the endocervical swab is described on p. 414. Specimens for chlamydia must contain endocervical cells, not pus or discharge.

Treatment

Doxycycline 100 mg orally twice a day for seven days or azithromycin 1 g stat. If pregnant or lactating, erythromycin 500 mg four times a day for 7 days or 250 mg four times a day for 14 days may be given.

It is vital that the woman's sexual partner is treated to prevent reinfection. She should be advised not to have sex with him until he can show her his empty bottle of tablets. In most cases the patient should also be referred to the genitourinary clinic for follow-up and contact tracing and given a clinic leaflet.

A test of cure is only needed if there is a risk that the patient or her partner may not have complied with treatment, reinfection may have occurred, or a less effective antibiotic such as erythromycin was used. It should be done 2–4 weeks after completion of treatment. It also provides an opportunity for further patient education.

Gonorrhoea

Neisseria gonorrhoea is unusual in general practice (Table 13.1). Symptoms, signs, and sequelae are similar to those of chlamydia infection, but patients with gonorrhoea are less likely to be asymptomatic. Rarely, gonococcal bacteraemia may produce skin lesions or septic arthritis.

Diagnosis

An endocervical swab in Stuart's transport medium will diagnose 90% of cases (Adler 1995). In genitourinary clinics urethral and rectal swabs are also taken to increase sensitivity.

Treatment

Amoxycillin 3 g with probenecid 1 g in single oral dose (Corcoran and Ridgway 1994), but the large number of tablets may cause problems with compliance. Alternatively, ciprofloxacin 500 mg orally in a single dose may be used. This is contraindicated in women who are pregnant or have a history of fits.

Since some strains of gonorrhoea are resistant to penicillin (penicillinase-producing *Neissera gonorrhoea*=PPNG) it may be necessary to consult the local laboratory about appropriate antibiotic treatment.

If the patient has signs of pelvic inflammatory disease longer treatment is required, for example, an additional 10-day course of co-amoxiclav 375 mg three times a day (or erythromycin 500 mg four times a day in patients allergic to penicillin). Since contact tracing and screening and treatment for other sexually transmitted infections such as chlamydia are vital, referral to a genitourinary clinic is strongly recommended. A test of cure is advised (Thin *et al.* 1995).

Table 13.3 *Diagnosis and management of infective causes of vaginal discharge*

	Candida	Bacterial vaginosis	Trichomonas	Chlamydia	Gonorrhoea
Introduction	Test for glycosuria	Associated with pre-term labour	STD Screen for other STDs	STD Can cause PID, infertility, ectopic preg.	STD Can cause PID, infertility, ectopic preg.
Symptoms (unreliable for diagnosis)	Itchy discharge	Fishy smell	Sore, frothy discharge	Mucopurulent discharge, pelvic pain, dysuria	Mucopurulent discharge, pelvic pain, dysuria
Diagnosis	HVS or cervical swab	HVS or cervical swab	HVS or cervical swab	Special endocervical swab-need cells not discharge	Cervical swab in Stuart's medium
Suggested treatment	If symptomatic: clotrimazole pessaries 200 mg *PV nocte* for 3 nights	If symptomatic: metronidazole 400 mg twice a day for 5 days. Avoid alcohol	Metronidazole 400 mg twice a day for 5 days. Avoid alcohol	Doxycycline 100 mg twice a day for 7 days. Additional Rx required for PID	Amoxicillin 3 g and probenecid 1 g stat. Additional Rx required for PID
Treat partner	If symptomatic	If recurrent infections	Yes	Treatment of partner vital. Refer to GUM for follow-up	Treatment of partner vital. Refer to GUM for follow-up

NB. Microbiological tests are essential for effective diagnosis and management of vaginal discharge

Pelvic inflammatory disease (see Chapter 15)

There is overwhelming evidence that sexually transmitted micro-organisms play a major role in the pathogenesis of pelvic inflammatory disease (PID). Despite this many women are still treated for PID without their contacts being screened and treated. In England and Wales over the past decade the increase in the number of new cases of uncomplicated sexually transmitted infections in women has been paralleled by a rise in the prevalence of PID (Bevan *et al.* 1995). Currently up to 50% of acute PID has been shown to be due to chlamydia and many episodes are 'silent' or subclinical. More than 10% of women who have had one episode of PID, and over 50% of those who have had three episodes develop tubal infertility. The risk of ectopic pregnancy is increased ten fold after an episode of PID.

Symptoms and signs

Patients may have pelvic pain, dyspareunia, malaise, dysuria, purulent vaginal discharge, or be asymptomatic. In practice, PID is notoriously difficult to diagnose clinically with any degree of accuracy. In a recent study from a London teaching hospital of 147 women presenting with abdominal pain and clinical signs of acute salpingitis (cervical motion pain, adnexal tenderness, and one of the following: pyrexia >38°C, ESR >15 mm/hour, WCC >10 000/ml), only 70% had acute PID diagnosed at laparoscopy (Bevan *et al.* 1995). Of these 45% had chlamydia infection, 14% had gonorrhoea, and 8% had both.

Diagnosis

Endocervical swabs for chlamydia and gonorrhoea are vital in all women with suspected PID.

Treatment

If the patient is ill hospital admission may be considered. Otherwise treatment should be started immediately after swabs have been taken with a 2-week course of both metronidazole 400 mg twice a day and doxycycline 100 mg twice a day. Erthromycin may be used instead of doxycycline if the patient is pregnant or lactating (Thin *et al.* 1995). If gonorrhoea is suspected ciprofloxacin 500 mg stat may be given (or amoxycillin 3 g and probenecid 1 g if the patient is pregnant).

Rest and sexual abstinence are recommended. It is vital that the patient returns after 1 week for the swab results so that treatment for gonorrhoea and contact tracing can be arranged if required.

Viral sexually transmitted infections

Genital warts and herpes are unpleasant, viral sexually transmitted infections for which treatment is unsatisfactory. The infections can only be suppressed, not cured. Once infected, people may transmit the virus to others even when they themselves are asymptomatic, and we do not know whether they remain infectious for ever. Using condoms reduces the risk but does not always prevent infections.

Women with first attacks of either genital warts or herpes need screening for coexistent infections, especially chlamydia, and contact tracing. Therefore in many cases the best option may be referral to the local genitourinary clinic.

Genital warts

Genital warts are common, usually sexually transmitted, and difficult to treat. They are caused by human papilloma virus, and some types are strongly associated with cervical cancer (Krieger 1995) (see Chapter 12).

Symptoms and signs

Genital warts are often asymptomatic, but may be associated with itching or discharge. They are usually noticed on the vulva or introitus. They may enlarge during pregnancy.

Diagnosis

This is clinical. However, subclinical human papilloma virus infection is much commoner than clinical warts and is often diagnosed on a cervical smear or colposcopy. No treatment is required for subclinical infection but visible cervical warts are an indication for cytology and colposcopy (Thin et al. 1995).

Treatment

As with common warts this is laborious and not very effective. Patients find the fact that treatment is so inadequate very difficult to deal with. The aim is merely to remove obvious lesions as no therapy has been shown to eradicate the virus (Krieger 1995). Treatment is more effective for warts that are small and have been present for less than a year. Provided the patient is not pregnant, local 25% podophyllin paint may be used. It is usually applied weekly to the warts by a doctor or nurse using vaseline to protect the surrounding skin. It must be washed off by the patient after 4 hours. Care must be taken as podophyllin is irritant and can cause severe burns. It is teratogenic.

If treatment is ineffective after 4 weeks, or the patient is pregnant and the warts are causing problems, cryotherapy or electrocautery may be offered, either in the practice or in the genitourinary clinic. Recurrence rates are at least 25% after 3 months. Warts may regress or reappear spontaneously and condoms should be used until at least 3 months after apparent cure.

Present policy is that the frequency of cervical smears depends on the degree of dyskaryosis. However, this may change when we can routinely type human papilloma virus (see Chapter 11). Partner notification and screening for coexistent infections are recommended.

Genital herpes

Genital herpes is the commonest cause of genital ulcers. Unfortunately, in England the incidence is increasing (Table 13.1). Most cases are transmitted by persons who do not know they are infected, or who are asymptomatic at the time of sexual transmission. Herpes simplex virus (HSV) is classified into types 1 and 2. Both can cause genital infection, but type 1 more often causes cold sores on the face and lips. It may be transmitted by orogenital contact. Since herpes is an unpleasant, chronic, incurable, emotive condition, diagnosis should always be confirmed by culture.

Genital ulcers may also be due to primary syphilis, tropical conditions such as lymphogranuloma venereum and chancroid, or Behcet's syndrome. If the patient has a history of foreign travel, a partner from abroad, or there is doubt about the diagnosis, referral to a genitourinary clinic is advisable.

Symptoms and signs

Primary herpes usually presents with multiple painful genital ulcers less than a week after sexual contact, although it may be asymptomatic. Skin lesions evolve through redness, vesicles, ulcers, and crusting, often associated with inguinal lymphadenopathy. The illness lasts about 3 weeks. Pain and malaise are variable but may be severe. Uncontrollable pain or acute urinary retention may warrant hospital admission. In pregnancy, active genital herpes at term is an indication for caesarian section to reduce the risk of neonatal herpes encephalitis.

Over 80% of women infected with HSV 2 develop recurrences, but in many cases these will be trivial (Patel and Barton 1995). Treatment of recurrences should be considered if physical or psychological symptoms are severe.

Diagnosis

Diagnosis is by viral culture which may not be available in many general practices. A special cotton wool swab is rubbed over the lesion and put in viral transport medium. Since serum is required it may be necessary to puncture some vesicles.

Treatment

Acyclovir 200 mg orally five times daily for 5 days is used for a primary attack of herpes. It reduces the overall duration of the episode by at least a third but does not reduce recurrence rates. Topical treatment is much less effective, and a combination of topical and oral treatment is no better than oral treatment alone (Patel and Barton, 1995). If the patient is pregnant specialist advice should be obtained (Thin et al. 1995).

Sexual intercourse should be avoided while lesions are present. Since asymptomatic infection and viral shedding can occur between attacks, regular condom use should be discussed. Long-term suppressive treatment may be considered for patients with more than five attacks annually. Over 80% of patients can be maintained recurrence free on acyclovir 400 mg twice a day, but such expensive treatment should probably be initiated by a specialist and be reviewed every 6 months. Lower doses of acyclovir are less effective. Simple analgesics, saline baths, and ice packs are useful.

Since accurate diagnosis, screening for other sexually transmitted infections, and contact tracing are vital, women with a first attack of genital herpes are probably best managed by a genitourinary clinic. In addition, they often benefit from counselling from the health advisers. However, women with recurrent attacks can be greatly helped by support and advice from their GP, practice nurse, or self-help groups (See Information for patients p. 430).

Genitourinary clinics

These are much more user-friendly than in the past. Thus older patients and GPs may find any anxieties unfounded. It is very helpful if there are good relations between GPs and local genitourinary physicians. A patient is much more likely to attend if the GP gives her a clinic leaflet and letter and reassures her that the doctors are sympathetic and understanding.

Genitourinary clinics have positive advantages. Treatment is free with no prescription charge. There are experienced health advisors with time for counselling and contact tracing (see below). The clinics will screen for other sexually transmitted infections, including HIV if requested. All details are totally confidential and, unless the patient agrees, will not be released to the GP where they could affect any future requests by the patient for life insurance. The tests used may be more sensitive (e.g. for *N. gonorrhoea* and *C. trachomatis*) or more extensive (e.g., for herpes) than those available in most general practices. Finally, the clinics can review compliance with treatment and perform a test of cure if required.

Contact tracing/partner notification

For each infected woman (index case) there are at least two people affected – her sexual contact and the person who infected her contact. Often it is more complicated. Thus contact tracing requires time and sensitivity. In genitourinary clinics it is done with the assistance of health advisors. After discussion the patient telephones or visits her partner and urges him to attend a genitourinary clinic for examination and treatment. The partner is given a contact slip which includes the original patient's note number and a code for the diagnosis. When he goes to a genitourinary clinic for treatment he hands in the contact slip which is then returned to the clinic of origin so that accurate contact tracing records can be kept. Health advisers prefer not to inform contacts themselves unless the patient is unable to do so. Confidentiality is paramount and no information will be given to anyone outside the clinic, including partners or other doctors, without the patient's permission.

In general practice, if a woman with a sexually transmitted infection is reluctant to attend a genitourinary clinic for contact tracing, she could be given a letter similar to a contact slip to give to her partner for him to take to a genitourinary clinic. The letter could state the woman's diagnosis and treatment given. If the partner hands this in at a clinic and gives consent for information to be released to the GP, the clinic will reply with details of his diagnosis and treatment. Both partners should be advised not to have sexual intercourse until they have completed their courses of treatment.

Sexual health promotion

One of the *Health of the Nation* targets, highlighted by the advent of AIDS, is to reduce the incidence of sexually transmitted infections. Strategies include encouraging safer sex, increasing screening, and improving treatment and contact tracing among people found to be infected. For primary prevention, increasing condom use in women with multiple partners is likely to be beneficial. However, since barrier methods are unreliable in preventing pregnancy, the Pill should also be used – the 'double Dutch method'.

Several safer sex campaigns have been shown to increase condom use (Olivarius *et al.* 1992; Oakeshott and Hay 1995). However, although condom promotion schemes in general practice are popular with both GPs and patients, there is as yet little evidence of their effectiveness (Curtis *et al.* 1995). My own data on over 1000 women attending inner city general practices for cervical smears found along with other studies (Johnson *et al.* 1994) that about 30% of women aged <35 reported that their partner used a condom last time they had sexual intercourse. However, although practices offering condoms were more likely to give them to patients and to advise on avoiding sexually transmitted infections, this did not significantly increase subsequent condom use (even among women reporting two or more sexual partners in the previous year). Despite this, it would seem sensible to consider offering advice about how to avoid sexually transmitted infections to all sexually active young women, especially when they attend for speculum examinations.

Secondary prevention of sexually transmitted diseases and their consequences is just as important. In the USA and Sweden screening programmes have been shown to reduce the prevalence of both cervical chlamydia infection and of sequelae such as pelvic inflamatory disease (Scholes 1996, Ripa, 1990). GPs and practice nurses have a vital role to play in screening women at risk of sexually transmitted infections, and ensuring that those found to be infected are managed appropriately.

Controversies

Which women should be screened for chlamydia infection?

The potentially devastating but preventable consequences of cervical chlamydia infection have generated much debate about the value of screening. Calculations of the cost-effectiveness of testing women for chlamydia depend on many factors including the prevalence in the population, the specificity and sensitivity of the tests used, the risks of complications, and the costs of treatment at every stage (Fig 13.2).

In order to decide if routine or selective screening is appropriate, GPs need to have some idea of the prevalence of chlamydia infection in their local community. This could be done by using 'spotter' practices. If the prevalence of infection is >6%, as in some inner city practices, it will probably be cost-effective to test all women of childbearing age when they attend for speculum

Fig 13.2 *Potential costs and benefits of screening for cervical chlamydia infection in general practice*

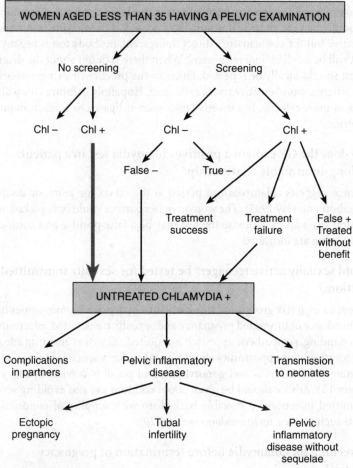

Chl – = Chlamydia negative
Chl + = Chlamydia positive

examinations. In populations with lower prevalences screening might be targeted at women with risk factors: age less than 25, recent change of sexual partner, absence of barrier contraception, mucopurulent vaginal discharge, friable cervix, sterile pyuria (Oakeshott and Hay 1995) (see Box 13.2). It is obviously less important to screen women for chlamydia once they are past childbearing, although it may be important for overall control of the infection.

How reliable are chlamydia tests?

Unfortunately, antigen detection tests used in general practice are not totally reliable and this may be exacerbated by poor technique in collection of endocervical specimens. The specificity and sensitivity of the direct fluorescent antibody test are >98% and >90%; and of the enzyme immunoassay (confirmed by direct fluorescent antibody) >98% and 67–91% respectively (Oakeshott and Hay 1995). Thus false positives and false negatives do occur, and the false positive rate will be higher in populations with a low prevalence of infection. In addition, when the enzyme immunoassay is used, if the enzyme immunoassay is positive but the confirmatory direct fluorescent antibody test is negative the result will be labelled 'indeterminate'. When there is doubt about the diagnosis the test should ideally be repeated, either in the practice or in a genitourinary clinic where a more sensitive test may be used. Hopefully in future GPs will have access to more reliable, less invasive tests such as ligase chain reaction on first pass urine.

How does the GP explain a positive chlamydia test in a patient in a long-term stable relationship?

Evidence suggests chlamydia can persist at the cervix for years, or disappear (Oakeshott and Hay 1995). The woman or her partner could have picked up the infection years ago. Otherwise the test may be a false positive and counselling and retesting are indicated.

Should sexually active teenagers be tested for sexually transmitted infections?

These are a high risk group, and those who live in deprived communities have a high incidence of unwanted pregnancy and sexually transmitted infections. An understanding, sympathetic approach is required. As well as ensuring adequate contraception, the opportunity should be taken for a speculum examination, screening for chlamydia and gonorrhoea, and possibly cervical cytology (see Chapter 12). Advice should be given about condom use and avoiding sexually transmitted infections, if possible backed up with supplies of condoms and leaflets such as *Wise up to condoms* (see p. 429).

Is screening for chlamydia before termination of pregnancy essential?

Women requesting termination of pregnancy have a high prevalence of chlamydia infection and up to 60% risk of developing post-abortal pelvic inflammatory disease if they have untreated chlamydia infection at the time of operation (Blackwell *et al.* 1993). For some women who then develop tubal infertility this may be their only pregnancy. Despite these risks many hospitals performing terminations still fail to screen or treat women for chlamydia infection. GPs should ensure that women awaiting termination are aware of the risks and the need for screening (which could be done either at the surgery or at the local genitourinary clinic). Women found to have chlamydia infection need antibiotic cover with doxycycline 100 mg twice a day or tetracycline 500 mg four times a day before or at the time of operation and for 10–21 days afterwards, and their partners should be notified (Blackwell *et al.* 1993).

Chlamydia testing is also recommended before insertion of an IUCD, especially when this is fitted as emergency contraception. If the patient is thought to be at high risk of sexually transmitted infection, after taking a chlamydia swab, antibiotic cover may be given as described above.

Do asymptomatic bacterial vaginosis or trichomoniasis need treating?

Recent research suggests treatment is indicated if the patient is more than 3 months pregnant and has a history of previous miscarriage or premature rupture of the membranes (McGregor *et al.* 1995), though the risk of teratogenicity should be remembered. Otherwise current evidence suggests treatment for bacterial vaginosis is not vital (MacDermott 1995). However, women with trichomoniasis should be treated to prevent symptoms and offered screening for other sexually transmitted infections.

Patients' views and information for patients

Symptoms – not diagnostic

'A bit more discharge and it's smelly and embarrassing.'
'It burns when I have sex.'
'I don't know why I haven't got pregnant as we haven't really used anything and we've been together for over 2 years' (17-year-old)
'I get shooting pains when we have sex.'

Management of women with a sexually transmitted infection

'We've split up since then and I don't see him anymore.'
'How could I have got it?'
'How do I know if the pills have worked?'

Referral to the genitourinary clinic

'I'm not going there. I might meet someone I know.'
'Oh yes, I went there last year and they did all the tests and said I was OK.'
'I got checked up at the clinic before I had the abortion. They were very kind.'

Information for patients

There is an excellent series of booklets on sexually transmitted infections published by the Health Education Authority and available from health promotion units and genitourinary clinics. These include: *Vaginal infections; Thrush; Chlamydia and NSU; Genital herpes; Genital warts;* and *Guide to a healthy sex life.* 'Healthy sex-first time' and 'condoms and the pill' are available free for up to 50 copies from:

> Customer Services, LRC Products Ltd, London International House, Turnford Place, Broxbourne, Herts EN10 6LN.

Practices should also have available a supply of local genitourinary clinic leaflets and the telephone number of the clinic health advisors.

There is an active self-help group for herpes sufferers:
The Herpes Association,
42 North Road, London N7 9DP.
Tel: 0171 6099061.

Key points

1. All GPs and practice nurses performing speculum examinations should have appropriate equipment available and know how to take endocervical swabs for chlamydia and gonorrhoea.
2. Women with chlamydia, gonorrhoea, or a first attack of genital herpes or warts need
    - appropriate treatment
    - contact tracing
    - screening for other sexually transmitted infections
    - referral to a genitourinary clinic.
3. Good relationships with local genitourinary physicians are very helpful. The practice should have a supply of genitourinary clinic leaflets to hand to patients.
4. The important bacterial causes of vaginal discharge which should not be missed are chlamydia and gonorrhoea because of their potential sequelae of pelvic inflammatory disease, tubal infertility, and ectopic pregnancy.
5. All sexually transmitted infections can be asymptomatic.
6. Indications for testing young, sexually active women for chlamydia and gonorrhoea include:
    - vaginal discharge, especially mucopurulent cervicitis
    - suspected pelvic inflammatory disease
    - suspected sexually transmitted infection
    - sexually active teenagers
    - before termination of pregnancy or IUCD insertion.

Acknowledgements

I would like to thank Dr P. Hay for advice, The Communicable Disease Surveillance Centre for preparing Table 13.1 and the South Thames R&D Project Grant Scheme for support.

References and further reading

Adler, M. (1995). *ABC of sexually transmitted diseases* (3rd edn). BMJ Publishing Group, London.

Bevan, C., Johal, B., Mumtaz, G., Ridgway, G., and Siddle, N. (1995). Clinical, laparoscopic and microbiological findings in acute salpingitis: report on a United Kingdom cohort. *British Journal of Obstetrics and Gynaecology*, **102**, 407–14.

Blackwell, A. L., Thomas, P. D., Wareham, K., and Emery, S. J. (1993). Health gains from screening for infection of the lower genital tract in women attending for termination of pregnancy. *Lancet*, **342**, 206–10.

Corcoran, G. and Ridgway, G. (1994). Antibiotic chemotherapy of bacterial sexually transmitted diseases in adults: a review. *International Journal of Sexually Transmitted Diseases and AIDS*, **5**, 165–71.

Curtis, H., Hoolaghan, T., and Jewitt, C. (1995). *Sexual health promotion in general practice*. Radcliffe Medical Press, Oxford.

Dimian, C., Nayagam, M., and Bradbeer, C. (1992). The association between sexually transmitted diseases and inflammatory cervical cytology. *Genitourinary Medicine*, **68**, 305–6.

Hay, P., Lamont, R., Taylor-Robinson, D., Morgan, D., Ison, C., and Pearson, J. (1994). Abnormal bacterial colonisation of the genital tract and subsequent preterm delivery and late miscarriage. *British Medical Journal*, **308**, 295–8.

Hilton, C., Isenberg, H., Alperstein, P., France, K., and Borenstein, M. (1992). Ingestion of yogurt containing *Lactobacillus acidophilus* as prophylaxis for candidal vaginitis. *Annals of Internal Medicine*, **116**, 353–7.

Hopwood, J. and Mallinson, H. (1995). Chlamydia testing in community clinics – a focus for accurate sexual health care. *British Journal of Family Planning*, **21**, 87–90.

Johnson, A. M., Wadsworth, J., and Wellings, K. (1994). *Sexual attitudes and lifestyles*. Blackwell Scientific Publications, Oxford.

Krieger, J. (1995). New STD treatment guidelines. *Journal of Urology*, **154**, 209–13.

Macdermott, R. (1995). Bacterial vaginosis. *British Journal of Obstetrics and Gynaecology*, **102**, 92–4.

McGregor, J., French, J., Parker, R., Draper, D., Patterson, E., Jones, W., *et al.* (1995). Prevention of premature birth by screening and treatment for common genital tract infections: results of a prospective controlled evaluation. *American Journal of Obstetrics and Gynecology*, **173**, 157–67.

O'Dowd, T. C. and Bourne, N. (1994). Inventing a new diagnostic test for vaginal infection. *British Medical Journal*, **309**, 40–2.

Oakeshott, P. and Hay, P. (1995). General practice update: chlamydia infection in women. *British Journal of General Practice*, **45**, 615–20.

Office of Population Censuses and Surveys (1995). *Morbidity statistics from general practice: fourth national study 1991–92*. HMSO, London.

Olivarius, F., Worm, A., Peterson, C., Kroon, S., and Lynge, E. (1992). Sexual behaviour of women attending an inner city STD clinic before and after a general campaign for safer sex in Denmark. *Genitourinary Medicine*, **68**, 296–9.

Owen, P., Hughes, M., and Munro, J. (1991). Study of the management of chlamydial cervicitis in general practice. *British Journal of General Practice*, **41**, 279–81.

Patel, R. and Barton, S. (1995). Antiviral chemotherapy in genital herpes simplex virus infections. *International Journal of Sexually Transmitted Diseases and AIDS*, **6**, 320–8.

Ripa, T. (1990). Epidemiologic control of genital chlamydia trachomatis infections. *Scandinavian Journal of Infectious Diseases*, **69**, 157–67.

Scholes, D., Stergachis, A., Heidrich, F., Andrilla, H., Holmes, K., Stamm, W. (1996). Prevention of pelvic inflammatory disease by screening for cervical chlamydia infection. *New England Journal of Medicine*, **334**, 1362–66.

Thin, R., Barlow, D., Bingham, J., and Bradbeer, C. (1995). Investigation and management guide for sexually transmitted diseases (excluding HIV). *International Journal of Sexually Transmitted Diseases and AIDS*, **6**, 130–6.

CHAPTER FOURTEEN

Cystitis

Sally Hope

What is man, when you come to think upon him, but a minutely set, ingenious machine for turning, with infinite artfulness, the red wine of Shiraz into urine?

Karen Blixen. *Seven Gothic Tales* (1934)

Consultations with a woman for a urinary tract infection can sometimes be the quickest and easiest, or the most complex; involving all the issues of that woman's lifestyle, diet, contraception, and sexual activity (Johnson and Stamm 1989; MRC Bulletin 1995). Cystitis is an extremely common problem in women. Estimates vary but it is thought that between 10–20% of women are affected by a lower urinary tract infection at some point during their lifetime. There are 5.2 million consultations per year in the US for urinary tract infections in women, with a billion dollar cost implication. In the UK 1–3% of all consultations to general practitioners (GPs) are for urinary tract infections.

Definitions

Cystitis

Cystitis is an inflammation of the lining of the bladder. It can be produced by an infection from bacteria, viruses, or fungi. Inflammation of the trigone area can also be produced by certain chemicals. In a bacterial infection the bladder elicits an inflammatory response which can be identified by the excretions of polymorphonuclear leukocytes in the urine (Nicolle 1990).

Bacteriuria

The presence of bacteria in the urine is abnormal, as bladder urine is sterile.

Significant bacteriuria

To differentiate an infection from contamination (see Controversies at end of chapter) an arbitrary cut-off point has been uniformly recognized. This was adopted after the work of H.E. Kass in the 1950s. He quantitatively assessed the predictive value of colony-forming bacteria in urine. From his work it has been

Table 14.1 *Risk factors of occult upper urinary tract infection*

Physiological
  Pregnancy
  Diabetes mellitus

Anatomical
  Urinary tract abnormality
  Urinary stone
  In-dwelling catheter
  Recent instrumentation

Past medical history
  Previous recurrent urinary tract infection
  Previous urinary tract infection as a child
  Previous pyelonephritis
  Symptoms present for more than 7 days before presentation
  Any immunosuppressive condition

Urogenital ageing in the post-menopausal woman

established that 10^5 colony-forming units (CFU) of bacteria per ml of voided urine is a highly specific threshold for acute pyelonephritis, but it has a low sensitivity. Recently, Stamm has argued that the threshold should be reduced to 10^2 CFU for coliforms as a sensitive indicator for infection in symptomatic women, men, and children (Johnson 1991).

Asymptomatic bacteriuria

Some women have been found to have significant bacteriuria without any symptoms. This is defined as asymptomatic bacteriuria.

Uncomplicated urinary tract infections

An uncomplicated urinary tract infection (UTI) is an infection of the bladder only, in an otherwise fit and well woman with no abnormality of her urinary tract, and no other major predisposing factors. (see Table 14.1).

Complicated urinary tract infections

Patients who have functional, anatomical or metabolic abnormalities are defined as having complicated urinary tract infections, (Stamm and Hooton 1993). All infections of the kidneys (upper urinary tract), or any infection of any part of the urinary tract in children or men should also be regarded as a complicated infection.

Relapse or reinfection?

Recurrence of bacteriuria with a different organism from the original one is defined as a reinfection. This implies acquisition of a new pathogen. This is in distinction to the recurrence of bacteriuria with the original isolate, which is termed a relapse and implies persistence of the bacteria in the urinary tract. A true, chronic urinary tract infection is the persistence of the same organisms in the urinary tract for months or years. Reinfection is a much more common clinical entity than relapse.

The urethral syndrome

In about 50% of all cases of women who present with acute dysuria and frequency, the urine culture is less than 10^5, and so is reported as 'sterile'. This is the definition of the 'urethral syndrome', also known descriptively as the frequency and dysuria syndrome. It is a topic fraught with controversy (see end of chapter), over aetiology, diagnosis, and treatment. Stamm feels that most of the women with symptoms have a true bacterial cystitis and should be treated accordingly (Stamm *et al.* 1980). Maskell feels that there are fastidious bacteria infecting these women (Maskell *et al.* 1979), whereas O'Dowd feels that this group have more in common with irritable bowel sufferers (O'Dowd 1995). Some women may have a chlamydia infection (Oakeshott and Hay 1995). In the context of a 'sterile' pyuria, chlamydia, gonococcal urethritis, and tuberculosis of the urinary tract should be considered.

Presentation of cystitis

Women often present in an agony of acute dysuria, frequency, and urgency. They may have been up all night, needing to void urine every half-hour to an hour. They may also have haematuria, which they may find alarming. Suprapubic pain occurs in 10% of cases.

Women with these symptoms may either have acute cystitis, acute urethritis, or acute vaginitis. The history makes the diagnoses in 90% of cases. If the woman is asked to describe the site of the pain, in acute cystitis the inflammation of the trigone area causes 'inside' dysuria (Komaroff and Friedland 1980) whereas with acute urethritis or vaginitis the dysuria feels more on the 'outside'.

If the woman presents with flank pain, low back pain, abdominal pain, fevers, rigours, sweating, headache, nausea and vomiting, malaise, or prostration, an overt upper urinary tract infection is probable. This may need in-patient, hospital, intravenous antibiotic treatment if she has complicating factors (see Table 14.1) or is unable to take antibiotics by mouth.

The problem with lower urinary tract infections is that about one-third of characteristic cases of acute cystitis also have an unrecognized infection of the upper urinary tract (Johnson and Stamm 1989). The risk factors of occult infection shown in Table 14.1 are considered.

Investigations

Leukocyte esterase and nitrite dip sticks

It is not helpful nor cost-effective to send routine mid-stream samples of urine (MSUs) prior to therapy on healthy, non-pregnant women presenting with acute cystitis. It is reasonable, however, to test the urine with a leukocyte ester-ase and nitrite dipstick (Hiscoke *et al.* 1990). This has a sensitivity of 75–95% predicting culture-proven infection (Stamm and Hooton 1993). Antibiotics should then be prescribed to those patients who have a positive test. MSUs should only be sent from women with complicated urinary tract infections (see Table 14.1), or those women who have failed to respond to first-line therapy.

Mid-stream sample of urine (MSU)

For many years nurses have spent much time and energy collecting mid-stream urine specimens from patients. In hospital they have used the modified nursing procedure from the Royal Marsden which requires cleansing of the external genitalia and urethral meatus with three sterile wipes before the patient is required to void the urine into a sterile bowl. The patient is asked to micturate and the midstream part of the urine flow is sampled. In non-ambulatory patients who did not have perineal cleaning, the urine specimens are heavily contaminated with mixed faecal and skin flora. However, no difference was found between using a sterile MSU pack and non-sterile wipes in a group of women over the age of 65 (Jones 1992).

In young, ambulatory patients, a study using either sterile bowls or non-sterile paper cups as a receiver for the MSU was carried out. There was no difference in the contamination rate from using an easy to handle, cheap paper cup (White 1992). In evaluating bacterial contamination from urine sampling techniques, it has been found in a prospective study that holding the labia apart is actually the most significant action when trying to obtain a 'clean' mid-stream urine sample (Baeheim *et al.* 1992) This decreased bacterial contamination from 31.1% to 13% (p <0.01) in healthy young women. This is not surprising since the urine leaves the female urethra orifice in a broad stream splashing on the labia, hosing down vaginal squamous cells, hairs, and bacteria into the receptacle for catching the urine. A full, clean-catch, mid-stream urine technique is difficult and time-consuming to understand and perform. The simple procedure of asking the patient to hold her labia apart whilst catching the urine in a paper cup significantly decreases contaminated specimens.

Having gone to all the trouble of obtaining a reasonably reliable MSU, the urine inevitably then spends 8 hours on a hot treatment room shelf awaiting collection! This ruins the specimen by bacterial overgrowth. Ideally, the specimen needs to go to the laboratory within 2 hours. In general practice this is rarely possible, and so the urine sample should be refrigerated until transportation to the laboratory.

What follow-up is required of women with urinary tract infections?

No follow-up and no post-urine cultures are required for a simple, acute, un-complicated cystitis in a well woman. If she remains symptomatic by the third day of treatment an MSU should be sent for culture and sensitivity. Any woman with a complex UTI, or during pregnancy, should be closely followed. Similarly,

2 weeks after finishing treatment for a proven pyelonephritis a further MSU should be sent for follow-up culture.

In the small percentage of women who have recurrent UTIs (greater than two UTIs in 6 months or more than three in a year) there is concern that these women may have a stone or an obstructive uropathy as an underlying aetiology. However, on ultrasound, intravenous pyelography, or cystoscopy, fewer than (5%) have a demonstrable abnormality (Hooton and Stamm 1991).

It is advisable for women on continous prophylaxis to send an MSU if they become symptomatic as this implies a reinfection with a resistant organism. It is imperative to know the culture and sensitivity to make the correct antimicrobial decision.

Causes of cystitis

In 1894, Escherich cultured 'Bacillus coli' in the urine of children with UTIs and described pyelitis as the disease of childhood. He gave his name to the bacteria which caused 85% of acute UTIs. *Escherichia coli* are facultative anaerobes from the bowel flora. They ascend via the short urethra. Women who have proven *E. coli* urinary tracts infections can be shown to have colonization of their vaginal introitus with *E. coli* bacteria of the same serotype. A small percentage of community-acquired infections are from other Gram-negative bacteria, *Proteus and Klebsiella. Staphylococcus saprophyticus* is the most important of the Grampositive pathogens. Rare causes of acute cystitis in the community are fungi and viruses, but these obviously play a more important part in hospital acquired infections, or in people who are immunosuppressed (Measley and Levison 1991) Genital herpes may be a cause of frequency, dysuria, and even acute retention.

Bacteria can theoretically gain access to the bladder by three possible routes: ascending the very short female urethra, or by lymphatic or haematogenous spread. The overwhelming number of bacterial infections are due to a local ascending infection. Infection is determined by the size of the innoculum, the host resistance or defence factors, and the virulence of the pathogen. For example, if the host defences are compromised only a small innoculum of bacteria is required to produce an infection. In the normal woman with no abnormalities of anatomy or function, a large innoculum of virulent bacteria are acquired to produce a symptomatic urinary infection. Indeed, the frequent flushing of the bladder by urine is thought to defend a woman from frequent small innocula of bacteria that never proceed to actual infection. The urine itself inhibits bacteria due to its high osmolarity, high urea concentrations and low pH. Tamm-Horsfall proteins competitively inhibit the attachment of *E.coli* to the mucousal surface of the bladder and aggregate bacteria in the urine.

Much research has gone into the virulent factors that might change *E. coli* from a harmless commensal in the bowel flora to a virulent uropathogen (Sobel 1991). In order to facilitate the ascent of bacteria from vaginal introitus and the periurethral skin up into the urethra and into the bladder, the *E.coli* needs to stick to the uroepithelial cells. There are various bacterial surface structures called adhesins and complementary components, the host receptors, which allow binding to the epithelial surface. An interesting observation is that in normal women the bacteria have to be virulent in order to cause an infection, whereas if there is gross underlying structural abnormality the patient falls prey to a variety of normal bowel flora. The bacterial adhesins take the form of fimbriae which are peptide subunits that can probe the epithelial surface for receptors. The normal vaginal bacterial commensal lactobacilli interfere with *E.coli* adherence to uroepithelial cells and therefore must have a protective effect in normal women. There is a thin mucopolysaccharide coating of the transitional epithelial cells of the bladder mucosa which also inhibit *E.coli* fimbrial attachment. It has also been suggested that antibiotic prophylaxis may work at subtherapeutic doses because the antibiotics inhibit fimbrial production, thus reducing the *E.coli's* virulence and allowing the normal host defence mechanisms of phagocytosis and mechanical flushing to prevent the bacteria seriously colonizing the bladder.

Treatment

Not all women presenting with the symptoms of acute dysuria and frequency have cystitis (see Controversies). It is reasonable to offer antibiotics to those women who have a positive leukocyte esterase and nitrite dip stick test (Hiscoke *et al.* 1990).

Self-help

Cystitis has been a major subject for self-help remedies over the years. Many women find that measures such as drinking large quantities of fluid, avoiding coffee, and taking agents that can alkalinize the urine may be effective. These may be effective because some episodes of cystitis are self-limiting. There has been no evidence-based data for any self-help measures; please see Controversies at the end of the chapter.

Cranberry juice

Recently, there has been a great interest in cranberry juice. Some women have been taking this as an alternative therapy for years, believing it to sterilize the urine. Recent work (Ofek *et al.* 1991) has shown that components in the juice may prevent urinary tract infection by inhibiting fimbrial adherence of pathogenic *E.coli*. Of seven juices (blueberry, cranberry, grapefruit, guava, mango, orange, and pineapple), only those from the vaccinium genus (family, *Ericaceae*) contained the high-molecular weight inhibitor of adhesin. More work is being done at present to try to isolate the active agent from cranberry and blueberry juices. Women may prefer this natural remedy which has fewer side-effects to taking courses of antibiotics (see Chapter 20).

Self-help groups

Angela Kilmartin set up the 'U and I' clubs in the 1970s to help fellow sufferers gain support, knowledge, and understanding. She also wrote *Understanding*

Table 14.2 *Percentage of strains fully sensitive from GP isolates*

	1971	1991
Trimethoprim	94	78.1
Nitrofurantoin	85.6	88.4
Co-trimoxazole	96.6	80.3
Ciprofloxacin	–	91.5
Cephradine	87.5	87.5
Cefuroxime	–	89.1
Co-amoxiclav	–	87.5
Ampicillin/amoxycillin	88.2	59.7

cystitis, and *Cystitis: a complete self-help guide.* Although the national self-help group is no longer in existence, there are still local groups. There are also a number of free information leaflets which give basic information about the causes of cystitis and preventive measures.

Which antibiotics work?

As a GP, the primary aim is to choose the most effective antibiotic. Other considerations are side-effects, safety in potentially pregnant women, and cost. Practitioners also need to be aware of local patterns of sensitivity regarding the prevalence of resistant bacteria to antibiotic changes (Table 14.2 and 14.3).

Specific antibiotics

Trimethoprim

Trimethoprim is still the antibiotic of choice. It is cheap and effective and is just as effective as co-trimoxazole but has fewer side-effects. Seventy-eight per cent of community-acquired, acute urinary tract infection will be sensitive to it. This does mean, however, that 22% will not when treated blind. It should also be remembered that data generated from urine specimens sent to laboratories should be interpreted with caution since many simple UTIs are treated successfully without recourse to an MSU. Those specimens analysed by laboratories may represent a more complicated patient group, with a higher incidence of resistant flora.

Cephalosporins

Most community-acquired infections are still sensitive to the cephalosporins. However, they are more expensive than trimethoprim and also disrupt the major gut flora more, thus giving potentially more side-effects to the woman (vaginal thrush, etc.).

Table 14.3 *Urinary pathogens 1993–94 Oxfordshire general practice Isolates sensitive (%)*

	Prevalence %	Trimethoprim	Ampicillin	Co-Amoxiclav	Cephalosporin	Ciprofloxacin
E. Coli	72	76	58	94	89	99
Proteus	6	20	67	88	82	98
Coliforms	6	57	50	71	58	95
Enterococci	6	58	99	99	R	R
Klebsiella	3	76	0	89	86	97
Pseudomonas	2	R	R	R	R	92
S.saprophyticus	2	92	7	95	95	93
CONS	1	39	21	76	76	78
Gp B Strep	1	21	100	100	100	R
S.aureus	1	80	21	94	94	83

Key: CONS Coag Negative Staph; R Inherently resistant

Ampicillin/amoxycillin

Unfortunately, as 40% of *E.coli* are now resistant to these drugs they are no longer recommended for treatment of acute UT unless the bacterial sensitivities are known. Amoxycillin is safe in pregnancy and whilst breast-feeding.

Co-amoxiclav

The addition of the beta-lactamase inhibitor clavulanic acid to amoxycillin has improved its effectiveness against *E.coli*. At present, bacteriologists prefer this drug to be left as a second-line agent when the sensitivities are known, or in complicated UTIs. There is no evidence of teratogenicity, but manufacturers advise avoiding co-amoxiclav in pregnancy unless essential.

Nitrofurantoin

This is returning to popularity as a first-line treatment for UTIs as 88% of community-acquired UTIs must be sensitive to it. It is also useful for long-term prophylaxis. A further advantage is that it can be given safely to pregnant women, although it may cause neonatal haemolysis if used at term. It does not induce bacterial resistance in the bowel. The major problem with nitrofurantoin is compliance, since it does cause nausea and vomiting (which of course is worse in pregnancy).

The quinolones

These new agents can be used as second-line treatment if trimethoprim has failed or in complicated UTIs. Unfortunately *no* quinolone can be used in pregnancy (arthropathy in animal studies). 4-quinolones should be used with caution in patients with epilepsy or a history of fits, patients with hepatic or renal impairment, diabetics, and patients taking theophylline or NSAIDS (see *BNF*). The cost for a course of a 4-quinolone is approximately 10 times that for trimethoprim.

Special situations

Pregnancy

Pregnant women have a higher prevalence of asymptomatic bacteriuria. In the non-pregnant woman asymptomatic bacteriuria appears to be more intermittent and self-limiting: 4–7% will have bacteriuria throughout pregnancy. It is thought that pregnant women are more prone to asymptomatic bacteriuria because the higher urinary pH allows more rapid colonization by *E.coli*. The progestogen effect on smooth muscle allows relaxation of the urethral meatus, giving both easier ascent of uropathogens into the bladder and more frequent reflux up to the kidneys, causing a high percentage of complicated upper urinary tract infections (Johnson 1991; MRC bulletin 1995). For women with asymptomatic bacteriuria in pregnancy, there is a significant risk that they will experience a symptomatic UTI, with obstetric complications of possible premature labour, small-for-dates babies, and an increased perinatal mortality.

Routine screening of pregnant women for asymptomatic bacteriuria is

Fig 14.1 *Algorithm for the management of simple UTIs in non-elderly females*
(MRC Bulletin (1995). 6. Reproduced with permission)

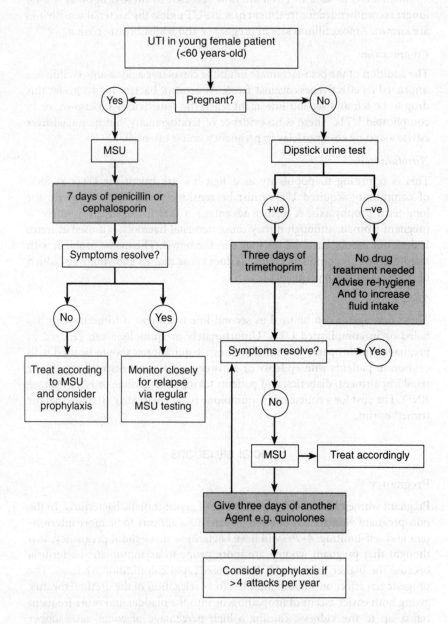

advised in the 16th week of pregnancy. If asymptomatic bacteriuria is found in these women, treatment should be given to prevent acute pyelonephritis. Pregnant women with asymptomatic bacteriuria should receive at least 7 days' treatment with an antibiotic. Most pregnant women are heavily indoctrinated not to take any drugs during pregnancy. The GP must explain to the woman why she needs to be treated for an asymptomatic condition in the pregnancy or compliance may be low, with disastrous results. Nitrofurantoin (except at term), amoxycillin, and the older cephalosporins are thought to be relatively safe in pregnancy and are commonly used as first-line agents, depending on the sensitivity of the uropathogen and the allergies of the patient. Various antibiotics are *not* recommended in pregnancy (the quinolones; co-amoxiclav) as the potential risk to the fetus is thought to be more harmful than the potential benefit to the woman. Trimethoprim has a theoretical teratogenic risk as it is a folate antagonist, and should be avoided in the first trimester. If there are problems with bacterial sensitivities of UTIs in pregnant women, specialist advice from the local bacteriology department should be sought. Tetracycline should be avoided in pregnancy as they colour the fetal teeth and bones in the second and third trimesters. There is also evidence in animal studies that tetracyclines may effect skeletal development in the first trimester; (see *BNF*). A pregnant woman with signs of an acute pyelonephritis should be referred for hospital admission as she will probably require intravenous antibiotics.

Diabetes mellitus

Asymptomatic bacteriuria is 40 times more common in the diabetic woman than the non-diabetic (Measley and Levison 1991). Fungal urinary tract infections are also slightly more common as the glycosuria encourages fungal and bacterial growth. The high urinary glucose also impairs leukocyte phagocytosis. There may be an autonomic neuropathy in long-term diabetics which impairs bladder emptying, predisposing to recurrent infections.

Up to 50% of diabetics have upper renal tract involvement. Long-term prophylaxis may be required in this group if there are proven underlying anatomical abnormalities, including significant residual urine due to a neurogenic bladder. Certainly diabetics should be treated immediately if there is a symptomatic infection, and some would argue for routine screening and treatment of asymptomatic patients in this subgroup. (Zhanel *et al.* 1990).

Urinary tract calculi

Stones in the urinary tract irritate the mucosa, which promotes bacterial adherence and colonization. The stone itself also acts as a focus for bacterial persistence. Urinary tract infections, in the presence of calculi, are more often caused by *Proteus mirarbilis, Ureaplasma urealyticum, Klebsiella pneumoniae,* and *Pseudomonas aeruginosa.* The flora may give the clue to reveal an occult urinary tract calculus. It is impossible to cure a UTI with antibiotics whilst there is a stone present. Bacteria are released from secluded sites deep in the stone, so a relapse is inevitable. Treatment requires a urological referral to disrupt the stone by ultrasound or surgical removal.

Urogenital Ageing

There is a rapid rise in the prevalence of UTIs in post-menopausal woman. Women over the age of 60 have an incidence of 15% UTIs per year. In the post-menopausal woman lactobacilli disappear from the vaginal introitus, and the pH of the vagina rises. This favours colonization by enterobacteria. Entry of uropathogens into the urethral meatus may be facilitated by a urethral caruncle, and bladder and uterine prolapse cause a stagnant pool of residual urine after voiding. The vaginal and urethral mucosa is atrophic and more vulnerable to *E.coli* colonization.

In a double-blind, placebo controlled trial of intervaginal oestriol cream in post-menopausal women, episodes of bacteriuria were measured. Over an 8-month period there was considerable reduction in the frequency of asymptomatic episodes in the women using oestriol cream (nightly for 2 weeks and then twice-weekly for 8 months) (Raz and Stamm 1993). Of the 50 women in the treated oestriol group there were 12 episodes of bacteriuria, the 43 in the placebo group had 111 episodes of bacteriuria (p <0.005). Some women withdrew from the treatment group because of pruritis and burning from the oestriol cream. The mean vaginal pH fell from 5.5 to 3.6 in the treated group, and the re-oestrogenized women become recolonized with lactobacilli. Lactobacilli produce lactic acid which lowers the pH of the vagina and discourages growth of uropathogens. If the vaginal pH is less than 4.5, *E.coli* do not colonize the mucosa. It has also been found in *in vitro* experiments that fragments of lactobacilli cell wall actually prevent attachment of *E. coli* to epithelial cells. At present it is not known whether this is by stearic hindrance or specific blocking of potential attachment sites.

Although urogenital ageing has been an entity for as long as there have been women that have survived to the post-menopausal period, this is a renewed area of interest at present due to the sudden profusion of local oestrogen treatments (oestrogen pessaries, creams, and rings). There is also full, systemic hormone replacement therapy without the necessity of monthly withdrawal bleeds; a factor that had previously discouraged many post-menopausal women from continuing on HRT. (Hope and Rees 1995). The use of HRT in post-menopausal women who do have recurrent urinary tract infections should be considered and the pros and cons discussed with the patient.

Recurrent urinary tract infections in pre-menopausal women

This group of women can have their lives made miserable be recurrent infection. Twenty per cent of women with UTIs have more than two UTIs in 6 months or three or more UTIs in 12 months. For a woman with persistent recurring infections an ultrasound of the urinary tract to exclude a stone or an obstructive uropathy may be reasonable, and a referral for cystoscopy if she has persistent haematuria. However, a cause is rarely found. Excretory urography and cystoscopy in women with recurrent UTIs demonstrates anatomical abnormalities in less than 5%, with extremely few correctable lesions (Stamm and Hooton 1993). There are three management strategies for women with recurrent UTIs:

(1) post-coital prophylaxis;
(2) intermittent self treatment;
(3) continuous prophylaxis;

Post-coital prophylaxis

This is effective in women who have a very clear temporal relationship between an episode of cystitis within 12 hours of sexual intercourse. Retrospective and prospective studies have shown that sexual intercourse has a mechanical effect in introducing uropathogens into the bladder. Sexually-active women have a greater risk (times 40) of infection than non-sexually active women. Some diaphragm-users have a higher rate than women using other methods of contraception. There is debate whether this is due to a mechanical effect of the diaphragm in the vagina altering the angle of the bladder neck (from urodynamic studies), or due to the change of vaginal pH from the spermicidal cream or jelly. If a woman gets recurrent post-coital dysuria and uses a diaphragm it is certainly worth considering either checking the diaphragm for its size and fitting, changing the spermicides, or discussing the use of another form of contraception.

A residual pool of urine in the bladder may act as a reservoir for infection. The woman may be advised to empty the bladder before and after intercourse. Early post-intercourse micturition has a proven protective effect (Hooton and Stamm 1991).

In women who do develop post-coital dysuria a single dose of trimethoprim can prevent an attack if taken immediately prior or post-intercourse. The issue of antibiotics causing less-effective contraception from the oral contraceptive drugs must also be considered in this group.

Intermittent self-treatment

Most women do not like taking drugs continuously. They may only get three attacks of cystitis a year and resent having to take daily medication for this unlikely event. From their symptoms 92% of women can correctly self-diagnose a UTI (Stamm and Hooton 1993). This is because acute cystitis usually presents with the same symptoms each time. When giving women antibiotics to start treatment on their own, they should be told that if the symptoms have not completely resolved within 48 hours they should seek medical attention. Women prefer this method as they feel more in control of their body and their medication.

Continuous prophylaxis

A low-dose, nightly antibiotic, or even twice-weekly, can reduce the recurrence of UTIs by 95%. If the woman relapses on prophylaxis the uropathogen is inevitably a reinfection with a different bacteria that is resistant to the antibiotic being used. Urinary cultures must be made to identify the uropathogen and define its sensitivity to antimicrobial agents.

Controversies

From ignorance our comfort flows
The only wretched are the wise

Matthew Prior (1664–1721)

Any topic in medicine can be controversial. Either the ideal prospective trials have never been done, or studies have been performed but various methodological problems call into question the validity of the data. In this part of the chapter some hot controversies on the area of cystitis will be highlighted. By the time the next edition of this chapter is written, hopefully some of these may be resolved.

When should cystitis be treated?

GPs are in an extremely difficult position because women with cystitis require immediate treatment. However, half of all non-pregnant women with the symptoms of urgency, dysuria, and frequency will have no detectable bacterial infection (but see What is significant bacteriuria, below). In about 50% of cases with proven bacteriuria symptoms may resolve through natural host defences without drug treatment in 3 days. It could therefore be argued that no woman should be treated for a lower urinary tract infection until they have had 3 days' symptoms. However, this is putting a large number of women potentially at risk from ascending infection, together with the misery of 3 days' illness (MRC bulletin 1995).

Many women try to avoid taking antibiotics for recurrent urinary infection since they know from bitter experience that the eradication of pathogenic bacteria from their urinary tract has an effect on their commensal flora of bowel and vagina. The broad-spectrum penicillins in particular destroy the commensal flora including the lactobicilli, so facilitating the colonization of the urethral entroitus with resistant Gram-negative organisms, and also allowing *Candida albicans* to gain dominance in the vagina. Many women know that they get thrush after antibiotics, but still 75% of women do not realize the link. Trimethoprim does not usually select resistant bowel organisms and leaves the urethral flora undisturbed, protecting the patient against Gram-negative colonization (Maskell 1992).

It would seem reasonable to only treat those symptomatic women with a dipstick positive for leukocytes and nitrites. It is also reassuring to know that the weight of evidence favours the conclusion that although UTIs can produce severe impairment of renal function, this is rare in the absence of major predisposing factors such as obstruction, stones, reflux, abnormalities of the voiding mechanisms, or diabetes mellitus (Kunin 1990).

What is significant bacteriuria?

The whole topic of UTIs is fraught with problems of definitions. The work by Kass in defining significant bacteriuria as $>10^5$ colony-forming units (CFU) per ml of voided urine was based on two groups of women, with asymptomatic bacteriuria and acute pyelonephritis. This has been widely generalized to all patient populations with UTIs but has never been evaluated for cystitis. The only reliable urine specimens are obtained by bladder aspiration or sterile catheterization; but these are invasive, uncomfortable, and not feasible in general practice. Voided urine is easy to collect but is inevitably contaminated with periurethral flora. The quest for a truly significant bacteriuria is almost like that of the Holy Grail.

A GP needs a test that distinguishes true bladder bacteriuria from contaminated specimens. On the Kass definition of 10^5 CFU per ml, many women with the symptoms of dysuria and frequency are told 'there's nothing wrong'. Stamm and Hooton (1993) argue that a new significant bacteriuria threshold should be agreed of >10^2 uropathogens per ml. This proves to be far more sensitive for *E.coli* (0.95) and only slightly less specific (0.85). This threshold of 10^2 CFU coliforms is a very sensitive indicator of infections since if these women are followed they will invariably reach a count of 10^5 over the succeeding days (Johnson 1991). At present, laboratories have not taken up this revised >10^2 CFU suggestion.

Should women be screened for asymptomatic bacteriuria?

The first problem is what is true asymptomatic bacteriuria and what is contamination (see above and section on MSUs, p. 436). Of true asymptomatic bacteriuria 30% will become symptomatic in time and then seek treatment. However, most women with true asymptomatic bacteriuria appear to experience it as a transient phenomenon. Women therefore get intermittent asymptomatic bacteriuria which can resolve without treatment (Zhanel *et al.* 1990). Since women with asymptomatic bacteriuria either present sooner or later with an acute urinary tract infection, or self-cure, there seems at present no good argument for routine screening of the whole sexually-active population of women. However, there are a few subgroups that should be considered: antenatal women, women with known abnormalities of their urinary tract, and diabetics.

When should an MSU be sent?

Given that voided urine in the general practice setting is almost inevitably contaminated (Baeheim *et al.* 1992; Jones 1992; White 1992), is there any point in sending one at all? The other major problem with sending urine for culture and sensitivity is that one has to make an immediate therapeutic decision when seeing the patient about treatment and the results from the laboratory will come back 3 days later when 80–90% of the patients seen and treated should be completely better.

At present, samples for urine microscopy and culture are the commonest requests received in the laboratory, accounting for 50% of all specimens. If leukocyte esterase dipsticks were adopted routinely there would be a marked drop in workload for laboratories, allowing for more resources to be allocated to the positive specimens. In a survey of Danish GPs, microbiologists, and urologists, 48% of GPs but only 24% of Danish microbiologists would routinely send a urine for culture on a previously-fit, 30-year-old woman (Olesen and Oestergaard 1995).

What length antibiotic course?

The literature is full of studies varying from single-dose antibiotics to a full 6-week course for acute UTIs (Stamm *et al.* 1987; Johnson and Stamm 1989;

Bailey 1990; Nicolle 1990; Stamm and Hooton 1993; MRC bulletin 1995). The advocates of a single-dose therapy argue that this is the treatment of choice for uncomplicated UTIs in general practice since a single dose insures compliance, and cures simple cystitis. There will be an immediate relapse in the 30% who have occult upper UTI. This can be looked on as a useful clinical guide to those patients that need further investigation, intensive treatment, and supervision. Other workers in the field are concerned that the single-dose regimes are less effective; further validation with large controlled trials are still needed. The 3-day course is now in vogue. It has the advantage of fewer side-effects than the previously favoured 7–14 day treatment schedules, and a lower relapse rate than a single dose.

If an upper renal tract infection is suspected there is evidence that a 14-day course of antibiotics is as effective as a 6-week course, with fewer side-effects (concomitant thrush, drug reactions such as rashes and diarrhoea, and patient compliance). There is also less likelihood of reinfection with resistant organisms.

In all uncomplicated, non-pregnant, female patients with a lower UTI a 3-day course seems reasonable. There is still controversy as to whether complicated UTIs (including those of pregnant women) should be treated with 7, 10, or 14-day courses.

Does the urethral syndrome need treatment?

There seems little doubt that the urethral syndrome has several possible causes, and should be reclassified by the various aetiologies. Since 55% of patients with acute dysuria and frequency do not have significant bacteriuria, how should they be treated? Many women with acute symptoms are told by the receptionist that there is nothing wrong when they telephone for their MSU result. This leaves the patient confused and angry.

As previously discussed, many women have counts of 10^2 which should be considered as significant (Stamm *et al.* 1980). However, this level of bacteria would be reported as 'no growth' by a laboratory using the Kass criteria. Stamm is a strong advocate that many of these women actually have a bacterial infection, despite a 'negative' culture. He argues that women with less than 10^5 CFU per ml should not be ignored if they have symptoms. Often they have low counts because they are early in the infection, and can be shown to achieve counts of 10^5 over the following few days. Other reasons for a low bacterial count are a rapid urine flow because the women are drinking so much; a low urine pH <5 decreases the ability of *E. Coli* to multiply; and possible bacteriostatic agents in the urine from over-the-counter preparations. Stamm claims that 95% of dysuric women with proven pyuria have treatable infections.

Chlamydia trachomatis is certainly an under-diagnosed cause of urethritis in sexually-active women with pyuria (Oakeshott and Hay 1995). The prevalence of chlamydia infection varies between 2–12% in general practice populations. The at-risk groups are women under the age of 25 with a recent change of sexual partner, who do not use barrier contraception, and may present with a mucoprolent vaginal discharge. On examination the cervix is friable and there is sterile pyuria. The difficulty of detecting chlamydia in general practice is one that needs to be addressed, as many of these women go undiagnosed and untreated. The long-term sequelae of possible pelvic inflammatory disease, and atopic pregnancy, must be avoided. The actual risk to an individual from one episode of chlamydia has not yet been quantified.

There is still a group of women who have dysuria and pyuria but do not have chlamydia or more than 10^2 uropathogenic *E.coli*. Rosamund Maskell advocates that these women have 'fastidious' micro-organisms that need to be grown in CO_2-dependent cultures. There is still controversy about these fastidious bacteria, and her work has not been supported by other researchers in the field (Maskell *et al.* 1979; Brumfitt and Hamilton-Miller 1990). O'Dowd feels that the syndrome has much more in common with the irritable bowel syndrome than it does with urinary tract infection. They may coexist within the same patient and he feels that these women may receive unnecessary courses of antibiotics without being given support and understanding to the psychological aspects that may be causing somatization in those who have no clear infective aetiology for their urethral symptoms (O'Dowd 1995).

As there has really been no satisfactory explanation for this group of women with symptoms but no isolated causative agent, some women have naturally given up on conventional medicine and turned to self-help. They have tried changing their diet to a ketogenic one on the understanding that this might change the local environment and pH of the urethra; as well as excluding caffeine (tea, coffee, and cola drinks) which excites the detrusor muscle of the bladder. Women have also tried making their urine alkaline, or acid, since the optimal pH for *E.coli* is pH 6.0–7.0. If the pH is changed some women find symptomatic relief. However, there remains an unhappy, untreated, symptomatic group of women who have the diagnosis of urethral syndrome with (at present) no underlying aetiological factor. This group need to be studied further.

Should women be advised to drink a large quantity?

One of the few things everyone seems to know about cystitis is that the sufferer should increase their fluid intake, anecdotely women say this can help. This is based on the normal urine osmolarity of 300–1200 mosmol/l; if urine becomes very dilute (<200 mosmol/l) growth of bacteria is reduced. A diuresis also helps bladder-emptying, theoretically allowing the pathogenic *E.coli* to be flushed out of the system (although this ignores the *E.coli's* ability to attach on to the bladder wall epithelium). Women also drink substances such as lemon barley, water, sodium bicarbonate, and over-the-counter potassium citrate preparations to change the pH of their urine to create a less favourable environment for pathogenic *E.coli* which further confuses the picture. However, some people argue that an excessive diuresis may actually enhance vesicoureteral reflux and in some cases actually facilitate bacteria reaching the kidneys. It also dilutes antibacterial substances in the urine which may decrease their therapeutic efficacy. There is no prospective trial on the beneficial or detrimental use of drinking fluids in women with uncomplicated urinary tract infections. This is distinct from the beneficial effects of drinking cranberry juice, which has been found to inhibit pathogenic *E.coli* fimbrial adherence.

Patients' experiences

During my first pregnancy my GP diagnosed cystitis. Later in that pregnancy I had 7 days in hospital with pyelitis. I felt really ill, and was frightened that my baby would be damaged.

For the last 40 years I have experienced bouts of cystitis. I have times when I constantly want to wee, and have bladder irritation. When I get an attack I cannot concentrate on my job. My boss stopped being understanding and started getting angry. I also feel too tired to go shopping or cook supper. I know where all the public toilets are from here to London – I'm always getting caught short. I often feel too embarrassed to go out to parties, and make excuses.

I had ignored my symptoms of cystitis for a few days, I felt I just couldn't go to my GP again; she was sick of seeing me! I then had what I thought was 'flu – pain in my hips and back, very cold and shivery, aching in my wrists and head. Then I started passing bright red blood and got really frightened. I wished I had got treatment sooner. It took months for me to feel well again.

Next time I'm coming back as a man; he doesn't get cystitis every time we have sex.

References and further reading

Baeheim, A., Asbjorn, D., and Hunskaar, S. (1992). Evaluation of urine sampling technique: bacterial contamination of samples from women students. *British Journal of General Practice*, **42**, 241–3.

Bailey, R. R. (1990). Review of published studies on single-dose therapy of urinary tract infections. *Infection*, **18**(2), 553–5.

Bowler, J. (1995). Urinary tract infections acquired in the Oxfordshire community. [Unpublished data]. Dept. of Bacteriology, John Radcliffe Hospital, Oxford.

Brumfitt, W. and Hamilton–Miller, J. M. T. (1990). Urinary infections in the 1990s. The State of the Art. *Infection*, **18**(2), 534–9.

Hiscoke, C., Yoxall, H., Greig, D., and Lightfoot, N. F. (1990). Validation of a method for the rapid diagnosis of urinary infection suitable for a general practice. *British Journal of General Practice*, **40**, 403–5.

Hooton, T. M. and Stamm, W. E. (1991). Management of acute uncomplicated urinary tract infections in adults. *Medical Clinics of North America*, **75**(2), 339–57.

Hope, S. and Rees, M. (1995). Why do British women start and stop hormone replacement therapy? *Journal of British Menopause Society*, **1**(2), 26–8.

Johnson, C. (1991). Definitions, classification, and clinical presentation of urinary tract infections. *Medical Clinics of North America*, **75**(2), 241–52.

Johnson, R. J. and Stamm, W. E. (1989). Urinary tract infections in women: diagnoses and treatment. *Annals of Internal Medicine*, **111**, 906–17.

Jones, E. (1992). In search of a fine specimen. *Nursing Times*, **88**(6), 62–3.

Komaroff, A. L. and Friedland, G. (1980). The dysuria–pyuria syndrome. *New England Journal of Medicine*, **303,** 452–3.

Kunin, C. M. (1990). Natural history of 'lower' urinary tract infections. *Infection*, **18**(2), 44–9.

Maskell, R. (1992). Antibacterial agents and urinary tract infection: a paradox. *British Journal of General Practice*. April 1992, 138–9.

Maskell, R., *et al.* (1979). The puzzle of the 'urethral syndrome': a possible answer? *Lancet*, May 19, 1979. 1058–9.

Measley, R. E. and Levison M. E. (1991). Host defense mechanisms in the pathogenesis of urinary tract infections. *Medical Clinics of North America*, **75**(2), Medicine's Resource Centre (August 1995) *Urinary tract infection*, Bulletin **6**, No.8.

Nicolle, L. E. (1990). The optimal management of lower urinary tract infections. *Infection*, **18**(5), 50–2.

Oakeshott, P. and Hay, P. (1995). General practice update: *Chlamydia* infection in women. *British Journal of General Practice*, **45,** 615–20.

O'Dowd, T. (1995). *Women's problems in general practice* (3rd edn) (ed. A. McPherson), pp.288–9. Oxford University Press, Oxford.

Ofek, I., *et al.* (1991). *Anti-Escherichia coli* adhesin activity of cranberry and blueberry juices. *New England Journal of Medicine*, **324,** 1599.

Olesen, F. and Oestergaard, I. (1995). Patients with urinary tract infection: proposed management strategies of general practitioners, microbiologists and urologists. *British Journal of General Practice*, **45,** 611–13.

Raz, R. and Stamm, W.E. (1993). A controlled trial of Intravaginal estriol in post-menopausal women with recurrent UTIs. *New England Journal of Medicine*, **329,** 753–6.

Sobel, J. D. (1991). Bacterial etiologic agents in the pathogenesis of urinary tract infection. *Medical Clinics of North America*, **75**(2), 253–73.

Stamm, W. E. and Hooton, M. (1993). Management of urinary tract infections in adults. *New England Journal of Medicine*, **329,** 1328–34.

Stamm, W. E. *et al.* (1987). Acute renal tract infection in women: treatment with trimethoprim, sulfamethoxazole or ampicillin for two or six weeks. *Annals of Internal Medicine*, **106,** 341–5.

Stamm, W. E. *et al.* (1980). Causes of the acute urethral syndrome in women. *New England Journal of Medicine*, **303,** 409–15.

White, S. (1992). Choosing the right container. *Nursing Times*, **88**(6), 64.

Zhanel, G. *et al.* (1990). Asymptomatic bacteriuria. Which patients should be treated? *Archives of International Medicine*, **150,** 1389–96.

CHAPTER FIFTEEN

Chronic pelvic pain

Stephen Kennedy and Julie Parkes

What is chronic pelvic pain?

Chronic pelvic pain (CPP) affects millions of women worldwide and causes considerable disability and suffering. However, the clinical problem is poorly understood and often inadequately managed. Unfortunately, the epidemiological characteristics of CPP are unclear principally because researchers have failed to use a consistent definition of the problem. The three most commonly used definitions are:

'Any type of pelvic pain that has lasted 6 months or longer'
'Chronic pelvic pain that lacks apparent physical cause sufficient to explain the pain', and
'Pain accompanied by significantly altered physical activity, including work, recreation, sexual life, as well as disturbance of mood'.

These definitions are all unsatisfactory for a number of reasons. Firstly, long-standing pelvic pain may be well-tolerated without affecting a woman's physical activity or quality of life; secondly, an apparent physical cause, such as endometriosis, may not actually be the cause of the pain; and lastly, it may be that a disturbance of mood arises for reasons unrelated to the pain.

The principal problems in producing a working definition of CPP are whether to exclude cyclical symptoms and dyspareunia, and whether to set an arbitrary threshold for the duration of symptoms such as 3 or 6 months. The broadest possible definition would undoubtedly be 'constant or intermittent cyclic or acyclic pain that persists for 3 months or more and includes dysmenorrhoea, deep dyspareunia, and intermenstrual pain'. However, if these different types of pelvic pain are actually manifestations of different pathologies then the distinction between cyclical and non-cyclical pain may be very important.

The concerns about an adequate definition are of practical relevance. From an epidemiological perspective, the few published studies on CPP in the UK are of limited value because a consistent definition has not been used which makes it difficult to calculate incidence and prevalence rates. In addition, all the studies

---

Box 15.1 *Causes of chronic pelvic pain*

Endometriosis
Irritable bowel syndrome
Chronic PID

Pelvic adhesions
Trapped ovary syndrome
Ovarian remnant syndrome
Pelvic congestion
Psychosomatic

---

have lacked population denominators and have been based on patients referred for hospital care and are therefore not representative of the general population. Therefore, it is extremely difficult to plan the allocation of health care resources for this clinical problem and to make recommendations about management.

For the purposes of this review, we wish to recommend the use of a definition devised by Howard (1993) as 'non-menstrual pain of 3 or more months' duration that localizes to the anatomic pelvis and is severe enough to cause functional disability and require medical or surgical treatment'. The only potential disadvantage in using this definition is that it excludes dysmenorrhoea which is generally accepted as one of the major symptoms associated with endometriosis/adenomyosis. Otherwise, it seems to encompass well the clinical problem that we describe below.

History

Some of the causes of CPP are shown in Box 15.1. The three major differential diagnoses are undoubtedly endometriosis, chronic pelvic inflammatory disease (PID), and irritable bowel syndrome (IBS). There is considerable overlap in symptomatology between these conditions. To try to distinguish between them it is important to take a detailed history from the woman, and her partner if at all possible, to assess the severity of the pain, its characteristics, and association with the menstrual cycle, and to estimate the effect of the problem on the physical and emotional well-being of the woman. The woman should be asked:

How long has she had the pain?
Has she ever had pain like this in the past?
Is there any association with the menstrual cycle?
Where is the pain maximally located?
Where does it radiate, i.e. into the back, down the thighs?
Is the pain exacerbated by movement (including sexual intercourse)?
Do simple remedies provide any relief, i.e. herbal teas, painkillers, local heat?
Is there deep pain on intercourse, and if so, in all or only some positions?
Is there pain in the 24 hours following intercourse?

Are her periods also painful?
If so, how incapacitated is she by the pain?

453

How many days of dysmenorrhoea does she have?
Is the pain relieved by simple remedies?
How severe is the pain in terms of emotional and functional disability?
How sympathetic is her partner?

Does the woman perceive that she has gynaecological disease?
Does she associate her symptoms with any specific event, i.e. a traumatic vaginal delivery?
Does she wish to conceive?

Does she have a relevant family history, i.e. malignancy or endometriosis?
Has she had gynaecological surgery in the past, i.e. a hysterectomy with ovarian conservation?

Has she taken hormonal contraception in the past and, if so, was she asymptomatic then?
Is she currently taking a hormonal contraceptive?
Has she taken hormonal medication in the past, i.e. danazol, which has relieved the pain?
What side-effects were experienced on hormonal medication/contraception?
Has she ever used an IUCD?
Has she had vaginal discharge?
Has her partner been symptomatic?
Does she or her partner have a past history of a sexually-transmitted disease?
Does she suspect that her partner has been unfaithful?
Has she had episodes of acute pelvic pain in the past, associated with fever?
Has the pain successfully been treated with antibiotics in the past?
Has she had problems conceiving?

Has her bowel habit changed?
Are the stools well-formed?
Is there pain associated with defaecation, and if so is the pain worse around the time of a period?
Does she have abdominal bloating?
Does she pass mucus or blood per rectum?

Examination

Passing a speculum and a bimanual examination are mandatory. There may be tenderness that is generalized or localized to one anatomical position. There may be vaginal discharge (see Chapter 13) and cervical excitation, suggestive of infection. The uterus may feel enlarged, as is sometimes the case in adenomyosis; it may be retroverted and fixed, especially if the pouch of Douglas has become obliterated by severe endometriosis. There may be thickening of the uterosacral ligaments due to endometriosis or a tender endometriotic nodule to be felt in the pouch of Douglas or rectovaginal septum. It may be possible to palpate adnexal masses, i.e. ovarian endometriomas or tubo-ovarian masses. Conversely, abdominal and pelvic examination may be entirely normal.

Specific causes of chronic pelvic pain

Endometriosis

The pain associated with endometriosis is traditionally described in very characteristic ways. Dysmenorrhoea commences 1–2 days before the onset of, and lasts throughout, the menstrual flow. It tends to be bilateral lower abdominal pain that radiates to the lower back and down the thighs. Pain on intercourse is common, especially on deep penetration: the pain is caused, it is believed, by pressure on endometriotic nodules in the uterosacral ligaments, pouch of Douglas, or rectovaginal septum. Pain may also be experienced up to 24 hours after intercourse has occurred. If the rectum or sigmoid colon is involved, women may complain of rectal pressure, an urgency to defaecate, and pain on defaecation, especially during the menses; suprapubic discomfort and dysuria may occur with bladder involvement. Haematuria and pain in the flanks or iliac fossae may occur secondary to ureteric involvement. The pain of endometriosis should be cyclical in nature, although many women describe the gradual onset of symptoms throughout the menstrual cycle which may progress to constant pain. Not surprisingly, this often causes a state of emotional despair and anxiety.

There may be a family history of endometriosis: first-degree relatives have a six to nine times increased risk compared to the general population and there is current research aiming to identify genes conferring susceptibility to the disease. There is no evidence that endometriosis has a predilection for middle-aged, upper class, ambitious, white women as suggested in many gynaecology textbooks: this stereotype probably only demonstrates that such women have greater access to medical care and a laparoscopic diagnosis. *Current* use of the combined oral contraceptive (COC) is believed to be protective. Possible risk factors include heavy and frequent periods, *past* use of the COC, Müllerian anomalies, tampon use, and sexual intercourse during menses.

The occurrence of any one of the above symptoms should alert medical practitioners to the possibility of endometriosis. It seems extraordinary, therefore, that patient self-help groups emphasize how frequently doctors in both primary and secondary care delay in making the diagnosis, either because they fail to consider endometriosis as a diagnostic possibility or because there are insufficient resources in the health service to allow all symptomatic women to be laparoscoped. Even in the US, where women have arguably greater access to laparoscopy, 27% of women with endometriosis in a retrospective study had been symptomatic for at least 6 years before a diagnosis was finally made. Not surprisingly, many women believe that a delayed diagnosis leads to increased personal suffering, more prolonged ill health, and a disease state that is more difficult to treat.

Chronic pelvic inflammatory disease

Inadequately treated, acute PID, leading to hydrosalpinges, pelvic adhesions, tubo-ovarian abscesses, and anatomical distortion, is one of the major causes

Table 15.1 *Symptoms associated with irritable bowel syndrome*

Common GI symptoms	Other GI symptoms	Non-GI symptoms
Abdominal pain	Nausea	Dysmenorrhoea
Bowel disturbance	Vomiting	Dyspareunia
Passage of mucus	Heartburn	Urinary frequency
Sense of incomplete evacuation	Dyspepsia	Loin pain
Abdominal distension	Globus hystericus	Back and thigh pain
Feeling of 'wind'		Depression

of infertility throughout the world. However, whether chronic PID actually causes CPP is unknown and it is also unclear whether the pelvic damage in chronic PID results from a state of ongoing, active infection or recurrent, acute episodes.

PID is usually diagnosed clinically on the basis of: (1) symptoms, such as unilateral or bilateral pain and dyspareunia; (2) the sexual history; and (3) the pelvic findings, which may include generalized tenderness, cervical excitation, and an adnexal mass, with or without tenderness. Infection screening tests of the woman and her partner(s) should be performed (see Chapter 13), but negative results do not exclude the diagnosis.

Many women who are found at laparoscopy to have chronic PID do not give a history of previous acute episodes, presumably because they have had *Chlamydia* infections which are frequently asymptomatic: this highlights the difficulty of managing the condition. Nevertheless, given the disastrous consequences of not making the diagnosis and not treating PID adequately, there is a strong case for empirically treating all patients with a suspected diagnosis of PID. Provided that the treatment has been adequate, this may be the only way of excluding PID as a component of the problem. Aside from possible side-effects associated with antibiotic treatment, the only potential disadvantage is the anxiety and anger that can be generated between doctor and patient and between the woman and her partner(s) by making this diagnosis inappropriately.

Irritable bowel syndrome

IBS has been defined as a 'functional bowel disorder in which abdominal pain is associated with defaecation or a change in bowel habit, with additional features of disordered defaecation and abdominal distension'. The principal symptoms are shown in Table 15.1. The following diagnostic criteria have been advocated – at least 3 months of continuous or recurrent symptoms of:

Abdominal pain or discomfort which is:
- relieved with defaecation, and/or
- associated with change in frequency of stool, and/or
- associated with a change in consistency of stool

Two or more of the following on at least a quarter of occasions or days:
- altered bowel frequency (>3 bowel movements per day or <3 per week)
- altered form of stool (lumpy/hard or loose/watery stool)
- altered passage of stool (straining, urgency or feeling of incomplete evacuation)
- passage of mucus
- bloating or feeling of abdominal distension.

There may or may not be an association with the menstrual cycle.

There are a few reports of the prevalence of IBS in a gynaecological setting. For example, at least three symptoms associated with IBS were reported by 60% of women who had had a negative laparoscopy to investigate CPP (Hogston 1987). In a survey of 798 women aged 18–70 attending out-patients for a variety of gynaecological problems, the prevalence of IBS was 37.3%, but IBS was present in 50% of the women referred with abdominal pain, dysmenorrhoea, or dyspareunia (Prior *et al.* 1989). A positive diagnosis was made only if there were all the following complaints: abdominal pain more than once per month, abdominal distension at times other than menstruation, and an abnormal bowel habit (constipation, diarrhoea, or alternating). Constipation was defined as three stools or less per week or frequent straining at stool, diarrhoea as three or more loose stools per day. In addition, an abnormality of consistency of stool was sought (thin, pellety, mushy, or slimy). Women were classified as IBS negative if they complained of all the above symptoms but were passing blood pr or had a past history of organic bowel disease. These studies are quoted in detail because they illustrate how commonly such symptoms can occur in women with pelvic pain being investigated by gynaecologists who may not be fully aware of all the manifestations of IBS. These studies are hospital-based; however, there are very few data available from community-based studies.

Trapped ovary and ovarian remnant syndromes

Trapped ovary syndrome occurs in 1–3% of women who have had a hysterectomy with ovarian conservation. Women typically present with pelvic pain, dyspareunia, and a fixed, tender ovary at the vaginal vault. At laparoscopy, the residual ovary or ovaries are found adherent to the vaginal vault and are usually covered by extensive adhesions. Ovarian remnant syndrome is defined as the presence of functioning ovarian tissue despite an apparently complete bilateral oophorectomy. It usually occurs following surgery for severe endometriosis or PID. The ovarian remnant may be difficult to locate at laparoscopy, but the diagnosis should be suspected if the FSH level is in the pre-menopausal range. Surgery remains the most effective treatment for both these conditions; ovarian remnants must be removed by an experienced surgeon because of the high risk of ureteric damage.

Pelvic congestion syndrome

The existence of a syndrome characterized by CPP associated with dilated pelvic veins and venous congestion is still disputed. Women are typically in the reproductive years and complain of a dull ache in one or both iliac fossae that may have acute exacerbations. The pain is often relieved on lying down and made worse on standing or bending forwards. It is usually accompanied by dysmenorrhoea, backache, vaginal discharge, headache, urinary symptoms, deep dyspareunia, and post-coital ache. On abdominal examination, deep pressure over the 'ovarian point' (the junction of the upper and middle third of a line drawn from the umbilicus to the anterior-superior iliac spine) is said commonly to elicit pain in the iliac fossa. The vagina may appear congested and the whole pelvis may be tender. At laparoscopy, large, dilated, pelvic veins may be seen in the absence of other pathology; although pelvic venography is supposed to be the definitive diagnostic test it is still only employed as a research tool.

Psychological disorders

It is quite common to hear comments expressed by women with CPP like: 'One of the problems is doctors' attitudes towards women complaining of this sort of pain – they always seem to think "She is neurotic, therefore she says she is in pain". They never think "She is anxious because she *is* in pain".' On the other hand, psychological or psychosexual disorders may be the underlying cause of CPP or may alter the perception of chronic pain. A history of childhood sexual abuse is perhaps the best example. However, it is very difficult to dissect out such problems and deep offence may be caused in the process. We have no simple solution as specialized counselling skills are undoubtedly required.

Who should be referred to hospital?

It would seem sensible to refer any woman who has:

(1) pelvic findings, i.e. pelvic mass, tender uterosacral nodule;
(2) failed to respond to a course of antibiotics and/or simple therapies, i.e. painkillers or COC;
(3) infertility as well as pelvic pain;
(4) pain sufficient to restrict her daily activities;
(5) extreme concerns and anxiety herself about the possibility of pelvic pathology.

Thereafter, the decision to refer for a hospital opinion will depend upon the severity of the woman's symptoms, her own personal wishes, and the general practitioner's (GP's) philosophy of medicine. There appear to us to be two points of view: (1) the primary objective is to treat the woman's pain and if that is successfully achieved then the diagnosis is irrelevant; and (2) it is essential to establish a diagnosis in every woman with CPP and then treat the pathology that is found.

Unless adnexal pathology is detected on bimanual palpation, there would seem to us to be no need whatsoever to arrange a pelvic ultrasound scan 'just in case something might be detected'; however, there is no evidence as yet from randomized controlled trials to substantiate the statement.

Whether the woman is referred to a gynaecologist, gastroenterologist, or genitourinary medicine clinic will depend entirely upon which symptoms are predominant. As there is so much overlap between these disciplines, there is a strong argument for a 'one-stop' pelvic pain clinic where patients can be counselled by doctors from all three specialities and from pain-relief services and liaison psychiatry.

Laparoscopy

What is the value of a diagnostic laparoscopy?

Despite evidence that endometriosis can be diagnosed using magnetic resonance imaging and suspected on the basis of an elevated serum CA-125 level taken during menstruation, the diagnosis can reliably be made only on visual inspection of the pelvis.

Unfortunately, however, even laparoscopy may not be the gold standard. The accuracy of diagnostic laparoscopy depends greatly upon the experience of the gynaecologist, and upon other factors such as the quality of laparoscopic equipment, the thoroughness of the examination, and the presence of coexisting pelvic adhesions. Even if conditions are optimal, a negative laparoscopy may not exclude the disease as microscopic endometriosis can exist in visually normal peritoneum, although there is no evidence that this type of disease is of any clinical significance. Nevertheless, it is conceivable that laparoscopy may be too primitive a tool for accurate diagnosis and women with pelvic pain who have a negative laparoscopy may be falsely reassured.

It is also possible that we may be doing some women with pelvic pain a disservice by performing a diagnostic laparoscopy. Firstly, laparoscopy has associated morbidity and a mortality rate of 1 in 10 000. Secondly, if only microscopic disease is present or if the procedure is performed by an inexperienced surgeon, unfamiliar with the non-pigmented forms of endometriosis, the woman will be discharged from hospital believing that her pelvis is normal and she will be told that the cause of her pain is non-gynaecological. Lastly, and most important of all, finding 'pathology' such as endometriosis or adhesions, in the pelvis of a woman with CPP may not prove that the pathology is the cause of the pain.

Is pain more common in women with abnormal laparoscopy findings?

Although adhesions are found in approximately 20% of women being investigated for CPP, there is very little evidence of a causal relationship between the two. In fact, adhesions are quite commonly found in asymptomatic women having a laparoscopy for infertility. It has been argued, without much evidence to substantiate the claim, that the location of the adhesions and the nature of the adherent organs determines whether a woman experiences pain or not. Thus, an ovary that is adherent to the pelvic side wall because of endometriosis will cause pain whereas bowel that is stuck to the broad ligament will not.

The association between pelvic pain and endometriosis is standard teaching in gynaecology textbooks and is based upon a traditional view of the disease that antedates the widespread use of laparoscopy for the investigation of pelvic pain and infertility. It is also based upon the assumption that only blue-black spots and chocolate cysts constitute disease. Since the mid-1980s, however, more numerous manifestations of the disease have been recognized such as: white opacification of the peritoneum; glandular excrescences on the peritoneal surface, which in colour, translucency, and consistency closely resemble normal endometrium; red flamelike peritoneal lesions; unexplained adhesions between the under surface of the ovary and the peritoneum of the ovarian fossa. The question now arises, therefore, as to whether the association between pelvic pain and endometriosis is genuine given how commonly endometriosis can be found at laparoscopy and given the poor correlation between the severity of a woman's symptoms and the extent of the disease.

Three of the largest studies in the literature demonstrate how weak the association may in reality be. In a study of 1000 consecutive diagnostic laparoscopies, the incidence of endometriosis was only 8.2% (11/135) in women with pelvic pain or dyspareunia and 7.4% (2/27) in those with dysmenorrhoea or mid-cycle pain, and in a series of 515 laparoscopies, endometriosis was found in only 12.5% (15/120) of women with pelvic pain. Mahmood *et al.* (1991) investigated the prevalence of menstrual symptoms in women with endometriosis in a prospective study of 1200 women undergoing laparoscopy or laparotomy. Although dysmenorrhoea, dyspareunia, and pelvic pain were reported more frequently in women with endometriosis than in those without the disease, dysmenorrhoea, the most commonly reported symptom, had a positive predictive value (PPV) for the diagnosis of endometriosis of only 28%, with a negative predictive value (NPV) of 85% (sensitivity=68% and specificity=50%). Therefore, the authors concluded that menstrual symptoms were poor predictors of endometriosis.

The problem may be that gynaecologists have simply used inadequate means of assessing the severity of pelvic pain in such observational studies. When a more intensive assessment is made, there is some evidence of a greater association between endometriosis and pain. For example, in a study of 192 infertile women, using a multi-dimensional scoring system and a 10-point linear scale, Fedele *et al.* (1992) showed that dysmenorrhoea was as common in women with endometriosis as controls without the disease, but it was significantly more intense in moderate-severe disease than in minimal-mild disease or controls. Deep dyspareunia was reported more often in women with endometriosis than controls, regardless of disease severity; pelvic pain occurred more frequently only in women with moderate-severe endometriosis. Using a similar detailed pain history, Overton *et al.* assessed the predictive value of clinical criteria for the diagnosis of endometriosis in a prospective study of 100 consecutive diagnostic laparoscopies for pain and/or infertility (unpublished data). Severe dysmenorrhoea, i.e. pain sufficient to interfere with a woman's ability to perform daily tasks, was found to be highly predictive of endometriosis with a PPV of 95% (NPV=63%, sensitivity=41%, and specificity=98%).

Given the uncertain correlation between pain symptoms and endometriosis, only two logical conclusions are possible. Endometriosis may not be a cause of pelvic pain; in other words, finding the disease at laparoscopy may merely be coincidental – an irrelevance in the absence of coexisting infertility. Alternatively, different types of endometriosis may exist, only some of which cause pain. There is some evidence in the literature for the existence of different types of endometriosis. A research group in Leuven has described a type of disease that infiltrates deeply beneath the peritoneal surface and that is strongly associated with pelvic pain. However, they found no correlation between intensity of pelvic pain and any of the parameters traditionally used to assess disease severity such as the total area of endometriosis, the total volume of subtle endometriosis, or the presence of endometriomas. Philippe Koninckx, who heads the Leuven group, feels that two important clinical lessons emerge from the analysis of their data: (1) pelvic examination during menstruation is the best time to detect deeply infiltrating disease; and (2) deeply infiltrating endometriosis can be missed at laparoscopy, because even a large volume of disease can manifest itself at the peritoneal surface as only a small lesion.

Treatment

General principles

There are a number of measures provided by the GP that may provide pain relief and reassurance, without necessarily establishing a definitive diagnosis; for example:

(1) simples remedies such as herbal teas, or alternative practices such as acupuncture;

(2) advising a woman to avoid those positions that cause pain during intercourse;

(3) the use of the COC taken continuously to treat dysmenorrhoea (see below);

(4) exploring relevant past events such as a traumatic vaginal delivery or a termination;

(5) addressing problems associated with infertility;

(6) dispelling fears about malignancy, especially if there is a family history.

The traditional approach to CPP, however, is to establish a diagnosis and then offer treatment on the basis of the pathology found. Once a surgical diagnosis has been made, the treatments offered for endometriosis are given below. It is beyond the scope of this chapter to consider in detail the treatments available for IBS and chronic PID. There is little evidence that long-term antibiotic treatment for the pain associated with chronic PID is effective. It may be, as in endometriosis, that a total abdominal hysterectomy with removal of the tubo-ovarian masses is the only sensible option in a woman with extensive pelvic damage.

Endometriosis

Hospital-based treatment for endometriosis varies greatly. It depends upon the severity of the disease, the woman's symptoms, and desire to conceive. It will also be influenced by an individual gynaecologist's experience and the facilities available in that hospital.

Radical surgery is the best advice for a symptomatic woman over the age of 40 who wants a permanent cure for the pain associated with endometriosis. This implies resection of all endometriotic tissue, a total abdominal hysterectomy, and bilateral salpingo-oophorectomy, as there is a 50% likelihood of further surgery being needed if endometriotic ovaries are conserved at hysterectomy. Most cases, however, involve much more complex management decisions, especially in young symptomatic women with severe disease. The decisions must be taken after lengthy discussion as years after a surgical cure, some women forget their past pain and deeply regret the decision to be castrated. In such circumstances, it may be beneficial to attempt a therapeutic trial of a gonadotrophin-releasing hormone (GnRH) agonist before a final decision about surgery is made.

For young women, conservative surgery performed laparoscopically, with or without adjuvant medical treatment, is increasing being advocated. However, there is no evidence as yet that laparoscopic surgery is as effective as its proponents would have us believe. Studies reporting figures for pain relief have been largely uncontrolled, non-comparative, and have employed inadequate means of evaluating efficacy. It is bizarre that in an age when intensive clinical testing is required before a new drug can be marketed, novel and expensive surgical techniques can be introduced without well-controlled studies to demonstrate their safety and efficacy. Of interest, therefore, are the results of the first double-blind, randomized study comparing expectant management after diagnostic laparoscopy with laser laparoscopic treatment plus uterine nerve ablation, in the management of pain associated with minimal-moderate endometriosis (staged according to the American Fertility Society classification system, which depends upon the volume of endometriosis and extent of adhesions present). Better pain relief (63% v. 23% of patients) was reported in the active treatment group compared to the expectant group at 6 months follow-up (Sutton *et al.* 1994).

Hormonal treatments for endometriosis have traditionally attempted to mimic pregnancy or the menopause, based upon the clinical impression that the disease regresses during these physiological states. There is scanty evidence of a therapeutic effect for pregnancy; however, the hypo-oestrogenic state induced by lactation may, like the menopause, be beneficial. The modern aim of hormonal treatment is still to induce ovarian suppression in the hope this will lead to atrophy of endometriotic implants.

The options include a progestogen such as dydrogesterone (Duphaston) or medroxyprogesterone (Provera) or the COC (usually one with a high progestogen content, i.e. Eugynon 30) taken continuously. The COC is our suggestion for first-line treatment. The principal disadvantage of taking it continuously is that it can cause irregular spotting; some clinicians argue that this can be prevented by using a tricycle regimen of three packets taken continuously followed by a 1-week break. Unfortunately, there are very few randomized controlled trials assessing the use of these drugs in endometriosis related pain and one is forced to rely upon clinical anecdote. Nevertheless, if fertility is not an issue and if PID has been excluded clinically, then there is an argument

Table 15.2 *GnRH agonists*

	Drug	Proprietary name	Dose
Nasal spray	Buserelin	Suprecur	2 sniffs three times a day
	Nafarelin	Synarel	1 sniff twice a day
Injection	Goserelin	Zoladex	1 every 28 days
	Leuprorelin	Prostap	1 every 28 days

for a therapeutic trial of any of these drugs *without a definite laparoscopic diagnosis.* The COC, for example, will provide excellent symptomatic relief for many women and it has been shown, in a small study, to be as effective as a GnRH agonist. The role of non-hormonal therapy such as non-steroidal anti-inflammatory drugs, i.e. mefenamic acid (Ponstan) or naproxen (Naprosyn), has not been properly evaluated.

The drugs that are most commonly used in the treatment of endometriosis, danazol and GnRH agonists, are associated with numerous side-effects and should ideally not be used until laparoscopy has been performed. Danazol (a derivative of 17α ethinyl testosterone) has several modes of action but its principal effects are to raise free testosterone levels via testosterone displacement from sex hormone-binding globulin (SHBG) and SHBG suppression. Danazol is typically given at a dose of 200 mg three times a day until amenorrhoea is achieved, following which the dose can be titrated against the side-effects and reduced to 200 mg twice-daily/once daily, although it would appear that amenorrhoea is not a prerequisite for effective treatment. Its side-effects are largely androgenic and barrier forms of contraception are advisable as there are case reports of female pseudohermaphroditism in fetuses conceived on the drug. Despite low oestrogen levels during treatment, danazol does not induce bone loss because its androgenic properties are bone sparing.

GnRH agonists induce hypo-oestrogenism by reversible suppression of gonadotrophin secretion – a form of medical oophorectomy. At present, they are taken by nasal spray or subcutaneous injection (the different formulations are listed below in Table 15.2); the choice depends upon the patient's own wishes and cost considerations. The first action of these drugs is agonistic; therefore, some women will notice an exacerbation of their symptoms caused by an initial rise in gonadotrophin levels that results in high oestradiol levels for the first few days of treatment.

There have been a large number of randomized trials comparing GnRH agonists and danazol, all of which have demonstrated that the two types of drug are equally effective at relieving pain but their side-effect profiles differ. The side-effects associated with danazol and GnRH agonists are shown in Table 15.3. It is important to know in counselling patients that the voice changes associated with danazol can be irreversible whereas all the other side-effects tend to

Table 15.3 *Side-effects associated with danazol and GnRH agonists*

Danazol	GnRH agonists
Weight gain	Hot flushes
Bloating	Headaches
Hirsutism	Vaginal dryness
Acne	Decreased libido
Deepened voice	Irritability
Oily skin	Depression
Muscle cramps	Palpitations
Headaches	Joint stiffness
Hot flushes	Insomnia
Irritability	Bone loss
Depression	
Decreased libido	

disappear off treatment. In general, GnRH agonists tend to be associated with more hot flushes and headaches, and danazol with greater weight gain.

Treatment is usually given for 6 months after which most patients would expect to have their first period within 6–8 weeks. Although there are no specific data available to substantiate this claim, it is our experience that many women who have taken both types of drug express a dislike of the side-effects associated with danazol and prefer taking a GnRH agonist. Menopausal side-effects and the additional problem of bone loss may be resolved by the use of 'add-back therapy', an androgenic progestogen such as norethisterone, taken orally at a dose of 5 mg daily with or without low-dose oestrogen during GnRH agonist treatment.

The limitations of medical therapy should be obvious to all clinicians and **should be communicated to the patient**: a cure is unlikely as symptoms often return once treatment has ended. Women with endometriosis frequently complain that doctors provide them with insufficient information about the nature of the disease and the implications of treatment.

Some women feel so much better on treatment that they have no desire to stop taking the medication for fear of the pain returning. The use of GnRH agonists beyond the licensed period of 6 months has been advocated with the use of 'add-back therapy' but the practice is not common, principally because of the cost involved. Danazol can be taken beyond the manufacturer's recommended duration of 6 months but it is important to counsel patients about the small risk of developing hepatic tumours with long-term use. Long-term therapy is also theoretically inadvisable as danazol reduces high-density lipoprotein levels. The current practice in Oxford for such patients is to recommend 6 months' treatment with a GnRH agonist followed by a COC taken using a tricycle regimen. We recommend that therapy beyond the recommended duration, with drugs such as Provera, danazol and GnRH agonists, should not be initiated in general practice because of the uncertainties regarding long-term effects, especially on bone and blood lipids.

Alternative treatments include selenium, magnesium, calcium, vitamin E, zinc, and evening primrose oil, a rich source of gamma-linolenic acid, which blocks leukotrine production and is said by endometriosis sufferers to be effective treatment for pelvic pain. There are also anecdotal accounts of pain relief from acupuncture, homeopathy, hypnosis, and aromatherapy.

Chronic pelvic inflammatory disease

There is little evidence that long-term antibiotic treatment for the pain associated with chronic PID is effective. It may be, as in endometriosis, that a total abdominal hysterectomy with removal of the tubo-ovarian masses is the only sensible option in a woman with extensive pelvic damage. A protocol for the treatment of PID in current use in Oxford is Doxycycline 100 mg twice a day for 14 days (reduced to 50 mg twice a day if not tolerated well) and metronidazole 400 mg twice a day for 5 days. Review after 2 weeks – continue treatment for further 2 weeks if still symptomatic. If the woman is pregnant or breast-feeding, erythromycin 500 mg four times a day for 14 days (reduced to three times a day if not tolerated well). All contacts should be screened and tested.

Problems associated with making a diagnosis

It is easy to forget that CPP is a chronic condition and to ignore its full impact upon the lives of affected women. Pain impinges upon every aspect of a woman's life. For example, sex becomes unenjoyable and something to be avoided, which may not be appreciated by a partner; a boss may not relish constant absenteeism because of symptoms or visits to the doctor, etc. Many women are embittered by the treatment they receive from the medical profession, without realizing the difficulties inherent in making an accurate diagnosis and in treating the condition. Therefore, patient education is a vital part of the management of a chronic problem such as CPP and it is preferable to avoid the problem of women being shunted from one specialty to the next. Many women seem to benefit from a multi-disciplinary approach involving anaesthetists specializing in pain relief, gastroenterologists, liaison psychiatrists, and specialized nursing staff, but such resources are in limited supply. Advising women to join a self-help group such as the Endometriosis Society may be helpful.

Open dialogue is required to manage CPP effectively, we believe more than in virtually any other field of medicine, because the problems are often of such an intimate nature and difficult to confront for both the doctor and patient. The doctor must display as sympathetic an approach as possible and an open mind is essential as the medical literature cultivates some extraordinary misconceptions; for example:

'[Dysmenorrhoea] . . . may be a focus of complaints, self-pity, and hypochondriasis and may lead to frequent medical consultations . . . This syndrome seems to be particularly common in introverted, intellectualized, neurotic women of obsessive personality'.

The woman must be prepared to report her symptoms in as uninhibited a way as possible. Inadequate input from either party will often lead to inappropriate management, and it is not surprising that many women make repeated visits to their doctor before there is even mutual consent about the existence of a problem. Women are understandably embarrassed by questions about the most intimate details of their life. The point is well-illustrated by analysing the frequency with which women report dyspareunia to their GP. In a survey conducted by the Endometriosis Society in 1988 of 726 of its members, 55% suffered from dyspareunia but only 13% reported the symptom.

Women with endometriosis in particular contend they are adversely affected by a delay in making the diagnosis. They believe the disease becomes progressively more severe and therefore harder to treat the longer it is left undiagnosed. Consequently, their general health is affected and they suffer unnecessarily. As so little is known about the natural history of the disease, it is unfortunate that such criticisms cannot be answered. We simply do not know whether all women with severe disease had minimal endometriosis at some earlier stage and whether progression could have been prevented by medical intervention.

Useful addresses

The Endometriosis Society,
Suite 50, Westminster Palace Gardens, 1–7 Artillery Row, London SW1P 1RL.
Tel: 0171 222 2776.

References and further reading

Fedele, L., Bianchi, S., Bocciolone, L., Di Nola, G., and Parazzini F. (1992). Pain symptoms associated with endometriosis. *Obstetrics and Gynecology*, **79**, 767–9.

Hogston, P. (1987). Irritable bowel syndrome as a cause of chronic pain in women attending a gynaecology clinic. *British Medical Journal*, **294**, 934–5.

Howard, F. M. (1993). The role of laparoscopy in chronic pelvic pain: promise and pitfalls. *Obstetrics and Gynaecology Survey*, **48**, 357–87.

Mahmood, T. A., Templeton, A. A., Thomson, L., and Fraser, C. (1991). Menstrual symptoms in women with pelvic endometriosis. *British Journal of Obstetrics and Gynaecology*, **98**, 558–63.

Prior, A., Wilson, K., Whorwell, P. J., and Faragher, E. B. (1989). Irritable bowel syndrome in the gynecological clinic. Survey of 798 new referrals. *Digestive Diseases and Science*, **34**, 1820–4.

Sutton, C. J., Ewen, S. P., Whitelaw, N., and Haines, P. (1994). Prospective, randomized, double-blind, controlled trial of laser laparoscopy in the treatment of pelvic pain associated with minimal, mild, and moderate endometriosis. *Fertility and Sterility*, **62**, 696–700.

CHAPTER SIXTEEN

Urinary incontinence

Jacqueline V. Jolleys

Definitions

Prior to 1988, when The International Continence Society defined incontinence as 'the condition in which the involuntary loss of urine is a social or hygienic problem and is objectively demonstrable', there were many definitions of incontinence, each involving different timescales and degrees of wetting. Despite international agreement, the ICS definition has not achieved universal acceptance in that the Royal College of Physicians' Working Party on incontinence (1995) defined urinary incontinence as 'involuntary or inappropriate loss of urine which may be demonstrated objectively' and The US Department of Health and Human Services adopted the Agency for Health Care Policy and Research (1992) definition 'incontinence is the involuntary loss of urine which is sufficient to be a problem' as it was thought more relevant to clinical practice. Whatever the definition, most women know what they mean by incontinence – wetting themselves when they don't want to.

Prevalence

Urinary incontinence in women is a common symptom. The literature exhibits considerable variability in reported prevalence but differences between surveys are due to definition and method of inquiry used and population studied (Jolleys 1994). The exact prevalence of women suffering from incontinence is not known since reticence and embarassment mean that for many sufferers the condition is not volunteered and remains unrecognized by doctors.

Thomas *et al.* (1980), in a study of over 22 000 people on the practice lists of 12 general practitioners (GPs) in London, showed that the prevalence of urinary incontinence in women patients aged 15–64 years was 8.5%. This rose to 11.6% in women aged 65 and over. The health care and social services agencies were aware of approximately one-quarter of these sufferers. Similarly, the results of a MORI poll survey of 4000 men and women aged 30–70 years, published by Brocklehurst (1993), showed that 14% of women interviewed suffered from incontinence (N=2980); however, only one-third had sought medical advice at the onset of the complaint and a further third subsequently had consulted a doctor.

Several studies have shown the incidence of urinary incontinence to be very high in selected populations: Brocklehurst in 1972 in a community-based study of women aged 45–64 years found a prevalence of 57% (N=454); Milne *et al.* (1972) studied women in Edinburgh aged 62–90 and found a prevalence of 42% (N=272); Nemir and Middleton (1954) looked at nulliparous American students and found a prevalence of 52% (N=1327); Wolin (1969) studied nulliparous women and found a prevalence of 51% incontinence; whereas Crist *et al.* (1972) reported an incidence of 30% in his study of nulliparous women aged 21–63 years. These apparent variations may in part be explained by differing definitions and methods of eliciting the presence of incontinence. Osborne (1976) looked at working women aged 35–60 years and found a prevalence of incontinence of 26% (N=600). Incontinence is usually thought to be associated with ageing as the prevalence increases with age (Thomas *et al.* 1980; Jolleys 1988). However, these studies indicate that urinary incontinence is common not only in the elderly, but also in the middle-aged and young female. Thomas *et al.* (1980) in their community prevalence study showed the incidence of urinary incontinence (inappropriate loss of urine twice or more per month) to be high in all age groups. The study showed that once over the age of 25 years women have a 30% chance of suffering incontinence. In a prevalence study of women aged 25 years and over registered with my practice, 43% were regularly incontinent (Jolleys 1988).

Mechanism of continence

Continence depends on the effective function of the bladder in storing and voiding and the integrity of the neural systems which allow voluntary control of micturition. Continence is maintained, in dynamic terms, when the pressure in the bladder is lower than the urethral resistance and urine is voided when this is reversed. There are several aspects of bladder and urethral function which are essential for maintaining continence. The bladder is a highly compliant organ and can fill with only a small rise in internal pressure in the detrusor muscle (<10 cm water). The urethral sphincter contracts to impart a positive pressure sufficient to ensure urethral closure. The urethral sphincter should not relax inappropriately or incontinence may occur.

Voluntary inhibition of the voiding reflex is continued between voids. During coughing, sneezing, and physical exertion which result in a rise in the intra-abdominal pressure, sensory information is also transmitted to the proximal urethra and peri-urethral skeletal musculature of the pelvic floor to initiate further contraction in order to prevent a pressure differential occurring and possible leakage of urine.

Damage to the structures of the lower urinary tract, the urethral mucosa, the bladder neck, dyssynergism causing increased pressure to be exerted by the detrusor muscle, or from within the abdominal cavity, deficient proximal and distal urethral sphincter mechanisms can all result in incontinence. Incontinence can also result from disturbances to the neurological control of micturition. Afferent information is relayed back from the lower urinary tract to the central nervous system (CNS) at all levels between the spinal cord and the cerebral cortex, but especially the medulla and thalamus, by sensory nerves in the posterior columns and the lateral spinothalamic tracts. Bladder sensation of fullness and voiding is perceived bilaterally in the spinal thalamic tracts, so that damage to both tracts must occur before normal bladder awareness is lost. Any disturbance of the CNS may cause disorders of micturition. The hypothalamus controls autonomic nervous function and the higher centres suppress detrusor contractions. The main influence of the brain is to inhibit micturition but it also allows coordination of the voiding mechanisms in the pons and voluntary inhibition of the reflex in the cerebral cortex.

Mechanism of micturition

The normal micturition cycle comprises the storage of urine until it can be voided at a convenient time in a suitable place. Normally the higher centres of the brain inhibit reflex voiding until it is socially appropriate, and control the voiding reflex to initiate micturition. As the bladder fills the sensory stretch receptors in the bladder wall are stimulated, the first sensation occurring at approximately 150–200 ml. This sensation of filling is transmitted to the spinal cord via afferent nerves which in turn synapse with motor nerves which stimulate the reflex contraction of the detrusor muscle, initiating micturition. Reflex information is transmitted in the normal patient to and from the cerebral cortex and pons via pathways in the spinal cord, allowing inhibition of the reflex between voids. This also coordinates the reflex, preventing dyssynergia. As the higher centres reduce or cease inhibition of the reflex, micturition is initiated. This occurs normally during voluntary voiding but may possibly be a cause of incontinence. The initiation of micturition involves a coordinated relaxation of the the pelvic floor, relaxation of the urethral sphincter, and then contraction of the detrusor muscle. In women, voiding in the absence of detrusor muscle contraction is possible with merely the relaxation of the pelvic floor and urethra.

Factors associated with the onset of incontinence

Incontinence is often an age-related complaint with the majority of these patients suffering from urge incontinence. Many young women develop stress incontinence during pregnancy or after vaginal delivery. Although there is evidence to suggest that partial denervation of the pelvic floor is responsible (Snooks *et al.* 1984), the cause is probably multifactorial. Community studies using postal questionnaires have proposed factors (Yarnell *et al.* 1982; Jolleys 1988) by associating the onset of incontinence with obesity, the type of delivery, vaginal suturing, parity, previous gynaecological surgery, etc. Unstable bladder and urgency have been reported following hysterectomy and pelvic surgery has been shown to predispose to genuine stress incontinence (RCP 1995).

The multifactorial aetiology of the different types of incontinence has still to be established, and the varying degree to which women are susceptible to the development of incontinence explained.

Classification of incontinence

Classifying incontinence on the basis of presentation is useful since it helps the clinician identify the possible cause of incontinence and consequently the appropriate management plan. In order of decreasing prevalence the causes of incontinence in women are:

(1) stress incontinence;
(2) urge incontinence
   (a) motor urge incontinence
     (i) detrusor instability
     (ii) detrusor hyperreflexia
   (b) sensory urge incontinence
     (i) detrusor hypersensivity;
(3) overflow incontinence secondary to acute or chronic retention;
(4) continuous (passive or reflex) incontinence;
(5) fistulae (worldwide, genitourinary fistulae result from obstructed labour whereas in the UK pelvic surgery, cervical cancer, and radiotherapy are the usual causes);
(6) enuresis;
(7) miscellaneous, e.g. faecal impaction, urinary tract infection, confusional states, oestrogen deficiency.

Stress incontinence

Stress incontinence is the term used to describe the symptom of involuntary loss of urine on exertion in the absence of bladder contraction – associated with laughing, coughing, physical exertion, or sneezing. The cause is the overstretching or laxity of the supporting structures of the urethra or bladder neck and the weakness of the pelvic floor muscles.

It can be observed as loss of urine from the urethra when the patient raises the intra-abdominal pressure by straining or coughing. If this does not occur when the patient is lying on the couch, it may be demonstrated with the patient standing. Genuine stress incontinence, as defined by the International Continence Society, is the involuntary loss of urine which occurs when the intravesical pressure exceeds the maximum urethral pressure in the absence of detrusor contraction. Without conducting urodynamic studies it is impossible to determine who has stress incontinence with detrusor muscle contraction occurring on coughing, and who suffers from genuine stress incontinence.

Genuine stress incontinence is associated with urethral sphincter defect. It may occur during intercourse on penetration. Giggle incontinence is a form of stress incontinence which occurs when laughing.

Urge incontinence

Urge incontinence is the condition characterized by the involuntary loss of urine accompanied by the strong desire to void. It can be subdivided into two types.

Sensory urge incontinence

This is the involuntary loss of urine associated with urgency, and a strong desire to void urine immediately due to hypersensitivity of the bladder and urethral sensory receptors which may prevent the bladder filling normally. The cause may be infection (cystitis), irritation of the lining of the bladder or its outlet, e.g. calculus, diuretics, and emotions, e.g. anxiety and excitement.

Motor urge incontinence (unstable bladder)

This is when urgency, bladder contraction, and leakage occur simultaneously due to unstable detrusor muscle contractions, and is the common cause of urge incontinence. It is characterized by urgency, frequency, nocturia, and incontinence. The cause may be cerebrovascular atherosclerosis, a cerebrovascular accident, diseases affecting the nervous system, e.g. multiple sclerosis and Parkinson's disease, or injury to the higher nervous centres. Diuretics will often precipitate this form of incontinence. Detrusor instability can also occur at orgasm, causing incontinence during intercourse.

Although an unstable bladder cannot be demonstrated clinically, it can, using cystometry, when it is shown to contract spontaneously, or on provocation during filling (International Continence Society definition). In a stable bladder the volume of urine filling the bladder increases without causing a significant rise in pressure and no voluntary contraction of the bladder wall is seen on the cystometry tracing. The incontinent patient experiences the unstable bladder contractions as urgency – an excessive desire to micturate – or may be unaware until leakage occurs.

Overflow incontinence

Overflow incontinence is the over-distention of the bladder resulting in involuntary loss of urine and constant dampness due to dribbling. Incontinence occurs when the intravesical pressure exceeds the maximum urethral pressure. Long-standing obstruction to the outlet of the bladder results in bladder distention and loss of compliance. Effective detrusor muscle contractions can no longer occur and continuous leakage of urine results. This retention with overflow can occur when uterine fibroids or uterine prolapse obstruct urine outflow.

Raised intravesical pressure can lead to impaired renal function if not corrected since the high pressure causes obstruction of the upper urinary tract.

The neurogenic bladder can also present like this due to detrusor failure following trauma to or lesions of the cauda equina. Faecal impaction is a common cause of overflow incontinence in the elderly, often immobile patient. Diabetic neuropathy and tabes dorsalis also cause overflow incontinence, as can multiple sclerosis and Parkinson's disease.

Enuresis

Although this means incontinence it is generally understood to apply to nocturnal enuresis, or bed-wetting. Bed-wetting is very common in children; however, all but 1% have gained total bladder control by puberty. Urodynamic assessment usually reveals bladder instability.

Continuous (passive or reflex) incontinence

Continuous incontinence can occur due to a variety of conditions. If the patient is conscious of the loss (rare) it may be due to sphincter damage or degenerative changes. More usually the patient is unaware of the loss and emptying of the bladder occurs with no conscious awareness. Neuropathic bladder usually results from damage to the CNS due to illness, an accident, spinal injuries, spina bifida, or cerebrovascular atherosclerosis or stroke. Functional passive incontinence can also occur in the absence of neurological or urodynamic disorder due to psychiatric and emotional disorders, chronic immobility, physical disability, or drug inducement (sedatives and tranquillizers), drowsiness, and confusion states.

The effects of incontinence on patients and their lifestyle

Incontinence causes embarassment and anxiety. Patients fear 'accidents' and worry about smelling of urine. As a result people who suffer from incontinence lose their confidence, socialize less, reduce their fluid intake, and cease participating in sports. Patients who suffer from urinary incontinence may make dramatic changes to their lifestyle, often planning their entire lives around fears of having an accident in public or even confining themselves only to their own home. For some, the expense of pads and additional washing causes hardship.

Lois, aged 28 – suffers stress incontinence and sensory urge incontinence

'After my daughter was born – she is now two and a half – I couldn't even walk without wetting myself. It was so embarrassing. Sometimes I could not get out of the bed quickly enough to get to the loo. Things are a bit better now but I still need to wear a sanitary pad all the time. If I cough, sneeze, or jump I wet myself . . . Occasionally the sound of running water is enough to cause trouble.'

After several months of pelvic floor exercises and use of vaginal cones –

'They've helped a bit. I am not wet half so often. When I forget and lift heavy shopping I still leak.

I could not begin to consider going to step classes which I used to enjoy before having Verity. I still wear some protection.'

Dorothy, aged 67 – suffers from urge incontinence

I've had a bit of problem for as long as I can remember – probably since I went through the change. It's worse now than it was. I used to go to out to friends' houses for a drink and a chat. Three evenings a week I played whist. I hate this problem for the loneliness it brings. I'm forever going to make water and unless I am near the toilet I don't always make it. At first I used to drink less tea in the hope that it would help. But it didn't help. I still got caught short when out. I would go before I left home and even on the bus less than an hour later I would need to go. I'd get the stomach cramps and I'd be desperate to go. I held myself, stood up and walked around, fidgeted and cursed until I could hold myself no more. I gave up wearing slacks and plain coloured skirts because it showed. I was wet, felt dirty, and was embarassed. I felt everyone would smell me. As soon as the bus stopped I made a beeline for the toilets to clean myself up as best as I could. I just wanted to get home. It happens so much now I wear padding and I stay at home. You don't get embarassed there.'

The British Association of Continence Care MORI poll (Brocklehurst 1993) found that 13% of incontinence sufferers said their lifestyle had been greatly affected, 23% said a fair amount, 37% not very much, and not at all in another 23% of cases. Although only 3% had had to cease employment through incontinence, 15% of people with incontinence stated that they went out less as a result, and it had made 4% housebound. Incontinence can affect personal relationships as the sufferer may socialize less, and indeed, 2% reported seeing less of their friends, and one in 100, less of the family owing to incontinence. Five per cent said that they had given up sporting activities such as aerobics or running, and 4% social activities such as dancing. One in 10 had reported restricting lifting activities. One-third drink less when going out, and one in three made a conscious effort to locate public toilets in advance.

Worryingly, only 46% of people with incontinence said that they were very confident about going to the supermarket with 12% not very or not at all confident. For going on a long car journey, the proportion of those sufferers who were very confident fell to one in three with 28% not confident to do so. Similar percentages were able to go to the cinema or theatre and use public transport with one in four unable to do so. Less than half felt very confident about visiting friends or going out to dinner, and only one in three felt very confident about going to work.

Those with incontinence reported carrying spare underwear (10%), wearing pads (16%), wearing incontinence underwear (3%), using sanitary towels or nappies (8%), self-medicating (3%), learning pelvic floor exercises (11%), and reading information (6%). Similarly, 6% of women registered with my practice permanently wore protection against urine leakage, and 15% when participating in sporting activities. (Jolleys 1988). The frequent use of self-care measures by incontinent women has been reported in other studies which also confirmed that many of the products used were not designed as continence aids, and may therefore not be as effective as pants and pads designed for the purpose. However, the former are more easily purchased and are less indicative of a continence problem.

Moreover, the MORI poll revealed the extent of perceived stigma in that only 10% of patients with incontinence tell their spouses and less than 10% tell a close friend or relative. Encouragingly, two-thirds of sufferers had consulted their family practitioner although nearly one-third had consulted their GP after they had had the problem for some time.

Incontinence frequently affects sexual relationships. Women who are embarassed and ashamed often feel dirty and lose their sexuality. Not uncommonly, women who have stress incontinence fear intercourse since they may experience leakage of urine with orgasm. For the elderly, incontinence may jeopardize the chance to live in the place of one's choice, be it sheltered housing, an old people's home, with the family, or at home.

The role of primary care

There is a place for the management of urinary incontinence in primary care within the setting of family practice. This is complementary to the service of gynaecologists, urologists, and continence clinics. The prevalence of urinary incontinence is such that specialist continence services in England are already fully stretched, even though probably the majority of women with incontinence problems do not present to the family doctor.

Even in this day and age, when people talk readily and openly about sex, patients are still embarassed to talk about bodily functions. Patients do not readily volunteer incontinence symptoms so it falls to GPs and practice nurses to encourage patients to discuss these sorts of personal problems with them. Screening and clinic appointments provide opportunities for sensitive enquiry, e.g. well woman clinics, pre-conception counselling, antenatal and postnatal appointments, to help identify sufferers. Displaying posters on incontinence in the waiting room may facilitate this process at the same time as raising patient awareness of services available in the practice.

Incontinence is rarely presented as a dominant symptom and it may be introduced by a query relating to a physical symptom, e.g. 'something is coming down in front'. Presenting symptoms may also be frequency, urgency and associated urge incontinence, leakage/stress incontinence associated with posture change or physical exertion, and incontinence during intercourse.

Having elicited a continence problem, the GP can take a history and medically assess the patient. In the majority of cases the doctor will be able to diagnose the continence condition and offer a management plan in the form of treatment and advice. If he is unable to provide the necessary treatment at the practice, feels the patient needs urodynamic investigations, or is unable to reach a diagnosis, he can then refer the patient to the appropriate health care professional – urologist, gynaecologist, continence advisor, or a nurse with an interest in incontinence.

GPs can use their unique doctor-patient relationship to give support and understanding, encourage self-help, and restore the patient's self-esteem and self confidence. Patients can be given lifestyle advice literature which reinforces the doctor's explanation of the common causes of incontinence, its prevalence, and treatability. Since continuing care of the incontinent patient is an important part of the GP's role, doctors and practice nurses needs an understanding of current therapies, e.g. clean intermittant catheterization for a neurogenic bladder, in order to be able to support and advise their patients.

The diagnosis and management of urinary incontinence in the primary care setting

History

The majority of diagnoses can be reached from the history alone and confirmed by examination. The history should elicit:

1. *The exact nature of the incontinence*, the onset, e.g. after pregnancy, vaginal delivery, gynaecological surgery, etc., related or precipitating factors to the incontinence episode, e.g. loss of control with a full bladder, when coughing, sneezing, lifting, etc.

Take, for example, the patient who describes classical stress incontinence. This can be confirmed by asking appropriate questions and examining the patient. The following questions on incontinence can be used for diagnosis. They are validated and offer a means of reaching a clinical diagnosis on which a primary care management programme can be based. It will not be necessary to ask all the questions in every case. Often mixed incontinence is present so it is advisable to ask the questions relating to both stress and urge incontinence. Symptoms vary from patient to patient so for a minority the clinical diagnosis reached will not be the same as the actual diagnosis, which will only become apparent on urodynamic investigation.

Questions relating to control of micturition

- Do you normally get a feeling of warning to pass urine? (Absence of feeling may indicate neuropathy.)
- Will the first feeling go away before you eventually pass water? (The first feeling usually comes and goes. Persistent feeling before and/or after voiding suggests bladder pathology, e.g. cystitis.)
- Does the feeling disappear after passing water? (The feeling should disappear or there is a suggestion of bladder pathology.)
- Is there is any pain associated with urine leakage? (Pain is indicative of urinary tract infection, atrophic vaginitis/urethritis and occasionally of obstruction.)
- When you are ready to pass water does it come straight away? (Hesitancy indicates dysfunction or neurological problems of multiple sclerosis.)
- Do you feel you empty your bladder completely? (Negative response may indicate obstruction or residual urine volume.)

Questions relating to the severity of the incontinence

- How bad is your leakage? How much do you lose? How often?
- Do you have to change your under/outer clothes or wear pads? If so, how many?

Questions to confirm stress incontinence

Replies in the affirmative indicate stress incontinence.

- Do you leak urine when you cough, sneeze, or laugh without having the feeling of wanting to pass urine?
- Do you leak urine when you play sport, run, or jump without having the feeling of wanting to pass urine?
- Do you leak if you make a sudden movement?
- When you leak do you lose small amounts of urine?

Questions to confirm urge incontinence/detrusor instability

Replies in the affirmative indicate urge incontinence/detrusor instability.

- Do you go to the toilet more than six times a day?
- Do you have to hurry to reach the toilet in time?
- Do you leak before you can get there?
- Do you wet the bed in your sleep or do you leak before you can get to the toilet?
- Do you have to get up to pass water three or more times at night?

Questions to confirm passive incontinence

Replies in the affirmative indicate passive incontinence.

- Have you ever passed water without knowing it?
- Do you have accidents when you are in bed at night?
- Do you have frequent accidents?

Questions to confirm overflow incontinence

Replies in the affirmative indicate overflow incontinence.

- Do you have to strain to pass water?
- Do you dribble after you have passed water?
- After you have passed water do you ever feel as if your bladder is still full?

2. *Fluid intake history – volume and type.* Alcohol and coffee can actually have diuretic effects. In some cases the balance between continence and incontinence can be altered simply by cutting down on liquid intake.

3. *Drug history.* A drug history is important since diuretics, antidepressants, hypnotics, tranquillizers, anti-parkinsonian drugs, and anti-oestrogens can all affect continence.

4. *Medical history.*

Examination

Included in the physical examination should be the height and weight of the patient, abdominal and where appropriate rectal or vaginal examination; a urinalysis for sugar, protein, and nitrites; and a neurological examination of the patient if indicated. Further examination of the urine is indicated if urinary tract infection is suspected.

Abdominal examination, particularly of the elderly patient, may reveal a palpable loaded colon, treatment of which may alleviate the incontinence. Alternatively there might be a palpable, enlarged bladder after micturition retention. If there is also a palpable bladder after micturition the patient needs urgent referral to a urologist. It is useful to pass a catheter post-micturition and establish the residual volume of urine.

On vaginal examination there may be atrophic vaginitis which can result in urge incontinence. Stress incontinence may be demonstrated on cough voiding. Ability to contract of the levator ani muscle can be confirmed by asking the patient to squeeze your finger. Presence of a large prolapse, cystocoele, fibroids, or rectocoele, which can be associated with either urge or stress incontinence, would suggest the need for referral to a gynaecologist.

Exclusion criteria for primary care management

The following conditions are unsuitable for primary care management and require specialist opinion:

(1) vesico-vaginal fistula – refer to a urologist or gynaecologist;
(2) palpable bladder after micturition. Large residual volume of urine post-micturition – refer to a urologist;
(3) disease of the CNS – refer to a urologist or continence clinic;
(4) certain gynaecological conditions, e.g. fibroids, procidentia, rectocoele, cystocoele, and fibroids of a size requiring surgical intervention – refer to a gynaecologist;
(5) Failure to reach a diagnosis – refer to a continence clinic or urologist.

Who to refer for urodynamic investigation

Many female patients present not only with stress incontinence but also with urge incontinence or frequency and nocturia. These patients ideally require urodynamic assessment to establish the diagnosis and select a suitable treatment. For example, apparent stress incontinence may be found on urodynamic investigation to be due to bladder instability. It is not necessary to refer patients with stress incontinence alone for urodynamics as they generally have genuine stress incontinence due to pelvic floor weakness. If, however, after a 3-month trial of pelvic floor exercises they have not improved, they should be considered for referral.

Indications for urodynamic assessment

(1) Stress incontinence complicated by coexistance of other symptoms;
(2) Failure to improve incontinence with primary care management;
(3) Incontinence, following previous unsuccessful surgery;
(4) Voiding problems – difficulty with emptying the bladder and retention;
(5) Neurological problems, spinal injuries.

Jarvis *et al.* (1980) looked at the correlation between clinical diagnosis and cystometric diagnosis in 100 incontinent women. Cystometry confirmed the clinical diagnosis in 68% of cases. The confounding problem in 25% of cases was that women who were later diagnosed as having genuine stress incontinence presented with urgency. The authors concluded that accurate diagnosis based on clinical symptoms alone is difficult since patients with either detrusor instability or stress incontinence often present with symptoms indicative of both disorders. Even though it is agreed the correlation between clinical and urodynamic diagnoses could be better, experience of treating incontinent women in general practice without access to urodynamic tests, with treatment chosen on the basis of a diagnosis reached through history and examination alone, has shown that continence is promoted in the majority of cases.

Furthermore, since many patients requiring urodynamic assessment have to wait to be seen, it may be appropriate and beneficial to commence management of the condition prior to the diagnosis being confirmed since pelvic floor exercises, frequency – volume charts, and habit retraining cannot have deleterious effects.

Management

Management of stress incontinence

Conservative management

Physiotherapy in the management of stress incontinence is well-documented (Mandlestam 1980; Mohr *et al.* 1983). A programme of pelvic floor exercises is an effective treatment for stress incontinence irrespective of the age of the patient and duration of incontinence.

Since the treatment of incontinence is quite time-consuming and requires various skills, it is appropriate that management of the incontinent patient is conducted by the primary health care team. After the doctor has diagnosed the patient and counselled her, depending on availability and interest, a joint approach to management may be adopted by the doctor, practice nurse, physiotherapist, dietitian, and community nurse. Initially an explanation of stress incontinence is required so that the patient fully understands the condition and is highly motivated to be compliant with instructions. The overweight patient is put on a **reducing diet**. Having checked the patient's current understanding of pelvic floor exercises, the patient is instructed on how to do them (Laycock 1987), i.e. a programme of isolated contraction of the levator ani muscle while breathing normally (Box 16.1). This means that there should be no simultaneous contraction of the abdominal or gluteal muscles. Confimation of active contraction of levator ani can be obtained on vaginal examination if necessary. It is essential to explain that initially the exercise may be difficult to do for 4 seconds owing to the weakness of the muscles, but that with practice the exercise programme will become easier to execute with time. Offering patients written instructions improves compliance and reinforces the information given, since many patients forget the content of the consultation after leaving the surgery.

Fig 16.1 *Female patients with urinary incontinence who wish to be treated*

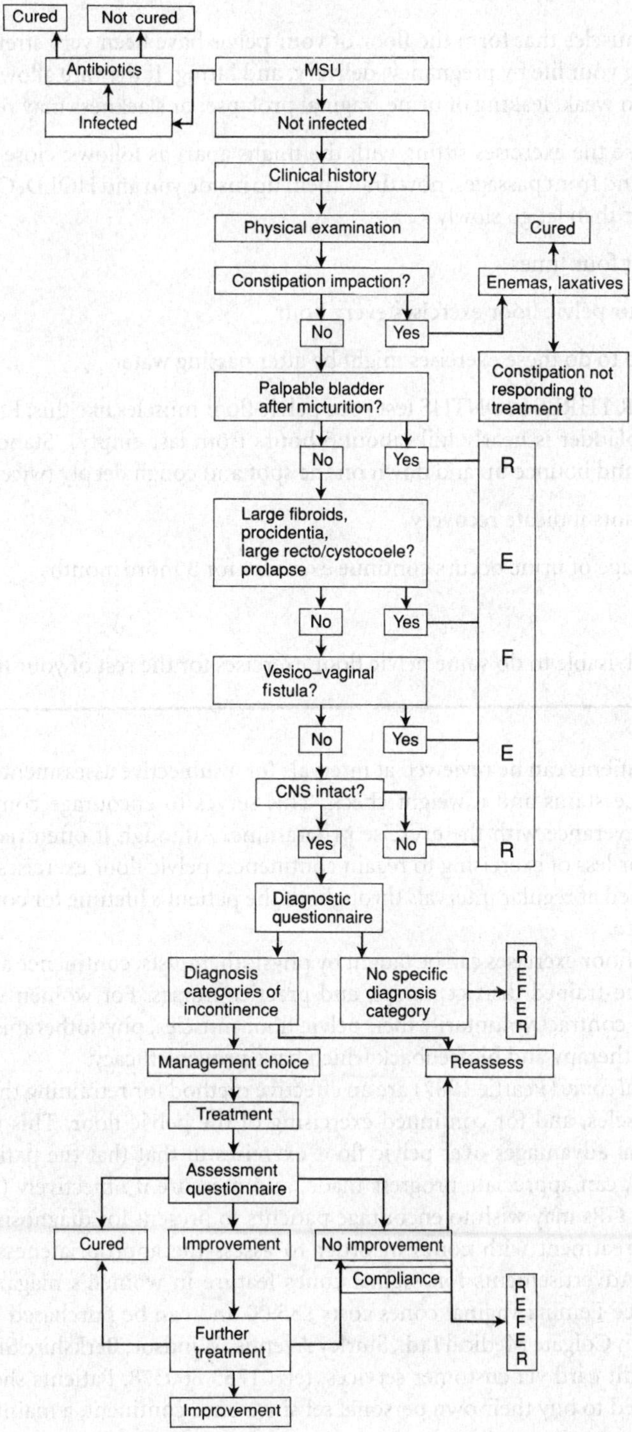

```
Cured        Not cured
   │            │
   └─── Antibiotics ───┐         MSU
              │        │          │
          Infected ◄───┴──── Not infected
                                  │
                             Clinical history
                                  │
                             Physical examination           Cured
                                  │                           │
                             Constipation impaction? ──► Enemas, laxatives
                                  │                           │
                              No     Yes                      │
                                       │                 Constipation not
                                       │                 responding to
                                       │                 treatment
                             Palpable bladder
                             after micturition?
                                  │
                              No     Yes ────────────────┐ R
                                                         │
                             Large fibroids,             │ E
                             procidentia,                │
                             large recto/cystocoele?     │ F
                             prolapse                     │
                                  │                       │
                              No     Yes ─────────────────┤
                                                         │ E
                             Vesico-vaginal              │
                             fistula?                     │
                                  │                       │ E
                              No     Yes ─────────────────┤
                                                         │
                             CNS intact?                  │ R
                                  │                       │
                              Yes    No ──────────────────┘
                                  │
                             Diagnostic
                             questionnaire
                                  │
                    ┌─────────────┴──────────────┐
              Diagnosis                      No specific      REFER
              categories of ──────────────►  diagnosis ─────►
              incontinence                    category
                    │
              Management choice              Reassess
                    │                           ▲
              Treatment                         │
                    │                           │
              Assessment                        │
              questionnaire                     │
                    │                           │
         ┌──────────┼──────────────┐            │
      Cured    Improvement    No improvement ───┘
         ▲         │          Compliance ──────────► REFER
         │    Further
         │    treatment
         │         │
         └─── Improvement
```

Box 16.1 *Pelvic floor exercises*

The muscles that form the floor of your pelvis have been very stretched during your life by pregnancy, delivery, and lifting. If they are allowed to remain weak, leaking of urine, vaginal prolapse, or slackness may result

Practise the exercises sitting with the thighs apart as follows: close your back and front passages, now draw them up inside you and HOLD. Count to four then let go slowly

Repeat four times

Do four pelvic floor exercises every hour

A time to do these exercises might be after passing water

AFTER THREE MONTHS test your pelvic floor muscles like this: Ensure your bladder is nearly full (about 3 hours from last empty). Stand feet apart and bounce up and down on the spot and cough deeply twice

Dry pants indicate recovery

If leakage of urine occurs continue exercises for 3 more months

Retest

It is advisable to do some pelvic floor exercises for the rest of your life

The patients can be reviewed at intervals for a subjective assessment of their continence status and a weight check. This serves to encourage compliance and perseverance with the exercise programme. Although it often requires 3 months or less of exercising to regain continence, pelvic floor exercises should be practised at regular intervals throughout the patient's lifetime for continued continence.

Pelvic floor exercises can be taught by physiotherapists, continence advisors, continence-trained district nurses, and practice nurses. For women who are unable to contract voluntarily their pelvic floor muscles, physiotherapists offer electrical therapy and biofeedback which have proven efficacy.

Vaginal cones (Peattie 1987) are an effective method for retraining the pelvic floor muscles, and for continued exercising of the pelvic floor. This method has several advantages over pelvic floor exercises in that that the patient can self-teach, can appreciate progress made, and measure it objectively (Wise *et al.* 1993). GPs may wish to encourage patients to present for diagnosis before starting treatment with cones in order to assess the appropriateness of the therapy. Advertisements for vaginal cones feature in women's magazines. A set of three Femina vaginal cones costs £35.00 and can be purchased by mail order from Colgate Medical Ltd., Shirley Avenue, Windsor, Berkshire SL4 5LH, or by credit card via customer services, tel: 01753 860378. Patients should be encouraged to buy their own personal set since once continent, a maintenance exercise programme is recommended for sustained effect. Usually cones need only be washed and dried after use although they may be boiled if preferred.

Some continence advisors and GPs may wish to loan patients sets of cones until their effectiveness is demonstrated, at which time patients may be encouraged to buy a set. Vaginal cones are made from heat-resistant plastic so that they can be autoclaved after use by one patient before being issued to another.

Along with exercise programmes it is essential to give advice on lifting correctly and avoidance of heavy lifting since this increases the intra-abdominal pressure and stretches the muscles of the pelvic floor. For this reason, it is advisable to instruct the patient to avoid the activities which precipitate incontinence until total control of urine flow has been regained.

There are **two new products**, neither of which is on the drug tarif as yet, available for the effective management of stress incontinence. One is the Coloplast sponge which supports the bladder neck and the second is a urethral plug 'Reliance'. Both have been shown to significantly reduce leakage and are suitable for women when active conservative treatment has failed, for women who are awaiting surgery, as well as those for whom surgery is not an option at the present time or who do not want surgery. Continence advisors have detailed knowledge of these innovations in conservative management as well as information on all containment products.

Surgical treatment

Conservative management will not significantly improve the symptom of incontinence or fail to cure it, if:

(1) the diagnosis is incorrect;
(2) the patient is not compliant with the management programme;
(3) severe damage to the pelvic floor muscles exists.

The patient requires referral to a specialist for urodynamic assessment and for a surgical opinion. There is no one surgical procedure which is suitable for treating all women with stress incontinence even though the principal indication for surgery is urethral sphincter incompetence. Surgery aims to elevate the bladder neck, correcting any anterior vaginal wall prolapse while raising bladder resistance. The choice of procedure is affected by the following considerations:

(1) surgeon's expertize in the procedures;
(2) surgical history of the patient;
(3) fitness of the patient;
(4) the need to treat other pathology;
(5) success rates for the different operations;
(6) incidence of post-operative bladder instability;
(7) mobility of the bladder neck at operation.

If childbearing is not complete, although it is appropriate to refer the patient and have a urodynamic assessment to confirm the diagnosis, it is appropriate to warn the woman that surgery is likely to be deferred until such time as her family is completed, as a subsequent vaginal delivery is likely to produce a recurrence of the incontinence.

There is no consensus as to the procedure of choice. Vaginal procedures are simpler with less morbidity and a short hospital stay, yet the beneficial effects of complicated retropubic procedures last longer. First surgery is likely to be the most successful, therefore selection of the right procedure at that time is essential.

The main procedures for the treatment of stress incontinence are suprapubic urethrovesical suspension operations (e.g. Burch colposuspension, whereby the vaginal fornices are used to support the bladder base in a sling procedure and the Marshall–Marchetti–Krantz operation) and endoscopic bladder neck suspension such as the Stamey procedure. In the Stamey procedure sutures are passed under endoscopic guidance on both sides of the bladder neck and tied anteriorly to the rectus sheath. The long-term prognosis for this procedure is poor although it is effective in the short term. It is used for older patients and those with poor anaesthetic risk. The vaginal approach anterior repair is often used but is less successful than the other procedures, and in many centres has been replaced by the suprapubic approach procedures.

Marshall–Marchetti–Krantz, Burch, and sling operations are carried out via an abdominal incision (a sling procedure also requires a vaginal incision) and are major procedures; more major than an anterior repair. The operation is usually followed by a brief period of catheter drainage and the patient may expect to remain in hospital for 7–10 days. Reported cure rates vary, depending on the centre, from 35–75%.

If there is vaginal wall prolapse as well as incontinence, a variation on the Burch procedure, when additional sutures inserted alongside the bladder base between the paravaginal fascia and ileopectineal ligaments provide additional support for the anterior vaginal wall, is particularly effective. Stanton and Cardoza (1979) reported an 86% overall cure rate at 2-year post-operation follow-up.

Patients need to be informed that post-operatively a gradual return to normal activity within 3 months is recommended, but that heavy lifting is to be avoided permanently. Intercourse should not be resumed until healing is complete, 2 months post-surgery.

A new minimally invasive surgical procedure offered by both gynaecologists and urologists is collagen implantation. Collagen is injected periurethrally under local or general anaesthetic to produce a physical reduction in the lumen of the urethra. Success rates and 2-year follow-up results are encouraging. In particular, collagen implantation could be a useful treatment for women who are unable to undergo surgery due to age, illness, etc. and use of collagen does not prejudice future surgery.

Finally, mention must be made of a non-surgical option for the management of incontinence due to uterine and/or vaginal wall prolapse and bladder neck descent. A ring pessary, accurately fitted, may relieve the symptoms of prolapse and incontinence. Some patients are so pleased with the result that they elect to continue wearing a ring pessary long term. For patients who present a poor surgical risk the ring pessary provides a safe, effective, alternative therapy which is changed every 3 months. Other women choose to wear a pessary temporarily while completing their family or awaiting surgery.

Management of urge incontinence

Conservative treatment

Getting the patient to complete a frequency/volume urinary output diary (Fig 16.2) for a period of 3 days to a week is an excellent way of clarifying the complaint since it establishes the frequency and pattern of voiding, as well as providing information relating to the volume of urine in the bladder prior to micturition (assuming complete voiding).

Subsequently, bladder retraining and psychological support is the treatment of choice (Jarvis 1980). In bladder retraining the patient is encouraged to void increasingly larger volumes of urine, gradually increasing the intervals between micturition, so relearning inhibition of abnormal detrusor muscle contractions. A rigid toileting regime should not be imposed on patients who are commencing habit retraining as too frequent emptying of the bladder (more than 2-hourly) without adjustments to suit the individual need may mitigate against restoration of continence by reducing the effective capacity of the bladder. The starting interval between voiding is taken from the frequency/ volume chart. If a patient is able to go 2 hours between voids then this would be a suitable interval between voids; however, if the chart shows that the bladder is usually emptied at hourly intervals or less, then hourly micturition would be appropriate.

On introduction of the toileting schedule, the patient is instructed to go the toilet to pass urine every half-hour or hour initially, depending on the severity of the condition. She must go to the toilet whether or not she needs to, even if she is already wet. The patient is instructed not to go to the toilet in advance of this time even if she fears an incontinence episode. She is instructed to keep to this toileting schedule until 2 whole days have elapsed without an incontinence episode. The micturition interval is then increased by half an hour and the process repeated until an interval of 4 hours is achieved. Patients are seen at regular intervals to assess progress which is recorded on micturition charts (Fig 16.3).

The unstable bladder is most successfully treated by a combination of retraining and drug therapy. Drug therapy aims to inhibit involuntary detrusor contractions in the bladder. Since the bladder has complex innervation no one single drug may be entirely effective. Available drug therapy lacks specificity and the unwanted anticholinergic side-effects limit their use. As with other drug therapy there may be initially a placebo response with apparent success, which rapidly falls off after several weeks as this placebo effect wanes.

Bladder retraining combined with anticholinergic pharmacological treatment aims to increase the time between micturitions by suppression of the reflex motor output to the bladder, thereby stabilizing the detrusor muscle. Drug treatment may be particularly helpful during the initial weeks of therapy

Fig 16.2 *A chart record of the frequency/volume of urine passed*
(*Reproduced with permission of Leicester General Hospital Continence Clinic*)

Go to the toilet when you want to go.
Measure the amount passed each time.

Date:													
Time	Vol.	Time	Vol.	Time	Vol.	Time	Vol.	Time	Vol.	Time	Vol.	Time	Vol.

when the patient's confidence is low and the clinical benefits of the training programme have not yet become apparent. The anticholinergic/smooth muscle relaxant oxybutynin 2.5–5 mg twice-daily or three times a day is the treatment of choice. Once continence has been regained many patients are able to sustain the improvement without the continued requirement of medication. All overweight patients benefit from weight reduction. An alternative but less fre-

Fig 16.3 *Daily chart record of micturation*
(Reproduced with permission of Leicester General Hospital Continence Clinic)

Go to the toilet every .... hours,
whether you want to or not, and whether you
are wet or dry.

Date: Day:	Wet or dry	Was urine passed	Wet or dry	Was urine passed	Wet or dry	Was urine passed	Wet or dry	Was urine passed	Wet or dry	Was urine passed	Wet or dry	Was urine passed	Wet or dry	Was urine passed
12 midnight														
1 am														
2 am														
3 am														
4 am														
5 am														
6 am														
7 am														
8 am														
9 am														
10 am														
11 am														
12 noon														
1 pm														
2 pm														
3 pm														
4 pm														
5 pm														
6 pm														
7 pm														
8 pm														
9 pm														
10 pm														
11 pm														

quently used adjuvent drug therapy is, for example, antidepressant imipramine 25 mg *nocte* or twice-daily.

Surgical treatment

The management of detrusor instability is medical, combining pharmacotherapy with physiotherapy. Only in the most severe intractable cases where conservative management has failed is sugery considered. Referral to a specialist urological centre is advised since the only reliable procedure is augmentation ileocystoplasty, when a section of the ileum is used to enlarge the bladder capacity.

Management of stress and urge incontinence

The treatment is a combination of pelvic floor exercises, bladder retraining, psychological support, and weight reduction.

Management of atrophic vaginitis

Treatment with local oestrogen preparations in the form of pessaries or cream, or with hormone replacement therapy is most successful in curing this complaint and the resulting urge incontinence.

Management of nocturnal enuresis

It is estimated that 10% of the adult population have an unstable bladder, of whom 1–2% adult females will have nocturnal enuresis. The enuresis may be (1) primary – the patient has never consistently been dry at night; or (2) secondary – the patient has relapsed after being dry for at least 1 year.

Prior to commencing treatment the following factors should be considered:

(1) Has the patient a urinary tract infection?
(2) Are physical or emotional problems involved? (Mobility, senility, neurological factors)
(3) Is there obstruction or a fistula?

The treatment of choice is desmopressin, a synthetic analogue of antidiuretic hormone, which may be administered nasally (Terho 1991) or orally. If this is ineffective, patients with detrusor muscle instability may be helped by treatment with oxbutynin or imipramine, but referral to a specialist is advised if a trial of therapy is ineffective.

Controversies

The diagnosis and management of incontinence causes much heated debate. Commonly raised issues include:

1. Discussion between gynaecologists and urologists as to whom are best trained to treat incontinent women. There is a subspecialist group of urogynaecologists who are experts in this field, but as yet very few are in post.
2. Is the management of incontinence a specialist or a generalist responsibility? Who should give advice and who is trained to? A centrally-funded working party has been set up to look at this and make recommendations with respect to the role and training of continence advisors and indeed the training of all health professionals in the management of incontinence. In the meantime, practice nurses could, with benefit, be encouraged to attend the short training courses organized for district nurses. Continence

advisors and clinics are usually pleased to have health professionals sit in on sessions.

3. Different procedures are offered by consultants to treat the same condition – which is the most effective in the short term and long term? There are long-term outcome studies in progress relating to the different surgical options for stress incontinence; however, interpretation of the results is further complicated by the variance in outcomes according to the expertize of the individual surgeons.

4. Is there primary prevention for urinary incontinence? This is being investigated by several centres. It is known that vaginal delivery causes stress incontinence and puts women at risk of faecal incontinence, but is the risk sufficient to suggest that elective caesarian section should be preferred? A risk–benefit profile of LSCS is needed. Can pelvic floor exercises prevent stress incontinence? Trials of pelvic floor exercises, commenced pre-conception, are in progress to see whether they may prevent the development of stress incontinence due to pregnancy and delivery.

5. When should a surgical treatment be recommended in preference to medical therapy? Medical therapy is the treatment of choice for urge incontinence. For stress incontinence the choice is less clear and cases need to be assessed individually.

6. How easy is it to distinguish between the different types of incontinence? In practice there may be some difficulty in clinical terms as one type of incontinence may coexist with another or indeed the symptoms overlap. Urodynamics is the only sure way of distinguishing between the types.

7. Are leaflets about pelvic floor exercises effective and useful? Can they be used as a substitute for instruction? There is a school of thought that they are of limited use unless it can be ascertained that the woman has control over her levator ani muscles and knows how to undertake isolated contraction, i.e. they are an effective reinforcement of instruction.

8. When should incontinence pads be used in preference to catheterization? Containment measures are only recommended when active treatment has failed. Ideally, the choice of method and product should be made in consultation with the patient and carer. Increasingly intermittant (self-) catheterization is taught to patients with long-term problems for comfort, mobility, etc. Advancing age is not a contraindication although lucidity and a degree of dexterity is required. Permanent catheterization, with its high risk of urinary infection, should rarely be used except in situations such as terminal care.

9. Women do not volunteer the symptom of incontinence so should health professionals be proactive and enquire after it or are they only discovering morbidity about which they can do little? General practice has a lot to offer sufferers of incontinence – it can be cured. Health promotion is a feature of general practice and there are many opportunities to ask women about continence, e.g. with having a smear, postnatally, and elderly health checks. Additionally, women welcome the chance of unburdening themselves,

gaining relief from knowing that they are not the only ones to suffer, that the condition is treatable, and that they need not be ashamed.

Conclusion

Currently incontinence is believed to consume 2% of health care funding, with projected spending in the future set to rise as the population becomes weighted towards the elderly. General practitioners are ideally placed to elicit and alleviate continence problems, which are the cause of much human misery and embarassment and may affect and restrict family relationships. Since the prevalence of incontinence increases with age, projected changes in population demographics mean that in future GPs will care for increasing numbers of incontinent patients. Fortunately, many patients can be treated satisfactorily by GPs using non-invasive interventions. As GPs gain expertize in the management of incontinence, unnecessary referrals can be avoided and consultant referral for urodynamics and management can be reserved for those patients with more complicated or serious problems.

Useful addresses

Age Concern,
60 Pitcairn Road, Mitcham, Surrey CR4 3NT.
Tel: 0181 648 5792)
Advice on special problems of the elderly.

Association for Continence Advice,
Winchester House, Kennington Park, Cranmer Road, The Oval, London SW9 6EJ.
Tel: 0171 820 8113.
List of continence advisers; product range information.

The Continence Foundation,
The Basement, 2 Doughty Street, London WC1 2PN.
Tel: 0171 404 6875.
A continence resource centre. Information on publications, management, aids, and special clothing. Directories of professionals and services.

Enuresis Resource and Information Centre (ERIC),
65 St Michaels Hill, Bristol BS2 8DZ.
Tel: 01179 264920.
Advice and information on bedwetting for patients, carers, and professionals.

Newcastle Council for the Disabled: continence advisory service,
The Dene Centre, Castles Farm Road, Newcastle upon Tyne NE3 1 PH.

Royal Association for Disability and Rehabilitation (RADAR), 25 Mortimer Street, London W1N 8AB.
Holidays for the disabled. Toilet-for-the-disabled keys.

References and further reading

Brocklehurst, J. (1993). Urinary incontinence in the community – analysis of a MORI poll. *British Medical Journal*, **306**, 832–4.

Jarvis, G. J. (1980). An assessment of urodynamic assessment in incontinent women. *British Journal of Obstetrics and Gynaecology*, **87**, 893.

Jolleys, J. V. (1988). The reported prevalence of urinary incontinence in women in a general practice. *British Medical Journal*, **296**, 1300–2.

Jolleys, J. V. (1989). Diagnosis and management of female urinary incontinence in general practice. *Journal of the Royal College of General Practitioners*, **39**, 277–9.

Jolleys, J. (1994). Incontinence: Diagnosis and management in general practice. Royal College of General Practitioners clinical series, London.

Jones, E. G. (1965). Non-operative treatment of stress incontinence. Obstetrics and Gynaecology, **6**, 220–35.

Kegel, A. H. (1951). Physiologic therapy for urinary stress incontinence. *Journal of the American Medical Association*, **146**, 915–17.

Laycock, J. (1987). Graded exercises for the pelvic floor muscles in the treatment of urinary incontinence. *Physiotherapy*, **73**(7), 371–3.

Mandelstam, D. (1980). Stress incontinence. *Nursing*, **18**: 787–8.

Mandelstam, D. (1986). *Incontinence and its management* (2nd edn). Crook Helm, London.

Mohr, J. A., Rogers, J., Brown, T. N., and Starkweather, G. (1983). Stress incontinence: a simple and practical approach to diagnosis and treatment. *Journal of the American Geriatric Society*, **31**, 476–8.

Peattie, A.B., Pleunik, S., and Stanton, S. (1987). Cone: a conservative method for managing genuine stress incontinence. *British Journal of Obstetrics and Gynaecology*, **89**, 1026–30.

Royal College of Physicians Working Party (1995). *Incontinence causes, management, and provision of services*. RCP, London.

Snooks, S. J., Setchell, M., Swash, M., *et al.* (1984). Injury to innervation of pelvic floor scphincter musculature in children. *Lancet*, **ii**, 546–50.

Stanton, S. and Cardoza, L. (1979). The colposuspension operation for incontinence and prolapse: clinical aspects. *British Journal of Obstetrics and Gynaecology*, **86**, 693–7.

Terho, P. (1991). Desmopressin in nocturnal enuresis. *Journal of Urology*, **145**, 818.

Thomas, T. N., Plymat, K. R., Blannin, J., and Meade, T. W. (1980). Prevalence of urinary incontinence. *British Medical Journal*, **281**, 1243–5.

Wise, B., Haken, J., Cardozo, L., and Plevnik, S. (1993). A comparative study of vaginal cone therapy, Kegel exercises and maximal electrical stimulation in the treatment of female genuine stress incontinence. *Neurology and Urodynamics*, **12**(4), 436–7.

Yarnell, J. W. G., Voyle G. J., Sweetnum P. M. *et al.* (1982). Factors associated with urinary incontinence in women. *Journal of Epidemiology and Community Health*, **36**, 58–63.

CHAPTER SEVENTEEN

Emotional disorders

Susanna Graham-Jones and Fiona Duxbury

How do you cope with your patients' emotional problems? Helping anxious and depressed patients is a daily challenge in general practice; for many doctors it is a significant source of stress. In this chapter we have drawn on our experience of dealing with vulnerable women, men, and their families in rural and inner-city practices. We describe some common presentations of emotional distress, illustrating some of the coping strategies which we have found useful.

Much of the stress is associated with a group of patients described by O'Dowd (1988) as 'heartsink' patients, 'a disparate group of individuals whose only common thread seems to be the distress they cause their doctor and the practice'. Some of these patients may also be classified by the practice as 'frequent attenders' who present often, sometimes with minor illness, often with a cluster of troublesome and recurrent symptoms. Women are over-represented in both these groups. It has recently been shown that general practitioners (GPs) who think they have many 'heartsink' patients report 'a greater *perceived* workload and less job satisfaction than other GPs, and fewer postgraduate qualifications and training in counselling and/or communication skills' (Mathers *et al.* 1995).

Family doctors detect around 60% of the psycho-social problems of their patients in routine consultations; the detection of depression has been the subject of many studies using waiting-room questionnaires to screen attenders (Goldberg *et al.* 1988). There are many factors contributing to this stalemate, including the stigma associated with 'mental illness'.

We hope that this chapter will help GPs to reflect on how emotional disorders present in general practice, and enable them to negotiate appropriate management plans for patients. Mathers and Gask (1995) point out that a positive outlook lightens the perceived burden of 'heartsink' patients.

The range of emotional disorders

The patterns of psychological morbidity most commonly encountered in general practice are outlined below. Eating disorders are discussed in Chapter 18 and psychosexual problems in Chapter 19; see also Chapters 8, 9, 10, and 11 for discussion of distress associated with gynaecological problems. We have not included any discussion of psychotic disorders.

The emotional disorders discussed here are extremely common; the fourth national collation of Morbidity Statistics from General Practice (MSGP4) puts consultation rates for mental disorders second only to those for acute respiratory infections. Over 7% of the population consult a GP for this reason each year; women have the highest prevalence rate: 944 per 10 000 woman-years at risk. Recent guidelines emphasize that up to 50% of general practice attenders may have some depressive symptoms, with 5% fulfilling criteria for major depression (see below).

Emotional disorders are far from distinct, and often overlap. The MSGP4 study suggests a 15–20% reduction in consultations by women for mental disorders in the last decade; this was associated with a shift in diagnosis away from such terms as 'anxiety state' and 'hysteria', towards symptoms classified as 'neurasthenic'. Vexed questions of diagnosis can be addressed with the help of the *Diagnostic and statistical manual of mental disorders* (DSM-IV 1994) of the American Psychiatric Association; as this is compatible with the current version of the *International classification of diseases* (ICD 10) it is relevant and useful in UK practice. As for severity, we note that symptom severity often seems to vary inversely with the amount of social and emotional support available to the sufferer.

Anxiety

There are many different manifestations of anxiety:

1. *Free-floating or generalized anxiety* impairs concentration and memory, and is characterized by restlessness, irritability, muscle tension, headaches, sleep disturbance, and fatigue. Patients are aware that they worry excessively. Some label themselves as depressed because they are prone to crying; but this may be a way of dealing with tension, as pointed out in DSM-IV.

2. *Phobic anxiety*: claustrophobia (fear of being confined), agoraphobia (fear of going out), phobic avoidance of certain stimuli such as spiders or reptiles; the patient may or may not be aware how the symptoms have arisen. The symptoms often take a similar form to:

3. *Panic attacks*: the experience of the 'fight or flight' physiological response to danger. Hyperventilation is often part of a panic attack with air hunger ('I can't get enough air'), palpitations (from adrenergic tachycardia), light-headedness and faintness, and paraesthesiae and occasional muscle spasms in hands, feet, and face, due to shifts in intracellular calcium associated with carbon dioxide wash-out from lungs in hyperventilation. Feelings of depersonalization ('I'm outside myself') and derealization ('everything feels unreal') are not uncommon. The attacks can be terrifying, and some sufferers actually think they are going to die.

4. *Post-traumatic stress disorder*: this can occur at any age, and can occur soon after the precipitating events or remain dormant for many years. It may

Box 17.1 *Post-traumatic stress disorder diagnostic criteria, from DSM-IV*

1. Exposure to a traumatic event involving threat of death or serious injury to self or others, with reaction including intense fear, helplessness, or horror (includes agitated behaviour in children)

2. *Intrusive symptoms*
   The traumatic event is persistently re-experienced, with
   distressing intrusive recollections or images, recurrent dreams or nightmares
   reliving the experience with flashbacks
   intense distress and somatic symptoms on exposure to relevant 'cues'

3. *Avoidance symptoms*
   avoidance of associated thoughts/feelings/anything arousing recollections of trauma
   inability to recall important aspects of trauma
   loss of interest in significant activities, detachment or estrangement from others
   restriction of normal feelings (may be incapable of love)
   sense of foreshortened future (lacks normal expectations)

4. *Increased arousal (anxiety)*
   difficulty in falling asleep or staying asleep, irritability or outbursts of anger
   poor concentration, increased vigilance, exaggerated startle response

To fulfil DSM criteria, symptoms must last for at least 1 month and cause clinically significant impairment in social, occupational, or other important areas of functioning. PTSD is described as 'chronic' when it lasts for more than 3 months, and 'delayed onset' if symptoms first occur 6 months or more after the traumatic events

be triggered by domestic violence, assault, childhood sexual abuse, rape, torture, wartime atrocities, or witnessing disaster in any form. Survivors often feel 'numb', unable to talk about their experiences (see Box 17.1). They may also feel ashamed, humiliated, and even guilty; they feel they ought to be able to cope (Dunn and Gilchrist 1993).

Adjustment reactions

These follow life events at work or in the family, and include the effects of job loss, illness, retirement, marital breakdown, moving house, culture shock, and bereavement (Parkes 1986). Adjustment disorders may present with depressed mood, anxiety, conduct disorders, or a mixture of any of these.

The stages of bereavement are now widely recognized (Box 17.2); these apply to other losses too. Most people go through family bereavement without needing medical help; but those with poor coping skills, lack of social support,

> **Box 17.2** *The five stages of bereavement (after Kubler-Ross 1970 and Parkes 1986)*
>
> *Stage 1:* denial, disbelief: 'this isn't really happening to me'
>
> *Stage 2:* anger and guilt, especially after abrupt losses: 'how could he do this to me?' or 'this would never have happened if I had . . .'
>
> *Stage 3:* anxiety is pronounced, with longing and yearning which can include pseudohallucinations: 'I saw her just ahead of me in the street' or a sense of unreality
>
> *Stage 4:* the penultimate stage is that of a depressive reaction, with feelings of deep sadness and loss
>
> *Stage 5:* acceptance of the loss, resignation, and recovery of near-normal social functioning

or a history of mental illness may be more at risk for atypical or severe grief reactions. Bereavement may also be complicated when it follows a long terminal illness, or a very sudden and unexpected death.

Psychosomatic problems

Various manifestations of stress and arousal come under this heading, such as 'tension' headaches, migraine, exacerbations of eczema and asthma, irritable bowel, and premenstrual tension.

Somatization disorder (Mayou 1991; Wilkinson and Bass 1994) is now recognized in DSM-IV as a specific entity; these patients present repeatedly, starting before the age of 30 years, with one or many symptoms for which no organic cause can be found. The range of symptoms is limitless and may include various bizarre syndromes. The symptoms usually distress the patient, and are not intentionally produced. Some somatizers are keen on hospital investigations and may be willing to undergo invasive tests or operations, rather than coming to terms with psychological explanations for their symptoms. Munchhausen's syndrome appears to be a severe manifestation of somatization disorder.

Problems of dependence

Drugs of addiction include alcohol, benzodiazepines, opiates, and other 'street' drugs, as well as nicotine (Kemp and Orr 1996; Women in Medicine 1996). Most patients using opiates keep their drug habit secret from their GP for years, fearing rejection by the doctor. Others ask for support in various ways; they may request 'something to help me come off the drugs', i.e. detoxification. Some request maintenance prescribing, usually of methadone (see p. 521).

Depression

Depression is often accompanied by anxiety, and may come on gradually or episodically as in 'dysthymic disorder' (DSM-IV).

Major depression is present in about 5% of attenders in general practice. It is twice as commonly diagnosed in women as in men, with a 10–25% lifetime risk. It is commonly associated with physical illness, which may delay diagnosis (Tylee *et al.* 1993). The incidence is higher in first-degree relatives. Criteria for major depression include a constantly depressed mood or loss of interest or pleasure and at least four of the other symptoms below, all present during the same 2-week period and representing a change from previous functioning:

(1) weight loss or weight gain, eating disturbance;

(2) sleep disturbance, with early morning waking or excessive sleep;

(3) low energy or fatigue;

(4) psychomotor disturbance (can be restless, agitated, or retarded);

(5) poor concentration, difficulty making decisions, memory failure (pseudo-dementia);

(6) low self-esteem, worthlessness, guilt, self-blame;

(7) recurrent thoughts of death, suicidal ideas, plans, or attempts.

Bipolar affective disorders include manic episodes as well as major depressive episodes, often with psychotic features. The distinction between 'reactive' and 'endogenous' depression is no longer regarded as useful, because all depressive episodes can be exacerbated by adverse circumstances. DSM-IV uses a multi-axial classification for the range of 'mood disorders' with reference to severity, natural history, familial patterns, and culture-specific features. It is worth noting that it is incorrect to diagnose an affective disorder without first excluding general medical disorders, drugs and toxins, other organic causes such as dementia, and thought disorder.

Self-harm and parasuicide

Parasuicide is attempted suicide, often by drug and alcohol overdose, and often an impulsive action in the context of relationship difficulties. Commoner in young women than in men, it is commonly called 'a cry for help'. It carries a significant recurrence rate and risk of successful suicide, particularly within a year of a previous attempt. 40% of those who kill themselves have seen a doctor within the month before their death (Gunnell and Frankel 1994).

Self-harm includes cutting, typically on the forearms, or burns from lighted cigarettes. Misuse of alcohol or drugs may also contribute to a recognizable pattern of self-harm. Such patients have low self-esteem and may indeed feel completely worthless, although there may be no other signs of depression. There may be a history of sexual abuse (Cahill *et al.* 1991).

Personality disorders

GPs are reluctant to diagnose personality disorder; it feels like passing sentence. It involves labelling people as potentially antisocial, difficult, aggressive, lacking in respect for the boundaries or conventions within which we practise. The very term 'personality disorder' has in the past implied that such people are untreatable.

Box 17.3 *Borderline personality disorder: diagnostic criteria (abbreviated from DSM-IV)*

A long-lasting pattern of unstable personal relationships and self-image with five or more of the following characteristics:
* frantic efforts to avoid abandonment, real or imagined
* unstable and intense relationships, swinging between idealizing and devaluing others
* persistently low self-esteem, unstable and denigrating self-image
* potentially self-damaging impulsivity, e.g. reckless spending, substance abuse, sex, binge-eating
* recurrent self-harming or suicidal behaviour or threats
* intense mood swings and irritability
* chronic feelings of emptiness
* inappropriate intense anger and difficulty controlling it
* transient, stress-related, paranoid thinking or dissociative symptoms, 'blanking out' and appearing numb and unfeeling at times when others would show strong emotions

---

Clearly, people with 'personality disorders' do have disturbed relationships: they may be unable to nurture others, emotionally cut off, emotionally over-dependent, manipulative, paranoid, obsessional, or rigid. Although GPs are not likely to be concerned with the niceties of psychiatric diagnosis, we include here (see Box 17.3) a description of 'borderline personality disorder', which is now being recognized as a possible consequence of child sexual abuse as well as experience of early parental loss or separation (Browne and Finkelhor 1986; Briere and Runtz 1987).

Where do heartsink patients fit in?

'Heartsink' is a manifestation of stress and unhappiness in doctors, particularly GPs (Mathers *et al.* 1995). Different patients will provoke 'heartsink' with different doctors, but there are some patients who make most of those who care for them feel hopeless and even angry. GPs are likely to suffer in this way because they cannot easily escape from their patients.

From the syndromes we have described, there are some that are particularly likely to be associated with heartsink. People with **borderline personality** can be very attention-seeking and manipulative. They, and others who are prone to **self-harm, problems of substance abuse and dependence**, and **eating disorders**, are certainly anxiety-provoking for carers and GPs. Their lack of 'boundaries' is evident; they may appear to invite rejection by missing appointments, turning up late, or calling inappropriately for home visits; with the consequence that they are ejected from one doctor's list after another.

Post-traumatic stress disorder (PTSD) is classified with the anxiety disorders. However, patients will differ as to how much they can recall of the trauma (see Box 17.1), and often 'avoidance' features will obscure the diagnosis. Sufferers from PTSD, like **chronic somatizers**, may present puzzling patterns of symptoms to the GP, taking years to disclose the trauma which has distorted their lives. The importance of enabling GPs to recognize such behaviour patterns has become clear to us in clinical practice.

Causes of emotional disorders

Individuals develop as a result of a complex interplay between genetics, gender, personality, and social support systems. Events, family circumstances, and styles of interaction contribute to early and later experience, and influence feelings and behaviour. Research has demonstrated **strong associations between environmental events and patterns of emotional disorders**. We feel that the recognition of these links is often helpful to patients, countering the stigma attached to the 'disease' labels used in the past. Moscarello (1991) notes 'the reluctance on the part of many workers in the field of women's mental health to acknowledge the diagnosis of post-traumatic stress disorder. The woman becomes identified as a patient, then a psychiatric patient, both of which are viewed as imposing a **second injury** or wound; [whereas] the experience of health care workers [caring for survivors of sexual assault] is that when women are informed about the diagnosis of post-traumatic stress disorder, they experience a feeling of relief'.

What is it, apart from the degree and type of trauma, that determines whether or not a victim of rape or trauma experiences post-traumatic stress disorder? The capacity to survive unharmed may originate in a supportive family; according to Nemiah (1995) 'stable family origins and a favourable childhood upbringing provide adults . . . with the psychological strength to master such traumatic [war] experiences'. Winnicott (1965) makes a general link between 'good enough' parenting and a child who develops a positive self-image and is 'robust enough to weather these storms' (see also Ashurst and Hall 1989).

In general practice we are well-placed to identify at-risk patients before they succumb to emotional strain. Brown and Harris (1978) linked several social factors to an increased vulnerability to depression amongst urban women. The relevant factors, picked out from a wide range of variables, were:

(1) loss of mother before age 11;

(2) being from a working-class background;

(3) having three or more children under the age of 14 at home;

(4) being unemployed;

(5) lack of a confiding, intimate relationship with spouse.

This research backs up the common-sense conclusion that that the more social problems a woman has to deal with, the more vulnerable she is to additional life stresses and events. Disease gradients across the socio-economic classes have worsened in recent decades, such that many diseases are more prevalent in people with fewer economic resources. Primary care teams, with their knowledge of family circumstances, will continue to be aware of the need to target care to vulnerable individuals and families whose emotional reserves are drained by poverty.

Sex differences: nature or nurture?

Women certainly have no monopoly on psychological distress. Several studies confirm that 'when rates of all types of mental disorders are examined, including alcoholism, drug abuse and . . . antisocial behaviours in addition to . . . subjective distress, women and men evidence similar disorder rates' (Dohrenwend and Dohrenwend 1976). Clare and Jenkins (1985) found that in comparable groups of childless men and women (students and civil servants) there was no difference in prevalence or outcome of depression or minor psychiatric morbidity.

Women do, however, present symptoms of anxiety and depression to GPs twice as often as men do (MSGP4). Why is this? Clare and Jenkins (1985) refute the myth of the 'weaker sex'. They conclude that emotional disorders in women are overwhelmingly caused by social factors. Most women have had lower social status than men; many are economically dependent on men. We have referred already to Brown and Harris's (1978) study of factors associated with vulnerability to depression in urban women. Another study suggested that marriage is associated with better mental health for men but not for women (Gove 1979).

Schwartz (1991) believes that the preponderance of women in psychiatric statistics is not attributable only to 'role stress', nor to the necessity for women to play several different roles. 'Morbidity' statistics reveal a gender difference in the way men and women are conditioned to seek help. The socially sanctioned way for women to react to stress is to carry on at home and at work but to manifest psychological or psychosomatic symptoms. When these symptoms become too severe for them to behave normally, many women come to expect help from doctors, medication, and, increasingly, counselling.

Boys and men experience different social pressures from those of women, and as a result are less inclined to 'medicalize' their problems. Instead, when stressed, they are inclined to drink more alcohol, to become less communicative (Rout 1996), and to 'act out' in physical ways. The combination of alcohol and domestic violence is a well-known and distressing example. Violent behaviour lands some men in prisons, where untreated depression and anxiety are rife and suicide rates are high. Even if they consciously feel 'stressed', men are less likely than women to come to doctors; the 'macho image' promotes denial, and does not sanction such help-seeking. The problem is not perceived as an illness, and doctors are not therefore sought out as helpers.

These gender differences are, of course, not absolute. Particularly under conditions of extreme social stress in deprived inner-city areas, women too may resort to release of intolerable tension through violence towards themselves and others.

Hormonal and neurochemical causes

Premenstrual tension, dysmenorrhea, and pregnancy can be accompanied by emotional distress. This ground is covered elsewhere in this volume. The relationship between serum hormone levels, neurochemical pathways, and psychological symptomatology is far from clear, as yet, though postnatal depression seems a likely candidate for a hormonally-triggered state; premenstrual tension seems capable of merging into overt depression; and the irritability, weepiness, and insomnia of some menopausal women has obvious links to depressive symptomatology. Recent use of neurochemical modulators such as fluoxetine in premenstrual mood disorders has met with some success, whilst increasing use of hormone replacement therapy symptoms may reduce the volume of antidepressant-prescribing for older women.

Traumatic life events

Child sexual abuse

Adult survivors of child sexual abuse (CSA) are more depressed and anxious than other women (Cahill *et al.* 1991). The nature and severity of CSA survivors' symptoms is very variable, some adults escaping relatively undamaged, whilst others have all the full-blown features of post-traumatic stress disorder. Factors identified as tending to result in greater damage following CSA include (Browne and Finkelhor 1986):

(1) perpetrator being a family member;

(2) abuse occurring over a long period of time;

(3) abuse accompanied by threats or violence or both;

(4) disclosure is not believed, or the victim is blamed;

(5) absent or unsupportive family.

In an American study, 66% of a group of children who had been sexually abused developed PTSD (Kiser *et al.* 1991). Other patterns of symptoms which have been shown to be associated with CSA include 'borderline personality disorder', psychosexual difficulties, phobic symptoms, panic disorders, bulimia, obesity, self-harm, parasuicide, and somatization (Dolan 1991).

A woman who has experienced severe CSA may be amnesiac in relation to part or all of her childhood; the traumatic memories are effectively repressed from consciousness (Ashurst and Hall 1989). In some women, bizarre presentations such as multiple personality may be understood as the survival strategies of abused children. Diagnosis is therefore difficult, especially since even obvious stress-related symptoms are diminished with the course of time, and may only recur when precipitated by environmental cues that 'reconnect' the patient with the traumatic events of the past, triggering panic attacks and phobias (see Box 17.1). Many CSA survivors have relationship problems, arising from very low self-esteem. They may dash into early marriage or cohabitation as an escape from abuse at home; unfortunately many, particularly incest victims, experience further physical and/or sexual abuse. Past abuse is associated with homelessness and with prostitution (Cahill *et al.* 1991; Dolan 1991).

Recognition of the **chronic nature of PTSD** is recent and has been triggered by growing recognition of the prevalence and impact of CSA and other forms of previously undisclosed trauma.

499

Domestic violence

About 25% of assaults reported to the police are domestic violence – well over 1 million incidents are reported in Britain each year, with an estimated 3 million more incidents going unreported (Home Office 1995). Of female murder victims, 40% are victims of domestic violence. For the age group 16–29 years, domestic violence is as common for women as pub-related violence is for men. According to the Women's Aid Federation, about 150 000 women and children seek help from women's refuges each year. Heath (1992) offers guidelines to help GPs care for women for whom 'the diagnosis of domestic violence emerges over time'.

Sassetti (1993) describes a cyclical pattern of domestic violence, with three phases. The **tension-building phase** is characterized by the batterer's increasingly unreasonable demands for complete acquiescence and obedience. The battered wife is not allowed any autonomy and is constantly berated and belittled. The batterer behaves more and more irritably until his anger erupts into **explosive violence**. Almost immediately, the tension is defused and the **honeymoon phase** begins. The batterer is typically doting, apologetic, and filled with remorse; until the **tension** begins to mount again as he strives to assert control over his partner and family.

Domestic violence and marital rape are less likely to be reported than other crimes; women who manage to escape from domestic violence may live in fear of their lives for years. Psychological sequelae for the battered woman include sleep disorders or hyperalertness, mood swings, depression, attempted suicide, and PTSD (Richardson and Feder 1996). Caring for children's physical and mental needs is disrupted when safety and survival are at stake; GPs should be aware of the tendency for battered women, overwhelmed by their own distress, to underestimate how much their children have witnessed. Whole families can become dysfunctional; behaviour patterns can be transmitted down through the generations; abused children may later participate in abusive relationships as adults.

Rape

The psychosexual consequences of rape are discussed more fully in Chapter 19. To summarize: an acute stress reaction to the trauma of rape, with emotional shock and disbelief, may be followed by post-traumatic stress disorder, particularly when there is rape by strangers or with violence or use of weapons, and if the woman is injured (Bownes et al. 1991). Feelings of self-blame, shame, and anger are common (Dunn and Gilchrist 1993), and may be followed by long-lasting depression and sexual dysfunction.

Cultural change

First-generation immigrants to Britain face enormous change as they move from deeply-rooted support networks with extended family ties into social isolation and alienation in British inner cities. Immigration has brought both well-off and impoverished individuals and families into Britain; all may be subject to racist assumptions and attacks, discrimination, unemployment, and poverty. Ethnic minority families in Britain are currently experiencing an exaggerated 'generation gap', given the differing expectations of young women from those of their parents and grandparents. Language barriers emphasize differences within and between communities, and there may be huge gulfs in understanding symptoms and feelings. Concepts such as 'depression' may be unfamiliar in some communities; any kind of recognizable mental illness is seen as shameful and stigmatizing for the entire family. Women from such communities will often present with somatic symptoms, however, and GPs will recognize, for example, the 'total body pain' of the Indian Asian community which serves as the expression of depression or difficulty in coping. A lay health worker found herself interpreting a Bangladeshi client's distress thus: 'My heart is screaming'.

The importance of diagnosis

There are several reasons why accurate diagnosis by GPs may be helpful in the therapeutic alliance between patient and doctor. Having found a professional ally who helps them to 'name' the problem, patients may be able to explore therapeutic options for themselves – including self-healing over time without specific intervention. Arriving at a shared diagnosis improves the doctor–patient relationship and reduces the likelihood of heartsink; and, once problems are accurately classified, work can proceed more effectively on therapeutic choices and outcome assessment.

Pattern recognition – spot the 'ticket'

Reaching a diagnosis brings its own rewards in every field of medicine; all GPs will have recognized anxious parents bringing their children's sore throats as 'openers' for a discussion of their own anxieties. Headaches and other 'physical' symptoms often serve the same purpose for a couple with relationship or psychosexual difficulties, as shown by Balint (1957) in his seminal work on the diagnostic and therapeutic potential of the GP consultation. Some patients are not aware of the extent of their emotional turmoil when they first see the GP; the doctor may, consciously or unwittingly, help to bring the underlying problem into the open where it can be dealt with. Both doctor and patient can be disconcerted when the patient suddenly bursts into tears in response to a sensitive question. Disconcerting this may be, but it can lead to a significant therapeutic breakthrough.

Meet the patient's expectations

Patients expect doctors to take a history, examine the patient, and arrive at a diagnosis before embarking on treatment; the conventions of standard clinical method have obvious logic. The 'laying-on of hands' has great significance to most patients whereas the baleful complaint 'the doctor never even examined me' often follows an unsatisfactory encounter.

Excluding an organic cause, even when an emotional cause is suspected, is a delicate task. With somatizers in particular, the doctor may be aiming at reattribution of the symptoms to 'anxiety', 'stress', or 'nerves', rather than pursuing detailed physical investigation of a symptom; but the proper examination of the 'affected part' should not be neglected. Explanation of the normal findings help to reinforce the non-organic diagnosis, and the confidence of the patient in her doctor. If the doctor seems dismissive about the patient's symptoms, or her theories about causation, the patient may be left confused and resentful.

Become an expert listener

Starting the interview with 'open' questions and letting the patient tell her story in her own way is usually productive. Throughout the consultation, listen for clues about help-seeking, considering both wants and needs. 'Why has the patient come? Why now?' 'Closed' questions may be useful towards the end of the interview, for completeness and clarification.

Active listening

This technique is used by many counsellors; it involves listening to what the patient says and then summarizing, reflecting feelings, and interpreting underlying meanings. 'You seem quite upset now, talking about your daughter.'

Non-judgemental acceptance

Stressed professionals find this difficult! But in the best interests of communication, we can try to avoid 'labelling' and denigrating patients. Being aware of feelings stirred up by previous encounters with the patient can help to prepare for the next consultation. Counsellors and therapists make time to consider such feelings deliberately, in the context of supervision sessions.

The angry reaction 'Not another panic attack – what on earth am I supposed to do about it?' can, with practice, be converted to: 'Panic attacks, they must feel very scary. Maybe I should look for something in her history? It's not *her* fault; perhaps I can help her unravel the cause'. In other words, the 'label' needs to be discarded because it stops us seeing the patient. She's not neurotic, she just exhibits neurotic behaviour. The patient who lets us down by failing to turn up for an appointment is not bad; she just cannot meet her own or others' expectations of her at this time.

Making 'mind–body' links

GPs become adept at spotting these links, in individuals and in families. They occur in all age groups, from the child with recurrent abdominal pain (periodic syndrome) to the sleeplessness and heartache of the recently bereaved.

The frequent attender

A woman in her late twenties, with a mask of make-up and a doll-like exterior, in her second marriage. She came repeatedly with abdominal pain (irritable bowel?), chest pain (Tietze's syndrome?), paraesthesiae (slept awkwardly?). We rotated through all parts of the body.

Why was she coming and why now? After a year of repeated consultations, I said I felt that I hadn't got to the bottom of her problems. She agreed, and volunteered that she had difficulties in her current marriage; she wondered whether she should see a counsellor. I suggested she wrote a problem list, to help me and the therapist understand her better.

At the top of her list, brought at the next consultation, was sexual abuse by the lodger in her mother's house, when she was 9 years old. She cried as she handed me the list. My eyes were opened. She had finally been able to write what she couldn't say. She entered therapy and over the next 2 years I saw her blossom. She became more self-assured, stopped dressing like a doll, and removed the mask of make-up. When anxious she still sometimes somatized. She'd say, 'I've got this numb feeling in my arm, doctor. I know it's just my nerves really, but I need you to check it out'. I'd check it out, and then we could talk about what had made her unduly anxious at this point in her therapy.

How can we help patients to make mind–body links for themselves, if they have not already done so? Careful history-taking (and diary-keeping) may help, looking out for obvious precipitants such as anniversaries in relation to previous losses. Investigating purposefully for a linking event could be worthwhile when the patient announces 'worst ever' symptoms.

The GP can reiterate that the mind and body are not two separate entities, but a united whole. Events can set off mental as well as physical pain. Tell the patient about the injured tennis player who only notices her pain after the match, when her pain threshold returns to normal; or the weekend migraines suffered by people who are stressed but too busy to take time off during the working week. The mind affects the body; this is a reality.

Why the panic attacks in the night?

A middle-aged woman had had a traumatic time in the dermatology out-patient clinic. When she returned for excision of another minor lesion, her heart raced alarmingly, she became sweaty, and felt faint. It was suggested that she should be referred for cardiac investigations. She also revealed that she sometimes felt she 'couldn't get her breath' in the middle of the night. I could find nothing abnormal on examination, and guessed that the episode had been a panic attack related to the previous treatment.

I explained the connection as I saw it, using a non-judgemental approach: 'When you're having a panic attack, it's extremely unpleasant and scary. You have no conscious control of it. If you had, you'd stop it. It's not your fault; but maybe your subconscious mind is trying to tell you something. I think you had a panic attack at the second visit to the hospital, activated by danger signals from the environment in which you suffered so much before'. I also asked about the night-time attacks, wondering, 'Has there been some past trauma, something at night perhaps?' She made the link at once, starting to cry as I spoke. She had been repeatedly beaten up by her husband after closing time at the pub; and he had died around the time of her first dermatology appointment.

In 15 minutes a diagnostic link was made that saved us months of investigations and worry. She recovered, slowly and with support, as she worked through a complicated bereavement.

Making the connection, for somatizers and others with emotional disorders hidden behind a physical 'ticket' symptom, can relieve the guilt and shame which is associated with psychological distress. The reward to GPs who make these diagnostic links for their patients is often immense gratitude and significantly less heartsink.

'Granny has to sit near the door'

When Phyllis, in her mid-sixties, came to discuss her impending admission for hip replacement, she asked if she could keep the door open during our consultation. She talked about her claustrophobia. I had not realized that this was why she hardly ever came to surgery. She couldn't bear being shut in a room with someone. Buses and trains were impossible; she felt she could not go through with the operation because she could not, ever, enter a hospital lift. She described all the symptoms of severe panic attacks.

Phyllis asked if I could think of any solutions. She thought she might be alright near a door or a window in a ground-floor ward. We laughed. 'But what are you escaping from?' I asked. She didn't know. She'd lived with this for years, had a family and grandchildren who all accepted Granny's peculiarities.

I said that in my experience panic attacks and phobias could be linked with past traumatic experiences, that subconscious mechanisms – not her fault – gave rise to symptoms of this kind. I wondered aloud whether some trauma in her past, even childhood perhaps, had involved confinement and a need to escape? She knew immediately. She had never told a soul how she had been tied up and raped by her elder brother over a period of 3 years before he finally left home in his teens. Phyllis looked astounded, excited. 'Do you think that's it?' she said. 'All this, going back all these years?' I nodded. Privately, I wasn't sure how much she'd be able to undo the patterns of a lifetime, but she was ready to have a go. She entered therapy and had her operation.

Needless to say, it may take several consultations or in some cases years of therapy for patients to gain such insights; the diagnostic link may still be resisted by the patient who is not ready. This will certainly be so for some adult survivors of child sexual abuse, rape, or assault. The linking of symptoms of distress with such traumatic events may be the most useful intervention the GP can make; but timing and sensitivity are vital.

Planning the follow-up care of the patient

Make a management plan

If an emotionally-laden consultation has had to be squeezed into an ordinary 5- or 10-minute appointment, the management plan at this point may simply take the form of a formal acknowledgement of the patient's distress, a very brief summary of what has been revealed, and the assurance of a proper and prompt response by the doctor. A further appointment with the same doctor will usually be required, and should be offered sooner rather than later. This will emphasize the doctor's commitment to 'getting to the bottom of the problem'. Although an inexperienced doctor may feel confused and unconfident at this point, being unsure what she or he has to offer, the patient is likely to feel both unburdened and supported.

Don't rush into referrals

Unless there is clear evidence of an immediate need for in-patient care, discussion about referral is best dealt with at a subsequent, planned consultation. A short interval allows the interested doctor to review the notes, digest the new information, and perhaps ask advice from colleagues; the patient needs time to think too. A doctor who takes one look at the patient's emotional burden, and immediately proposes referral to someone else, may be seen as rejecting the patient. The patient, who has by the end of the first interview exercised a choice to reveal significant information, is likely to be experiencing some new hope in relation to the investment made. This hope will be reinforced by the offer of another appointment.

Investigations

Laboratory investigations such as thyroid function tests, hormone levels, blood count, and urinary drug screening may be used to aid differential diagnosis, but it may be sensible to delay these tests until the patient's needs and priorities are clearer. Excluding an organic cause for important symptoms (such as fatigue or palpitations) is part of the GP's role; but the pursuit of investigations may do more harm than good if psychological issues are neglected.

Investigation of **psychological morbidity**, using standardized question-naires for screening, diagnosis, or monitoring of progress, is now routine in mental health care; several of these have been used by GPs and counsellors (see Wilkin *et al.* 1992).

Follow-up appointments with the GP

When the patient attends for a follow-up appointment, her thoughts since the first consultation deserve careful attention. She may express satisfaction or disappointment, or neither. Her symptoms may have improved or worsened; she may have been consciously preoccupied with the problem as described in the first interview or she may have reformulated or 'buried' it. The doctor's feelings about the patient are also a valuable resource at this stage. Indeed, Balint (1957) took the view that what the doctor feels is part of the patient's condition. Some patients evoke a definite feeling of, say, protectiveness, or perhaps irritation or despair. Recognition of such communications can help GPs as well as psychotherapists in their work with patients (see Brown and Pedder 1991 on therapeutic relationships).

The patient's motivation is a key factor at this stage. Missed appointments may testify to patients' misgivings about having revealed too much about themselves too early. Many doctors will leave it up to the patient to rebook a further appointment if they so wish; sometimes, on the other hand, it feels appropriate to send an invitation for a further appointment.

Non-drug treatments for uncomplicated stress reactions

Patients who can see the connection between their symptoms and anxiety or stress may be able to use direct advice about stress reduction, exercise or relaxation routines, and lifestyle changes such as cutting down tea and coffee (which exacerbate tension symptoms such as heartburn, diarrhoea, and trem-or). If they feel able to embark on a self-help routine straight away, so much the better. Relaxation video- and audio-tapes and stress-management booklets are available commercially, can be distributed by staff in the health centre, and can help patients motivated enough to use them regularly. Therapies such as massage and aromatherapy can promote self-care and dispel tension and distress.

Short-term counselling and the problem-solving approach

If the patient herself expresses a desire to work through the problem, or 'to sort myself out', then the GP may consider taking on a counselling role as an alternative to referring the patient to a counsellor or therapist. This can be seen as an extension of the information-gathering phase, a process of learning together. A central task is to identify problems and address them step-by-step so that they no longer seem overwhelming. Problem-solving has been shown to be as effective as medication for selected patients in primary care (Catalan and Gath 1985; Mynors-Wallis *et al.* 1995).

Cognitive analytic therapy (Ryle 1990) is an example of a structured framework which GPs or counsellors can use, with training and supervision. The patient is encouraged to use a workbook or 'psychotherapy file' to identify problems to work on, and the counsellor/GP then helps with goal-directed discussion for an agreed number of sessions.

The GP as counsellor

It helps to be honest with patients. Say you hope to learn together; you don't have answers, but you can provide support and you believe that in this sense two heads are better than one. If your patient can be helped to explore the problem, relax enough to set feasible goals, and work in a step-by-step way towards them, her self-esteem will rise and she may feel less tense or depressed. Some people think that GPs cannot be effective as counsellors (Cocksedge 1989; Rowland et al. 1989) because of conflicting demands of the two roles. It is important, for example, not to allow the patient to become too dependent on you. That is one of the central issues in psychotherapy, where the therapist makes use of dependency issues (the transference) to explore the emotional consequences of events and relationships in the patient's early life.

In general practice we muddle along, and some patients do become dependent on us. If we don't have the insight and supervision to deal with this, patients can get worse rather than better. Balint groups provide ongoing support for this kind of work, but individual supervision from an experienced counsellor or psychotherapist is best.

The family background

The first interview is unlikely to have included much family history. You will need to fill in this background later. But patients may perceive systematic questioning about their family background as intrusive or time-wasting, unless it is obviously relevant to the consultation. So do not insist on a full history by cross-examination.

In time you may start to look at themes such as sibling rivalry, parenting, or reactions to losses or deaths in the family. The patient's feelings about family relationships can be explored using the family circle (see Fig 17.1) – this is quicker and simpler than a genogram to do (Asen and Tomson 1992), and often eye-opening for both patient and doctor. The patient is encouraged to draw a circle and to mark herself somewhere in the circle. Then she is asked to draw in other important members of her family in her circle, deciding for herself where each should go.

The drawing in Fig 17.1 shows a 24-year-old's feeling of distance from her parents. She became quite upset explaining how her younger sister was, in contrast, very close to her mother. This family circle was used as a tool to explore a repetitive pattern of under-achievement; she was a graduate but had only ever worked in unskilled, low-paid jobs. Her presenting symptom had been a feeling of lethargy and tearfulness 'for no reason'. She returned, as planned, 2 weeks after drawing the family circle, saying that she had been 'in a daze' after thinking about it all day: 'it really made me think!' She was subsequently offered

Fig 17.1 *A family circle*

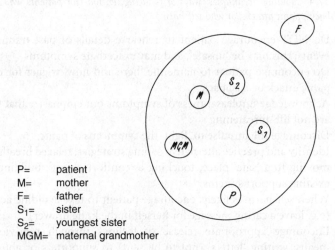

P=   patient
M=   mother
F=   father
S_1=   sister
S_2=   youngest sister
MGM=   maternal grandmother

counselling to help unravel her personal problems with relationships and work situations. Drawing the 'family circle' seemed to have unlocked her motivation to take herself seriously. It also spared her from undertaking a conventional but usually unhelpful series of investigations to exclude organic causes for her malaise. She continues to have symptoms, but regards them now as part of the 'pleasure and pain' of therapy.

Advantages and disadvantages of medication

Patients and doctors vary enormously in their attitude to the use of medication in depression, anxiety and life crises. Prescribing a pill for every ill is not good practice, and is habit-forming and harmful for doctors as well as patients. But medication can be very useful in a crisis, and where there is a high risk of suicide, antidepressants in sufficient dosage can save lives. Patients may need specific and repeated reassurance that antidepressants are not addictive. An update on psychotropic medication can be found at the end of this chapter.

The holding role

What can GPs do for patients whose problems are chronic or seemingly intractable? In earlier sections of this chapter we have suggested that some of these people will have a history of sexual abuse or other traumatic events. Whether or not this is known to their doctors, they may be 'diagnosed' as having antisocial or challenging behaviour and/or 'personality disorder'.

Such patients are extremely vulnerable, sensitized by rejection and abuse. A GP who can accept such a person, warts and all, can play a vital role as a 'good-enough parent' figure (Winnicott 1965) who is reliable and non-judgemental. In this 'holding role', the doctor can help the patient set boundaries for herself and discover what is 'safe' as opposed to 'unsafe'. Regaining a measure of self-esteem reduces both internal and external chaos; gradually she

Box 17.4 *'Holding' techniques: ways of reducing tension (for patients who have flashbacks, panic attacks, or who self-harm)*

1. Do NOT encourage patient to rehearse details of past traumatic events; this may be 'unsafe', and may exacerbate symptoms
2. Do encourage patient to name the 'here and now' trigger for each panic attack or flashback
3. Acknowledge unpleasantness of symptoms but emphasize that they are not life-threatening
4. Discourage the impulse to 'fight' the symptoms of panic
5. Identify and practice alternative coping strategies; relaxed breathing, moving to a 'safe' place, touching a 'comfort object'; building on existing support systems
6. When self-harm is likely, encourage patient to take avoiding action (e.g. leave a caring message for herself in the knife drawer)
7. Encourage appropriate release of feelings through non-violent means: writing 'letters' (not to be sent) to supporters or abusers, hitting cushions when angry, exercising, crying. Taking 'time out' to avoid situations which exacerbate symptoms. All these are better than lashing out at self, or at people who happen   to be near at hand
8. Encourage positive statements about herself: 'I'm doing OK today'; 'I'm strong'; enable her to praise herself and celebrate successes
9. Do not spend time with patient on trying to understand or forgive an abuser. Concentrate on the survivor's experience and needs
10. Self-help manuals may help some patients, once long-term therapy has commenced (e.g. Bass and Davis 1990)

may find the confidence to keep planned appointments, and to set goals for herself.

On the other hand, the GP should not pretend to be an idealized, perfect parent – or analyst! The aim of the holding role is to help patients deal with the here-and-now, rather than to uncover the details of past trauma (see Box 17.4). Specialists in the field of child abuse emphasize that it can take months or years of therapy to establish a safe therapeutic alliance; until this is achieved, it can in fact be damaging for patients to rehearse the details of their trauma. So: look for further help as soon as you start to feel that a patient's problems are draining your resources.

Referrals: the networking role of the GP

The GP has access to many agencies with expertise in handling psychosocial problems. Because of the vulnerability of people suffering with emotional problems, however, referrals need to be handled with care. The GP, in the 'holding' role described above, is often able to sustain the patient through periods of uncertainty; if a referral is needed, it will ideally be to a person known personally to the practitioner. It therefore helps to have a named contact within each agency.

GPs and community mental health teams

Most NHS psychiatry and psychology referrals are now channelled through locality-based, multi-disciplinary community mental health teams. The team includes community psychiatric nurses, clinical psychologists, psychiatrists and social workers. Services provided may include day care provision or drop-in facilities. There may be stress management sessions, group therapy using behavioural or interpretive techniques (e.g. psychodrama, art therapy), social skills or assertiveness training, as well as individual casework with patients under the general heading of 'supportive psychotherapy'. There is considerable overlap between the roles of the different professionals.

Except in the case of emergency admissions, there will be a significant delay before a member of the team sees a patient referred by a GP. The wait may be a matter of weeks or months; the GP's management plan must therefore include a strategy for this 'holding' period, and must nowadays take account of the possibility that the referral will not be accepted.

Community mental health teams (Corney 1996) are required to prioritize their workload to address the needs of those with defined psychiatric illness, especially those discharged from psychiatric beds into the community. Because of constrained resources and pre-set priorities, they are increasingly having to turn away GP referrals which do not meet their criteria. This new situation is worrying for GPs. Although we know that some emotional crises will resolve spontaneously and fairly rapidly, there are others which end in tragedy. GPs should therefore be familiar with local teams; specifically, it helps to know when the CMHT intake meetings are held each week, and to be prepared to argue forcefully for a patient to be seen urgently by a specialist, in time of need.

Referrals to specialist mental health services within the NHS can often be discussed in advance with local CMHT members. Such services will include child and family psychiatry, psychotherapy services, psychosexual counselling, forensic psychiatry, drug dependency teams and clinical psychology services for children. It may also be worth enquiring about liaison psychiatry services linked to hospital services such as obstetrics, transplant surgery, oncology and palliative care.

The purpose of a referral should be made clear to both specialist and patient; it is helpful to audit correspondence to check whether clear requests have been made and responded to. The quality of these communications varies widely. In general, the maximum benefit for patients will derive from a rapid referral for a straightforward problem for which a reliable treatment is known to be available. Treatment for severe depression or puerperal psychosis can be lifesaving; prompt treatment of severe phobic anxiety can prevent years of disability. For many other problems, however, the outlook for our patients seems to depend largely on the quality of relationships with family, carers, and professionals.

Even in the best-served areas, NHS resources available to patients suffering from emotional disorders are severely constrained. The interfaces between primary, secondary and community-based care are far from seamless. For these reasons, practices – fundholders and non-fundholders – are doing ever more in-house work in the field of mental health, despite the current situation in which fundholding budgets are not intended to cover mental health referrals.

Counselling in general practice

Some practices have a long history of employing counsellors, social workers, community psychiatric nurses or clinical psychologists, or inviting psychiatrists to run 'shifted out-patients clinics' in health centres (Ferguson and Varnam 1994). Under successive stages of the NHS reforms, incentives for such arrangements have varied enormously. The 1990 'health promotion clinic' payments resulted in the employment of counsellors in up to 40% of practices (Sibbald et al. 1993), with stress management being recognized as a form of health promotion.

Counsellors proved very popular with patients. Since this form of funding was withdrawn, many fundholding practices have opted to employ counsellors. Non-fundholding practices have had less financial flexibility, with the result that the provision of counselling 'on the NHS' is now very patchy. Some FHSAs have earmarked funds for counselling on the basis of pilot studies showing its acceptability to patients and GPs (Speirs and Jewell 1995); others have refused to do so, partly because of the dearth of conclusive evidence on the cost-effectiveness of practice counsellors.

Does counselling work?

This is an interesting debate analogous to that over the efficacy of psycho-therapy. Randomized, controlled studies, designed to avoid 'selection bias', are required in order to draw unambiguous conclusions about the efficacy of any therapy (King et al. 1994). Most studies to date have been well-intentioned but have not had adequate sample sizes or have not dealt adequately with confounding variables such as variations in therapist style and method, case-mix, and severity. There has been no consensus on outcomes, partly because of initial reluctance to use patient questionnaires and audit. The need for evaluation is now more generally accepted by counsellors, and more rigorous studies are being undertaken to address the issue of efficacy.

One of the arguments against funding counselling in general practice has been that the needs of neurotic patients constitute a bottomless pit. With regard to particular costs and benefits of counselling in the general practice setting, there have been several relevant evaluations, reviewed by Corney and Jenkins (1993). GP workload can be estimated using consultation rates; patients who take up counselling have been shown to seek fewer consultations with the GP in the post-counselling period than prior to counselling. Further studies are required to confirm these findings to the satisfaction of purchasers; interpreta-tion is dependent on the relative value placed on GPs' versus counsellors' time (Waydenfeld and Waydenfeld 1980, Trepka and Griffiths, 1987).

Counselling provision does not seem to reduce expenditure on medication, however (Fletcher *et al.* 1995; Sibbald *et al.* 1996). This is a blow to the argument that if GPs 'prescribe' counselling they will not need to prescribe antidepressants; but given the small numbers of patients who actually see a counsellor, such a reduction in overall prescribing costs is very unlikely.

The Counselling in Primary Care Trust encourages a 'brief intervention' model, with an average of 6–7 sessions per patient, for cost-effective practice. This means careful selection of patients, to avoid blocking counsellors' slots with the more vulnerable patients who need long-term support. Identifiable problems suitable for effective, brief counselling interventions will often be 'crises of limited severity or duration' (Curtis-Jenkins, 1995). Other problems which counsellors may address include:

(1) adjustment disorders, recent post-traumatic stress, recent diagnosis of major illness;
(2) behaviour problems, anger, relationships, substance abuse;
(3) anxiety, depression, grief, and loss reactions;
(4) somatic fixation;
(5) psychosexual problems;
(6) collaborative management of chronic pain.

How to find a counsellor or therapist for your practice

Until recently there has been no standard accreditation for counsellors and psychotherapists; now there are two such professional bodies concerned with training and accreditation and minimum standards. These are the British Association for Counselling (BAC), with its section for counselling in medical settings, and the UK Council for Psychotherapy (UKCP), founded in 1993 (see resource list).

Both BAC accreditation and UKCP full registration require 3 years of coursework (for UKCP this is at Master's level) and supervised work with clients, and counsellors will be expected to follow a code of ethics which emphasizes confidentiality. Counsellors in training can apply for individual membership of BAC. Only psychoanalytic and psychodynamic therapists will be required to have personal experience of individual or group therapy as a condition of accreditation.

A third body, the Counselling in Primary Care Trust (CPCT), has been established to deal specifically with counsellors working in primary care teams (see Curtis-Jenkins 1995; and resource list). CPCT recommends UKCP registration for counsellors in general practice, with full BAC accreditation as a basic minimum. Advice and support are available from CPCT for practices considering appointing a counsellor for the first time. It is vital that the practice team has clear and realistic expectations of a counsellor. When drawing up a job description and interviewing candidates, it is useful to involve an experienced counsellor who is aware of the particular roles and responsibilities involved in the setting of general practice (Rowland *et al.* 1989). After interview and induction, the new practice counsellor needs to be made to feel part of the practice team; effective liaison between referring GPs and counsellor requires protected time for face-to-face meetings.

What is the difference between counselling and psychotherapy?

There is much confusion amongst lay people as well as doctors as to the practice and definition of counselling and the many different forms of psychotherapy and psychoanalysis. For an overview, see Brown and Pedder's *Introduction to psychotherapy* (1991).

Much of what is offered by GPs, counsellors, and general psychiatrists amounts to **supportive psychotherapy**. This includes emotional support, opportunities to ventilate pent-up feelings, and attempts at problem-solving. These are used for coping with life crises and problematic relationships; a more or less 'directive' approach can be chosen. Counsellors in general practice or in community settings might offer 2–6 sessions of 30–50 minutes for a patient experiencing such a crisis, such as bereavement or divorce, often using a person-centred approach rather than giving direct advice. GPs may offer support over a much longer timescale, but with shorter appointments.

The **humanistic and integrative section of the UKCP** represents a group of therapies such as gestalt, transactional analysis, encounter, meditation, and psychodrama which have emerged from the **'human potential' movement** and interest in the psychodynamics of group behaviour. These therapies are not generally available on the NHS. They emphasize the exploration of emotional reactions, sometimes through role play, body work, and guided imagination. Therapists choose approaches ranging from giving support, reflecting on feelings, through to challenging 'action' therapies which encourage creativity in the client, but may involve emotional 'flooding'. Patients may seek GPs' views before seeking therapies such as these; it may be helpful to obtain consent to make contact with the therapist by telephone, to find out what the therapy involves.

Behavioural psychotherapy methods are based on experimental learning theory, and focus on attempting to modify maladaptive behaviour. Learning to relax is often a first step. Clinical psychologists are the principal practitioners in this field, working nowadays with community psychiatric nurses in community as well as hospital and day-hospital settings. **Cognitive therapy** (Gask 1996) combines a problem-solving approach with behaviour modification; patients are taught to identify and challenge 'automatic' thoughts such as 'I always fail', or 'nobody will ever like me'.

NHS psychotherapy departments usually offer a range of services which vary from one unit to another. Patients will be assessed for suitability for group or individual treatment. Cognitive and behavioural therapies may be offered, as well as training and supervision for counsellors and CMHT members in more exploratory, psychodynamic techniques. Some units offer **cognitive analytic therapy** (Ryle 1990) which allows for a range of therapeutic strategies.

Dynamic or analytic psychotherapy uses the therapist – patient relationship as its main focus, using this as a window through which to explore the influence of past relationships on present behaviour and attitudes (e.g. transference). This requires an extended timescale (varying between 6 months and 3 or more years) in which to develop a high degree of trust, and sensitive and selective interpretation by the therapist of emotions and defences which the patient is barely aware of. Personal experience of therapy is regarded as essential to equip the therapist with the self-understanding and poise to guide the patient's own explorations safely. To quote Brown and Pedder (1991), 'The aim of treatment at this deeper level is therefore more than symptomatic relief; it is reintegration and change in personality functioning, both intrapsychic and interpersonal, towards greater wholeness, maturity, and fulfilment'.

Referral to underfunded NHS psychotherapy units may involve intensive individual assessment of patients, with screening questionnaires followed by a wait for an assessment interview. Patients accepted for treatment will then have a further wait – for months, if not years – before being offered sessions individually or in a group. GPs are wary of referring patients for psychotherapy, knowing that they may have to handle the feelings of rejection in patients who are not accepted for treatment. If private referral seems the only option, for patients who will be further damaged by a long wait, the Association for Psychoanalytic Psychotherapy, the UKCP, or the BAC may be able to help in choosing a therapist. It is helpful for the GP to get to know a range of therapists personally, for consultation purposes as well as referral.

Teamwork for mental health

Variation in GP workload

GPs vary, and patients select their doctors. Nearly half the adult patients in one study (Fennema *et al.* 1990) had a preference as to the gender of their doctor, 43% of women and 31% of men preferring a doctor of their own gender. Two-thirds of all primary care attendances are by women; consultations with women doctors tend to be longer; and twice as many women as men present to their GP with emotional problems (MSGP4); these consultations are longer than those for other causes. In the field of mental health as in other areas, only a small proportion of patients are referred. Less than 10% of cases of depression are referred for specialist care; although men with depression tend to be referred to psychiatrists more often than women.

Women GPs, whether working full-time or part-time, may thus carry much of the psychological workload of the practice, seeing many of the more time-consuming patients. Workload issues are important, and these findings warrant discussion between partners (Chambers and Campbell 1996).

The primary care team

Many different members of the practice team are aware of the emotional difficulties of patients; referral and discussion within the practice team is often very fruitful, if time-consuming. Health visitors are equipped to work with families and especially with women at risk of depression; social workers may be involved with at-risk families in the context of fostering, adoption, or child protection procedures. The emergence of the nurse practitioner role means that practice nurses now carry a caseload of women with emotional problems, particularly in practices without a woman GP. Indeed, some practice nurses have been trained to incorporate mental health risk scores into their routine health promotion consultations with new patients (Armstrong 1995a), in the interests of early detection of such problems. Guidelines for assessment and management of a range of problems, from anxiety and depression to problem drinking and dementia, are now available from the National Primary Care Facilitation Programme and should promote multi-disciplinary work within practices (Armstrong 1995b).

Stress management within the practice

Practices aware of a high burden of psychosocial ills are also likely to be aware of stress amongst staff, especially in inner-city deprived areas. Indicators of stress, such as staff time off sick, or the frequency of confrontations between patients and reception staff, may be worth monitoring. It is becoming more common for practices to have occasional 'away days' for team members in work time, to help the team to put their work in perspective and prevent them from being overwhelmed by such front-line work. Issues of control and communication often need to be addressed; for example, all the members of a team will benefit from having clear job descriptions and being involved in setting goals and objectives for the work of the team. These strategies are well-established in industrial and other professional settings. Health professionals have been slow to undertake self-care and to practise what they preach.

Skill-sharing and continuing professional development

How can primary care teams make the best use of their skills, improve the quality of the care they deliver, and avoid 'burn-out'? The skill-sharing model may have much to offer here. This involves experienced counsellors, therapists, psychiatrists, and other members of the CMHT working on a consultation basis with primary care teams, as well as seeing individual patients (Wilson and Wilson 1985; Ferguson and Varnam 1994). One-off or regular visits from specialists can be arranged at a time suitable for a team meeting. The aim might be a problem-solving case discussion, focusing on an individual or family known to the team, and the outcome an agreed management plan which the practice team would try to implement, with support from the specialist as necessary. Working together in this way can improve the confidence of the individuals in the team in dealing with similar problems, and help them to recognize each other's strengths.

The skill-sharing model requires commitment to meetings, and ideally to practising new skills and evaluating the results. The same is true of a range of opportunities which can stimulate GPs and others to develop their skills: Balint

---

Box 17.5 *Self-help groups and community resources (examples)*

AGE CONCERN – support and befriending for the elderly

ALCOHOLICS ANONYMOUS

BRITISH ASSOCIATION FOR COUNSELLING – for list of local accredited counsellors

CITIZENS ADVICE BUREAU – trained volunteers backed up by information resources

COMMUNITY VOLUNTEER SERVICES – may produce a directory of local resources

COUNCIL FOR INVOLUNTARY TRANQUILLIZER ADDICTION – Also TRANX groups

CRUSE – Phoneline, support groups, and individual help for the bereaved

DEPRESSIVES ANONYMOUS – self help for depressed patients

GINGERBREAD – support for single-parent families

MENCAP – help for people with learning disorders

MIND – support and information for people with mental illness

RAPE CRISIS CENTRES – for women who have been sexually abused

RELATE – for relationship and psychosexual problems

SAMARITANS – telephone help line

SANDS – (Stillbirth and Neonatal Deaths) – support for parents after death of a baby or miscarriage

SCHIZOPHRENIA FELLOWSHIP – for patients and families

WOMEN'S AID – refuges for families fleeing domestic violence

VICTIM SUPPORT – after-care for victims of crime

(See other chapters for further details of self-help groups; Citizens Advice Bureaux can provide local addresses.)

---

groups, psychosexual medicine training groups, and individual supervision sessions. Time for these new activities must be found, and CME approval should be forthcoming (Tylee 1996). The results may pay dividends in terms of increased job satisfaction, a willingness to experiment with new approaches to care, and effective support for the practice team.

Reaching out: community resources

Community and voluntary resources are changing rapidly in response to the privatization of the welfare state. Voluntary, private-sector agencies are now encouraged to bid for contracts with health authorities, purchasing commissions, or social services departments to provide services which were previously the responsibility of the state. This is changing the pattern of local provision and – inevitably – reducing the independence of these 'providers'.

Some voluntary agencies, however, have retained their independent status and autonomy. Many of these (see Box 17.5) have their origin in small self-help groups, specializing in the provision of accessible client-centred support and continuing care. They can reduce the sense of isolation which many patients, carers, and families suffer, by providing personal contact, practical help, and information. **Self-help groups** can be empowering for consumers, but they can also be problematic. For example, there may be no assurance of confidentiality, the help available may vary over time, and the group may have its own ups and downs.

The selection and start-up process for **professionally-led groups**, on the other hand, is extremely time-consuming. Many patients are reluctant to join a group, although this is obviously an economical way of providing support to a number of people with similar problems. Some practices have set up successful stress-management groups, but in general CMHTs and NHS psychotherapy departments, drawing on a large population, are in a better position than individual practices to set up groups for a range of needs. Group psychotherapy is notoriously difficult to evaluate, but numerous attempts have been documented (Bloch 1988, McCallum and Piper 1990).

A practice folder containing details not only of addresses, telephone numbers, and contact people at local agencies, but also response times, is useful and time-saving. Ideally the folder – which could include guidelines for management of mental health problems (Armstrong 1995b) – would be used and updated by the entire practice team.

Using psychotropic drugs in general practice

Many doctors share with their patients a distaste for using drugs to 'medicalize' distress which is clearly related to life-events. However, drugs can help patients cope with overwhelming symptoms. Drugs used for the range of emotional problems discussed in this chapter consist mainly of antidepressant and anxiolytic drugs. Other relevant drugs are antispasmodics for gastrointestinal and bladder symptoms, anti-migraine drugs, and anticonvulsants which may be used synergistically with antidepressants and analgesics for persistent pain syndromes. We have not attempted to discuss major tranquillizers for psychotic symptoms.

The GP needs to be thoroughly familiar with a few drugs, in the mental health field as in any other. Drawing up a practice formulary provides an opportunity for sharing information and experience with particular drugs, in an attempt at consensus.

Antidepressant drugs

Evidence-based guidelines state that antidepressants perform better than placebo in helping people recover from depression in terms of both severity and duration of symptoms. They recommend that courses of antidepressants should last at least 4 months to prevent relapse, and that doses should be adequate (Effective Health Care Bulletin 1993; Edwards 1995). Table 17.1 gives a basic menu from which to choose an antidepressant.

One area of controversy is the non-evidence-based use in general practice settings of tricyclics in relatively low dosage for dysthymic patients with insomnia. The sedative action of the tricyclics has a faster onset than the mood-elevating effects, and there is no danger of addiction as there is with benzodiazepines. According to current guidelines for treatment of major depression and prevention of suicide, this amounts to inadequate dosage for inadequate lengths of time. Nevertheless it is common practice, and patients and doctors continue to view it as a successful coping strategy for preventing a patient with insomnia and a mood disorder from sliding into major depression.

Selective serotonin reuptake inhibitors (SSRIs) are now established as being as effective as tricyclic antidepressants in the treatment of depression. SSRIs are safer in overdose, but much more expensive than tricyclics. Besides fluoxetine, which has been successfully marketed by the pharmaceutical industry as the 'happy pill' of the 1990s, sertraline and paroxetine are in common use, and others including noradrenaline and serotonin-uptake blockers are available. Guidance for cost-effective prescribing in the UK emphasizes that any advantage to patients of SSRIs over tricyclics stems from the more favourable toxicity profile and simpler dosage, rather than from any major difference in efficacy as regards antidepressant action, or in compliance by patients (Effective Health Care Bulletin 1993). However, evidence about the usefulness of SSRIs in controlling anxiety symptoms and panic attacks and post-traumatic stress disorder has given these drugs a high profile (Vargas and Davidson 1993; Melvor and Turner 1995). The advantages of serotonin and noradrenaline reuptake inhibitors (SNRIs) over SSRIs are unclear as yet (MEREC Bulletin 1996). Unfortunately, few of the studies on drug therapy continue for longer than 18 months; long-term outcome studies in general practice are badly needed.

Anxiolytic drugs

Non-medical management of anxiety is now attempted by a majority of GPs; where medication is needed, the tricyclic antidepressants and fluoxetine may provide relief. The sedative benzodiazepines are well-known to be addictive, and have now been shown to be *less* effective than SSRIs in the treatment of panic attacks and anxiety (McIvor and Turner 1995). Because of their rapid-onset sedative action, however, benzodiazepines are still prescribed (in short courses of 5–10 days) for bereavement and other crises, and for mitigation of anxiety at the start of SSRI treatment in post-traumatic stress disorder (PTSD) (see Table 17.1).

Beta-blockers such as propanolol have a limited role in performance anxiety and palpitations and are probably less effective than SSRIs in PTSD (Vargas and Davidson 1993).

Neuroleptics such as phenothiazines are sometime used as a second-line treatment for refractory, severe anxiety, aggression with overwhelming anger, and flashbacks of trauma with visual and auditory hallucinations; they may be of some use in countering self-harming behaviour. Clonidine, methadone, and naloxone are occasionally used in specialist units for self-mutilatory, stress-related behaviours.

Table 17.1 *Choosing an antidepressant*

Drug	Cost of 28 days treatment at full dosage (Feb 1996)	Pros and cons	Uses
Trycyclics			
Amitriptyline (150 mg daily)	£1.50	Sedating, with cardiotoxic, cholinergic side-effects. Postural hypotension. Weight gain. Sexual dysfunction. Cognitive impairment. Drivers beware. Beware in CVS disease, glaucoma, and obstructive uropathy. Non-addictive. Anxiolytic; no real mood-elevating benefit during first 3 weeks of treatment. Affects noradrenaline (NA) and serotonergic (5HT) neuro-chemical systems. High risk of death in overdose	Depression. Promoting sleep and reducing anxiety. Effective for *avoidance* symptoms of PTSD only, e.g. flat affect, feeling detached, avoiding reminders, psychogenic amnesia
Imipramine	£2.00	Less sedative – otherwise as amitriptyline. Affects NA and 5HT pathways	Depression where sedation not required, e.g. if apathetic or withdrawn. *Intrusive* symptoms of PTSD only e.g. nightmares, hypervigilance, flashbacks, poor impulse control
Lofepramine	£10.00	Genuine advantages over imipramine and amitriptyline in that it is less sedative, less anticholinergic, less cardiotoxic. Low risk in overdose	Depression, especially if suicidal risk. Elderly

Table 17.1 Continued.

Drug	Cost of 28 days treatment at full dosage (Feb 1996)	Pros and cons	Uses
Clomipramine	£6.50	Sedative – otherwise as amitriptyline. Medium risk in overdose. Affects NA and 5 HT pathways	Depression. Obsessive/compulsive disorder
Trazodone	£12.00 (tablets)	Very sedative – less anticholinergic, less cardiotoxic. Medium risk in overdose. No weight gain	Depression needing sedation and in those who cannot tolerate other drugs. Sometimes combined with an SSRI at low dose to promote sleep
SSRIs (Serotonin re-uptake inhibitors)			
Fluoxetine (20 mg daily)	£20.77	Not sedative, not cardiotoxic, and no weight gain. Less anticholinergic effects than tricyclics. Side effects nausea, dyspepsia, headaches, restlessness, insomnia, dizziness. Increased anxiety. Caution in epilepsy. Relatively safe in overdose – low risk. Strong hepatic enzyme inhibitor – beware plasma elevation of other drugs, e.g. haloperidol, lithium, phenytoin, warfarin. Half-life of active metabolite is 1 week. Do not start tricyclic until 3 weeks after stopping SSRI, nor MAOIs until 5 weeks after stopping SSRI. Selective decrease in uptake of 5HT	Depression. Bulimia nervosa, Obsessive/compulsive disorder. *Avoidance* symptoms of PTSD Poorly compliant patients. Long half-life overcomes some of the effects from erratic doses and allows initial alternate day dosage which avoids initial increase in anxiety

Table 17.1 *Continued*

Drug	Cost of 28 days treatment at full dosage (Feb 1996)	Pros and cons	Uses
Sertraline (100 mg daily)	£39.77	As for fluoxetine but fewer drug interactions	
RIMA (MAOI) (reversible monamine oxidase inhibitor)			
Moclobemide (600 mg daily)	£31.50	Unlike older MAOIs, this does not have significant interactions with food (even so, advise to avoid tyramine excess). Interacts with sympathomimetic amines and opiates. Non-sedating. No anticholinergic or cardiotoxic actions. May cause nausea, insomnia. Monitor liver function. Relatively safe in overdose	Atypical depression. Panic disorders, e.g. agoraphobia. *Intrusive* symptoms of PTSD

Helping drug-dependent women

GPs are still engaged in weaning a generation of women off benzodiazepines, prescribed for them in good faith in the 1970s, following the epidemic of iatrogenic barbiturate addiction from earlier decades. Benzodiazepines are still used for managing withdrawal symptoms from alcohol, although there are newer alternatives (Kemp and Orr 1996).

GPs are often reluctant to get involved in prescribing for opiate users, perhaps because of fear or unfamiliarity. Practitioners who see drug-users regularly rarely encounter aggression; they are aware that users, especially those injecting heroin, may be very frightened of withdrawal symptoms, which include insomnia, tremor, diarrhoea, dry mouth, and irritability. Patients who come to the surgery for help will include an important group who are trying to get away from the uncertainties of relying on street drugs. Methadone maintenance may be a worthwhile harm-limitation strategy for these patients, some of whom can be helped to reduce their habit. Benzodiazepines are in any case contraindicated for these patients as they can be traded in on the black market. The Home Office Drugs Unit guidelines require notification of all opiate users, and it is unwise to prescribe any opiates or opiate-like drugs to new patients. Instead, the first consultation, as with any new patient, can be used to ask about general health needs and to build rapport. It is worth obtaining local drug dependency unit guidelines and following their recommendations; a common approach to management brings benefits for patients, doctors, and all in the primary care team. Women, especially those with children and those who are pregnant, are usually given a high priority by drug dependency units, so help from a community psychiatric nurse or specialist should be at hand in case of difficulty.

Are women's needs being met?

Attempts are being made in the new NHS to make closer links between consumer needs, evidence about the effectiveness of treatment, and service provision. It remains to be seen whether factors which are particularly important to women patients are acknowledged by purchasers and providers in future health care provision. There are pragmatic requirements to be met before women can even be said to have full access to health care. Interpreters and link workers are needed as a minimum requirement to help the many urban women whose first language is not English. Women with young children, at high risk for depression and economically dependent, often have difficulty finding the time and money to attend for appointments. Free child care in hospitals and health centres might help.

Women are more likely than men to express a preference for a female doctor or therapist (Fennema *et al.* 1990, Meeuwesen *et al.* 1991). The reason may be simply a preference for relating to someone of the same gender; there may be religious reasons; or there may be anxiety about disclosure of important but sensitive material such as a history of childhood sexual abuse or a drink problem, with worries about whether they will be understood and supported.

Women may take longer to 'engage' in therapy than men. Ashurst and Hall (1989) have reviewed 'the special ingredients of women's distress'.

Women mental health workers and doctors have expressed discomfort about the aims and means of psychiatric treatment; about possible collusion in labelling and treating women who, through their psychiatric symptoms, seem to be rebelling against oppression or abuse, past or present, in their family or work situation (Women in Medicine 1991). The increasing recognition of links between traumatic life events and their late sequelae opens up a Pandora's box for practitioners in primary care, too. We are feeling our way, in this chapter, towards a positive role for GPs in relation to emotional disturbance in individual patients: we have focused on the importance of 'mind–body' links in explaining behaviour, on the 'holding' role of GPs in relation to long-standing emotional disturbance, and their networking role in locating sources of help.

The demand from patients for counselling and psychotherapy is constantly rising, as patients seek a deeper understanding of their problems as well as symptom relief. Purchasers are reluctant to divert limited resources to meet demand unless there is hard evidence that such therapies are cost-effective. There is, unfortunately, a dearth of such evidence. Evidence-based guidelines for medical treatment of major depression have been produced, but even here the quality of the studies involved is variable and many important questions remain unanswered (Dowrick and Buchan 1995). The situation as regards cost-effectiveness of psychotherapy and counselling is even more ambiguous. Well-designed studies to evaluate the efficacy of counselling are now underway (King *et al.* 1994), but even if they yield convincing and generalizable results, NHS provision is likely to be patchy for years to come.

Feminist psychotherapy has developed from a sense that classical psycho-analysis and the post-Freudian and counselling traditions of male-dominated societies often miss, or distort, the conscious and unconscious material brought by women patients. Feminist therapists working both in and alongside es-tablished NHS psychotherapeutic practice are attempting to offer models of understanding and care which give women a wide choice of therapeutic styles and recognize the many-faceted conflicts they must survive. For example, a woman may be helped in therapy to reinterpret her individual struggle to de-velop as a daughter, as an economically-disadvantaged woman in a patriarchal society, and as a mother, through understanding that 'mothering is not simply an individual relationship, it is a social institution' (Eichenbaum and Orbach 1987). The Women's Therapy Centre in London offers individual and group therapy as well as workshops on aspects of society which affect women's health (Ernst and Maguire 1987).

Acknowledgements

We hope that this chapter will encourage GPs to feel more positive about managing their 'heartsink' patients. We would like, in our turn, to thank Sue Gerhardt, Helen Stewart, Erica Whitfield, Jackie Ferguson, and Linda Bloch for their thoughts while we were writing this chapter.

Useful addresses

Association for Psychoanalytic Psychotherapy in the NHS, c/o Tavistock Clinic, 120 Belsize Lane, London NW3 5BA.

British Association for Counselling, (Counselling in Medical Settings Division), 1 Regent Place, Rugby CV21 2PJ.
Tel: 01788 578328/550899. Ask for: factfile on counselling in primary care; and guidelines for the employment of counsellors in general practice.

British Association of Cognitive Analytic Therapists, Munro Clinic, Guy's Hospital, London SE1 9RT.
Tel: 0171 955 4822.

Cochrane Collaborative Review Group on Depression and Neurosis: possibilities for forming a Review Group are being explored.
Facilitator: Dr Per Bech, Psychiatric Institute, Fredericsborg General Hospital, Dyrehavevej 48, DK 3400 Hillerr'd, Denmark.
Tel: 0045 5226 3877; Fax: 0045 42263877.

Counselling in Primary Care Trust, Director: Dr Graham Curtis Jenkins, Suite 3a, Majestic House, High Street, Staines TW18 4DG.
Tel: 01784 442601/441782.

Defeat Depression Campaign, c/o Royal College of Psychiatrists, 17 Belgrave Square, London SWIX 8PE.
Tel: 0171 235 2351. Ask for: training package for primary care teams.

Mental Health Foundation, 37 Mortimer Street, London W1N 7RJ.
Tel: 0171 580 0145.

MIND (National Association for Mental Health), Granta House, 15–19 Broadway, Stratford, London E15 4BQ.
Tel: 0181 519 2122.

National Primary Care Facilitation Programme, Mental Health Training Officer: Elizabeth Armstrong, Division of General Practice and Primary Care, St George's Hospital Medical School, London SW17 ORE.
Tel: 0181 725 2773.

UK Council for Psychotherapy, 167–169 Great Portland Street, London W1N 5FB.
Tel: 0171 436 3002.

Women in Medicine, c/o 21 Wallingford Avenue, London W10 6QA.

Women's Therapy Centre
6–9 Manor Gardens, London N7 6LA.
Tel: 0171 263 6200.

References and further reading

Armstrong, E. (1995a). *Mental health issues in primary care: a practical guide.* Macmillan, Basingstoke.

Armstrong, E. (1995b). *Getting your act together: brief guidelines for the primary care of mental health.* National Primary Care Facilitation Programme, St George's Hospital Medical School.

Asen K. and Tomson, P. (1992). *Family solutions in family practice.* Quay Publishing, Lancaster.

Ashurst, P. and Hall, Z. (1989). *Understanding Women in Distress.* Tavistock/Routledge, London.

Balint, M. (1957). *The Doctor, the patient and the illness.* Pitman, London.

Bass, E. and Davis, L. (1990). *The courage to heal.* Cedar, London.

Bloch, S. (1988). Research in group psychotherapy. In *Group therapy in Britain* (ed. M. Aveline and W. Dryden). Open University Press, Milton Keynes.

Bownes, I. T., O'Gorman, E. C., and Sayers, A. (1991). Assault characteristics and post-traumatic stress disorder in rape victims. *Acta Psychiatrica Scandinavica,* **83,** 27–30.

Briere, J. and Runtz, M. (1987). Post sexual abuse trauma: data and implications for clinical practice. *Journal of Interpersonal Violence,* **2,** 367–79.

Brown, D. and Pedder, J. (1991). *Introduction to psychotherapy: an outline of psychodynamic principles and practice* (2nd edn.) Routledge, London.

Brown, G. W. and Harris, T. O. (1978). *Social origins of depression.* Tavistock, London.

Browne, A. and Finkelhor, D. (1986). Impact of child sexual abuse: a review of the research. *Psychology Bulletin,* **99,** 66–77.

Cahill, C., Llewelyn, S., and Pearson, C. (1991). Long-term effects of sexual abuse which occurred in childhood. *British Journal of Clinical Psychology,* May 30, 117–30.

Catalan, J. and Gath D. H. (1985). Benzodiazepines in general practice. *British Medical Journal,* **290,** 1374–6.

Chambers, R. and Campbell, I. (1996). Gender differences in general practitioners at work. *British Journal of General Practice,* **46,** 291–3.

Clare, A. and Jenkins, R. (1985). Women and mental illness. *British Medical Journal,* **291,** 1521–2.

Cocksedge, S. H. (1989). [Letter] *Journal of the Royal College of General Practitioners,* **39,** 347.

Corney, R. and Jenkins, R. (1993). *Counselling in general practice.* Routledge, London.

Corney, R. H. (1996). Links between mental health care professionals and general practices in England and Wales – the impact of GP fundholding. *British Journal of General Practice,* **46,** 221–4.

Curtis-Jenkins, G. (1995). Counselling in general practice. *Pulse*, June 3, 65–73.

Dohrenwend, B. D. and Dohrenwend, B. P. (1976). Sex differences and psychiatric disorders. *American Journal of Sociology*, **81,** 1447.

Dolan, Y. (1991). Resolving sexual abuse. W. W. Norton and Co., London.

Dowrick, C. and Buchan, I. (1995). 12-month outcome and depression in general practice: does detection or disclosure make a difference? *British Medical Journal*, **311,** 1274–6.

DSM-IV (1994). *Diagnostic and statistical manual of mental disorders.* American Psychiatric Association, Washington DC.

Dunn, S. and Gilchrist, V. (1993). Sexual assault. *Primary Care*, **20,** 358–73.

Edwards, J. G. (1995). Suicide and antidepressants. *British Medical Journal*, **310,** 205–6.

Effective Health Care Bulletin no. 5 (1993). *The treatment of depression in primary care.* School of Public Health, Leeds University.

Eichenbaum, L. and Orbach S. (1985). *Understanding women.* Penguin, London.

Ernst, S. and Maguire, M. (ed.). (1987). *Living with the Sphinx: papers from the Women's Therapy Centre.* Women's Press, London.

Fennema, K., Meyer D. L., and Owen N., (1990). Sex and physician: patient's preferences and stereotypes. *Journal of Family Practice*, **30,** 441–6.

Ferguson, B. G. and Varnam, M. A. (1994). The relationship between primary care and psychiatry: an opportunity to change. *British Journal of General Practice*, **44,** 527–30.

Fletcher, J., Fahey, T., and McWilliam, J. (1995). Relationship between the provision of counselling and the prescribing of antidepressants, hypnotics and anxiolytics in general practice. *British Journal of General Practice*, **45,** 467–9.

Gask, L. (1996). Understanding cognitive therapy. *Practitioner*, **240,** 290–6.

Goldberg, D., Bridges, K., Duncan-Jones, P., and Grayson, D. (1988). Detecting anxiety and depression in general medical settings. *British Medical Journal*, **297,** 897–9.

Gove, W. (1979). Sex differences in the epidemiology of mental disorders: evidence and explanation. In *Gender and disturbed behaviour* (ed. Gomberg, E. and Franks, V.). Brunner/Mazel, New York.

Gunnell, D. and Frankel, S. (1994). Prevention of suicide. *British Medical Journal*, **308,** 1227–33.

Hampton, H. L. (1995). Care of the woman who has been raped. *New England Journal of Medicine*, **332,** 234–7.

Heath, I. (1992). *Domestic violence: the GP's role.* RCGP member's reference book, pp. 283–5.

Home Office (1995). *Domestic violence: Don't stand for it.* Interagency circular.

Jenkins, R., Newton, J. and Young, R. (ed.) (1992). *The prevention of depression and anxiety: the role of the primary care team.* HMSO, London.

Kemp K. and Orr, M. (1996). Managing drug misusers – a guide. *Practitioner,* **240,** 326–34.

King, M., Broster, G., Lloyd, M., and Horder, J. (1994). Controlled trials in the evaluation of counselling in general practice. *British Journal of General Practice,* **44,** 229–32.

Kiser, L. J., Heston, J., Millsap, P. A., and Pruitt, D. B. (1991). Physical and sexual abuse in children; relationship with post-traumatic stress disorder. *American Academy of Child and Adolescent Psychiatry,* **30,** 776–83.

Kubler-Ross, E. (1970). *On death and dying.* London Tavistock.

McCallum, M. and Piper, W.E. (1990). A controlled study of effectiveness and patient suitability for short-term group psychotherapy. *International Journal of Group Psychotherapy,* **40,** 431–52.

McIvor, R. and Turner, S. (1995). Drug treatment in post-traumatic stress disorder. *British Journal of Hospital Medicine,* **53,** 501–506.

Mathers, N. and Gask, L. (1995). Surviving the heartsink experience. *Family Practice,* **12,** 176–83.

Mathers, N., Jones, Hannay, (1995). Heartsink patients: a study of their GPs. *British Journal of General Practice,* **45,** 293–6.

Mayou, R. (1991). Medically unexplained physical symptoms. *British Medical Journal,* **303,** 543–53.

Meeuwesen, L., Schaap, C., and van der Staak, C. (1991). Verbal analysis of doctor–patient communication. *Social Science and Medicine,* **32,** 1143–50.

MEREC bulletin Vol 7, No. 2. February (1996). *Citalopram, netazodone and venlafaxine; three new antidepressants.*

Moscarello, R. (1991). Post-traumatic stress disorder after sexual assault: its psychodynamics and treatment. *Journal of the American Academy of Psychoanalysis,* **19,** 235–53.

MSGP4: *Morbidity statistics from general practice, 4th national study (1991–2).* OPCS/ RCGP, London.

Mynors-Wallis, L. M., Gath, D., Lloyds-Thomas, A. R., and Tomlinson, D. (1995). Randomised controlled trial comparing problem-solving treatment with amitriptyline and placebo for major depression in primary care. *British Medical Journal,* **310,** 441–5.

Nemiah J. C. (1995). A few intrusive thoughts on post-traumatic stress disorder. *American Journal of Psychiatry,* **152**(4), 501–3.

O'Dowd, T. C. (1988). Five years of 'heartsink' patients in general practice. *British Medical Journal,* **297,** 528–30.

Parkes, C. M. (1986). *Bereavement: studies of grief in adult life.* Penguin Books, London.

Richardson, J. and Feder, G. (1996). Domestic violence: a hidden problem for general practice. *British Journal of General Practice*, **46,** 239–42.

Rowland, N., Irving, J., and Maynard, A. (1989). Can general practitioners counsel? *Journal of Royal College of General Practitioners*, **39,** 118.

Rout, U. (1996). Stress among GPs and their spouses: a qualitative study. *British Journal of General Practice*, **46,** 157–60.

Ryle, A. (1990). *Cognitive analytic therapy: active participation in change.* Wiley, Chichester.

Sassetti, M. (1993). Domestic violence. *Primary Care*, **20**(2), 289–305.

Schwartz, S. (1991). Women and depression: a Durkheimian perspective. *Social Science and Medicine*, **52,** 127–46.

Sibbald, B., Addington-Hall, J., Brennerman, D. *et al.* (1993). Counsellors in English and Welsh general practices: their nature and distribution. *British Medical Journal*, **306,** 29–33.

Sibbald, B., Addington-Hall, J., Brennerman, D., and Freeling, P. (1996). Investigation of whether on-site GP counselling has an impact on psychotropic drug prescribing and costs. *British Journal of General Practice*, **46,** 63–7.

Speirs, R. and Jewell, J. (1995). One counsellor, two practices: report of a pilot scheme in Cambridgeshire. *British Journal of General Practice*, **45,** 31–3.

Trepka, C. and Griffiths, T. (1987). Evaluation of psychological treatment in primary care. *Journal of the Royal College of General Practitioners*, **37,** 215–17.

Tylee, A. T., Freeling, P. and Kerry, S. (1993). Why do general practitioners recognize major depression in one woman patient yet miss it in another? *British Journal of General Practice*, **43,** 327–30.

Tylee, A. (1996). A new era in mental health. *Practitioner*, **240,** 279.

Vargas, M. and Davidson, J. (1993). Post-traumatic stress disorder. *Psychiatric Clinics of North America*, **16,** 737–48.

Waydenfeld, D. and Waydenfeld, S. (1980). Counselling in general practice. *Journal of the Royal College of General Practitioners*, **30,** 671–77.

Wilkin, D., Hallam L., and Doggett, M. (1992). *Measures of need and outcome for primary health care.* Oxford University Press, Oxford.

Wilkinson, P. and Bass, C. (1994). Hysteria, somatisation and the sick role. *Practitioner*, **234,** 384–90.

Wilson, S. and Wilson, K. (1985). Close encounters in general practice: experiences of a psychotherapy liaison team. *British Journal of Psychiatry*, **146,** 277–81.

Winnicott, D. (1965). *The maturation processes and the facilitating environment.* Hogarth, London.

Women in Medicine (1991). *Mental health.* Women in Medicine newsletter, January.

Women in Medicine (1996). *Women and addiction.* Women in Medicine newsletter, March.

CHAPTER EIGHTEEN

Eating disorders

Deborah Waller

Eating disorders account for considerable hidden morbidity among young women in our society. It is difficult to know how many people suffer from such disorders because the majority will never seek medical help. Recent community studies suggest a prevalence of at least 4% for binge-eating problems in Britain. The general practitioner (GP) is in a special position to offer help to sufferers and to intervene early in the development of the disorder, but first, he/she needs to identify the problem, and second, have an effective management plan.

The aims of this chapter are to give an overview of eating disorders and their management, to help increase GP awareness and detection of eating problems among their patients, and to outline a simple treatment programme for binge-eating problems suitable for use in primary care.

A typical day in the life of a 20-year-old student with bulimia nervosa

Wake up with splitting headache, parched mouth, feeling sick and bloated. Memories of last night's binge fill me with remorse: I must not eat today. I'm so weak and pathetic. I hate myself. Can't face getting up so stay in bed and miss my morning lecture. Feel guilty and anxious about this and my essay. Dizzy when I get up – drink two glasses of water. Weigh myself: 9 stone 2 lbs. Oh no – I've gained 2 lbs since yesterday. Feel terrible. No food today. Put on baggy jumper and tracksuit bottoms to hide my disgusting thighs and stomach. Sit down at my desk to make notes for my essay. Drink another glass of water. Try to concentrate, but my mind keeps wandering back to thoughts of food. About 20 minutes pass – it's no good, I'll go out for a run. The cold air on my face makes me feel a little better. Force myself to run round the park five times. Chose a route back to my room which passes by a newsagent's. As I approach the shop I feel an overwhelming need for something sweet and comforting. Buy two flapjacks, a packet of biscuits, two chocolate bars, and a jar of peanut butter. Start eating as soon as I get out of the shop. The food tastes delicious and I feel strangely elated. Hurry back to my room where I gorge on the peanut butter straight from the jar – can't stop myself. When it's all finished I head for the toilet. Put my fingers down the back of my throat until I gag. It's disgusting, but so easy. Throw up repeatedly until I've got rid of everything in my stomach. I look at my face in the mirror: listless, puffy eyes, fat, 'hamster' cheeks. Hate myself, feel so ashamed by my lack of willpower. I must not eat again today. Decide to go to the library to write my essay. Will allow myself a diet coke at 3pm. Find it very difficult to concentrate, make slow progress. As lunch-time approaches I imagine my friends meeting at the canteen. Part of me would love to join them, but I certainly don't deserve to eat anything and it would be embarrassing to sit there while they eat. They might even suspect something. Force myself to read another page. Have diet coke as planned in library snack-bar. Feel an incredible urge to eat, but with a huge effort I return to the library and my books. The afternoon and evening stretch out before me. I ought to be writing my essay, but all I can think about is how fat and out of shape I am and how no one could possibly like me the way I look at the moment. Despite this, I keep dreaming about just the sort of foods I must not eat. I'm worried about bingeing tonight. I know there's a party in college and decide to go along. Feel nervous and awkward, avoid talking to anyone, and have several glasses of wine in quick succession. There's a buffet meal but I know I must get out of there before I give in and eat anything. Hurry back to my room. All that alcohol – so many calories. Feel lonely and depressed. What can I do now? It's only 9pm. Weigh myself: 9 stone 1 lb. Good. At least I've lost a pound today despite the binge. If I could only lose a pound every day for the next 2 weeks . . . Half-heartedly sit down at my desk, but can't get motivated. Feel tense and bored . . . I check the communal fridge at the end of the corridor. Pinch a yoghurt, consoling myself that it can't be that fattening. Eat it in my room. Well, now I've broken my resolve I might as well give in and binge. Hurry out to the late night shop and buy a packet of cornflakes, four pints of milk, a pound of sugar, a loaf of bread, half a pound of margarine, a chocolate cake, a jar of strawberry jam, a family-sized carton of ice-cream, two doughnuts, and a litre bottle of lemonade. As soon as I get back to my room I start. I eat rapidly, washing down the food with the lemonade. It's as if I'm in a trance. I start with the chocolate cake, then the ice-cream. I mix margarine and sugar and eat until it's all gone. I have slice after slice of bread and jam, bowl after bowl of cornflakes with milk. I eat steadily until I'm so full it hurts. The whole binge takes 45 minutes. Afterwards my stomach feels as if it's going to burst and every breath is painful. Time to get rid of all this. I go to the bathroom – it's easy to throw up. I vomit and vomit until the chocolate mixture reappears – now I've brought back everything. I'm exhausted. I lie down. I know I will have put on weight. Desperation and self-disgust flow over me. I wish I were dead.

Definitions

The term eating disorders generally refers to anorexia nervosa and bulimia nervosa as well as a wider group of eating problems with some of the features below (atypical eating disorders). Anorexia nervosa and bulimia nervosa have in common a characteristic preoccupation with shape and weight and most of their clinical features are secondary to this.

Diagnostic criteria for anorexia nervosa (DSM-IV 1994)

1. Characteristic over-concern with shape and weight with intense fear of becoming fat.
2. Active maintenance of an unduly low weight (less than 85% of expected weight for age, height, and sex), achieved mainly by strict dieting and excessive exercising, and in a minority, self-induced vomiting.
3. Amenorrhoea for at least 3 months (if not on the contraceptive pill).

Restricting type: no binge-eating or purging behaviour.

Binge-eating/purging type: regular binge-eating and self-induced vomiting or laxative/diuretic misuse.

Diagnostic criteria for bulimia nervosa (DSM-IV)

1. Characteristic over-concern with shape and weight.
2. Frequent 'binges' (bulimic episodes).
3. Use of extreme behaviour to prevent weight gain, such as self-induced vomiting, misuse of laxatives and diuretics, and fasting.
4. The binges and compensatory behaviours occur, on average, at least twice a week for 3 months.

Fig 18.1 *A schematic representation of the relationship between the diagnoses anorexia nervosa, bulimia nervosa, and eating disorders not otherwise specified (EDNOS)*

(From: (1993). Binge eating: nature, assessment, and treatment (ed. C. G. Fairburn and G. T. Wilson). Guilford Press, New York. Reproduced with permission)

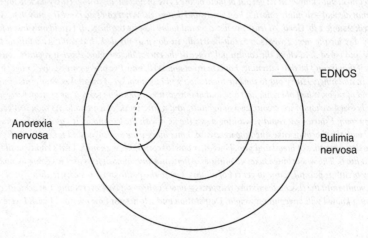

Purging behaviour (vomiting or laxative/diuretic misuse) is not essential for the diagnosis of bulimia nervosa as long as there is recurrent binge-eating and some compensatory behaviours to prevent weight gain.

Most cases are within the normal weight range for their height.

Definition of a binge

1. Eating, in a discrete period of time (e.g. within a 2-hour period), an amount of food that is definitely larger than most people would eat in a similar period and under similar circumstances.
2. A sense of lack of control during the episode (an aversive feeling that one cannot stop eating or control what or how much one is eating).

Atypical eating disorders or Eating disorders NOS

These terms are used for disorders of eating that do not meet the above criteria. Problems with binge-eating are particularly common, and the term **binge-eating disorder** has been coined to describe recurrent episodes of binge-eating in the absence of extreme weight-controlling behaviour (the majority of these people are overweight).

Prevalence and distribution

Epidemiological data show that eating disorders are Western illnesses, largely affecting young women in affluent societies with Western cultural ideals. Only 5–10% of sufferers are male. Certain occupations, such as ballet dancers and fashion models, have a particularly high prevalence of eating disorders, though it is not known whether these professions attract people prone to develop eating disorders or whether the occupation itself carries the increased risk. Cases of

Fig 18.2 *Rates of referral to an eating disorder centre in Canada (Clarke Institute of Psychiatry and the Toronto General Hospital)*

(From: Garner, D. M. and Fairburn, C. G. (1988). Relationship between anorexia nervosa and bulimia nervosa: diagnostic implications. In Diagnostic issues in anorexia nervosa and bulimia nervosa (ed. D. M. Garner and P. E. Garfinkel), p.60. Brunner/Mazel, New York. Reprinted with permission)

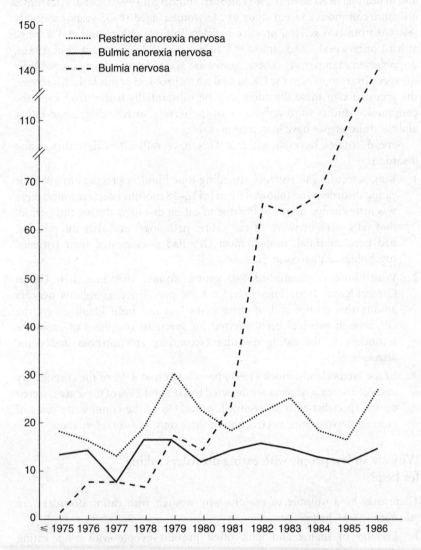

anorexia nervosa were described as long as 120 years ago, whereas bulimia nervosa is thought to have emerged as a disorder relatively recently, and was first described in 1979 (Russell). Fig 18.2 shows rates of referral to a leading eating disorder centre in Toronto since 1979. While the anorexia nervosa referral rates have remained relatively constant, there has been a dramatic rise in the number of reported cases of bulimia nervosa. Similar trends have occurred in New Zealand and England. In London the annual referral rates for bulimia nervosa increased from 2.8 to 10.1 per 10 000 females aged 15–40 years between 1980 and 1989 (Lacey 1992).

Prevalence studies, based on community studies and using strict diagnostic criteria, suggest a prevalence of anorexia nervosa among young women of 0.2% and of bulimia nervosa of 1–2% (Fairburn and Belgin 1990). Partial syndromes are more common: a recent study of 243 women, aged 16–35 years, randomly selected from two general practice registers in Oxfordshire, found 4% binge at least once weekly, and almost 9% at least monthly (Fairburn *et al.* 1992*a*, unpublished manuscript). These figures are alarming; we clearly do not have the specialist resources in the UK to deal with a problem of this scale. Moreover, the prevalence of these disorders may be substantially higher than even the community studies suggest, because of the secrecy surrounding binge-eating and the difficulty we have in detecting cases.

Several studies have shown that GPs have difficulties detecting eating disorders:

1. King screened 748 patients attending four London practices in 1989 for eating disorders and followed them up 12–18 months later. He found there was little change in morbidity due to eating disorders during this period, that GPs were unaware of the eating pathology, and that intervention had been minimal, though most GPs had documented their patients' psychological distress in the notes.

2. Whitehouse *et al.* studied 540 young women attending their GP in Cambridge in 1991. They found a 1.5% prevalence of bulimia nervosa among this group: half of these cases had not been identified by the GP, though two had been referred for specialist treatment of problems secondary to the eating disorder (secondary amenorrhoea and panic attacks).

3. In the Netherlands, Hoek (1991) has shown that 43% of the community cases of anorexia nervosa are detected by GPs and 79% of these are referred on for specialist care. In contrast, only 11% of the community cases of bulimia nervosa are detected, and of these only half are referred on.

Why are so few people with eating disorders asking for help?

There may be a number of reasons why women with eating disorders are reluctant to seek help:

1. Feelings of shame and guilt often prevent people with binge-eating problems from confiding in anyone.

2. They often hope the problem will go away on its own (and in some cases it does).

3. Chronic, low self-esteem is common; they feel the disorder is self-inflicted and that they do not deserve help, or that it is not severe enough to warrant help.

4. Many find it very difficult to tell doctors about their eating. They may have

consulted with problems secondary to the eating disorder in the past and feel awkward about admitting to the underlying problem.

5. If they do tell the doctor they may come across obstructive attitudes, often because the GP does not know how to help. The GP may trivialize the problem or act inappropriately, e.g. hand over a diet sheet.

6. They are often fearful that treatment will involve weight gain.

7. In some cases, particularly with anorexia nervosa, the sufferer does not view the eating disorder as a problem and does not want to overcome it.

How do women with eating disorders tend to present in general practice?

Women with eating disorders generally find it very difficult to admit to the problem and to ask for help. The GP will often be the first professional she approaches. The GP needs to be aware of this as well as being sensitive to any clues the patient might give alluding to an eating problem. Patients may present directly, but more commonly they will present indirectly with symptoms secondary to the eating disorder.

Presentation of bulimia nervosa

Directly:

-   loss of control over eating: wanting help to stop binge-eating/vomiting, but not usually to stop dieting

Indirectly:

-   requesting help with dieting (e.g. appetite suppressants or laxatives/diuretics)
-   gastrointestinal symptoms (e.g. irritable bowel symptoms, constipation, abdominal pain)
-   fluid retention with oedema of hands and, less commonly, feet; feeling bloated
-   menstrual irregularities/infertility
-   coexistent psychopathology, especially depression, anxiety, and self-inflicted injuries
-   fatigue
-   tooth sensitivity

Typical signs:

-   puffy face due to parotid gland enlargement
-   calluses or abrasions on the dorsum of the hand – due to repeated stimulation of the gag reflex
-   dental enamel erosion due to recurrent vomiting
-   they are usually within the normal weight range for their height (BMI 20–25)

Presentation of anorexia nervosa

Directly:

- cry for help
- pushed into seeking help by relative/friend

Indirectly:

- physical effects of starvation, e.g. feeling cold all the time, poor concentration
- gastrointestinal symptoms, e.g. constipation, abdominal pain
- fluid retention, intermittent oedema
- amenorrhoea, infertility
- coexistent psychopathology, e.g. depression, anxiety, obsessional and compulsive symptoms

Typical signs:

- emaciated: wearing layers of baggy clothing to conceal shape
- bradycardia
- resting and orthostatic hypotension
- mottled, cold extremities
- lanugo hair
- yellow discoloration (attributed to carotene pigmentation)
- alopecia
- dry, scaly skin
- sweet ketotic breath

Features of bulimia nervosa

Psychopathology

Bulimia nervosa has a profound effect on people's psychological well-being and the vast majority of sufferers will have some symptoms of depression and anxiety. Low self-esteem and feelings of guilt, helplessness, failure, and self-loathing are extremely common. Some may feel desperate at times and are driven to attempting suicide. Others resort to self-inflicted injury as a way of releasing tension after a binge. Of the women coming for treatment in the UK, 5% admit to having taking an overdose at sometime. However, in the majority of cases the anxiety and depressive symptoms disappear once the patient has regained control over eating, without the need for antidepressants.

Fluid and electrolyte disturbances

Vomiting and laxative or diuretic misuse lead to fluid loss and dehydration. Patients lose large amounts of potassium in the urine along with chloride in the vomitus, resulting in a metabolic alkalosis. Up to 50% of bulimia nervosa sufferers have electrolyte disturbances of this kind, though most are mild and asymptomatic. In patients taking large amounts of laxatives, there can be excessive loss of bicarbonate in the diarrhoea leading to a metabolic acidosis. The symptoms of electrolyte imbalance include thirst, dizziness, lethargy, fluid retention, muscle twitches, and spasms. Cardiac arrhythmias secondary to hypokalaemia are rare but potentially dangerous.

Gastrointestinal symptoms

Constipation is common due to dehydration and laxative misuse. Patients may also get intermittent abdominal pain. Rarely, chronic stimulant laxative misuse can cause permanent damage to colonic innervation. Mallory-Weiss (oesophageal) tears are also seen due to repeated vomiting.

Menstrual disturbances

Approximately 80% of women with bulimia nervosa have secondary amenorrhoea for over 3 months, and for 60% this will last for over a year. The amenorrhoea is related to the weight-losing behaviours rather than to loss of body fat. With recovery from the eating disorder, ovulation and menstruation return.

Features of anorexia nervosa

Psychopathology

Women with anorexia nervosa have a 'morbid fear of fatness'. They feel obese even though they are emaciated. When help is offered, they tend to react with anger, deception, and manipulative behaviour. As the disorder becomes more established, they retreat from society, becoming very restricted in their activities, and increasingly dependent on family or therapist. The psychological effects of starvation include depressed mood, irritability, loss of libido, preoccupation with food, obsessional rituals, reduced concentration, and drowsiness. These symptoms will usually improve with weight gain.

Gastrointestinal symptoms

Constipation, bloating, and abdominal pain are all common complaints, due partly to delay in gastric and whole gut transit times. Prokinetic drugs such as cisapride and domperidone may help during the early stages of refeeding.

Amenorrhoea and infertility

Amenorrhoea of at least 3 months duration is a mandatory diagnostic criterion for anorexia nervosa. Pre-pubertal levels of LH and FSH lead to hypogonadotrophic hypogonadism. In pre-pubertal girls this may result in failure of breast development. Menses and secondary sexual characteristics return with weight restoration.

Cardiovascular symptoms

Sinus bradycardia, with pulse rate as low as 30, hypotension, and mottled cold extremities are common. These lead to dizziness and syncope.

Haematological features

Normochromic, normocytic anaemia, mild leukopenia with relative lympho-cytosis, and low ESR are common findings. There is no increased risk of infection.

Thyroid function

T4 levels are in the low normal range whereas T3 levels are depressed and TSH levels are normal. These changes are seen in other starvation states and are presumably a means of conserving energy. There is clinical evidence of hypothyroidism, with dry skin, hypothermia, bradycardia, constipation, and delayed relaxation of deep tendon reflexes.

Osteoporosis

Osteoporosis and stunting of growth are serious and possibly irreversible consequences of anorexia nervosa. Peak bone density levels are reached in the late teens; adolescent girls with anorexia nervosa are unlikely to reach their potential peak bone density, putting them at increased risk of osteoporosis in later life. Chronic low oestrogen levels and raised cortisol levels may be responsible. Fractures have been reported in anorexia nervosa sufferers who have been amenorrhoeic for only a year. Exercise appears to have a protective effect, but there is clearly an important role for hormone replacement (usually in the form of the combined pill) in these women.

How do eating disorders affect social life?

Binge-eating is usually done in secret and is surrounded by feelings of guilt and shame, aggravated by self-induced vomiting and laxative abuse. Over-concern about shape and weight is a constant preoccupation, and if the sufferer is feeling fat she may withdraw completely from social situations so that no one sees her. Many social occasions revolve around eating and she is likely to find eating in public a stress she would rather avoid. As a result, women with eating problems frequently become socially isolated and relationships with family and friends often become strained.

Aetiology

Cultural pressures

In Western society today, thinness in women is seen as the ideal in terms of sexual attractiveness, health, and success. We are encouraged by the media to pursue the perfect body through special diets and exercise programmes. Cosmetic surgery is available to improve our looks. The inference is that anybody can have the perfect shape if they exercise and restrict their food intake sufficiently. In fact, genetic factors play a large part in body shape and weight and the body cannot be 'shaped' at will (Brownell 1991).

The exercise and weight loss needed to attain the aesthetic ideal are far in excess of what is recommended for healthy living. Models exercise as many as 35 hours a week in order to keep 'in shape'. It is not surprising that most women fail to achieve these goals. Regrettably, many judge themselves unfavourably as a consequence. Adolescent girls are particularly susceptible to these pressures with lower self-esteem among girls who regard themselves as unattractive.

Despite the great pressure to diet, only a small proportion of women develop full eating disorders. Genetic, psychological, and family factors may all influence the development of an eating problem. There is evidence to suggest that eating disorders increase in prevalence in rapidly developing countries as they take on the cultural values of the West, and that when immigrants move from less industrialized to more industrialized countries they are more likely to develop eating disorders.

Eating disorders are far commoner in females than males (approximately 10:1). This sex difference is substantially greater than for any other psychiatric disorder and can be explained by the disproportionate cultural pressure on women to be thin.

Ethnicity, social class, and occupation

Eating disorders appear to occur more frequently among white, middle to upper class women. However, recent studies suggest that as non-Caucasian groups in developing countries take on Western values, they too are beginning to experience eating disorders. Research in the US shows that recurrent binge-eating may be as common in black as in white women. It may be that women from higher social classes have better access to health care and are more likely to ask for help. Eating disorders are known to occur more frequently among people in certain occupations, e.g. ballet dancers, models, athletes, in which the need to conform to a certain body shape is heightened.

Personality traits

Women with anorexia nervosa tend to be unusually compliant and conscientious as children. They are often shy and solitary, emotionally restrained, and tend to be competitive. These traits seem to be the precursors of low self-esteem and perfectionism seen in anorexia nervosa sufferers.

Bulimia nervosa sufferers tend to be impulsive, sensitive, and low in self-esteem. They may exhibit dichotomous thinking with low frustration tolerance and acting-out behaviour. In a small minority, bulimic symptoms may be one feature of a multi-impulsive borderline personality disorder (problems with impulse control; e.g. substance abuse, promiscuity, gambling, reckless driving, as well as unstable relationships, recurrent suicidal threats, and fluctuating mood states).

Environmental and genetic factors

Several published studies have shown that eating disorders appear to run in families. This could be due to inherited factors and/or to environmental influences. Twin studies in which the concordance for eating disorders in monozygotic and dizygotic twin pairs was compared, showed concordance rates for both anorexia nervosa and bulimia nervosa to be substantially greater for the monozygotic twins (Kendler *et al.* 1991; Strober 1992).

There is also evidence to suggest that mothers with eating disorders have an effect on their children's eating habits. In Stein's controlled study (1994) of 1-year-old children of mothers with eating disorders, the mothers were observed to be more critical of their children and there was more conflict during meal times than in the controls. The mothers were more reluctant to let the infants feed themselves, concerned that the children would make a 'mess'. The children tended to weigh less than controls, and children's weight was inversely correlated to their mother's concern about her own body image. Pike and Rodin (1991) compared the responses of mothers of daughters with disturbed eating with a control group. The mothers differed from controls in that they had more disturbed eating themselves, they thought their daughters should lose more weight, and they were more critical of their daughter's appearance.

Psychiatric disorders within the family

There is now considerable data showing that relatives of patients with eating disorders have a higher incidence of clinical depression. The lifetime rates of depressive illness are two to three times higher than in the general population. The reason for this is unclear; it might be the effect on the child of being brought up by a depressed parent, or it might be due to a shared defect in serotonin metabolism (Cowen *et al.* 1992). Serotonin has been implicated in the mediation of satiety and food intake regulation, and dieting has been shown to affect serotonin levels, especially in women. Serotonin also plays an important role in the aetiology of depression. The suggestion is that an abnormality in serotonin metabolism might predispose families to eating disorders as well as to depression, and that dieting in women might increase this risk.

How genes may contribute to the development of eating disorders remains speculative, but possible explanations include their influence on personality traits and behaviour regulation.

Course and outcome

Anorexia nervosa

Follow-up data on patients with anorexia nervosa is largely limited to cases treated in specialist centres. There are no prospective population-based studies to date so the outcome data is subjected to selection bias and should be interpreted with caution. The results of 68 outcome studies of 3104 patients showed that, on average, more than 40% of cases recover, one-third improve, and 20% have a chronic course (Steinhausen *et al.* 1991). The mean crude mortality rate is 5% (range 0–21%). Early age of onset (though not childhood onset), histrionic personality, and early treatment are good prognostic factors.

Vomiting, bulimia, profound weight loss, and long duration of illness carry a bad prognosis. The effects of different treatments on recovery are unknown and it is difficult to give an individual patient an accurate prognosis.

Bulimia nervosa

The outcome data for bulimia nervosa show that 30% of cases have a previous history of anorexia nervosa, but that relapse into anorexia nervosa is extremely rare. Obesity is not common at follow-up compared to figures for the general population. Favourable prognostic factors include a short duration of illness prior to treatment, the absence of personality disorder, and, surprisingly, a family history of alcoholism. Fifty per cent of patients treated with cognitive behaviour therapy (p. 542) are asymptomatic 2–10 years later; 20% remain symptomatic and appear to have a chronic course; while the remaining 30% are not fully recovered, either with a partial binge-eating disorder or with relapses and remissions over time. There is insufficient follow-up data for other forms of treatment of bulimia nervosa. The mortality rate associated with bulimia nervosa is unclear, but it may be higher than in the general population (Hsu 1995).

Treatment

Drug treatments

There is no current evidence to support the use of any drug for anorexia nervosa. In particular, trials of antipsychotic drugs, tricyclic antidepressant drugs, and of lithium have shown no statistically significant benefit in anorexia nervosa. It has been suggested that fluoxetine may be of use in preventing relapse in patients who have gained weight, and a controlled trial to investigate this is currently taking place.

There is some evidence to support the use of antidepressant drugs in bulimia nervosa, though the longer-term effects of these drugs have been shown to be disappointing (Mitchell and de Zwann 1993). A series of short-term, double-blind, placebo-controlled trials using a range of different antidepressant drugs, showed that drugs proved superior to placebo in terms of reduction of binge frequency (by 50–60% within a few weeks of starting treatment), along with a general improvement in mood and decreased preoccupation with shape and weight. The drug effect occurred irrespective of whether or not the patient was clinically depressed, and this suggests that antidepressant drugs may have a specific 'anti-bulimic' effect, unrelated to their effect on mood. This finding is further supported by a study of almost 400 patients in which fluoxetine at a dose of 60 mg a day, but not at 20 mg a day, was superior to placebo in treating bulimia nervosa (Fluoxetine Bulimia Nervosa Collaboration Study Group 1992). The therapeutic dose for treating clinical depression is 20 mg, so this reinforces the idea of a separate anti-bulimic effect of fluoxetine which is only apparent at high dose.

Most of the antidepressant drug studies have been short term (only lasting

8 weeks). Walsh *et al.* (1991) looked at the longer-term effects of desipramine in bulimia nervosa. He found that although the binge frequency fell by 47% in the first 6 weeks of treatment, only a minority of patients managed to stop binge-eating and purging altogether and almost a third relapsed over the following 4 months. The relapse rate was high whether or not the patient continued to take the drug.

Psychological treatments are more effective in the treatment of bulimia nervosa than antidepressant medication. However, there may be a place for the concurrent use of antidepressants in patients who are failing to respond adequately to good psychological therapy, and in patients who have a severe depressive illness independent of the eating disorder. At present, fluoxetine at a dose of 60 mg daily may be the drug of choice in these situations.

Treatment of anorexia nervosa

Anorexia nervosa is a serious, potentially life-threatening disorder and requires effective intervention as early as possible in order to minimize psychological, social, and physical repercussions. The younger the patient, the more pressing the need. Family therapy, parental counselling, and individual therapy all have their place and there may be a need for a period of in-patient treatment. Treatment is likely to be prolonged and intensive and early referral for specialist help is indicated. There is little place for management in general practice, though the GP may be a valuable, ongoing support to the family.

Family therapy

There is substantial evidence to support family therapy as an effective treatment for anorexia nervosa in adolescence. A series of randomized controlled trials at the Maudsley Hospital demonstrated that patients with early-onset anorexia nervosa (under 19 years of age) and a duration of illness of less than 3 years did significantly better with family therapy than with individual supportive treatment, both at the end of the treatment programme and at 5-year follow-up (Dare *et al.* 1990). In this study, all cases were treated initially as in-patients and were randomly assigned to a 1-year course of family therapy or individual therapy at discharge. Family therapy is increasingly being used as an initial out-patient treatment for adolescent anorexia nervosa, leaving hospital admission for those with life-threatening complications.

A variety of theoretical approaches have been used, but as yet these different approaches have not been validated. Therapy is often based on the hypothesis that eating disorders originate from a specific pathological pattern of family structure and functioning and that they can be treated by tackling these causative factors within the family. However, research data point away from a family aetiological model which puts the 'blame' very much with the family, suggesting instead that the differences between eating disorder families and control families are more to do with the pressures of severe or chronic illness than with a distinctive dysfunctional entity (Le Grange *et al.* 1992). This model may be more helpful as it shifts the blame away from the family and enables all family members to consider themselves as a resource for effective treatment.

In-patient treatment of anorexia nervosa

It is generally accepted that patients with anorexia nervosa are unlikely to benefit from psychological treatment while their body weight is very low. The initial aim of therapy is therefore weight gain.

Indications for in-patient treatment

(1) very low body weight: BMI <13, or if weight loss has been very rapid;
(2) the patient or her carers feel out of control and request admission. Admission can serve to separate the patient from main carers, allowing problems to be tackled in a different way;
(3) serious physical complications (e.g. severe electrolyte disturbances, acute stomach dilatation) or significant suicidal risk;
(4) lack of response to out-patient treatment;
(5) severe behavioural disturbance.

In-patient treatment should be seen as a complement to out-patient treatment, and needs to be tailored to the patient's needs with as much continuity of care as possible.

A behavioural approach is usually adopted initially to induce weight gain. Patients are given support and encouragement to eat, with granting of privileges if they gain weight. Other treatment approaches include nasogastric feeding or total parenteral nutrition. Patients should be warned in advance of the possible transient adverse effects of weight gain, including dependent oedema and gastrointestinal discomfort.

In most in-patient programmes, the aim is to increase body weight until normal weight range is reached (BMI 19–24) and to stabilize at this weight. During the weight stabilization phase, patients are fully informed about healthy eating and eating disorders. This is often done in groups, and families are involved where ever possible.

The transition from in-patient to out-patient care is stressful for many patients. Continuity of care is important with regular, planned follow-up sessions.

Treatment of bulimia nervosa

Education

Education may be sufficient treatment in itself in helping people with binge-eating problems. Maladaptive beliefs and behaviour may develop out of incorrect or absent information and it follows that sufferers need to be fully informed about their disorder. Several excellent self-help books on eating disorders are now available in the UK containing clear educational material (see 'Useful reading' at end of chapter).

Olmsted and colleagues in Toronto (1991) studied the effectiveness of a group educational programme for women with bulimia nervosa. It consisted of five 90-minute lectures providing educational material and advice on how to overcome the disorder, but no personal guidance or support. The effects of the programme were compared with individual cognitive behaviour therapy

Table 18.1 *The core elements of cognitive behavior therapy*

Stage one
- Educating the patient about bulimia nervosa and explaining the cognitive rationale for the treatment
- Recording in detail all eating, vomiting, and laxative misuse at the time that it occurred, together with relevant thoughts and feelings
- Introducing a pattern of regular eating, thereby displacing many binges
- Using alternative behaviour to help resist urges to binge
- Educating patients about the ineffectiveness of strict dieting, self-induced vomiting, and laxative misuse, and informing them about their adverse effects

Stage two
- Introducing avoided foods into the diet and gradually eliminating other forms of strict dieting

Stage three
- Planning for the future, including having realistic expectations and strategies for use should problems recur

(CBT). The two treatments were found to be equally effective, except for those people with more severe bulimia nervosa who did better with CBT. Unfortunately, there was no long-term follow-up, so whether change is maintained with education alone is unclear. This study suggests that for many people with milder binge-eating problems, sound information and advice alone may be sufficient to help them.

Cognitive behaviour therapy

CBT for bulimia nervosa was first described in 1981 by Fairburn. It has been evaluated in over 40 randomized controlled trials and shown to be more effective than a variety of other treatments, including antidepressant drugs, behavioural therapy, and supportive psychotherapy (Fairburn *et al.* 1992*b*; Wilson and Fairburn 1993). For at least two-thirds of patients, individual CBT produced a substantial improvement in the frequency of binge-eating and purging, with a third to a half of patients giving up binge-eating altogether. Concerns about shape and weight are also reduced. Follow-up studies (up to 6 years post-treatment) suggest that changes are well-maintained and that relapse is uncommon.

The full treatment involves about 20 50-minute sessions over 4–5 months with a specialist therapist. The treatment is based on a cognitive view of the factors that perpetuate bulimia nervosa (Fig 18.3). According to this model, the disorder is maintained by a series of interlocking vicious circles; the key to the disorder is dieting. The bulimia nervosa sufferer tends to have low self-esteem and to judge self-worth almost exclusively in terms of shape and weight. This over-concern about weight encourages strict dieting. When she diets she adopts

Fig 18.3 *The cognitive view of the maintenance of bulimia nervosa*
(From: Fairburn, C. G., Marcus, M. D., and Wilson, G. T. (1993). Cognitive-behavioral therapy for binge eating and bulimia nervosa: a comprehensive treatment manual. In Binge eating: nature, assessment, and treatment (ed. C. G. Fairburn and G. T. Wilson). Guilford Press, New York. Reproduced with permission)

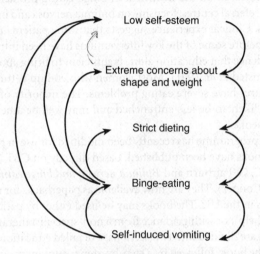

strict rules. As long as she keeps to these rules she feels in control; but if she breaks a rule, even in a minor way, she feels out of control and then over-reacts, abandoning all controls, and binges. In addition, if she has been starving herself in between binges, there is also a physiological drive to overeat. To break out of this vicious circle she needs to stop dieting. Another vicious circle is set up with vomiting encouraging overeating. This occurs because of the misconception that vomiting reduces calorie absorption, thereby removing one of the normal constraints against overeating. Emphasis is placed on breaking out of these vicious circles by changing behaviour as well as thinking.

Interpersonal psychotherapy

This is a form of short-term psychotherapy originally developed to treat depression. It focuses on interpersonal problems and does not attempt to tackle eating difficulties directly. There has been one study to date to evaluate interpersonal psychotherapy (IPT) for bulimia nervosa (Fairburn *et al.* 1993*a*; Fairburn *et al.* 1995). When compared with CBT, IPT was not as effective in the short term, but there were delayed benefits so that by 1 and 6-year follow-up IPT was found to be as effective as CBT. A much larger study is currently underway in the US to evaluate this treatment further.

Treating bulimia nervosa and binge-eating problems in primary care

It is estimated that up to 4% of young women in this country have binge-eating problems. Many of these women are not in treatment, and if more women did come forward for help the psychiatric services would not be able to cope with a problem on this scale. In any case, young people are often reluctant to see a psychiatrist because of the stigma attached. Full psychological treatment is costly and time-consuming. Treatment in primary care may be less threatening and easier in practical terms and therefore more attractive to women.

Most of the research on the treatment of binge-eating problems has taken place in tertiary referral centres, focusing on bulimia nervosa and involving specialist therapists. Clinical experience suggests that some patients respond very rapidly to CBT before some of the key interventions have been introduced, and there is also evidence that education alone is sufficient to bring about change in some cases (Olmsted *et al.* 1991). Most women who end up getting treatment in specialist centres have severe eating problems. The majority of cases in the community are likely to be less entrenched and may well be amenable to less intensive treatments.

The full CBT programme has recently been modified for use in primary care. Two self-help books have been published, based directly on CBT (*Overcoming binge eating* by C. G. Fairburn and *Bulimia nervosa and binge eating: a guide to recovery* by P. J. Cooper). They are now available as paperbacks for under £10 in most bookshops in the UK. The books may be used either by patients on their own ('pure self-help') or with guidance from a non-specialist therapist ('guided self-help'). Both are divided into two sections: a detailed educational section in the first half of the book, followed by a step-by-step treatment programme. The programme is designed to take between 12–16 weeks.

The advantage of 'pure self-help' is that the sufferer can treat herself without involving anyone else, and this may appeal to her if she wants to keep her eating problem a complete secret. However, 'pure self-help' needs great motivation and commitment, and for many women the encouragement and support offered with 'guided self-help' improves compliance. Guided self-help involves six to eight 20-minute sessions over 3–4 months. The therapist needs to be familiar with the structure of the self-help book, but no specialist training is required and it can be provided by any interested member of the primary health care team (e.g. GP, practice nurse, health visitor, practice counsellor, or community dietitian).

Each session has a similar format. The patient keeps detailed monitoring sheets (eating diaries; see Fig 18.4) and these are reviewed together during the sessions. Problems and possible solutions are discussed, drawing on the advice given in the programme. The therapist helps to set the pace through the programme, provides praise and encouragement as the patient progresses, and helps with difficulties as they arise. The therapist may also need to keep the patient focused on the eating problem rather than being distracted by other difficulties. The sessions can be largely patient-led. A simple step-by-step manual for therapists to use in conjunction with *Overcoming binge eating* is included in the Appendix of this chapter.

A recent pilot study (Waller *et al.* 1995) in general practice evaluated a brief form of CBT similar to 'guided self-help'. Eleven young women with bulimia nervosa were treated by their GP or practice nurse with a maximum of eight, weekly, 20-minute sessions. At the end of treatment, six of the women had improved substantially (four had stopped binge-eating completely). Only

Fig 18.4 *A typical monitoring sheet for use in conjunction with Overcoming binge eating. Asterisks signify eating viewed by the person as excessive; V/L signifies vomiting or laxative use*

Day... *Thursday* ...... Date... *7th July* ......

Time	Food and drink consumed	Place	*	V/L	Context and comments
7.45	Black coffee Yoghurt	kitchen			Didn't feel hungry but made myself eat this for breakfast as must keep to regular meal plan.
11 am	Black coffee	office			
1 pm	Rivita x2 with cottage cheese Yoghurt Black coffee	office			Ate lunch as planned. Pleased to be in control tempted to eat more – but resisted urge to go to canteen
4.30	Black tea Apple	office			
5.15	Chocolate biscuits x3	office	*		friend offered me a biscuit – felt guilty as soon as I'd taken it. Then ate another 2
5.35	Iced buns x2 Apple turnover	on the way home	* *		went into bakery out of control
5.50	2 bowls muesli with milk 6 slices bread/butter	kitchen	* *	V	raided the cupboard as soon as I get home – couldn't stop. HATE myself
6.30					went to gym to work out 11/2 hrs.
9 pm	Baked potato 1/2 tin baked beans	kitchen			Ate supper with boyfriend. Cooked him cornish pastry as well.
10 pm	1 glass wine	pub			Refused peanuts when offered – good.
11.30					went to bed – fed up by binge, but pleased I managed to regain control after this.

three needed to attend all eight sessions. Of the five patients who failed to respond, two were unable to commit themselves to the treatment due to major external events (one had final examinations, the other an accidental pregnancy), two had personality disorders, and one was very overweight and was more concerned with dieting than with overcoming the eating problem. The improvements were sustained at 6-month follow-up. The treatment was felt to be straightforward and rewarding by the GPs, and there was positive feedback from participants who found it convenient and relatively unthreatening. The study suggests that, provided patients are selected carefully, a simple form of CBT can be effective for the treatment of binge-eating problems in primary care.

Carter and Fairburn (1996) have recently completed a controlled trial comparing pure self-help and guided self-help, using the book *Overcoming binge eating*. They recruited 72 women with binge-eating disorder directly from the community. The findings indicated that both approaches produced substantial and sustained change (in about 40% of cases) compared to a waiting-list control group, with guided self-help being marginally superior. Follow-up data are awaited.

To date, there have been five published studies looking at the effectiveness of self-help literature in the treatment of binge-eating problems (see Carter and Fairburn 1995 for a review). The findings of these studies were positive with a significant number of patients benefiting from some form of self-help. However, with the exception of one study, the patients were recruited from specialist centres rather than the community, and there is very little follow-up data so the question of long-term maintenance of change is unresolved. Further studies are needed with appropriate patient samples if these simpler treatments are to be validated.

Controversies

Does dieting cause eating disorders?

It is clear that dieting precedes the development of anorexia nervosa and bulimia nervosa in young women, and epidemiological data support this. Patients with bulimia nervosa nearly always report that their binge-eating first started when they were on a diet. Eating disorders are more common in occupations and sports where a low body weight is required. There is a correlation between cultural pressure to be thin and prevalence of eating disorders, both across and within ethnic groups. The evidence is so strong that it has prompted some experts to rename these conditions 'dieting disorders'. Two prospective studies have linked dieting to the development of eating disorders. In a study of 15-year-old schoolgirls in London (Patton *et al.* 1990), girls who were dieting at the beginning of the study were eight times more likely than non-dieters to develop an eating disorder over the following year, though only 21% of the total dieters went on to develop an eating disorder. The second prospective study used data from over 1000 female twins located through the Virginia twin registry (Kendler *et al.* 1991). Self-reported weight fluctuation and current dieting status predicted the development of bulimia nervosa 1–3 years later.

However, dieting does not appear to be a risk factor for obese binge-eaters. People with binge-eating disorder do not practise the weight-controlling behaviours (e.g. self-induced vomiting) typical of bulimia nervosa sufferers and they report less dietary restraint. In obese binge-eaters the binge-eating usually precedes any attempts to diet, unlike bulimia nervosa. Cultural pressures in the West are such that most young women diet at some time or other. Yet the lifetime prevalence of bulimia nervosa is 1.5–2%. Some other factors must interact with dieting in susceptible subjects in order to precipitate eating disorders. Probable risk factors include certain personality traits, genetic susceptibility, and family influences (see p. 537–38).

Is binge-eating an addiction?

Terms like 'compulsive overeating', 'food addicts', and 'carbohydrate craving' have become popular and suggest that binge-eating is a form of addiction similar to alcohol or drug addiction. The self-help organization, Overeaters Anonymous (OA), models its approach on Alcoholics Anonymous and believes that certain foods, such as sugar, have addictive potential in susceptible individuals. OA argues that the only way to deal with the addiction is by lifelong avoidance of such 'toxic' foods. There are some obvious similarities between binge-eating and alcohol/drug dependence, but these are superficial. In the case of bulimia nervosa, the sufferer is continually trying to restrict her food intake. Binge-eating represents a loss of control and carries the risk of weight gain. In contrast, alcoholics have no inherent drive to restrict alcohol intake. They show no fear of getting drunk and do not have equivalent cognitive characteristics which interact in bulimia nervosa to maintain the disorder (see p. 543). In bulimia nervosa, the desire to restrict eating leads to binge-eating, whereas alcohol and drug addicts are not vulnerable to abuse of these substances because they wish to avoid them. It follows that the treatment of alcohol and drug dependence is based on increasing self-restraint and abstinence, whereas the key to treating bulimia nervosa is stopping dieting (Vandereycken 1990).

There have been several controlled studies which demonstrate that patients with bulimia nervosa do not 'crave' sugar or show a preference for simple carbohydrates during binges (Turner *et al.* 1991). The essential difference between the binges of bulimic patients and the 'normal' meals of controls is not in the nutrient composition but in the amount of food consumed. This also applies to obese binge-eaters.

In the case of binge-eating disorder, the situation is different again. Binge-eating is not driven by dieting in these people, many of whom are overweight. Here, binge-eating appears to be a way of relieving stress, and the mechanisms driving overeating may be similar to those involved in alcohol and drug abuse.

Involuntary hospital admission for anorexia nervosa

If a severely emaciated anorexic patient refuses treatment it may be possible to admit her to hospital for treatment against her will, under the Mental Health

Act, because of the risk of death. However, this is a complex area as it may be apparent that the individual is not suffering from a formal mental illness. Doctors face an ethical dilemma here: are some patients with anorexia nervosa truly incurable and is palliative care more appropriate in these cases? Or should it be argued that because of the effects of starvation on the brain, the severely anorexic patient is not able to make a rational decision about active treatment (Russell 1995)?

Can a minor with severe anorexia nervosa refuse consent to medical treatment? The ruling in the [1]Gillick case (1986) was that so long as the young person in question was competent, that is, of sufficient understanding and maturity, she could consent to medical treatment (in this case contraception) without the need for her parents to consent. The implication of this ruling was that if the minor was competent to consent to medical treatment, then equally, she was competent to refuse to consent to treatment. On this basis, it would seem that a mature minor could make a decision regarding her health, even if in the opinion of her parents and doctors it was not in her best interests. The crucial question then is how the court decides whether or not a minor is competent. Lord Scarman in 'Gillick' put this duty on the doctor.

There have been two cases subsequently which have overturned the liberal ruling in the Gillick case. The case [2]Re E (1990) involved a 15-year-old Jehovah's Witness suffering from leukaemia who, along with his parents, was refusing to consent to a blood transfusion. The boy was made a ward of court when the illness became life-threatening. The judge ruled that although the boy was obviously intelligent, he did not fully understand the issues involved and was not, therefore, competent to refuse consent.

The second case, [3]Re W (1992), involved a 16-year-old girl with severe anorexia nervosa, in the care of the local authority, who was refusing to consent to medical treatment. The initial ruling was that she had sufficient understanding to make an informed decision. The case went to the Court of Appeal. By the time the case was heard, her condition was life-threatening. The Court of Appeal conceded that anorexia nervosa is capable of destroying the ability to make an informed choice, that it creates a compulsion to refuse treatment. She was accordingly considered not competent to refuse consent.

In both these cases, the court considered firstly the outcome of the minor's refusal and, having concluded that the consequences were very serious, did not wish to be responsible for such drastic results. The court was able to override the minors' refusal on the grounds that they were not sufficiently competent to understand the full implications of their decision. It has been further argued by Lord Donaldson that even if the minor were deemed competent, his/her autonomy could still be over-ruled for the simple reason that it would be in the minor's best interests to undergo treatment.

Once a patient is in hospital, there is the question of how best to treat her.

---

1 Gillick v West Norfolk and Wisbech Area Health Authority (1986)
2 E (A minor) (Wardship: Medical Treatment) Re (1990)
3 W (A minor) (Medical Treatment: Court's Jurisdiction) Re (1992)

Although strict in-patient refeeding regimes achieve weight gain in the short term, more lenient treatments work as well for most patients. Anorexia nervosa sufferers lack a secure sense of self and have a great fear of being out of control. Inflexible refeeding regimes can reinforce these fears and limit recovery. Patients who refuse treatment and are then forced to gain weight in hospital may oppose all constructive therapeutic measures and stop eating, reverting to an anorexic state again as soon as they leave hospital. It is important that doctors do not engage in power struggles with their patients. Most would agree that compulsory admission should be avoided if at all possible for this reason.

Appendix

Treating binge-eating problems in primary care: therapist's manual for guided self-help to use in conjunction with *Overcoming binge eating*

Table 18.2 *Suggested time schedule for programme*

Week	Session	Step
0	Assessment	Homework: Read Part 1 of book
1	Session 1	Step 1
2	Session 2	Review Step 1 Introduce Step 2
3	Session 3	Review Step 2
4	Session 4	Review Step 2 Introduce Step 3
5		
6	Session 5	Review Steps 2 and 3 Introduce Step 4 (Problem-solving)
7		
8	Session 6	Review Step 4 (Taking stock) Introduce Step 5
9		
10	Session 7	Review Step 5 Homework: Step 6
11		
12	Session 8	Final session: review Step 6

Pretreatment assessment session (10 minutes)

1. *Does the patient have a binge-eating problem?*
   Ask about:

   (a) current eating habits
   - is she actively dieting?
   - does she have episodes of overeating:
     – objective binges?
     – how frequent? (episodes/week)
   - does she feels she loses control when she binges?

   (b) current methods of weight control

- dieting
- self-induced vomiting
- misuse of laxatives/diuretics
- extreme exercising

(c) attitudes to shape and weight
   - overconcern about shape and weight
   - current weight and height (as stated by patient). BMI
   - desired weight. Is this realistic?

2. *Inclusion criteria for Guided self-help*:
   Anyone with a binge-eating problem including those who fulfil criteria for bulimia nervosa.

3. *Exclusion criteria for Guided self-help*:
   (a) eating disorder present for over five years
   (b) previous treatment failure
   (c) very low weight (BMI <18).
   (d) substance misuse
   (e) severe personality disorder
   (f) significant medical problems, e.g. diabetes.

People with these problems are likely to need more intensive help and SPECIALIST REFERRAL is indicated.

4. *Is this the right time for the patient to embark on treatment?*
   The programme will take 12 weeks and needs commitment. She must make it her main priority over this period. If she can foresee other significant events occuring in this period (e.g. exams, house move), then she should defer the programme until she is ready to devote herself to it.

5. *If you agree treatment is appropriate*:
   Ask her to buy the book *Overcoming binge eating* (or order by phone: tel 01273 748427) and read Part 1 (educational section) before the next meeting.

Session 1 – Step 1: Getting started

1. *Outline goals of the programme*:
   (a) regain control over eating
   (b) help her to eat in a normal healthy fashion and, if relevant, to stop dieting. (Dieting and weight loss are NOT goals of the programme, though they may be important to the patient. Refer her to Chapters 4 and 6 where the vicious circle between dieting and binge-eating is discussed.)

2. *Explain what the programme involves*:
   (a) maximum of 8 sessions over 12–16 weeks
   (b) each session to last 20 minutes
   (c) sessions will focus exclusively on overcoming the eating problem.

3. *Introduce self-monitoring:*
   (a) explain briefly how to monitor (refer to completed monitoring sheet, p. 13)
   (b) explain the rationale for monitoring
      - it provides a detailed picture of her eating habits
      - it highlights circumstances under which problems arise
      - it will help her to change.

4. *Introduce weekly weighing:*
   (a) ask patient to weigh herself once a week at home and record her weight on the monitoring sheet each time she does so
   (b) explain the rationale for weekly weighing
      - it is reasonable to monitor weight since eating habits will change during treatment
      - weighing more frequently that once-weekly can lead to undue concern with inconsequential fluctuations in weight
      - It is only legitimate for a patient to conclude that her weight has changed if there is evidence of a consistent trend over 4 weeks.
   (c) she should decide on which day of the week to weigh herself (a weekday is best). If she is tempted to weigh herself more frequently, she should hide the scales in between weigh-ins.

5. *Stress key educational points (Chapters 4 and 5):*
   (a) explain the Body Mass Index (Appendix 1): BMI=weight (kg)/ height (m^2)
      - she should be advised against having a precise desired weight. Instead, she should accept a weight range of about 6 lbs (3kg). In practice, it is best if patients postpone deciding upon a specific weight range until they have regained control over eating
      - *for patients who are overweight,* overcoming their binge-eating problem may mean accepting a weight which is above their desired weight. At this stage they need to focus on overcoming the eating problem rather than on losing weight
      - *for patients within the normal weight range,* they should be reassured that overcoming a binge-eating problem is not generally accompanied by significant weight gain. They are unlikely to gain weight because binges, which are calorific, are replaced by normal meals.
   (b) physical consequences of binge-eating, self-induced vomiting, and laxative abuse (see Chapter 5)
      - electrolyte disturbance and oedema
      - salivary gland enlargement
      - erosion of tooth enamel
      - menstrual irregularities

(c) relative ineffectiveness of vomiting and laxative use as a means of weight control (Chapter 4, pp. 51–3)

- quote the Pittsburgh Human Feeding Laboratory study: self-induced vomiting resulted in the retrieval of less than half the food consumed during an average binge (calorie content of average binge=2131 kcal, calorie content of vomit=979 kcal).

Homework:

(1) self-monitoring – ask her to bring monitoring sheets to next visit

(2) Weekly weighing

(3) Summary sheet (pp. 114–15).

NEXT APPOINTMENT 1 WEEK

Session 2 – Review Step 1: Getting started

1. *Detailed review of monitoring sheets:*

   (a) 2 or 3 days' sheets should be chosen and discussed in detail (she should chose a 'good' day and a 'bad' day)

   (b) ask about accuracy of recording

   (c) aim to understand why she eats what she eats and what governs when she eats

   (d) pay particular attention to 'excessive eating' episodes (indicated by asterisks).

2. *Outline and personalize 'cognitive view of maintenance of bulimia nervosa' (p. 58, fig. 10) unless not applicable:*

   Points to emphasize:

   (a) Although dieting is undoubtedly a response to binge-eating, it also maintains binge-eating because:

   - the patient adopts strict and inflexible dietary rules; if she keeps to the rules she views herself as 'in control', but if she breaks the rules (even in a minor way) she views herself as 'out of control' and then overreacts, abandons all control, and binges. Once control has been relinquished, other factors actively encourage overeating. These include the pleasure that results from eating 'banned' foods, distraction from current problems, and a temporary allievation of feelings of anxiety and depression

   THE POINT THAT DIETING ENCOURAGES OVEREATING NEEDS TO BE MADE REPEATEDLY THROUGHOUT THE PROGRAMME

   - if the patient is effectively starving herself in between binges then there is a physiological drive to overeat.

   (b) Self-induced vomiting and, to a lesser extent, laxative and diuretic misuse also encourage binge-eating since belief in their effectiveness as a means of reducing calorie absorption removes normal constraints against overeating.

   (c) Over-concern about shape and weight, particularly the tendency to judge self-worth in terms of shape and weight, promotes extreme dieting and thereby maintains the eating problem.

EMPHASIZE THE NEED FOR BOTH BEHAVIOUR AND COGNITIVE CHANGE
(Return to this theme in subsequent sessions.)

3. *Is she ready to move to Step 2?*
   (a) Step 1 checklist (p. 15)
   (b) review of summary sheet: if she has had 6 or 7 good days, then she is ready to move to Step 2.

INTRODUCE STEP 2: REGULAR EATING

4. *Introduce a pattern of regular eating. THIS IS VERY IMPORTANT:*
   (a) restrict eating to 3 planned meals a day, plus 3 planned snacks
   (b) there should be no more than a 3-hour interval between eating times and the patient should always know when she is next due to eat
   (c) this eating pattern should take precedence over other activities
   (d) between these times the patient should do her utmost to refrain from eating
   (e) if necessary, this pattern can be introduced gradually, e.g. starting with breakfast and mid-morning snack
   (f) reassure that patient is unlikely to gain weight because binges will decrease in frequency.

Homework:
   (1) self-monitoring
   (2) Weekly weighing
   (3) summary sheet
   (4) move on to Step 2 (if appropriate).

NEXT APPOINTMENT 1 WEEK

Session 3 – Step 2: Regular eating

1. *Establishing a pattern of regular eating (see no.4 above for details):*
   Start by reviewing at least two monitoring sheets in detail:
   (a) pay particular attention to attempts to eat regular meals
   (b) emphasize behaviour that reinforces cognitive model
   (c) emphasize that dieting encourages binge-eating.

2. *Reassure her again that she is unlikely to gain weight* because regular meals will displace binges (p. 166).

3. *Advice on 'eating hygiene' (NOT VERY IMPORTANT):*
   (a) do not engage in other activities at the same time as eating
   (b) confine eating to one room in the house and have a set place to eat
   (c) supplies of food should not be left on the table while eating
   (d) practice leaving food on the plate

(e) throw away leftover foods

(f) limit exposure to 'danger' foods

(g) plan shopping and stick to a shopping list. Only take sufficient money to buy things on the list. Choose foods that require preparation rather than things that can be eaten immediately

(h) avoid preparing meals for others.

4. *Stopping vomiting and misusing laxatives and diuretics (refer to Chapter 4)*:

(a) advice regarding vomiting

- emphasis should be focused on changing eating habits rather than on stopping vomiting. If the patient stops overeating she is unlikely to continue vomiting (as outlined in cognitive view)

(b) advice regarding laxatives and diuretics

- reiterate ineffectiveness in preventing food absorption and suggest patient ceases to take them and discards supplies

- withdrawal schedule if necessary.

5. *Is she ready to move to Step 3?*

(a) Step 2 checklist, p. 168

(b) review of summary sheet.

Homework:

(1) self-monitoring

(2) weekly weighing

(3) keep to a regular pattern of eating

(4) summary sheet

(5) move on to Step 3 (if appropriate).

NEXT APPOINTMENT 1 WEEK

Session 4 – Step 3: Alternatives to binge-eating

1. *Start by reviewing at least two monitoring sheets in detail, stressing*:

(a) regular pattern of eating

(b) cognitive model.

2. *Introduce alternatives to binge-eating*:

(a) to help resist the urge to overeat/vomit

(b) to help avoid situations liable to result in binge-eating. Ask patient to draw up a list of pleasurable activities which might serve as a substitute for binge-eating (e.g. having a shower, phoning a friend, playing music, taking exercise). Whenever she feels the urge to binge she should engage in each possible activity.

Homework:

(1) self-monitoring

(2) weekly weighing

(3) regular pattern of eating

(4) introduce alternative activities

(5) summary sheet.

NEXT APPOINTMENT 2 WEEKS

Session 5 – Step 4: Problem solving

1. *Review at least two monitoring sheets in detail, stressing regular pattern of eating and use of alternative activities.*

2. *Is she ready to move to Step 4?*

    (a) See checklist, p. 175

    (b) review summary sheet.

3. *Introduce problem-solving:*

    (a) goal is to deal with problems that might otherwise trigger binges

    (b) the six steps of efficient problem solving (see p. 184 for example):

    - identify the problem as early as possible
    - specify the problem accurately
    - consider as many solutions as possible
    - think through the implications of each solution
    - choose the best solution or combination of solutions
    - act on the solution

Afterwards, review the entire problem-solving process.

Homework:

    (1) self-monitoring

    (2) weekly weighing

    (3) regular pattern of eating

    (4) introduce alternative activities

    (5) practise problem-solving

    (6) summary sheet.

NEXT APPOINTMENT 2 WEEKS

Session 6 – Step 4 continued

1. *Review at least two monitoring sheets in detail, looking at any examples of problem-solving.*

2. *Taking stock:*

    (a) Is the programme helping? By now, if the programme is going to help, there should be definite signs of improvement. Check:

    - If the frequency of binges has decreased (and, if applicable, the frequency of vomiting/laxative use) then CONTINUE
    - If the frequency of binges has not changed, but she is trying very hard to change – as reflected by the high proportion of 'Good days' on her summary chart – then programme is not helping. CONSIDER REFERRAL.
    - If the frequency of binges has not changed and she is not

following the programme as well as she could do, then question her commitment to change. Is this really right for her to be embarking on the programme? IF SO ABANDON THERAPY FOR TIME-BEING

- If the frequency of binges has not changed and she has features of clinical depression then CONSIDER FLUOXETINE AND/OR REFERRAL.

(b) Changes in weight: most people find little or no weight change during the programme. If weight has decreased by more than 2.5 kg (5 lbs):

- is she underweight (BMI <20)?
- is she eating too little (<1500 cal/day)? Stress this will limit progress

If weight has increased by more than 2.5 kg (5 lbs)

- was she underweight at the beginning of the programme? If so, now that she is eating more normally her weight will tend to return to her 'natural' weight. This is a good thing. Stress that it is best to concentrate on overcoming the binge eating problem and to accept any weight change that may occur.
- Is she now overweight (BMI >27)? If so, refer her to Appendix 2.

3. *Introduce Step 5: Dieting and related forms of food avoidance:*

(a) stress it is dieting that makes people prone to binge (refer to cognitive model, p. 58)

(b) abandoning dieting does not mean she will gain weight (much of her calorie intake has been from binges)

(c) aim now is to STOP DIETING.

The three types of dieting and how to deal with each:

(a) trying not to eat for long periods of time. Establish a regular pattern of eating (Step 2)

(b) trying to restrict the overall amount of food eaten. Ensure she is eating over 1500 calories/day. If eating below this she will have a strong physiological drive to eat and this will encourage binge-eating

(c) trying to avoid certain types of food. If she breaks her diet by eating 'forbidden' foods then this is a strong trigger to binge. To overcome this she needs to draw up a list of AVOIDED FOODS and to rank them in order of degree of reluctance to eat them; then categorize them into three groups of increasing difficulty. She can do this by going round a supermarket and noting down all the foods she normally avoids. She should then introduce group 1 (least avoided) foods into her diet deliberately, when she feels in control. The food should be eaten as part of a planned meal or snack. At first the amount of food eaten is not important, although the goal is that the patient is capable of eating normal amounts.

How to deal with related forms of avoidance:

(a) encourage patient to relax control over eating by eating foods with an uncertain calorie content, e.g. eating in a restaurant

(b) encourage patient to identify anything she avoids because it makes her anxious about her shape and weight and to do it repeatedly until she is no longer alarmed by it, (e.g. trying on clothes in a shop fitting-room, looking at her body in the mirror, going to the swimming pool).

Homework:

(1) self-monitoring

(2) weekly weighing

(3) regular pattern of eating

(4) introduce alternative activities

(5) practise problem-solving

(6) stopping dieting

(7) summary sheet.

NEXT APPOINTMENT 2 WEEKS

Session 7 – Step 5 continued

1. *Review at least two monitoring sheets, looking at:*

(a) regular pattern of eating

(b) use of problem-solving

(c) introduction of avoided foods

(d) exposure to anxiety-provoking situations.

Homework:

(1) self-monitoring

(2) weekly weighing

(3) regular pattern of eating

(4) alternative activities

(5) practise problem-solving

(6) introduce avoided foods

(7) read Step 6

(8) summary sheet.

NEXT APPOINTMENT 2 WEEKS

Session 8 – Step 6: what next?

1. *Review two monitoring sheets and summary sheet looking for introduction of avoided foods.*

2. *Preventing relapse:*

(a) Having realistic expectations:

- it is common for people who have stopped binge-eating to hope that they will never binge again. This is unrealistic. The eating problem will always be an 'Achilles heel', prone to recur at times of stress. The patient needs to be prepared for this
- patients often want to start dieting to lose weight as soon as they have stopped binge-eating. Warn her that strict dieting will put her at risk of binge-eating again. It is better for her to accept her 'natural' weight than to try and fight biology.

(b) Distinguishing a 'lapse' from a 'relapse':

- a lapse is a set-back or slip
- a relapse is returning to square one.
  Remind her that most people 'overeat' at times, and this is neither abnormal or a sign that control over eating is deteriorating. She would allow herself to overeat occasionally and not to view this negatively. To minimize the chance of relapsing, it is important not to label a lapse as a relapse. If she does have a lapse (and this may well happen at times of stress) she should use the skills she has developed during the programme to deal with the problem. Then review why the set-back occured and try to avoid it in future.

(c) Re-emphasize the risks of dieting in the future.

FOLLOW-UP: Suggest review appointment in 3 months.

Acknowledgements

I would like to thank Professor Christopher Fairburn for his guidance and comments in writing this chapter. The therapist's manual for use in conjunction with *Overcoming binge eating* is based on Fairburn, C. G., Marcus, M. D., and Wilson, G. T. (1993). Cognitive-behavioral therapy for binge eating and bulimia nervosa: a comprehensive treatment manual. In *Binge eating: nature, assessment and treatment* (ed. C. G. Fairburn and G. T. Wilson). Guilford Press, New York.

References and further reading

American Psychiatric Association (1994). *Diagnostic and statistical manual of mental disorders* (4th edn) (DSM-IV). American Psychiatric Association, Washington, D. C.

Brownell, K. D. (1991). Dieting and the search for the perfect body: where physiology and culture collide. *Behaviour Therapy*, **22**, 1–12.

Brownell, K. D. and Fairburn, C. F. (ed.). (1995). *Eating disorders and obesity: a comprehensive handbook*. Guilford Press, New York.

Carter, J. C. and Fairburn, C. G. (1995). Treating binge eating problems in primary care. *Addictive Behaviors*, **20**, 765–72.

Carter, J. C. and Fairburn, C. G. (1996). Self-help and guided self-help for binge eating disorder: a controlled study. Paper presented at the Ninth International Conference on Eating Disorders, New York, April 1996.

Cooper, P. J. (1995). *Bulimia nervosa and binge eating: a guide to recovery.* Robinson, London.

Cowen, P. J., Anderson, I. M., and Fairburn, C. G. (1992). Neurochemical effects of dieting: relevance to changes in eating and affective disorder. In *The biology of feast and famine: relevance to eating disorders* (ed. G. H. Anderson and S. H. Kennedy). Academic Press, New York.

Dare, C., Eisler, I., Russell, G. F. M., and Szmukler, G. I. (1990). The clinical and theoretical impact of a controlled trial of family therapy in anorexia nervosa. *Journal of Marital and Family Therapy,* **16,** 39–57.

Fairburn, C. G. (1981). A cognitive behavioural approach to the management of bulimia. *Psychological Medicine,* **11,** 707–11.

Fairburn, C. G. (1995). *Overcoming binge eating.* Guilford Press, New York.

Fairburn, C. G. and Belgin, S. J. (1990). Studies of the epidemiology of bulimia nervosa. *American Journal of Psychiatry,* **147,** 401–8.

Fairburn, C. G., Belgin, S. J., and Davies, B. (1992*a*). Eating habits and disorders amongst young adult women: an interview-based study. Unpublished manuscript.

Fairburn, C. G., Agras, W. S., and Wilson, G. T. (1992*b*). The research on the treatment of bulimia nervosa: practical and theoretical implications. In *The biology of feast and famine: relevance to eating disorders* (ed. G. H. Anderson and S. H. Kennedy), p. 317–40. Academic Press, San Diego.

Fairburn, C. G., Jones, R., Peveler, R. C., Hope, R. A., and O'Connor, M. (1993a). Psychotherapy and bulimia nervosa: the longer-term effects of interpersonal psychotherapy, behaviour therapy and cognitive-behaviour therapy. *Archives of General Psychiatry,* **50,** 419–28.

Fairburn, C. G., Marcus, M. D., and Wilson, G. T. (1993*b*). Cognitive-behavioural therapy for binge eating and bulimia nervosa: a comprehensive treatment manual. In *Binge eating: nature, assessment and treatment* (ed. C. G. Fairburn and G. T. Wilson), pp. 361–404. Guilford Press, New York.

Fairburn, C. G., and Wilson, G. T. (ed.) (1993*c*). *Binge eating: nature, assessment and treatment.* Guilford Press, New York.

Fairburn, C. G., Norman, P. A., Welch, S. L., O'Connor, M. E., Doll, H. E., and Peveler, R. C. (1995). A prospective study of outcome in bulimia nervosa and the long-term effects of three psychological treatments. *Archives of General Psychiatry,* **52,** 304–12.

Fluoxetine Bulimia Nervosa Collaboration Study Group (1992). Fluoxetine in the treatment of bulimia nervosa: a multicentre, placebo-controlled, double-blind trial. *Archives of Psychiatry,* **49,** 139–47.

Hoek, H. W. (1991). The incidence and prevalence of anorexia nervosa and bulimia nervosa in primary care. *Psychological Medicine,* **21,** 455–60.

Houghton-James, H. (1992). The child's right to die. *Family Law*, **550**.

Hsu, L. K. G. (1995). Outcome of bulimia nervosa. In *Eating disorders and obesity: a comprehensive handbook* (ed. K. D. Brownell and C. G. Fairburn), pp. 238–44. Guilford Press, New York.

Kendler, K. S., MacLean, C., Neale, M., Kessler, R., Heath, A., and Eaves, L. (1991). The genetic epidemiology of bulimia nervosa. *American Journal of Psychiatry*, **148**, 1627–37.

King, M. B. (1989). Eating disorders in a general practice population: prevalence, characteristics and follow-up at 12 to 18 months. *Psychological Medicine*, (suppl. 14).

Lacey, J. H. (1992). The treatment demand for bulimia: a catchment area report of referral rates and demography. *Psychiatric Bulletin*, **16**, 203–5.

Le Grange, D., Eisler, I., Dare, C., and Hodes, M. (1992). Family criticism and self-starvation: a study of expressed emotion. *Journal of Family Therapy*, **14**, 177–92.

Mitchell, J. E. and de Zwann, M. (1993). Pharmacological treatments of binge eating. In *Binge eating: nature, assessment and treatment* (ed. C. G. Fairburn and G. T. Wilson), pp. 250–69. Guilford Press, New York.

Olmsted, M. P., Davis, R., Garner, D. M., Eagle, M., Rockert, W., and Irvine, M. J. (1991). Efficacy of a brief group psychoeducational intervention for bulimia nervosa. *Behaviour Research and Therapy*, **29**, 71–83.

Parkinson, P. N. (1987). The Gillick case: just what has it decided? *Family Law*, **11**.

Patton, G. C., Johnson-Sabine, E., Wood, K., Mann, A. H., and Wakeling, A. (1990). Abnormal eating attitudes in London schoolgirls – a prospective epidemiological study: outcome at twelve month follow-up. *Psychological Medicine*, **20**, 383–94.

Pike, K. M. and Rodin, J. (1991). Mothers, daughters and disordered eating. *Journal of Abnormal Psychology*, **100**, 198–204.

Russell, G. F. M. (1979). Bulimia nervosa: an ominous variant of anorexia nervosa. *Psychological Medicine*, **9**, 429–48.

Russell, J. (1995). Treating anorexia nervosa. *British Medical Journal*, **311**, 584.

Stein, A., Woolley, H., Cooper, S. D., and Fairburn, C. F. (1994). An observational study of mothers with eating disorders and their infants. *Journal of Child Psychology and Psychiatry*, **35**, 733–48.

Steinhausen, H. -C., Rauss-Mason, C., and Seidel, R. (1991). Follow-up studies of anorexia nervosa: a review of four decades of outcome research. *Psychological Medicine*, **21**, 447–51.

Strober, M. (1992). Family-genetic studies. *In Psychology and treatment of anorexia nervosa and bulimia nervosa* (ed. K. Halmi), pp. 61–76. American Psychiatric Press, Washington, D.C.

Turner, M. St J., Foggo, M., Bennie, J., Carroll, S., Dick, H., and Goodwin, G. M. (1991). Psychological, hormonal and biochemical changes following carbohydrate bingeing:

a placebo-controlled trial in bulimia nervosa and matched controls. *Psychological Medicine*, **21,** 123–33.

Vandereycken, W. (1990). The addiction model in eating disorders: some critical remarks and a selected bibliography. *International Journal of Eating Disorders*, **9,** 95–101.

Waller, D., Fairburn, C. G., McPherson, A., Kay, R., Lee, A., and Nowell, T. (1995). Treating bulimia nervosa in primary care: a pilot study. *International Journal of Eating Disorders*, **19,** 99–109.

Walsh, B. T., Hadigan, C. M., Devlin, M. J., Gladis, M., and Roose, S. P.(1991). Long-term outcome of antidepressant treatment for bulimia nervosa. *American Journal of Psychiatry*, **148,** 1206–12.

Whitehouse, A. M., Cooper, P. J., Vize, C. V., Hill, C., and Vogel, L.(1992). Prevalence of eating disorders in three Cambridge general practices: hidden and conspicuous morbidity. *British Journal of General Practice.* **42,** 57–60.

Wilson, G. T., and Fairburn, C. G. (1993). Cognitive treatments for eating disorders. *Journal of Consulting and Clinical Psychology*, **61,** 261–9.

Useful reading for patients

Self-help books for binge-eating problems with a programme based on cognitive behaviour therapy

Cooper, P. J. (1995). *Bulima nervosa and binge eating: a guide to recovery.* Robinson, London.

Fairburn, C. G. (1995). *Overcoming binge eating.* Guilford Press, New York: (Order by phone: tel. 01273 748427.)

Schmidt, U. and Treasure, J. (1993). *Getting better bit(e) by bit(e).* Erlbaum, Hove.

Educational material for anorexia nervosa sufferers

Dally, P. and Gomez, J. (1990). *Obesity and anorexia nervosa – a question of shape.* Faber, London.

Palmer, R. L. (1989). *Anorexia nervosa – a guide for sufferers and their families.* Penguin, Harmondsworth.

Other recommended literature on dieting and eating disorders

Abraham, S. and Llewellyn-Jones, D. (1996). *Eating disorders: the facts* (4th edn). Oxford University Press, Oxford.

Burns, D. D. (1992). *Feeling good: the new mood therapy.* Avon, New York.

Orbach, S. (1978). *Fat is a feminist issue.* Paddington Press, London.

Rodin, J. (1992). *Body traps.* William Morrow and Company, New York.

CHAPTER NINETEEN

Sexual problems

Keith Hawton and Susan Harrison

This chapter is addressed in particular to those doctors who would like to offer help to their patients with sexual problems, but who feel they need further information in order to be able to help more effectively.

The main emphasis is on the sexual difficulties of women, but the difficulties of men are also discussed as it is almost invariable for a problem in one partner in a sexual relationship to be associated with some difficulty in the other partner, whether as a secondary effect or as a partial cause of the presenting problem. Most attention will be devoted to sexual dysfunctions (such as reduced sexual desire, vaginismus, and erectile dysfunction) arising in a heterosexual relationship, but female homosexuality and male sexual variations are also mentioned because these may come to the attention of the general practitioner (GP) and can be related to sexual dysfunction.

How common are sexual problems?

We have limited knowledge about the incidence of sexual dysfunction in the general population. Masters and Johnson (1970) made the surprising claim that as many as 50% of marriages in the US are troubled by sexual dysfunction at some time, and their estimate received support in 1978 from a small interview survey carried out in the US. A community survey in the UK of a random sample of women aged 35–59 years with partners indicated that approximately one-third reached criteria for a sexual dysfunction, the prevalence increasing markedly with age (Osborn et al. 1988). However, only one in 10 of all the women regarded themselves as having a sexual problem (a similar figure to that found in younger women attending family planning clinics) and less than half of these said they would like help if it were available.

Relatively little is known about how many women in the general population are homosexual or bisexual. In a recent extensive survey of sexual behaviour in Britain 3.4% of women reported having had some sort of homosexual experience, 1.7% genital contact with a woman, and 0.6% a female sexual partner within the previous 2 years (Wellings et al. 1994). Because of the reticence of some people to answer questions about homosexuality truthfully, these figures are likely to be an underestimate. However, on this basis the average GP with a list size of 2500 patients can expect to have approximately 15 women in the practice who have had recent homosexual experience, and many more who have had homosexual interest at some time. Most of these will not regard their homosexuality as a problem. However, homosexual women may present with sexual difficulties similar to those of other women.

All those, whatever their profession, who work with couples or families will know how often sexual problems are linked with marital disharmony, or with actual breakdown of a marriage, and will know also how in the absence of a happy sexual relationship one vital channel for the resolution of disharmony is removed from the partnership. Unfortunately, few statistics are available to confirm this clinical impression. It is impossible in a brief account to do justice to either the complexities of cause and effect between sexual difficulty and general tension in a relationship, or the depth of unhappiness that such difficulties may cause. However, the following case illustrates some of the effects:

Mary and Arthur married when he was 24 and she was 20. They knew at the time that he had a problem with premature ejaculation, dating back to his first hasty intercourse at the age of 16 in the back of a car after a party. Mary had been involved in several unhappy relationships before she met Arthur, and found that she was very slow to become aroused during lovemaking. They hoped that the problems would resolve once they were married, but they did not, and by the second year of their marriage Margaret and Arthur were on the verge of separating. They tried to make a fresh start and Mary became pregnant. During the pregnancy Mary felt very keen on sex, but Arthur found her unattractive, and when after delivery his interest in her returned, she felt sore and began to be repelled by the idea of sex. On the few occasions that they did try to make love, Arthur ejaculated so quickly that he began to feel 'a complete failure', and acquiesced in Mary's avoidance of sex. By the time they went to their doctor they had not had sex for 8 months, and the subject had become unmentionable. They were still determined to stay together for the sake of the child. Mary said, 'I want to sort things out but I feel it's impossible.'

Sexual dysfunction may also cause a woman to avoid forming further relationships, especially if a previous sexual encounter was unsuccessful. Such avoidance may lead to further unhappiness and lack of confidence, which in turn can add to the woman's conviction that she is 'sexually inadequate'.

How sexual problems may present to doctors

In spite of the drastic changes in public attitudes to sexuality that have occurred over recent years, many people still find it embarrassing to talk honestly about sexuality, especially their own. A very important part of the help that a doctor can give is in making it easier for patients to overcome this hurdle. Doctors need to be sensitive to clues that a patient has a problem that she (or he) wants to discuss, and be able to convey their willingness to enter into the discussion. Often patients have heard, through the press and elsewhere, of the availability and effectiveness of treatment of sexual problems, and such patients may come to the doctor with *direct requests for help*.

Other patients may be too shy to express their worry directly, or may not even realize that there is a sexual cause for the difficulty that they experience, and in these cases the doctor must be aware of the possible *covert presentation* of sexual problems. On the whole, such covert presentations take the form either of emotional or psychological symptoms (such as depression, marital disharmony, poor sleep), or gynaecological complaints (such as requests for a change of contraceptive pill, or the report of a vaginal discharge). The following case illustrates such a presentation.

Alicia was 35 and had been married for 9 years when she attended a cervical screening session at her doctor's surgery. The doctor found it almost impossible to take the smear and it then came to light that Alicia's marriage had never been consummated. For nine years she had allowed her husband to caress her but not to approach her genitals, while she had masturbated him. She had been too ashamed of her inability to have sex ever to confide in anyone else. Her doctor referred her for sex therapy, but she cancelled the appointment. However, a few months later she asked to be re-referred.

A gynaecological examination can provide a surprisingly helpful opportunity to enquire into a patient's sexual anxieties, and in which reassurance (e.g. about the normality of the genitals) can be given. Another common presentation is for the patient to *complain of the partner's sexual dysfunction.* This sometimes may be because the partner is unwilling to attend, but often it is because the patient has not recognized that the problem is at least partly her or his own.

Normal sexual function

Understanding of the different types of sexual problems is facilitated by a knowledge of normal sexual behaviour, and particularly of the events that occur during the various stages of sexual desire and response. Only a brief summary of such information can be provided here. This information is based largely on that provided by Masters and Johnson (1966) following their extensive study of sexual response in non-dysfunctional individuals of both sexes. For more detailed information the reader is referred to Bancroft's (1989) book *Human sexuality and its problems.*

Normal sexual behaviour can be divided somewhat arbitrarily into four phases:

1. *Interest or desire.* The background level of interest in sexuality, willingness to seek opportunities for sexual contact, and occurrence of sexual thoughts or fantasies outside as well as within times of actual sexual contact.

2. *Arousal or excitement.* The initial physiological responses to sexually stimulating activity or thought. This phase includes: (a) the *vascular* changes that produce genital engorgement and lubrication in the female, erection in the male, together with flushing of the face and body; (b) *neuromuscular* changes such as ballooning of the interior of the vagina and retraction of the clitoris in the female, elevation of the testes and tightening of the scrotum in the male. During this phase of arousal, thoughts and feelings also become increasingly focused on the sexual experience. It is normal for the subjective experience of arousal to intensify not gradually, but by a series of waves of arousal of increasing intensity.

3. *Orgasm.* This includes both the observable event of pubococcygeus muscle

contractions in the female or ejaculation in the male, and the subjective experience of orgasm. The male response may be divided into two phases: the first in which seminal and prostatic fluid enters the urethral bulb, and the second, beginning from the point at which the process becomes inevitable and irreversible, in which the seminal fluid is ejected from the urethra.

4. *Resolution*. During this phase the physiological events of arousal are gradually reversed. Descent of the uterus and resolution of vascular engorgement occur in women. In men a moderate immediate loss of erection is followed by a slower complete reversal to the flaccid state. In both sexes these changes are accompanied by subjective sensations of relaxation and languor. For the male this phase includes a *refractory period* of variable length (from 15–30 minutes for a 15-year-old, to 24 hours or more for an 80-year-old) before full sexual arousal can recommence; for the female there may be no corresponding physiological refractory period, and some women experience a series of orgasms in close succession. However, degree of satisfaction is not necessarily a function of the number of orgasms.

These four phases normally follow each other in sequence. It is said however that for many women there seems to be less 'need for orgasm' than for many men: but whether this is physiologically or culturally determined is not clear. In any case, many women enjoy sexual arousal, intercourse, and the ebbing of arousal without necessarily experiencing an orgasm on each occasion, or regretting its absence (see Hawton (1985) for further discussion of this).

The role of hormones in sexual behaviour is complex. Although *androgens* are essential for the development of full sexual functioning in men, their withdrawal, as occurs following castration, often does not cause loss of a man's ability to respond to sexual stimulation with erection, but sexual desire and the ability to ejaculate may be impaired. Androgens are important with respect to a woman's sexual interest or desire, although much lower levels of androgens are necessary in females than in males for this purpose. In women, *ostrogens* appear to be important in facilitating normal vaginal response to sexual stimulation, but have little or no direct effect on sexual interest. The role, if any, of *progesterone* in female sexual response is largely unknown.

Types of sexual problems

Sexual dysfunctions

In general terms a sexual dysfunction refers to a failure or impairment of sexual interest or response. The types of sexual dysfunction of women and men are listed in Table 19.1. The classification is based on the first three phases of sexual response; that is, sexual interest or desire, arousal or excitement, and orgasm. However, vaginismus and sexual phobias do not usually correspond to a particular response phase.

Table 19.1 *Sexual dysfunctions of females and males*

Phase of sexual response	Sexual dysfunction	
	Female	Male
Interest or desire	Low sexual desire	Low sexual desire
Arousal or excitement	Impaired arousal	Erectile dysfunction
Orgasm	Orgasmic dysfunction	Premature ejaculation
		Retarded ejaculation
		Pain on ejaculation
Other types of dysfunction	Vaginismus	
	Dyspareunia	Dyspareunia
	Sexual phobias	Sexual phobias

All the problems listed may be either *primary* or *secondary*. A *primary problem* is one that has been present since the onset of sexual activity. A *secondary problem* is one which occurs after a period of normal sexual function. The types of sexual dysfunction which occur in women and men will be described separately.

Sexual dysfunction in women

The general term 'frigidity' was in common use at one time to describe any female sexual dysfunction. The term is non-specific, incorrectly suggests a lack of emotional warmth, and is pejorative, so it should be avoided.

Low sexual desire

This is the most common sexual problem for which women seek help, although often without much hope of improvement. Commonly it is a woman's partner who insists on her obtaining help for this problem. The effect that low sexual desire will have on a woman's life will depend on the degree of the impairment and on other circumstances. Some women who experience no spontaneous interest in sex may choose to avoid sexual activity; but many others will choose to enter relationships in which they are expected to engage in sexual activity. In this latter category will be some women who also suffer from difficulties during the phases of arousal and orgasm, while others will find that, although they lack spontaneous sexual desire, they can respond to the partner's interest and experience orgasm during sexual activity. Primary low sexual desire is often related to an upbringing in which sexuality was regarded as unmentionable, dirty, or wicked, a view often reinforced by religions beliefs. On the other hand, secondary low sexual desire is more usually related to general difficulties in the relationship, or to an important event such as childbirth, or to depression.

Impaired arousal

Problems of the excitement phase are characterized by failure of the normal physiological responses which occur during arousal, especially vaginal swelling and lubrication, and by lack of the sensations usually associated with sexual excitement. Such problems are relatively uncommon in women with unimpaired sexual drive, except during later life when hormonal changes may cause impairment of the normal vaginal response so that intercourse becomes uncomfortable and willingness to engage in it is reduced.

Orgasmic dysfunction

It has already been noted that enjoyment of sexual activity without reaching orgasm does not necessarily constitute a 'problem'; the extent to which a woman feels she has a problem concerning orgasm will depend in part on her or her partner's expectations. These can change with time and because of information obtained from a variety of sources, including novels and magazines. Sometimes this may be misleading and cause unreasonable expectations.

Orgasmic dysfunction can be *total*, which means that orgasm is never experienced during sexual activity of any kind, or it can be *situational*, which means that orgasm can be achieved under some circumstances but not others, such as during masturbation but not with a partner, or with one partner and not another. It is important to establish which type of orgasmic dysfunction is present, because the choice of treatment will depend on the nature of the problem.

Vaginismus

This refers to spasm of the pubococcygeus muscles surrounding the entrance to the vagina, which makes sexual intercourse impossible or difficult or painful. Vaginismus is usually due to a specific fear about penetration, the ability to enjoy other aspects of sexual behaviour being largely unimpaired. Occasionally, however, it is part of a more general sexual problem. Vaginismus is a major cause of non-consummation of marriage. It mostly presents as a primary problem although it can occur following vaginal trauma such as an episiotomy, especially if this has not been satisfactorily repaired.

Dyspareunia

This refers to pain occurring during sexual intercourse. The pain may be localized to the entrance to the vagina (in which case it is usually related to mild vaginismus or a vaginal infection), or the pain may occur on deep penetration. This deep pain may result from lack of arousal and consequent absence of ballooning of the inner vagina, such that the cervix is buffeted during sexual intercourse. Deep dyspareunia may also be due to pelvic pathology, such as chronic salpingitis or endometriosis.

Sexual phobias

Some women are repelled by certain aspects of sexuality. These might be very specific, such as aversion to kissing, or to seminal fluid, or more generalized, such as aversion to foreplay. A sexual phobia need not necessarily inhibit a woman's enjoyment of the rest of sexual activity, but in many cases the phobia prevents arousal altogether. Sexual phobias are occasionally related to a past traumatic experience such as rape or incest.

Sexual dysfunction in men

Low sexual desire

It is common for most men to feel lessened sexual desire at some time. However, men are somewhat less likely than women to seek help because of long-standing low desire, although referrals of this problem to specialist services have increased in the past few years. Possibly the widely-held myth that men are always ready and able to have sex makes it difficult for a man to acknowledge that his desire for sex is lacking. Also, men with low sexual desire often have associated erectile difficulties for which they are more likely to seek help. In some cases the problem presents in the context of a depressive disorder. It may also be related to unacknowledged feelings of anger towards the partner.

Erectile dysfunction

Whereas impairment of arousal in women is not a very common complaint, erectile dysfunction is the male sexual problem most commonly encountered in clinical practice. The erectile response is extremely vulnerable to psychological influences, especially anxiety, and may also be affected by organic disorders, such as diabetes and multiple sclerosis, and by several forms of medication, especially antihypertensive agents.

Erectile dysfunction is often a secondary phenomenon and is particularly likely to occur in middle-aged and older men. Where psychological factors contribute to the dysfunction it is usually situational, in that the man is able to get and sustain an erection on his own through masturbation or wakes with an erection at night, but fails to get an erection with his partner or easily loses it – especially when he wishes to penetrate. Sometimes erection difficulties are complete, so that no erection occurs; in other cases a partial erection may be obtained.

Premature ejaculation

This is an extremely common problem among young men, and may be viewed as a relatively 'normal' phenomenon in many males having their first sexual relationships. There is no satisfactory definition of premature ejaculation. Probably the best guide is the extent to which a man and his partner feel that his ejaculatory control is sufficient. In its most severe form it includes failure to prevent ejaculation before vaginal penetration. More often the man ejaculates within a few seconds of the start of sexual intercourse or immediately he begins to thrust.

Retarded ejaculation

This disorder of ejaculation was relatively uncommon but appears to have increased recently. It includes a total failure of ejaculation under any circumstances, partial failure where ejaculation is not possible with a partner but does occur through masturbation, and difficulty in ejaculating where sexual stimulation or intercourse must be continued for an excessively long time for ejaculation to occur. It is sometimes associated with a sexual variation such as fetishism when the man is unable to ejaculate unless the fetishistic object (e.g. female clothing) is present. Some men with this problem have a history of forceful masturbation in which very vigorous stimulation is required for ejaculation to occur. Retarded or absent ejaculation can also be caused by some forms of medication, notably antidepressants, especially the recently introduced serotonergic drugs.

Pain on ejaculation

This is rarely encountered in clinical practice. However, some men do complain of acute pain in the perineum and penis during or following ejaculation. This is usually associated with an infection of the urethra or prostate, although in some cases it may be related to spasm of the perineal muscles.

Dyspareunia

Some men experience pain if they try to have sexual intercourse. This may be because of a tight foreskin when the penis is erect. It can also be related to genital infections.

Sexual phobias

Men rarely present complaining of aversion to specific aspects of sexual behaviour. However, phobias sometimes appear to be part of another sexual dysfunction. Thus among men with erectile dysfunction will be found some who experience aversion to extreme sexual excitement in their partners, others who are particularly averse to vaginal penetration, and others who dislike the touch and/or sight of the female genitals. This last cause can occur in men who have been actively involved in their partner's childbirth.

Sexual variations

The term 'sexual variation' refers to sexual interest or behaviour which varies from that experienced predominantly by the majority of the population, and in women it refers principally to homosexuality, transsexualism, and sado-masochism. 'Sexual variation' (or its alternative, 'sexual deviation') is a better term than the rather pejorative 'sexual perversion'.

Female homosexuality

Homosexual interest may range from simple feelings of attraction towards another woman, to full sexual activity with a female partner. Some women are exclusively homosexual, but many more experience sexual feelings towards both sexes, and some degree of attraction to other women among heterosexual women appears to be extremely common.

Occasionally, unacknowledged homosexuality turns out to underlie a complaint of sexual dysfunction such as low sexual desire (for a heterosexual partner). Therefore the doctor should routinely ask an appropriate question about homosexual interest during the course of a full assessment of a sexual problem, and be receptive to any sign that the patient wishes to discuss the issue further.

Other sexual variations

A *transsexual* is a person who feels that his or her gender is really that of the opposite sex. This leads in many cases to a wish to adopt the style of dress of the opposite sex and to undergo hormonal and surgical treatments in order to bring about appropriate anatomical changes. The greater general acceptance of masculine styles of dress for women than feminine styles for men may allow many female transsexuals to go relatively unnoticed. Occasionally a female transsexual will seek specialist help to obtain hormonal treatment and surgery. The latter can include mastectomy, hysterectomy, and genital reconstruction, although the last of these is unlikely to be successful.

Sado-masochism is the only other sexual variation likely to be found in women. Sadistic behaviour includes infliction of pain or restriction of the partner's mobility ('bondage'), while 'masochism' refers to the wish to be the recipient of such activities. It has been argued that a mild degree of sado-masochistic behaviour should be regarded as abnormal only when it consistently provides the main focus of a sexual relationship, and where sex cannot be enjoyed in its absence. It is unequivocally a problem either when one partner does not wish to take part, or where the sadistic or masochistic activities become dangerous.

Male sexual variations

Not uncommonly a woman will present to her doctor complaining directly or indirectly about her partner's sexual behaviour or desires because in her opinion these are abnormal. The behaviour may be of a kind which many couples ordinarily include in their lovemaking, such as orogenital sex, or anal intercourse, but sometimes the source of concern will be a sexual variation such as fetishism, transvestism, sado-masochism, or homosexuality, which the partner finds impossible to accept. Sometimes couples may only need reassurance that they can continue with a practice that they both enjoy, but usually the problem arises from the unwillingness of one partner to engage in a practice that the other wants. Where this is so, the doctor should try to see the partner and discuss this with him, not moralistically, but with the intention of helping the couple come to an arrangement that suits them both. Sometimes the woman can be helped to accept the practice, if this is what she wishes, in other cases it may be possible to encourage the man to restrict his interest in the variation to masturbatory activity or to fantasy alone. Sometimes the sexual variation seems to be maintained because of a sexual dysfunction in one or other partner and therefore this should be the focus of treatment. A fairly common problem presenting in general practice is some form of cross-dressing which has been tolerated by the partner until the children become of an age at which they might realize what is happening. This is a difficulty which may need referral

Table 19.2 *Some psychological causes of sexual dysfunction*

1. *Predisposing factors*
   Family attitudes to sexuality
   Inadequate sex education
   Traumatic sexual experiences

2. *Precipitants*
   Psychiatric illness
   Childbirth
   Infidelity
   Dysfunction in the partner
   General relationship problems

3. *Maintaining factors*
   Anxiety
   Poor communication
   Lack of foreplay
   Depression
   Dysfunction in the partner
   Poor sexual information
   General relationship problems

for specialist help. Some men with this problem and their partners may find it beneficial to contact the Beaumont Trust (see Useful addresses at the end of the chapter).

Causes of sexual dysfunction

In many cases there are multiple causes for sexual dysfunction. The range of possible causes is very wide but may be separated into *psychological* and *physical factors.*

Psychological factors

Factors which may lead to sexual dysfunction can usefully be divided into: (1) *predisposing factors*; (2) *precipitants*; and (3) *maintaining factors*. These will be considered separately and some of the more important are summarized in Table 19.2.

Predisposing factors

Often these are factors arising out of experiences early in life which either made a person vulnerable to developing a sexual problem at a later date or actually caused a sexual dysfunction to develop at that stage. Such factors typically occur in three areas of early experience: family attitudes to sexuality, sex education, and traumatic sexual experiences.

Family attitudes to sexuality. The attitudes to which a person is exposed during early development can have a profound effect on later sexual adjustment. In many families, sex is never discussed and to the children this can imply that sex is a taboo subject and must be in some way wrong or shameful. In other families, negative attitudes towards sex may be expressed openly. For example, a mother may tell her daughter that sex is a chore that must be undertaken in order to please her partner. Either type of experience is likely to make a young woman feel guilty about her sexual desires or enjoyment, and may contribute to the development of sexual dysfunction. Attitudes which suggest that sex is dirty or shameful may lead to difficulties in arousal or orgasm. Those which suggest that lovemaking is painful may contribute to the development of vaginismus.

The following case is an example of a mother's adverse attitudes that may have been important in causing a subsequent problem for her daughter:

Helen's parents had frequent rows and separated when she was in her early teens. She lived with her mother, a tense, nagging woman who had instructed Helen carefully from an early age in the 'facts of life', while conveying an idea of sex as something joyless and mechanical. When Helen began to go out with boys she repeatedly warned her to 'be careful', and when a few years later Helen got engaged and allowed her fiancé to persuade her to make love, it was her mother who first detected Helen's pregnancy. Helen had enjoyed lovemaking before marriage, but after the baby was born (after a difficult delivery), she enjoyed it no longer: she came easily to climax but was overcome by guilt afterwards. She enjoyed foreplay with her husband but would rarely agree to go on to intercourse.

Inadequate sex education. Inadequate or poor information about sexuality is a very important factor in the development of sexual dysfunction. For many people, especially those now of middle or older age, sex education has been either woefully inadequate or entirely lacking. Such information as they possess is likely to be based instead on 'dirty' jokes heard during childhood and adolescence, or on discussion with other children whose information may have been equally inadequate. This can lead to serious misinformation, and particularly to those incorrect beliefs which have been termed *sexual myths.* Some examples of these are given in Box 19.1. Belief in such myths can lead to false expectations concerning sexuality and therefore may cause dysfunction because of the anxiety that results. Lack of knowledge about sexual anatomy (e.g. the position of the clitoris, or even that it exists) can likewise lead to sexual dysfunction. Knowledge of sexuality is likely to be particularly poor with regard to that of the opposite sex. This may mean that a person does not know how to provide a partner with adequate stimulation.

Traumatic sexual experiences. It is now clear that the number of women who have had traumatic sexual experiences earlier in their lives, especially childhood sexual abuse (see p. 589), is considerable (Jehu 1988). Such a history is common in women with sexual dysfunction, especially low sexual desire, problems concerning sexual arousal, and specific sexual phobias. Traumatic experiences most likely to lead to problems are those that involved threat, force, or pain, which took place repeatedly, and which involved someone considerably older than the woman herself. Sexual assaults and rape (see p. 591) may cause sexual difficulties, especially if the woman has not received support following the trauma. The consequences of sexual traumas are often related to their damaging

---

Box 19.1 *Some common sexual myths*

1. A man always wants and is always ready to have sex
2. Sex must only occur at the instigation of the man
3. Any woman who initiates sex is immoral
4. Masturbation by either sex is dirty or harmful
5. Sex equals intercourse: anything else does not really count
6. When a man gets an erection it is bad for him not to use it to get an orgasm very soon
7. Sex should always be natural and spontaneous: thinking or talking about it spoils it
8. All physical contact must lead to sexual intercourse
9. Men should not express their feelings
10. Any man ought to know how to give pleasure to any woman
11. Sex is really good only when partners have orgasms simultaneously
12. If people love each other they will know how to enjoy sex together
13. Partners in a sexual relationship instinctively know what the other partner thinks or wants
14. Married partners with a good sexual relationship never masturbate
15. If a man loses his erection it means he does not find his partner attractive
16. It is wrong to have fantasies during sexual intercourse

---

effects on the victim's self-esteem and to confused feelings of guilt and anger about the experience.

As with the other remote factors, the extent to which such experiences lead to sexual dysfunction will often depend upon events which occur later, and particularly upon the type of relationships which are established. Some women have very adverse early experiences in terms of family attitudes, sex education, or early sexual relations, yet enjoy highly satisfactory sexual relationships in adulthood.

Precipitants

These are numerous and only some of the more common ones (listed in Table 19.2) will be dealt with here. Psychiatric disorder, as well as physical illness and medication, which can be particularly important precipitants, are discussed later.

Childbirth. Sexual problems in women are especially likely to develop after childbirth, particularly after the birth of a second or subsequent baby. Most women experience a decline in sexual interest and activity in the later stages of pregnancy and during the early puerperium. A number of factors may then inhibit the return of sexual interest which normally occurs during the 3 months after childbirth (see p. 593).

Infidelity. Discovery of her partner's infidelity may cause a woman to lose interest in continuing a sexual relationship with him, or infidelity on her own part may cause loss of interest because of anxiety resulting from guilt, or simply because her other sexual relationship is more rewarding. Sometimes a woman first discovers that she has a sexual problem, or that she has one only with her current partner, when she encounters a new partner who is perhaps more knowledgeable or sensitive than her regular one. This is illustrated in the following case example:

Sally and George had difficulties from the beginning of their marriage, mainly because of his premature ejaculation and her lack of enjoyment of sex. In the fourth year of the marriage they began to attend an infertility clinic where it was discovered that George had a moderately low sperm count. The sexual difficulty was not picked up then, nor when Sally became depressed and went into a psychiatric hospital for a month. After this they separated, and Sally had an affair with an older man. With him she discovered that she enjoyed sex and was orgasmic. A year later she and George decided to live together again, and at this point she came to her doctor to ask for help with their sexual difficulties.

Dysfunction in the partner. Where the male partner either already has a sexual problem or develops one this may cause the woman herself to suffer sexual dysfunction. For example, orgasmic dysfunction or reduced sexual desire in a woman are often associated with premature ejaculation or erectile dysfunction in her partner. Vice versa, it has been shown that many female partners of men with erectile dysfunction have themselves had sexual difficulties which preceded (and possibly contributed to) the erectile problem (Speckens *et al.* 1995). In such cases it is important to determine which dysfunction developed first because that should also be a focus of treatment.

Problems in the general relationship. Deterioration in the general relationship between a woman and man often, although by no means always, leads to problems in their sexual relationship. Where the partners' affection for each other has declined or disappeared then the sexual relationship is almost certain to be disrupted. Distinguishing between a sexual dysfunction which has *resulted* in general relationship difficulties and one which is *symptomatic* of problems in the general relationship is one of the most important tasks in the assessment of people with sexual dysfunction. However, often this is not easy and may be impossible.

Maintaining factors

It is the factors perpetuating a sexual problem which are most important for treatment purposes because only these perpetuating or maintaining factors are directly amenable to modification. Recognition of the predisposing factors and precipitants can provide the doctor with an understanding of the disorder, and explanations to the patient on this basis may be therapeutic in the sense of helping the patient see that the problem is explicable. However, one cannot change events that have already occurred; one can only try to deal with the consequences of such events. The following are some of the more common maintaining factors (listed in Table 19.2).

Anxiety. This is the main factor underlying most sexual problems. Anxiety may be due to a wide range of causes, including sexual inhibitions, poor self-image, fear of failure, fear of pain, a specific phobia concerning vaginal penetration, and ignorance. Whatever the cause of the anxiety, it can affect sexual function by leading to avoidance, causing lack of drive, inhibiting arousal, or preventing orgasm. Some women clearly recognize that they become anxious during sex. Others may notice a sense of detachment from the sexual activity, almost as if the woman had become an uninvolved observer. This experience has been termed 'spectatoring' by Masters and Johnson (1970).

Poor communication. If a woman fails to let her partner know about her sexual needs and anxieties it is very likely that difficulties will result. In addition, partners often become less communicative about sex once a problem begins, thus making the situation very much worse. This is illustrated in the following case example:

Andrew and Jackie were in their fifties when they came for help. They had married in their twenties, having known each other for a while before that. Sex was always enjoyable for Andrew; for Jackie it was less good at first, but improved as the years went by. Neither had ever read any books about sex, or discussed sex at all with friends, and their lovemaking was simple. Four years before they presented, Andrew came under a lot of stress at work. He became very tired, and on a couple of occasions he lost his erection. Jackie was upset but did not know how to help him, and Andrew refused to talk about it. On holiday things improved a little, but gradually Andrew's interest in sex declined and he found his erections becoming more transient. He became irritable if Jackie made tentative advances to him, and began to cut off all affectionate physical contact with her. Jackie felt very hurt and rejected, and dealt with this, as she had done with similar feelings in her rather neglected childhood, by withdrawing into silence.

When communication is impaired there is a danger that each partner will try to guess what the other is thinking, and this is likely to lead to further problems due to incorrect guesses. Two 'sexual myths' are likely to aggravate this situation. The first myth assumes that men should know all about sex and especially should know 'how to handle a woman', the implication being that if the man does not he is not a proper man. The second myth assumes that people who love each other, instinctively know what the other thinks and feels. On the basis of this myth, where communication is already hampered, people may begin to think 'He (or she) doesn't understand what I feel, he doesn't say what I need to hear; it must be because he doesn't want to, because he doesn't love me'.

Lack of foreplay. A sexual problem, such as impaired sexual arousal, orgasmic dysfunction, or vaginismus, may well be caused and also persist because there is little or no foreplay. This may of course be due to ignorance on the partner's part, especially about the longer amount of foreplay required by many women (although not at all times) in order to become aroused compared with men. In addition, where a problem has developed it is very common for the amount of foreplay to decline because one or other partner encourages this. Thus a woman who has lost interest in sex may hurry her partner through the sexual act because she knows it is not going to be enjoyable for her and so she would prefer to get it over with quickly. A man with erectile dysfunction may try to have sexual intercourse as soon as he gets an erection, for fear of losing the erection.

Depression. Loss of interest in sex is usually found in patients who develop depression, and may bring additional distress to the patient through the guilt she feels over the loss of affectionate feelings towards her partner. It is important to reassure such a patient that these are normal symptoms of depression, and that her interest in sex will return as her depression lifts, although sexual desire is often one of the last things to be restored to normal.

An episode of depression may have an important aetiological role in persistent low sexual desire, even though the psychiatric disorder may have resolved. Thus in an American study a much higher proportion of people (mostly women) with low sexual desire but not currently depressed were found to have a history of depression than were people with unimpaired sexual desire, the onset of the sexual dysfunction always following or accompanying the depressive disorder (Schreiner-Engel and Schiavi 1986). Furthermore, all the subjects with primary low sexual desire had a history of depression during adolescence. The nature of this association between low sexual desire and depression is unclear. It could reflect persistent psychological disturbance (e.g. with regard to self-esteem and/or self-image) or a biological factor (e.g. neurotransmitter abnormality).

Other factors mentioned already, as predisposing factors or precipitants, can also, if they persist, help to maintain the dysfunction.

Physical factors

Physical disorders and medication can have very profound effects on sexual function. They may directly interfere with physiological or anatomical mechanisms involved in sexual response, or cause secondary psychological reactions leading to sexual dysfunction, or, and not uncommonly, they may disrupt sexual function due to a combination of direct and psychological effects. Thus a woman who initially finds sexual intercourse very uncomfortable after a gynaecological operation may subsequently lack interest in sex because of secondary fear, in spite of complete healing at the surgical site.

The physical disorders and surgical procedures which may lead to sexual problems are listed in Table 19.3 and briefly discussed in the text. The reader who wishes to obtain more detailed information is referred to Bancroft (1989) and Hawton (1985).

Medical disorders

Endocrine. In men, *diabetes* very often causes erectile dysfunction. The sexual effects of diabetes in women are less clear. There have been conflicting results of studies in terms of whether Type I or Type II diabetes is more likely to affect sexual function. In one study many women with Type II diabetes experienced reduced sexual desire, ability to experience orgasm, vaginal lubrication, and sexual satisfaction (Schreiner-Engel *et al.* 1987). In addition to physical effects of diabetes, the psychological impact of the disorder on the women and on their relationship with their partner may also be an important determinant of any negative sexual consequences.

Both *hyperthyroidism* and *myxoedema* may affect sexual function, the former

Table 19.3 *Some medical disorders and surgical procedures which may cause sexual dysfunction in women*

Medical disorders

Endocrine	Diabetes
	Hyperthyroidism; myxoedema
	Addison's disease
Cardiovascular	Myocardial infarction
	Angina pectoris
Respiratory	Chronic obstructive airways disease; asthma
Arthritic	Osteoarthritis
	Rheumatoid arthritis
	Sjögren's syndrome
Neurological	Pelvic autonomic neuropathy
	Spinal cord disease or trauma
Renal	Dialysis
Gynaecological	Vaginitis
	Pelvic infections
	Endometriosis

Surgical procedures

Mastectomy

Colostomy and ileostomy

Gynaecological	Oophorectomy
	Surgery for cervical neoplasia
	Episiotomy
	Vaginal repair or prolapse

Amputation

---

because of anxiety and irritability, and the latter because of tiredness and menorrhagia. Reduced activity of the *adrenal glands*, as in Addison's disease, often affects sexual interest and performance, presumably due to impairment of androgen production.

Cardiovascular. At present there is a scarcity of information about the effects of *myocardial infarction* on female sexuality. However, it seems that many women reduce the frequency of their sexual activity after a heart attack. As with men who have had heart attacks, this may be because of an unfounded fear of precipitating further attacks. Depression, poor self-esteem, and medication may be other factors. Sexual difficulties, including erectile dysfunction or fear of resuming sexual activity, commonly occur in men after heart attacks. This is likely to cause sexual problems for their partners, who in addition may feel guilty about continuing to experience sexual desire. *Angina pectoris* may also limit sexual enjoyment if chest pain or palpitations occur during sexual activity. Prophylactic use of a nitrate preparation or a beta-blocking agent can help prevent these symptoms.

Respiratory. Severe chronic respiratory disease is likely to inhibit sexual activity because of limitations on sexual positions which can be tolerated, especially the 'missionary' position. Occasionally patients with *asthma* repeatedly experience asthmatic episodes during sex.

Arthritis. Joint pain, especially if this arises in the hip joints, may severely limit a woman's ability to enjoy or even participate in sexual activity. Chronic pain is likely to lead to tiredness and loss of interest in sex. In *Sjögren's syndrome* there may be impairment of vaginal lubrication.

Neurological. As sexual response is mediated largely through neural pathways it is obvious that disruption of such pathways will affect sexual performance. Thus damage to the pelvic autonomic nerves (e.g. through neuropathy, malignant disease, or surgery), or the spinal cord, is likely to interfere with genital swelling and lubrication and orgasm. Further discussion of the effects of spinal cord damage occurs later (p. 596).

Renal. Low sexual desire and difficulties in becoming sexually aroused are found in some women on *renal dialysis*. This may in part be due to tiredness and depression, and also to electrolyte and hormonal disturbances.

Gynaecological. Obviously many gynaecological disorders may be associated with sexual problems. Examples include *vaginitis*, due to infection (e.g. thrush) or oestrogen deficiency, which may cause soreness during sexual intercourse, and *pelvic inflammatory disease* or *endometriosis*, which can cause pain on deep penile thrusting.

Surgical procedures

Several surgical procedures in women are likely to affect sexual function (Table 19.3): some because they interfere directly with organs and structures involved in sexual activity and response; others because of their psychological effects.

Examples of surgical procedures which may cause organic damage are gynaecological operations such as *oophorectomy*, following which reduction in circulating oestrogens is likely to impair vaginal lubrication; *episiotomy*, which if poorly sutured may cause tenderness or tightness of the introitus; and *vaginal repair of prolapse*, which may have a similar effect if the repair is unsatisfactory. Finally, *amputation*, especially if a leg has been removed, can cause considerable mechanical difficulties during sexual activity.

Several surgical procedures are likely to have psychological consequences which may profoundly affect a woman's ability to enjoy her sex life. A common psychological sequel is an altered self-image leading to a decreased sense of sexual attractiveness. This is particularly likely after mastectomy. At least one-third of women who have had a breast removed suffer severe long-standing deterioration in their sexual relationships, and in many cases sex is abandoned altogether. Part of the problem may be revulsion experienced by the woman's

> **Box 19.2** *Some drugs which may have negative effects on female sexuality*
>
> Anticholinergics (e.g. probanthine)
> Anticonvulsants (phenytoin; carbamazepine; phenobarbitone)
> Antihypertensives and diuretics (beta-blockers; bendrofluazide)
> Anti-inflammatory drugs (indomethacin)
> Hormones (oral contraception; steroids)
> Hypnotics and sedatives (benzodiazepines)
> Antidepressants (especially serotonergic agents)
> Major tranquillizers (especially thioridazine)
> Alcohol
> Opiates

partner. Similar impairment of self-image may occur following amputation, or after colostomy or ileostomy, where, in addition, concern about possible odour or fear that discomfort or damage might result from sexual intercourse are likely to complicate the picture.

Although hysterectomy has been regarded as being associated with a high incidence of sexual problems, in a systematic prospective study this was not found to be so (Gath *et al.* 1982). Indeed, some of the women studied experienced an improvement in their sexual relations.

A diagnosis of cervical cancer or cervical intraepithelial neoplasm may precipitate sexual problems in many women. Difficulties in understanding a diagnosis of a pre-cancerous condition of the cervix may cause shock, panic, depression, and hopelessness. Media focus on an association between cervical neoplasia, genital warts, and having had several sexual partners may cause shame and guilt, leading to loss of interest in sex. There is some evidence that sexual problems are at least as common in women with cervical cancer as in those who have had cancer of the breast, with impaired self-image and the deleterious effects of both the cancer and treatments for it being important contributory factors (Horton 1991).

Depression, which commonly occurs following some operations (e.g. mastectomy), is likely to be an added factor contributing to impairment of sexual function following surgery.

Effects of medication

Unfortunately there is a paucity of information concerning the effects of medication on female sexuality. Largely by extrapolation from what is known about the effects in men, it seems that several types of medication may have important consequences for sexual interest and performance in women and that one should always enquire about medication when a woman presents complaining of impaired sexual desire or arousal, or difficulty in achieving orgasm.

The drugs which may affect female sexuality are listed in Box 19.2.

Anticholinergic agents may interfere with vaginal engorgement and lubrication. It is possible that *anticonvulsants* may in some cases have an adverse effect on a woman's sexual desire because of their induction of hormone-binding globulin which binds testosterone and therefore leads to a reduction in circulating free testosterone. It is worth considering as a cause of impaired libido where the decline in interest has developed after a long period of anticonvulsant therapy. Drugs used to treat hypertension, such as *beta-blockers* (e.g. propranolol) and *diuretics* (bendrofluazide), are known to have erectile dysfunction as a major side-effect (*Lancet* 1981), and can cause reduced sexual desire.

Controversy has surrounded the possible role of *oral contraception* in causing sexual dysfunction. However, with most of the modern, low-dose oral contraceptives most women experience no significant changes in their libido, and some even report enhancement of their enjoyment of sex.

Some *antidepressants* (notably the serotonergic agents and the mono-amine oxidase inhibitors) can cause delay or absence of orgasm in both sexes. Because the *major tranquillizers*, especially thioridazine, can have profound effects on male sexual performance, this suggests that they may also interfere with female sexual response. Although *benzodiazepines* (e.g. diazepam) are occasionally prescribed as treatment for sexual problems related to anxiety, it seems likely that they have an adverse effect in some patients because of their tendency to cause drowsiness. While *alcohol* is likely to enhance sexual desire and reduce inhibitions when used in moderation, chronic alcohol abuse often leads to loss of interest in sex because of its depressant effects, and to erectile difficulties associated with autonomic neuropathy, liver disease, and testicular failure. *Opiate* abuse often causes sexual dysfunction, especially reduced sexual desire, in both men and women.

If it is thought that a particular medication is having a deleterious effect on a woman's sexual interest then it will be necessary to weigh up the pros and cons of stopping or changing the medication and the likely effect on the physical or psychological condition for which the drug has been prescribed. Where an effective alternative drug is available this might be tried. However, it is important to be alert to the fact that changes in sexual interest or enjoyment are often blamed on medication when other factors, especially those of an interpersonal nature, are the real cause.

Some forms of medication can improve sexuality. *Androgens* administered for medical conditions can enhance sexual interest, and some attempt has been made to incorporate these drugs in the treatment of women with impaired sexual desire, though results of most studies suggest little or no effect. However, they are beneficial for many women who experience post-menopausal reduction in sexual desire (Sherwin *et al.* 1985). *Oestrogens* administered for menopausal symptoms may improve sexual arousability because of their beneficial effects on the post-menopausal vaginal mucosa.

How to assess patients with sexual problems

Help or advice should *never* be offered to anyone presenting with a sexual problem without first making a careful assessment and coming to a clear understanding of the full nature of the problem. Often the problem is very different from that suggested by the initial complaint. Sometimes the woman may believe that it is she who has the problem when in fact it is primarily her partner's, so that, for example, a woman whose husband has premature ejaculation may complain to her doctor of inability to achieve orgasm during intercourse.

Assessment of a sexual problem has in itself a very important therapeutic function:

1. It can begin to clarify and make intelligible a problem that, in the patient's mind, is obscure and associated with shame, bewilderment, and suffering.

2. It demonstrates that it is both respectable and feasible to talk effectively about sex, and that it may therefore be possible for the woman to talk to her partner about it too.

3. It demonstrates that sexual difficulty is regarded by doctors as a legitimate worry, and one that they are trained to deal with. The doctor can make it clear that the problem is neither extraordinary nor blameworthy, and that it can be helped.

4. It offers an opportunity for mistaken fears and beliefs to be dispelled. Much anxiety and self-blame is based on half-truths, muddled information, and 'sexual myths' (see Box 19.1).

Unfortunately many doctors have not received training in taking a sexual history. Two general points are important here. First, it is essential for the doctor to feel comfortable about the procedure, in order to concentrate on dispelling the patient's embarrassment and anxiety, and also so that accurate information can be obtained without the doctor feeling obliged to side-step any issues because of her or his own embarrassment. Secondly, there is a difficulty about the words used to discuss the problem. Doctors feel comfortable using medical terminology, but many patients will not comprehend words like lubrication, ejaculation, and so on; on the other hand, colloquial words do not always have a precise enough meaning, and also they may seem shocking or inappropriate to the patient when spoken in medical consultation. Often the only remedy to this problem is to discuss the difficulty openly with the patient, and then to come to a gradual agreement on the terms to be used in the interview, by translating frequently between the technical and the colloquial terms, and allowing the patient to select and to become accustomed to using the words that she prefers. For example, the doctor might say. 'Ejaculation is the technical word for the moment when the seminal fluid comes out of the end of the penis. In ordinary speech people often call that "coming", and they may call the seminal fluid "spunk". Do you know what I mean by that? Which words would you like to use? ... All right, now you were telling me that when your husband ejaculates, he ...'

There are other considerations, applicable to interviewing in general, that can help to make the interview less stressful for the patient, and more productive of information. Thus it is often a good idea to proceed from 'less painful' to 'more painful' topics, and to switch temporarily to less painful topics if the patient needs to recover herself at any time in the interview. Examples of 'less painful' areas are: simple factual information (times, places, events); information about other people; and happy or successful aspects of the patient's life. Examples of 'more painful' areas may be: details of the sexual difficulty; the patient's own feelings; and any discussion of marital or family tension. It is worth trying to use a judicious mixture of 'open-ended' questions that allow the patient to tell her story in her own words, uncontaminated by the doctor's presuppositions, and more 'closed', detailed questions that allow precise information to be established while relieving the patient of some of the burden of naming embarrassing things. Examples of open-ended questions are: 'Tell me more about the problem' and 'How did you feel when that happened?' A closed question might be: 'I think you are telling me that you feel that your vagina doesn't become wet enough, so that it feels uncomfortable when your husband wants to put his penis in. Is that what you mean? Or did you mean something different?'

It is particularly helpful to ask the patient to recall a *specific* occasion, as recent as possible, on which the sexual difficulty arose. If the patient can describe such an occasion, she can be asked to give a minute-by-minute account, which should include an idea of how her partner responded to anything she did, of her response to his actions, of her thoughts and what she imagined he was thinking at the time. Such a detailed account of a single episode, which is probably best obtained later in the interview when the patient is more relaxed, is much more informative than any general statements about the nature of the problem that the patient may have worked out for herself. Having established a picture of one occasion, the doctor should then ask whether other occasions have followed the same pattern, or, if not, how they have differed.

When a patient appears embarrassed it can be helpful if the doctor acknowledges this and then explains that she will get more confident with time. It is crucial not to side-step issues because they are embarrassing; they may be central to the problem.

If the woman has a partner and he is relevant to her difficulty it is important to try to see him. Apart from the possible necessity of involving him in subsequent treatment, the information obtained from him may cast a very different light on the problem. When a woman says she doubts if her husband will attend, the doctor might consider dropping him a note to encourage him, provided the patient gives her permission.

History-taking

The main points to be covered in carrying out a detailed assessment of a patient with a sexual problem are contained in the Appendix to this chapter (p. 598). A systematic assessment of this kind will take at least half an hour and therefore might be spread over two or three interviews. Certainly a detailed assessment is required if the doctor is considering treating the patient with some form of sex therapy. For other purposes a briefer assessment might be sufficient. If the doctor is short of time on the day when a woman first mentions that she has a sexual problem, she could be asked to return for a longer and more leisurely interview later. However, every effort should be made to ensure that at the *first* interview she has said enough and has received enough encouragement for her to want to attend for a second longer interview.

In making a *brief assessment* the doctor should cover the following points:

(1) what is the precise nature of the problem?

(2) what is the effect of the problem on the woman and her partner?

(3) is there a major problem in the couple's general relationship?

(4) has the patient had a satisfactory sexual relationship in the past?

(5) is the patient adequately informed about sex?

(6) is there any medical or psychiatric condition which might contribute to or cause the problem?

(7) is the patient on any medication and what is her level of alcohol consumption?

(8) what changes would the patient like to achieve in her sexual adjustment?

It will be clear that even a brief assessment must be far from cursory if the doctor is to obtain sufficient information to decide what help to provide, including whether or not to refer for specialist treatment.

Management of sexual problems

The variety of approaches available for dealing with sexual problems can be separated conveniently into two categories, distinguished by the intensity and scope of the treatment. These are (1) *brief counselling*, and (2) *sex therapy*. The first category, which includes the provision of simple advice and information, should be within the scope of all GPs. Some GPs will also want to practise sex therapy, in which a detailed step-by-step programme is used to help an individual or couple. However, this requires special training and is fairly time-consuming so that the majority of GPs are unlikely to carry this out themselves.

The important therapeutic function of the assessment interview must be re-emphasized here. Often a patient or couple will experience a great deal of relief from simply having the opportunity to talk about the problem and from the reassurance that the doctor can provide during the assessment. It is not always necessary to provide advice at this stage; often it is better to ask the patient(s) to return a few days later, when the doctor will have had time to think further about the problem and the best means of tackling it, and the patient(s) will have had time to discover whether they need any further help.

In this section the two categories of management in relation to couples with sexual dysfunction are considered. Then treatment of the individual woman without a partner, the management of problems related to sexual variations, and the referral of patients for specialist treatment are discussed. Finally, management of problems associated with childhood sexual abuse and rape are described.

Treatment of couples with sexual dysfunction

Brief counselling

This is most appropriate for those problems that arise from inadequate or muddled information, and for those which involve anxieties about sexual behaviour of a particular kind (e.g. oral sex) or at a particular time (e.g. pregnancy; after the menopause). Usually such problems can be managed over the course of only a few consultations. Sometimes only one consultation will be necessary, although the doctor should always try to assess subsequently whether the counselling has been effective. Brief counselling can include the following strategies:

Provision of information. As ignorance or misinformation are often shared by a couple, both partners should, if possible, be present when information is to be given by the doctor, so that they can both question it at the time, and discuss it together afterwards. The doctors can provide accurate information on sexual anatomy (especially using pictures), can describe what happens during sexual arousal in either sex, can convey an idea of the range of normal biological variation in anatomy and physiology, and the frequency (and therefore 'normality') of different types of sexual behaviour, such as oral sex or homosexual contacts during adolescence. The patient might also be recommended suitable reading material, *The Relate guide to sex in loving relationships* (Litvinoff 1992), *Women's experience of sex* (Kitzinger 1985), and *A woman's guide to loving sex* (Barnes and Rodwell 1993) being helpful examples.

Advice. For example, the doctor may give advice on the following: how to engage in more enjoyable foreplay, suitable positions for sexual intercourse during pregnancy or recovery from a physical illness, and means whereby a couple can come to a compromise over their differing levels of sexual desire. Advice should be given only after careful appraisal of what is likely to be acceptable for the couple. However, it is generally useful to encourage couples to make more time for this part of their relationship.

Permission-giving. Sometimes a patient feels needlessly guilty about some aspect of sexual behaviour (such as masturbation or the occurrence of sexual fantasy). Where such feelings are the legacy of repressive parental attitudes, they can be countered by the doctor adopting a different parental role, helping the patient to accept that the activity in question is not harmful or wicked and is shared by most other ordinary people. However, this must be done with caution and respect, to avoid putting pressure on patients to accept a value system that is alien to them.

Sex therapy

Masters and Johnson (1970) revolutionized the treatment of couples with sexual problems when they introduced their relatively brief but intensive therapeutic approach. This is based on the rationale that although sexual problems may arise from a wide range of causes, some of which are rooted in the past, nevertheless the problems are maintained by factors which operate in the present, and therefore are amenable to modification by techniques focused on present occurrences, feelings, and thoughts.

The methods of Masters and Johnson have proved very effective, with some modifications, within the setting of the NHS. This modified approach will be summarized here; anyone wishing to use the method will need to consult a fuller account (e.g. Hawton 1985) and obtain appropriate training.

After full assessment of each partner individually, the couple is presented with a *formulation* of the problem, setting out its nature, and the likely predisposing factors, precipitants, and maintaining factors that have contributed to it. The purpose of the formulation is to provide the couple with a better understanding of their problem and to provide a rationale for the treatment approach. The principal components of the treatment are (1) homework assignments: (2) counselling; (3) education.

Homework assignments. These have two purposes. The first is to provide a method by means of which couples can establish or re-establish the confidence and freedom in their sexual contact with each other that will allow unhindered sexual response to occur. The second is to assist the therapist and the couple to identify precisely the factors that are contributing to maintenance of the problem. In essence the programme of assignments consists of a graduated series of clearly-defined tasks in touching and being touched by each other in specific ways, so that the difficulty is broken down into manageable steps, in which room is made for discussion of obstacles arising at any stage. Where appropriate, additional specific techniques are used to tackle particular kinds of dysfunction.

The couple is first asked to agree to undertake the programme which includes an initial ban both on sexual intercourse and on touching of the genital areas and the woman's breasts. Instructions for *sensate focus* are then provided. The partners are asked to find a suitable time when they can concentrate on this exercise in a relaxed fashion. The exercise consists of each partner taking turns at caressing the other over all areas of the body, apart from the 'no-go' areas already mentioned. The purpose of this is for each to learn to accept pleasure from the other, for each to find out how and where the partner likes being caressed, and to help the partners feel relaxed and comfortable with each other without striving towards arousal. Through this they can begin to learn to communicate on sexual matters, and advice specifically addressed to this issue will also be given by the therapist. Sometimes it is necessary to suggest that the couple start their physical contact at an even earlier stage (e.g. holding hands, putting arms round each other), especially in cases whether either partner has become extremely adverse to sexual contact.

When this stage is satisfactorily established, the couple is asked to progress to *genital sensate focus*, during which both the genitals and breasts are included in caressing, but the emphasis is still on discovery of each other and on improving communication. Subsequently the couple moves from individual caressing, turn and turn about, to simultaneous mutual pleasuring. The next stage is a gradual progression to sexual intercourse via an intermediate stage of *vaginal containment* in which penetration occurs but there is no movement.

Specific techniques are used for particular types of dysfunction, only some of which can be mentioned here. Finger exploration of the vagina in a series of graded steps by both partners is suggested where the woman has vaginismus. This needs to be accompanied by examination of fears that the task may evoke. Masturbation exercises are often advised where the woman is unable to achieve orgasm. Heiman and LoPiccolo's (1988) self-help manual, *Becoming orgasmic*, provides useful step-by-step guidance for such women. Pelvic floor exercises (as advised for women following childbirth) are useful for both vaginismus and orgasmic dysfunction. The 'stop-start' or 'squeeze' techniques may be suggested where the man has premature ejaculation. In both of these the woman provides her partner with intermittent penile stimulation according to his level of sexual arousal. In the squeeze technique she also applies firm pressure with her fingers to the base of the glans penis when her partner feels he is near to ejaculation. Masturbation exercises are also suggested in the treatment of ejaculatory failure.

Counselling. As the couple moves through the graduated programme, discussion at each stage enables both the therapist and the couple to get a clearer idea of the factors maintaining the problem. In addition, at some stage almost every couple encounters a block to progress, which yields further valuable information. In order to help modify the factors maintaining the sexual problem and particularly to overcome blocks to progress, a considerable amount of counselling will be necessary. The components of such counselling include the following:

1. Helping the partners reconsider *attitudes* they hold and perhaps have never questioned (e.g. that sexual activity should always be the responsibility of the male partner, with the woman playing a passive role). As discussed in relation to brief counselling, the therapist should avoid imposing values on patients, but should help them to look at attitudes which clearly obstruct their progress towards the goals they have chosen for themselves.

2. *Confronting* patients when there appears to be a discrepancy between their stated aims and what they are actually doing in practice. Quite often partners say that they are keen to improve their sexual relationship but in fact fail to carry out the therapist's instructions.

3. Identifying and discussing *feelings* originating from other areas of the relationship but finding expression through the sexual relationship.

4. *Permission-giving*, as when a therapist encourages the partners to carry out sexual activity which they had not thought of, or regarded as taboo (such as masturbation), but which is likely to help overcome their problem.

5. Providing *reassurance*.

Some of the techniques employed in cognitive therapy for a variety of emotional problems are useful in sex therapy (see Hawton 1989), especially when trying to help a couple (and the doctor) understand the reasons why particular reactions and feelings occur in sexual situations and attempting to modify such factors.

Education. The educational aspects of sex therapy are similar to those involved in brief counselling. It is often advisable to devote part of an early treatment session to providing simple information about sexual anatomy and response. In the course of this it is helpful to address some of the common, often shared myths about male and female roles (Box 19.1).

The duration of sex therapy will vary from couple to couple but between eight and 16 sessions of treatment are usually required. Although Masters and Johnson use male and female co-therapists to treat couples, it seems that one therapist is just as effective and that the gender of the therapist is usually not important, except in some cases where there may be obvious benefits for the therapist to be of the same gender as the dysfunctional partner (e.g. a very timid woman with vaginismus).

The results of sex therapy originally reported by Masters and Johnson (1970) have proved to be far superior to those obtained by other workers. However, results obtained elsewhere are far from disappointing (for a review see Hawton 1995). Thus, in clinical practice in this country (Hawton and Catalan 1986) it appears that two-thirds of couples derive considerable benefits from treatment. Vaginismus and premature ejaculation respond particularly well. Results are less good for low sexual desire, partly because this problem often reflects general relationship difficulties. The long-term outcome of sex therapy suggests that while progress is maintained for many couples, especially those who originally presented with vaginismus, a considerable proportion will experience relapses, although the attitudes of partners to their problems may be more tolerant. Also couples often report having coped with setbacks by using the skills learned during therapy, such as not ignoring the problem, talking about it, and repeating some of the sensate focus exercises (Hawton *et al.* 1986).

Treatment of women without partners

It may happen that a woman will present asking for help, but have no partner, or be unwilling to involve her current partner in treatment. Fortunately there is much that can be done to help such women, especially those with vaginismus or orgasmic dysfunction. For some women brief advice can be given, e.g. concerning the use of a vibrator. For others, more detailed graduated programmes will be necessary.

A woman with vaginismus may first be asked to become familiar with her external gentalia, perhaps while in the bath. Subsequently, after a vaginal examination by the doctor, the woman will be encouraged to explore her vagina with a finger in order to become more comfortable with vaginal penetration. She can also be taught the pelvic floor exercises.

In primary orgasmic dysfunction the woman will be encouraged to learn to masturbate. During the course of such treatment she may require help to modify her attitudes to masturbation. She will also need advice on ways of subsequently showing a partner how to stimulate her appropriately. The results of such treatment of orgasmic problems are usually very good.

Treatment of problems related to sexual variations

It will be rare for the GP to be called upon to counsel a woman with established homosexual interest. Most such women do not feel they need help. However, a GP who is asked for help by a homosexual woman who wishes to come to terms with her sexual interest might be best advised to refer her to an organization such as Friend (p. 599) which provides a counselling service.

The female transsexual who asks for help will almost invariably require referral to a specialist.

When a woman complains about her husband's deviant sexual interest it will be most important to try to see the husband and to find out whether he is concerned about his sexual interest and whether he wishes to do anything about it. If he does, specialist referral will usually be necessary.

Referral of patients for specialist treatment

Only a rough guide can be given as to which patients with sexual problems should be referred for specialist attention. This will depend in part on how well equipped the GP feels to deal with the problem. Assuming the GP does not wish to undertake sex therapy, referral will be indicated for women who present with a sexual problem that appears to be the result of significant early experiences and where simple advice and reassurance do not have any effect. This applies to any type of sexual dysfunction. It is also particularly worth trying to arrange treatment where the man has erectile dysfunction, because a variety of effective treatments are now available.

Before initiating referral the partner should be seen if possible to assess his attitudes to the problem and particularly whether he is willing to do anything about it. A brief assessment, along the lines suggested earlier, should be made for both partners before making the referral. A physical examination should be carried out where indicated. This applies particularly to vaginismus and erectile dysfunction. Advice on what is likely to happen when the couple see the specialist may help to reassure them.

Sometimes a couple may say they would prefer not to be referred at present. They may already have been helped by their discussion of the problem with their doctor and therefore referral might be delayed a while to see whether this was enough to allow them to make further progress unaided.

The GP will need to know who runs the nearest sexual dysfunction clinic. Unfortunately the availability of such clinics varies greatly from area to area. Relate (formerly Marriage Guidance) has many counsellors specially trained in sex therapy. Likewise a number of family planning doctors undertake such training. Some sex therapy clinics are based in psychiatric hospitals and psychology departments. The doctor might enquire from any of these agencies locally. There may also be private (accredited) therapists in the area.

Sexual abuse

Increasing numbers of women from all social backgrounds are seeking help for the long-term consequences of being abused in childhood. It is unclear whether this is because childhood sexual abuse has become more common or because there has been a great deal of media attention to this problem which has encouraged women to reveal their traumatic experiences which otherwise they would have kept as a painful secret. It is very important for doctors to believe the story that is being told to them. Fear of not being believed, especially if that was the woman's experience as a child, makes a doctor's initial response crucial. The stories are often so shocking that a common defence is not to believe what is being said. If the abuser is known to the doctor and regarded as a 'pillar of society' it may be even more difficult to accept what is being said.

The extent to which sexual abuse by adults will have long-term consequences varies greatly. Characteristics of sexual abuse especially likely to have long-term effects include prolonged experience of abuse, early age at onset and abuse by the father or stepfather rather than a non-relative, actual physical contact, and the use of force. The most fundamental consequences of childhood sexual abuse are chronic low self-esteem and a lack of trust in men. As a result women are likely to suffer mood disturbances, interpersonal difficulties, especially with partners, and sexual dysfunction, particularly low sexual desire, sexual phobias, and problems of arousal. Sexual promiscuity is also sometimes found in young victims of abuse.

Many factors may contribute to sexual abuse of daughters by their fathers or stepfathers (this being the most common form of childhood sexual abuse), including personality disorder and alcohol abuse in the father, marital disharmony between the parents, and collusion of the girl's mother. Often a girl is drawn into an incestuous relationship because of her need to feel special and loved when she is too young to appreciate the implications of this behaviour. Only when older might she come to experience guilt and shame about the relationship, this then being likely to have implications for her subsequent sexual adjustment. In spite of all the attention to this problem in the media, often an abused woman will feel that she is the only person who has suffered such an experience.

It is common for a woman not to disclose childhood sexual abuse at initial presentation to a doctor, for fear of not being believed or because she feels guilty or ashamed about it (Hobbs 1990). It is not unusual for a woman to present for the first time when she has been in an intimate and safe relationship for a few years, perhaps when her children go to playschool and are less under her control (this may raise her anxieties for their safety). Paradoxically, it is fairly common for a woman to develop sexual problems after disclosure, in spite of not having had difficulties previously.

The following is a brief case vignette.

Mary, a 24-year-old mother of two children, disclosed her childhood sexual abuse to her health visitor when her older child was about to start playschool, because she found she could not leave her daughter alone at the school. After disclosure to her sister (who she had always felt was her mother's favourite) she discovered that her stepfather had also tried to abuse her but she had rejected him. Her feelings of despair and shame were overwhelming and she said 'how could I have let him, I am weak and bad'.

Sometimes the death of the abuser can prompt a woman to seek help.

Occasionally it may be because of rough handling by a doctor which reawakens an abused woman's sense of powerlessness.

When a history of abuse is revealed, the doctor's reaction is going to be an important initial step in any therapeutic process. It is important to begin by listening and allowing the woman to tell her story. The doctor should find out if she has ever told anyone else. It is crucial to convey a non-judgemental attitude and also not to try to take action quickly – this can result in the woman feeling rejected. It may be helpful to invite the woman back for a second appointment after she has had a chance to think about what she would like to do and what sort of help she might wish for. The doctor should not be misled by a woman displaying an appearance of capable coping, but listen carefully to what she is saying about her inner despair. Seeing the partner and helping him to understand the powerlessness of the woman when she was a child is very important as partners often cannot understand why women are unable to say 'no'.

Referral for specialist help, either for the woman on her own or with her partner, from a psychiatrist, clinical psychologist or counsellor will usually be necessary because considerable time and expertize are often required to help women overcome the effects of sexual abuse (Jehu 1988). The doctor can play a supportive role while the woman is waiting to receive help and also while therapy is in progress.

Rape

'Rape is not a sexual encounter in the usual sense. Instead, it is an event in which one person hurts another *by means of sex*' (Everstine and Everstine 1983). Rape represents many different kinds of assault simultaneously: on a person's sense of control over her own life, on her trustful assumptions about other people and her safety in the world, as well as a devastating invasion of her personal space. The victim's responses and her needs for help follow the same patterns as those of victims of other kinds of life-threatening trauma, especially those involving sudden overwhelming loss. Like them, she will experience an immediate period of *shock*, in which ordinary patterns of behaviour are wholly disrupted (in ways she may afterwards find difficult to understand or to accept), followed by a variable *post-traumatic phase* in which severe anxiety, depression, guilt, anger, somatic symptoms, sleep disturbance, sexual difficulty, feelings of isolation and worthlessness may all play their part.

These emotional consequences need to be kept in mind from the earliest moments in the aftermath of a rape, but the practical aspects must also not be overlooked. If the woman consents to report the rape to the police, the GP can give useful advice about what to do. She should expect to be seen by a police surgeon and examined if medical evidence is needed in court. She should not wash or change her clothing, nor have a drink nor take any medication, until she has been seen by a police surgeon. As she may be asked to leave her clothes behind at the police station she should take a change of clothing with her. She may be helped if she is accompanied by a supportive friend, especially if this friend saw her soon after the incident and can give evidence to the police.

Finally, she should be advised to make a note of details of the sequence of events associated with the rape to help her in making her statement to the police.

The main possible *physical* after-effects of rape are damage to pelvic organs and the rest of the body, venereal infection (including HIV), and pregnancy. Examination of a raped woman by a police surgeon for forensic purposes may not necessarily deal with these aspects, and the GP's help may be vital here. The psychological violation experienced by a raped woman can unfortunately be compounded by attitudes of suspicion or contempt encountered from doctors, lawyers, or police, or even from those closest to her. These attitudes arise partly as defences to the very powerful feelings provoked by the occurrence of a rape, and partly from the many myths that surround the subject. Such myths include the belief that a woman can always resist rape if she really wants to, that women lead men on and falsely cry rape afterwards. that respectable girls do not get raped, that a woman with sexual experience is not harmed by being raped, and that rape is subconsciously enjoyable. The feelings of guilt and self-questioning ('why me?') that are part of the woman's normal psychological response to acute trauma may further increase the impact of these attitudes on her and cause her to believe the myths to be true in her case.

The most immediate need of a raped woman is for sympathetic, informed, and gentle handling. Early support is thought to be very important in preventing long-term psychological damage, and it should be offered in a way that fosters the woman's sense of autonomy and her freedom to choose what help she wishes, so as to counter the feelings of enforced helplessness induced by rape. She should be encouraged but never pressurized to talk about the details of what occurred, and she may need to tell the story many times to the same listener before she gains the strength to recount its most distressing or humiliating aspects. The doctor has an important role in meeting the need, both of the victim and her family, to understand what has happened to them and the feelings they are experiencing. Simple explanations about the mechanism of shock, or of psychologic defences (such as denial), refutation of damaging assumptions based on myths, reassurance about the normality of feelings they may experience (including paradoxical and rapidly changing feelings) so as to dispel fears of insanity, and joint decisions about the kinds of support the family can most usefully give, will all form part of the psychological first aid that a GP can appropriately provide.

The woman is likely to have to cope with the feelings of those close to her, especially of her sexual partner. He may succeed in being supportive, or may instead be overwhelmed by his own feelings of rage, helplessness, or revulsion, which can in turn lead to sexual difficulties for him (especially erectile dysfunction). For her part, the victim may find it hard to accept her partner's support, because of her feelings (however irrational she knows them to be) of anger or despair at his failure to protect her when she most needed his help. It is advisable therefore for the doctor to give time separately to the family, and especially the partner, so that they can be free to say things which they might otherwise conceal for fear of hurting the victim further. It is useful, too, if at an early stage a suitable person close to the victim or a fellow professional (e.g.

a social worker) can be identified who will be able to continue the support through the weeks that follow.

Research on the long-term consequences of rape indicates that the commonest enduring consequences are probably depression and sexual dysfunction (especially fear of sex, lessened enjoyment, and arousal difficulties). The risk of long-term consequences seems to be greatest where the rape was associated with much violence, where the woman had pre-existing difficulties, either psychological or social, where early support was lacking or inadequate, and (perhaps) where an apparently rapid return to normal adjustment concealed a denial of feelings, or guilt, which prevented the acceptance of help. Where such risk factors exist, and in other cases as necessary, referral for specialist help should be considered.

Rape crisis centres are available in most areas. In some places, self-help groups for the victims of rape have been formed, with the object of providing emotional support, information on medical and legal matters, companionship at court hearings or other stressful times, and often with the additional and wider aim of educating the general public and encouraging a change in attitudes.

Sexuality and sexual problems at special times in a woman's life

There are certain times in a woman's life when sexuality is particularly likely to undergo change and these are times when sexual problems commonly occur. The most significant of these times are pregnancy and childbirth, the menopause, and older age.

Pregnancy and childbirth

Although there is some variation in the findings from different studies of the changes in sexual activity during pregnancy, all studies agree that for most women sexual interest declines during the third trimester, with a consequent decline in the frequency of sexual intercourse. Reduced frequency of intercourse may also be due to physical discomfort, awkwardness, sense of loss of attractiveness, and recommendations from doctors to avoid sex.

Although only limited information is available about the effects of intercourse during pregnancy, it appears that there are no specific complications of, or contraindications to, intercourse at any stage in normal pregnancy. Thus there is no evidence that coitus will cause physical damage to the fetus, or rupture the membranes, nor that orgasm might induce premature labour. Some clinicians may advise against sexual intercourse if there is a history of miscarriage, ante-partum bleeding, or pain during intercourse. Under such circumstances the doctor might recommend non-coital sex but female orgasm need not be avoided. However, orgasm should probably be avoided where there is either a history of premature deliveries or any evidence of premature labour.

Apart from providing reassurance to the woman who is concerned about her loss of sexual interest during pregnancy, the doctor might also advise a woman about positions for sexual intercourse that are likely to be comfortable for her. These include side-by-side and rear-entry positions.

Following childbirth, most women experience a reduction in their interest in sex, which may last for up to 3 months or even longer. In addition, soreness of an episiotomy scar and post-partum vaginal dryness associated with reduced levels of circulating oestrogens, particularly in breast-feeding mothers, may make intercourse uncomfortable and therefore lead to avoidance or reduced interest. Many other factors may contribute to sexual difficulties following childbirth, including the stress for both partners in adapting to their new roles as parents, a mother being emotionally close to the baby so that her partner may feel excluded, poor sleep and tiredness, and puerperal depression. In addition, a nursing mother may feel guilty about sexual arousal that can occur with breast-feeding. Finally, previous sexual maladjustment often manifests itself as frank sexual dysfunction following childbirth.

The GP can forewarn women about some of these problems and give appropriate advice if they actually occur. If post-partum vaginal dryness occurs the patient can be given an explanation and recommended to use a lubricant (such as KY jelly) during intercourse. Where soreness of an episiotomy scar prevents intercourse, a gradual return to non-coital sexual activity might first be recommended. It is important to reassure both women and their partners that loss of interest in sex is normal after childbirth and that it will gradually return. It is especially important to encourage the partners to maintain physical contact with each other over this period. Some couples may only want a loving cuddle; in other partnerships, the wife may wish to continue caressing her husband, though not yet wishing to be caressed by him.

Menopause

The onset of the menopause can provide a profound sense of liberation for some women and this may lead to enhanced interest in sex. However, in others there is a decline in sexual desire. A number of factors are likely to be influential at this time (Pearce *et al.* 1995). Reduction in circulating oestrogens will often cause decreased sexual arousability and may make sexual intercourse painful. Decline in androgen levels may have specific effects on sexual interest or desire. Other factors include, for example, children being about to leave home, a woman worrying that she is unattractive (especially by comparison with an attractive daughter), the increased risk of developing depression, and the partner possibly experiencing a decline in sexual performance.

Hormone replacement therapy may help alleviate sexual dysfunctions (see Pearce *et al.* (1995) for review). For example, vaginal application of hormonal cream, will benefit any vaginal dryness. While reduced sexual desire following the menopause is little affected by oestrogen or progestogen therapy, androgens will usually help restore sexual desire, especially when the menopause has been precipitated by oophorectomy. In addition to hormone administration the GP may be able to provide counselling, along the lines suggested earlier, which will assist the woman who is experiencing sexual difficulties. Whenever possible the partner should be included in such consultation. The management of problems of the menopause is discussed in more detail in Chapter 11.

Older age

Several studies have demonstrated that the majority of women and men remain sexually active beyond the age of 60, and, depending on the availability of a partner, as many as one in five are active at 80. For women in particular, it is very often the loss or disability of the spouse that determines the end of sexual activity.

'Sexual myths' affect the attitudes of both young and old and doctors towards sexuality in later life. These myths include the following: (1) because procreation is not possible after the menopause sexual activity should therefore cease; (2) sex is the prerogative of the young and attractive person; (3) sexual performance declines rapidly after middle age; (4) the problems associated with ageing preclude any interest in sexual activity. Belief in such myths may cause guilt in people who find that their sexual interest does not suddenly decline after middle age, and may contribute directly to problems such as loss of interest and impaired performance.

A number of physical and psychological difficulties may affect the sexual life of older women. First, the physical changes which occur with normal ageing, such as atrophic vaginitis, a decline in the vaginal response during sexual arousal, hypersensitive and tender labia, sagging breasts, impaired mobility, and weight gain, may impair the sexual interest and performance of both the woman and her partner. In addition, those physical illnesses which are likely to impair sexual function become more common in old age. These include cerebrovascular disease, especially strokes, degenerative joint disorders, maturity-onset diabetes, thyroid dysfunction, parkinsonism, malignant disease, especially of the breast and bowel, and amputations. In parallel with the increase in physical disorders, the numbers of women receiving medication, and the range of medication used, steadily increase with age. Some of the drugs used may have profound effects on sexuality (p. 580). Finally, psychiatric disorders, especially depression, anxiety, and dementia become more common, and all three, together with drugs used to treat them, are likely to be associated with impaired sexual interest and function.

Some of the difficulties will be amenable to brief counselling, particularly if the doctor has an understanding of sexuality during older age and is able to discuss the topic without embarrassment. Sexual dysfunction in older persons is often very amenable to sex therapy, provided the therapist is sensitive to the sexual value systems of older patients, which may be considerably more restricted than those of some younger people. On the other hand some couples welcome the change in social attitudes and the opportunity it gives them to discuss problems they may have uncomplainingly accepted for years. One of the changes for older women is how to adjust to their partner having a less firm erection. Many women feel that this is because of their failing looks. The doctor can help the partners through recommending that they adjust their lovemaking to include more foreplay and rather less emphasis on penetrative sex. Particular attention should be paid to physical aspects of therapy, including hormone replacement and the use of physical aids. Older men with erectile dysfunction may be helped by the use of a penile constriction ring (if the erections are at least partial), a vacuum constriction device, or intracavernosal injections of vasodilator substances such as papaverine or prostaglandin (Gregoire 1992).

Sexual problems associated with disability

Only in recent years have the sexual problems encountered by physically and mentally disabled people begun to receive appropriate attention. Several factors seem to have contributed to this neglect. Some people responsible for the care of the disabled have maintained the illusion that disabled persons somehow lack sexuality. Not only is this obviously untrue but it is also apparent that as many as three-quarters of persons who are disabled encounter problems in fulfilling their sexuality. Probably this attitude stems partly from the fact that both disability and sex are found by many people to be sensitive and difficult topics; the combination of the two therefore tends to provoke extreme discomfort which is dealt with by denial. This is reinforced by a general notion that to be sexy one must be able-bodied and attractive.

We can consider the problems of disablement in terms of (1) the woman who is disabled; (2) the woman with a disabled partner; and (3) management of sexual problems associated with disablement.

Sexual problems of the disabled woman

Although most of our information about sexual problems and physical disability concerns men, it is clear that disabled women are likely to suffer just as many problems as disabled men. Several aspects of a woman's sexuality can be affected. First, her image of herself as a physically desirable individual is likely to be precarious. Secondly, her awareness of the stigma attached to sexuality of the disabled may limit her interest in sex. Thirdly, the debilitating effects of the disorder from which she suffers, or of the medication she receives for it, may impair her drive. This particularly applies to chronic painful conditions. Fourthly, the condition may interfere with her mobility; thus, for example, severe arthritis or a spinal cord lesion may make coitus difficult or impossible. Fifthly, her capacity to receive the sensory input necessary for sexual satisfaction may be limited: this is particularly likely with neurological disorders. Finally, if she is being cared for by others (whether by relatives or in an institution) it is their attitude which will determine whether she has any opportunities for sexual activity, alone or with a partner.

Some of the conditions which may cause disability and affect sexuality have already been considered (see pp. 577–80). Others deserve mention in this context. Many neurological conditions, such as multiple sclerosis and cerebral palsy, are associated with sexual problems. The woman with a complete spinal cord transection will be unable to achieve an orgasm through genital stimulation, though she may well still be capable of pregnancy. She is also likely to have problems of urinary and bowel control. Often the woman with a spinal cord lesion develops new erogenous zones, especially at the level of the lesion. A woman who is blind may face taboos concerning learning about sexuality through touch, may be concerned about odour associated with sexual activity, embarrassed about nudity, frustrated due to the extra dependency she must have on her partner, and will completely lack the visual components of sexuality. Social isolation and difficulties in communication are likely to lead to poor sexual information for the woman who is deaf. Finally, mental retardation is associated with a whole range of further problems, particularly those arising from the attitudes of staff responsible for the woman's care, and especially from their concern about the woman's vulnerability to sexual exploitation and risk of pregnancy.

Sexual problems for the spouse of the disabled man

The woman whose partner is physically disabled is likely to face numerous difficulties concerning their sexual relationship. First and foremost there are the problems that arise because other people are often unable to accept a sexual relationship between an able-bodied woman and a disabled man. In addition, there are the problems arising out of role reversals that may be necessary in the general relationship, the concern the woman may have about hurting her partner, impairment of fertility (especially when the partner has a spinal cord lesion), difficulties the man may have in accepting his wife in a more sexually active role, and the attitude both partners have to non-coital sexual activity where sexual intercourse is impossible. The man may suffer considerable jealousy about the wife's ability to enjoy sex more than he does, and about the risk that she may develop another relationship. Furthermore, the woman may have great difficulty in accepting a role that combines the tasks of nurse (especially where excretory functions need to be looked after) and the feelings of a sexual partner.

Management of sexual problems of the disabled

Many of the sexual difficulties discussed here are straightforward and ideally should be dealt with by those who care for the disabled in the course of their everyday work. However, carers need education and support in order to do this. Many other sexual problems associated with disability are of a special nature, and will need referral for expert counselling. Until recently there were few people experienced in this type of work, but in some areas in the UK special clinics offering expert counselling have now been established and should receive every encouragement. The voluntary organization called SPOD (Sexual Problems of the Disabled) can offer advice and assistance to the disabled themselves, their partners and families, and also to those who care for the disabled (p. 599). The GP who wishes to learn more about sexual problems of the disabled and their management is recommended to contact this organization and request appropriate leaflets.

Conclusion

GPs are in the front line for presentation of most of the sexual difficulties discussed in this chapter. They should be able both to detect and assess patients with sexual difficulties, and provide counselling for at least the most straightforward cases. Teaching of human sexuality in medical schools should provide the necessary background knowledge for such work, but this needs to be supplemented by opportunities through general practice training schemes of experience in managing sexual problems. Most sexual dysfunction clinics can arrange further training for those who wish to improve their counselling skills in this area and some may be able to offer supervision to those who wish to treat their own patients with difficult or complicated sexual problems. Relate offers specific training courses for those wishing to learn how to do therapy. For the patient the most critical moment is when she first hints to her GP that she has a problem, and it is the GP's response which will determine whether she ever discusses this fully and receives appropriate help.

Appendix: assessment of a patient with a sexual problem – main points to be covered

1. *The problem.* Clarify in detail the nature of the sexual problem, its duration, any precipitants, and the way it has developed, including any factors that have made it worse and any that have led to improvement.

2. *Partner's response.* What has been the partner's response to the problem? Does he/she have a sexual problem? Are the couple able to discuss the problem, or talk about sex in general?

3. *Family history.* Parents' ages and occupations; nature of their relationship; nature of patient's relationships with both parents and siblings; was sex discussed in the home? – if so, in what context and what impression did this have on the patient? Is there any important family history of physical or psychiatric disorders?

4. *Early development.* Was patient happy during childhood? Did she encounter any problems in developing her sense of femaleness? What age did menarche occur, whether informed beforehand, and what was her reaction. What age did puberty (development of breasts, pubic hair, etc.) occur and what was patient's reaction?

5. *Sexual information.* How did patient acquire her knowledge about sex; does she feel she has adequate knowledge? (One should check on the patient's knowledge about sexuality throughout the interview.)

6. *Early sexual experiences.* Age at which sexual interest developed; masturbation (ask 'when did you find out about masturbation?') and reactions to it if she has masturbated; nature of early relationships with boyfriends including sexual experience; any homosexual interests or behaviour; any traumatic sexual experiences, including sexual abuse or rape?

7. *Current relationship.* Duration; how relationship developed; nature of general relationship, especially interests, friends, communication and friction; nature of sexual relationship; (if married) effect of marriage on sexual and general relationships; effect of pregnancy and childbirth on sexual relationship; relationships with children and attitudes to their sexuality.

8. *Schooling and occupations.*

9. *Religious beliefs.*

10. *Medical history.* Including menstruation, contraception, and medication.

11. *Psychiatric history.* Including medication.

12. *Use of alcohol and drugs.*

13. *Mental state examination.* In particular, is the patient suffering from depression or anxiety?

14. *Physical examination and investigations.* If appropriate (e.g. vaginal examination should be carried out, with care, if a woman complains of vaginismus).

15. *Goals of treatment.* What would the patient consider a satisfactory sexual relationship, and what would she like to change in her relationship (i.e what might be the aim of treatment)?

Useful addresses

British Association of Sexual and Marital Therapists,
PO Box 62, Sheffield S10 3TS.
Will give advice on sex therapists available in different parts of UK.

Lesbian Helpline,
Tel: 0171 837 2782, Sunday to Thursday 7.30–10 pm.

Relate (Marriage Guidance),
Herbert Gray College, Little Church Street, Rugby, Warwickshire CV21 3AP.
Tel: 01788 573241.
The majority of Relate centres now have trained psychosexual therapists.

SPOD (Sexual Problems of the Disabled), 286 Campden Road, London N7 0BJ.
Tel: 0171 607 8851.
The association to aid the sexual and personal relationships of people with a disability. It produces useful leaflets for different disabilities.

The Beaumont Trust,
BM Charity, London WC1N 3XX.
Tel: 0171 730 7453 and 01606 871 984.
This charity provides support for transvestites and their partners.

The London Friend Gay and Lesbian Helpline, 86 Caledonian Road, London N1. Tel: 0171 837 3337, every day from 7.30–10 pm

The London Rape Crisis Centre,
PO Box 69, London WC1X 9NJ.
Tel: 0171 916 5466.
Counselling line–tel: 0171 837 1600.

References and further reading

Bancroft, J. (1989). *Human sexuality and its problems* (2nd edn). Churchill Livingstone, Edinburgh. (Excellent authoritative account of all the major aspects of human sexuality.)

Catalan, J., Hawton, K., and Day, A. (1990). Couples referred to a sexual dysfunction clinic: psychological and physical morbidity. *British Journal of Psychiatry*, **156**, 61–7.

Everstine, D. S. and Everstine, L. (1983). The adult woman victim of rape. In *People in crisis: strategic therapeutic interventions*, pp. 177–200. Brunner/Mazel, New York. (Detailed guidance on the psychological effects of rape and its management.)

Gath, D., Cooper, P., and Day, A. (1982). Hysterectomy and psychiatric disorder: I Levels of psychiatric morbidity before and after hysterectomy. *British Journal of Psychiatry*, **140**, 335–50.

Greengross, W. (1976). *Entitled to love: the sexual and emotional needs of the handicapped.* Mallaby Press and National Marriage Guidance Council, in association with National Fund for Research into Crippling Diseases. (For patients and professionals: sensitive account with more emphasis on emotional and social aspects than on practical details of sex.)

Gregoire, A. (1992). New treatments for erectile impotence. *British Journal of Psychiatry*, **160**, 315–26.

Hawton, K. (1985). *Sex therapy: a practical guide.* Oxford University Press. (A detailed account of how to help people with sexual problems by sex therapy or counselling.)

Hawton, K. (1989). Sexual dysfunctions. In *Cognitive behaviour therapy for psychiatric problems: a practical guide*, pp. 370–405. Oxford University Press. (Focuses especially on the psychological components of sex therapy.)

Hawton, K. (1995). Treatment of sexual dysfunctions by sex therapy and other approaches. *British Journal of Psychiatry*, **167**, 304–14.

Hawton, K. and Catalan, J. (1986). Prognostic factors in sex therapy. *Behaviour Therapy and Research*, **24**, 377–85.

Hawton, K., Catalan, J., Martin, P., *et al.* (1986). Long-term outcome of sex therapy. *Behaviour Therapy and Research*, **24**, 665–75.

Hawton, K., Gath, D., and Day, A. (1994). Sexual function in a community sample of middle-aged women with partners: effects of age, marital, socioeconomic, psychiatric, gynaecological and menopausal factors. *Archives of Sexual Behavior*, **23**, 375–95.

Hobbs, M. (1990). Childhood sexual abuse: how can women be helped to overcome its long-term effects? In *Difficulties and dilemmas in the management of psychiatric patients* (ed. K. Hawton and P. Cowen), pp. 183–96. Oxford University Press.

Horton, B. (1991). Sexual outcomes arising from the diagnosis and treatment of cervical cancer and cervical intra-epithelial neoplasia: a review of the literature. *Sexual and Marital Therapy*, **6**, 29–39.

Jehu, D. (1988). *Beyond sexual abuse: therapy with women who were childhood victims.* Wiley, Chichester. (A detailed account of a psychological treatment approach for women experiencing various negative consequences of sexual abuse.)

Lancet (1981). Adverse reactions to bendrofluazide and propranolol for the treatment of mild hypertension. *Lancet*, **ii**, 539–43.

Leiblum, S. R., and Rosen, R. C. (1988). *Sexual desire disorders.* Guilford Press, New York.

Masters, W. H. and Johnson, V. E. (1966). *Human sexual response.* Little Brown, Boston. (A very detailed account of research concerning physiological and anatomical aspects of sexual response.)

Masters, W. H. and Johnson, V. E. (1970). *Human sexual inadequacy.* Churchill, London. (The original description of intensive sex therapy, but difficult to read.)

Osborn, M., Hawton, K., and Gath, D. (1988). Sexual dysfunction among middle aged women in the community. *British Medical Journal*, **296**, 959–62.

Pearce, J., Hawton, K., and Blake, F. (1995). Psychological and sexual symptoms associated with the menopause and the effects of hormone replacement therapy: a review. *British Journal of Psychiatry*, **167**, 163–73.

Schreiner-Engel, P. and Schiavi, R. C. (1986). Lifetime psychopathology in individuals with low sexual desire. *Journal of Nervous Mental Disorders*, **174**, 646–51.

Schreiner-Engel, P., Schiavi, R. C., Vietorisz, D., *et al.* (1987). Diabetes type and female sexuality. *Journal of Psychosomatic Research*, **31**, 23–33.

Sherwin, B. B., Gelfand, M. M., and Brender, W. (1985). Androgens enhance sexual motivation in females: a prospective, crossover study of sex steroid administration in the surgical menopause. *Psychosomatic Medicine*, **47**, 339–51.

Speckens, A. E. M., Hengeveld, M. W., Lycklama à Nijeholt, G. A. B., *et al.* (1995). Psychosexual functioning of partners with presumed non-organic erectile dysfunction: cause or consequence of the disorder? *Archives of Sexual Behavior*, **24**, 157–72.

Steketee, G. and Foa, E. (1987). Rape victims: post-traumatic stress responses and their treatment. A review of the literature. *Journal of Anxiety Disorders*, **1**, 69–88.

Wellings, K., Field, J., Johnson, A. E. M., *et al.* (1994). *Sexual behaviour in Britain: the national survey of sexual attitudes and lifestyles.* Penguin, London.

Further reading for patients

Barnes, T. and Rodwell, L. (1992). *A woman's guide to loving sex*. Boxtree, London. (A clear account of women's sexuality and tackling sexual difficulties.)

Greengross, W. and Greengross, S. (1989). *Living, loving and ageing*. Age Concern, Mitcham. (An easily read, pleasant, and short book.)

Heiman, J. and LoPiccolo, J. (1988). *Becoming orgasmic: a sexual and personal growth programme for women*. Piatkus, London. (An excellent self-help book for women with orgasmic problems, but also has a wider focus on female sexuality.)

Kitzinger, S. (1985). *Women's experience of sex*. Penguin, London. (An excellent account of female sexuality and the experience of being a woman, from many angles. Useful for women who may be inhibited, of low self-esteem, or feel they are 'different' from others. Fairly sophisticated.)

Lacroix, N. (1989). *Sensual massage*. Dorling Kindersly, London. (A tasteful practical guide to caressing. A good self-help book and also useful in the context of sex therapy.)

Litvinoff, S. (1992). *The Relate guide to sex in loving relationships*. Vermilion, London. (A book covering many aspects of sexuality and sexual relationships in a pleasantly simple and direct manner. Also a useful self-help guide for couples who wish to try and overcome their sexual difficulties themselves.)

London Rape Crisis Centre (1984). *Sexual violence: the reality for women*. Women's Press, London. (Good practical guide for rape victims.)

Parks, N. (1990). *Rescuing the inner child. Therapy for adults sexually abused as children*. Souvenir Press, London. (A self-help book for adults victims of childhood sexual abuse and their partners.)

Zilbergeld, B. (1978). *Men and sex*. Fontana, London. (An excellent self-help book for men and their partners.)

Books on sex education for young people

Fenwick, E. and Walker, R. (1994). *How sex works*. Dorling Kindersley, London. (A clear, factual, and non-threatening book for adolescents.)

Harris, R. H. (1994). *Let's talk about sex*. Walker Bros, London. (A gentle and humerous account of sexuality for young adolescents.)

CHAPTER TWENTY

Complementary medicine and women's health

Christine A'Court, Jacqueline Wootton
Adriane Fugh-Berman and Kim A. Jobst

Users of Complementary medicine

A consumer-led boom

One in four of the UK's general population now report use of Complementary medicine in the previous 12 months, compared with one in seven in 1986 (Francis 1995; Dickinson 1996). Between 1993 and 1995, a 25% increase in sales of Alternative medicines was noted (Mintel 1995). Australia has also witnessed an increase in usage, with twice as much public expenditure on Complementary as on conventional medicines (MacLennan *et al.* 1996). The trend has been described as a consumer-led boom (Dickinson 1996). Poor outcomes from conventional care, especially in chronic conditions, may drive patients to seek alternatives (Murray and Sheperd 1993; Francis 1995). However, patients are not always 'pushed' by dissatisfaction, they may also be 'pulled' by lifestyle and holistic beliefs towards alternatives (Francis 1995; Furnham and Vincent 1995; Dickinson 1996).

Users of Complementary medicine come from all socio-economic groups, although in the UK the majority of users tend to be young to middle-aged and of higher educational level and social class than average (Fulder 1996). In the US, high usage is seen in the wealthier white population but is also characteristic of minority communities, reflecting their rich, ethnic medical traditions (Eisenberg 1993). In developing countries, 80% of the population still rely on 'traditional' medicine, including herbalism, spiritual healing, and acupuncture (Bodeker 1994).

A debate continues as to whether various forms of unorthodox medicine are truly alternative, or complementary, to orthodox medicine (Fulder 1996). In this chapter we do not dwell on this issue, but use the term Complementary medicine to cover therapies which patients may choose to use in isolation, or as an adjunct to orthodox medicine. The most popular and widely-used methods on both sides of the Atlantic are: osteopathy, chiropractic, homeopathy, acupuncture, aromatherapy, reflexology, herbalism, healing, hypnotherapy, and naturopathy (Tables 20.1 and 20.2).

Table 20.1 *Widely-used complementary therapies*

Acupuncture
Treatment by the insertion of fine, filiform needles at specific sites along lines of '*Qi*' (energy flow) called 'meridians' linking certain organs. Manipulation of the needle is believed to stimulate or dissipate unbalanced energy and so improve organ function

Aromatherapy
Massage, baths, compresses, and inhalations employing distilled or pressed aromatic ('essential') oils derived from plants, flowers, herbs, spices, and woods. Individual oils typically contain up to 100 different chemical compounds

Biofeedback
The use of equipment to monitor physiological signals and to bring involuntary processes under voluntary control

Chiropractic
Chiropractic postulates that various mechanical stresses (called 'subluxations') occur around intervertebral and other joints, and affect the functioning of the nervous system and possibly other systems. These stresses may be the result of misuse of the skeleton; commonly bending and lifting, or prolonged adoption of poor postures at work, during recreation, or sleep. other causes include emotional stress and associated muscle spasm; trauma; or birth injury. Following diagnosis of the specific site of problems, manipulation of the spine and other joints is carried out

Healing
Transmission of psychic energy for therapeutic purposes

Herbalism
Use of whole plants and, in some cases, minerals for therapeutic purposes

Homeopathy
Detailed history-taking evaluating multiple symptoms, followed by treatment of symptom complexes with a substance (the 'simillimum') creating near-identical symptoms in a healthy person. Extreme dilutions are used (protentization), mixed in a prescribed way by violent agitation (succussion). In classical homeopathy, specific, tailored remedies are prescribed to an individual, in contrast with over-the-counter purchase of homeopathic remedies for common symptom complexes

Hypnotherapy
Based on the belief that the mind (conscious and unconscious) can influence organic diseases. After induction of a trance or deeply relaxed state, suggestions can be implanted. It aims to reduce general stress and unconscious disease-causing patterns but sometimes selective suggestions may be made. Practised either in the presence of a therapist, or in absence (self-hypnosis). Hypnosis subjects can control blood supply, sensitivity to injury, and pain tolerance

Table 20.1 *Continued*

Macrobiotic medicine
The macrobiotic philosophy attributes disease to heredity, climate, psychologi-cal states, behaviour, and an excessive intake of particularly 'yin' and/or 'yang' foods. Treatment emphasizes dietary manipulation, with reduction of intakes of excessively 'yin' foods such as sugar, food additives, tropical fruits, dairy products, refined flour, and commercial tea and coffee, and similar reduction of excessively 'yang' foods such as eggs, meat, salt, and salty varieties of cheese. The 'standard' microbiotic diet which is midway in the 'yin – yang' scale is recommended to form the basis of any diet. It is based on grains, legumes, and forms of soy, with emphasis on root vegetables in patients who are too 'yin', and leafy vegetables in patients who are too 'yang'

Naturopathy
A system aiming to promote self-healing. Diagnosis employs a detailed interview concerning lifestyle, nutrition, bodily functions, and iris diagnosis (iridology). Treatment aims to eliminate toxins by dietary restriction or fasting, heat, internal or external hydrotherapy, exercise, manipulation, mud packs, and so on. Nutrition therapy, the dominant subspeciality within naturopathy, advocates a wholefood, high-fibre diet, preferably using food grown organi-cally, and assumes that individual requirements vary according to genetic, physiological, and lifestyle influences. Some therapists advocate mega-vitamin and mineral supplements, whilst others adhere to the dietary approach

Osteopathy
Examination of musculoskeletal system, interpretation in terms of tension, adhesions, fibrosis, sprains, and circulatory stasis, then treatment by manipula-tion of soft tissues and joints. Many osteopaths believe this process affects not only the function of the musculoskeletal system, but other organ systems

Reflexology
The application of manual pressure to 'reflex' points on the ears, hands, or feet that somatotopically correspond to specific areas of the body. Believed to reduce stagnation in the system and encourage the healing process

Relaxation and imagery
Assumes the mind can influence organic disease. Induction of states of deep relaxation and often guided visualization. In these states, suggestions can often be fully absorbed as effectively as in hypnotherapy

Traditional Chinese medicine
Holds that man is an indivisible combination of mind, body, and spirit. Disease may be a consequence of hereditary or environmental influences, and physical or psychological activity, any of which can interrupt the free flow of 'Qi' or energy. Therapy involves acupuncture, Oriental herbal medicine, diet, and psychophysical exercise such as T'ai-chi or Qigong designed to promote the free flow of Qi

Table 20.2 *Usage of Complementary Therapies amongst members of the Consumers Association sent a postal questionnaire (Super Survey 1995). Of 8745 respondents, 2724 (31%) had used a therapy in the last 12 months (Francis 1995) . The type of therapy is shown*

Practitioner consulted in last 12 months	Percentage of respondents consulting practitioner
Osteopath	28
Chiropractor	17
Homeopath	16
Acupuncturist	12
Aromatherapist	12
Reflexologist	9
Herbalist	6
Spiritual Healer	5
Hypnotherapist	4
Alexander technique	3
Naturopath	2
Other practitioner	5

Women as users of Complementary medicine

Women's usage of Complementary medicine is generally found to exceed that of men's (Fulder and Munro 1985; Thomas *et al.* 1991; Dickinson 1996). Women comprise over two-thirds of the patients of Alternative practitioners (Thomas *et al.* 1991; Vincent and Furnham 1996). Surveys carried out on general practice patient populations find approximately a third of men to have used one Alternative medical therapy over the previous 10 years, compared with almost half of women (Murray and Sheperd 1993). The predominance of female usage may simply reflect the higher rates of consultation among women for medical care generally (Royal College of General Practitioners 1986). Prevalence of usage need not imply a difference in attitudes; one recent study found no difference in attitudes between men and women to Complementary medicine (Vincent and Furnham 1996). Nor is there a gender difference in reported satisfaction with the outcome of Alternative care (Francis 1995).

In two surveys, musculo-skeletal symptoms were by far the most common presenting problem amongst patients attending osteopaths, chiropractors, naturopaths, and acupuncturists (Fulder 1996). Headaches, migraine, pain at other sites, anxiety, and depression also feature prominently in surveys confined to manipulative therapies. How often women turn to Complementary therapy for specific 'women's problems' is more difficult to extract from the available data. While men often use massage, chiropractic, and osteopathy, women are more likely to consult herbalists and homeopaths (Murray and Sheperd 1993) or reflexologists and aromatherapists (Francis 1995). Women also favour a variety of lifestyle programmes, often used in combination.

These include: dietary changes, mega-vitamin and mineral supplementation, relaxation and imagery, and various forms of exercise. It has been argued that women appear to be attracted most to methods promoting general good health, whereas men tend to favour an emphasis on the management of an immediate condition (Dickinson 1996). Both men and women with cancer or AIDS frequently look to Complementary therapy. While Alternative 'cancer cures' may attract attention and controversy, Complementary therapies are more likely to be used as an adjunct to conventional treatment for the relief of symptoms or side-effects of treatment.

Paying for Complementary care: inside and outside the NHS

Most people who want Complementary medicine have to pay for it at the point of contact. This situation discriminates against those who cannot afford it. On the other hand, the need for direct payment might in some cases contribute to the therapeutic effect, since patients may be more likely to feel the benefit of something actively sought out and directly paid for.

In the UK, regional differences in use of Complementary therapies have been related to differences in amounts charged by practitioners (Fulder 1996). Healing, which is often free, and other relatively inexpensive therapies like herbalism and hypnotherapy, are used more in the north of the country while acupuncture, naturopathy, osteopathy, and chiropractic flourish in the more prosperous areas of the UK (Fulder 1996). In American society, high usage of some Complementary therapies in low-income, minority ethnic groups reflects not only their cost but ethnic practice.

In 1995, only 6% of Complementary therapy-users were having their treatment paid through the NHS (Dickinson 1996). However, this low figure belies a considerable increase in availability within the NHS. Indeed, it has been argued that Complementary medicine is already an established part of the NHS (Smith 1996). A nationwide survey in 1995 found 60% of health authorities and 40% of general practitioners (GPs) were routinely purchasing Complementary services. Most NHS referrals were for homeopathy or acupuncture. Fundholding GPs, in particular, were likely to commission Complementary therapies, often provided within the health centre. Half of the commissioning GPs offered Complementary treatments themselves (Thomas *et al.* 1995). One in 20 GPs employed a non-NHS therapist – often an osteopath. Out of the total NHS budget of £32 billion, an estimated £1 million is currently spent on Complementary medicine. The perception of Complementary medicine as low-tech, low risk, and relatively cheap may be promoting its integration into NHS practice, despite the paucity of objective evidence of efficacy (Smith 1996). There is as great a need for evidence supporting the use of Complementary medicine as there is for orthodox medicine; recent estimates of the evidence base for orthodox medical interventions ranging from 20–80% (Ellis *et al.* 1995; Gill *et al.* 1996).

Sickness certification, insurance fees, and compensation

The DSS has stated that non-registered medical practitioners can issue a sickness certificate (leaflet N1277). Many private medical insurance companies will reimburse the fees of registered (osteopaths and chiropractors) or medically-qualified and well-established Complementary practitioners, provided patients have been referred by a registered medical practitioner (Fulder 1996). Fees are also being reimbursed by the Criminal Injuries Compensation Board and the Industrial Injuries Board (Fulder 1996). Some firms and trade unions now consistently reimburse the charges of osteopaths and chiropractors.

Considerations for the referring or commissioning GP

Professional liability

Complementary therapists in the UK enjoy a common law freedom to practise. In other countries, as in much of continental Europe and most states of the US only registered therapists are permitted to practise. Although at one time a doctor's association with unregistered practitioners was deemed serious professional misconduct, the General Medical Council (GMC) now recognizes the valuable role of Alternative practitioners. The 1995 update of the GMC's professional guidance states that a GP can 'delegate medical care to nurses and other health care staff who are not registered medical practitioners'. . . 'but you must be sure that the person to whom you delegate is competent to undertake the procedure or therapy involved'. (GMC 1995). This is a tall order, given that few conventional doctors have an in-depth understanding of Alternative therapies. Indeed, GPs recommend a Complementary therapist in order to take advantage of an Alternative paradigm. It has been argued that without GPs possessing the skills involved, the situation cannot properly be described as delegation (Stone 1996). The GMC states that their guidance on this matter is under continuing review by the Standards Committee. Currently, 'referral' is not considered an appropriate term for a GP's recommendation to a patient to consult a Complementary therapist; a GP is expected to have sufficient under-standing of a Complementary therapy to 'delegate' professional care, whilst retaining overall clinical responsibility. This is also the case in most states in the US where certain Complementary therapists can only practise under medical supervision. When the GP cannot claim sufficient understanding of a therapy, the GMC view is that the GP runs the risk of not acting in the patients' best interests (GMC, personal communication). Use of a Complementary therapist will often be in situations where the problem is chronic or intractable, or where a patient exercises choice. The GMC view is that any practitioners involved are responsible for their own actions, but since the GP retains overall clinical responsibility for a patient, he or she must, throughout, provide, or at least offer, a reasonable standard of care.

Doctors may hope that they will avoid professional and legal liability provided they recommend practitioners who are suitably qualified, or have statutory registration, as obtained in the UK by the osteopaths in 1993 and chiropractors in 1994. Although the standards imposed by various Comple-mentary professional bodies vary greatly, the GMC takes registration as a good indication of professional competence. In the absence of registration, the GMC view is that the GP should take reasonable steps to ensure the competence of individual Alternative practitioners (GMC, personal communication).

Legal liability

In the event of a mishap directly resulting from an Alternative practitioner's intervention, UK medical defence bodies would, in general, resist any attempt to attribute liability to a GP. However, if the GP had referred the patient to a practitioner with a poor track record, then the GP might be deemed reckless, and liability might be shared (Medical Defence Union, personal communication). From the patient's point of view, the situation differs from that of referral to a specialist within the NHS (Stone 1996a). Although Complementary therapists have a legal duty of care towards a patient, allegations of negligence may be hard to prove in the absence of nationally agreed standards of care. Moreover, many Alternative therapists carry no indemnity insurance. The current unlicensed status of most herbal medicines in the UK protects the vendor from legal liability, and precludes systematic safety monitoring, a situation potentially hazardous for patients (De Smet 1995). The recent extension of the Yellow Card scheme to unlicensed herbal medicines is a welcome step (CSM/MCA, Oct 1996). A licensing procedure is still needed to assess and enforce product quality, provide comprehensive post-marketing surveillance and enable, if necessary, product recalls. However, the relatively low incidence of reported toxicity and side-effects relative to the enormous sales of herbal products, and recent public resistance to European Union licensing proposals, demonstrates the need for a separate herbal medicine licensing procedure, as in some other countries (e.g. France, Germany, Australia) (De Smet 1995, Fulder 1996).

Employment of Complementary practitioners

If GPs themselves wish to employ Complementary practitioners, they may be helped by guidelines from the West Yorkshire Health Authority, specifically drawn up to facilitate the employment of Complementary therapists within the NHS. They emphasize the need to ensure that practitioners have appropriate qualifications, belong to a professional body complying with a defined code of ethics, and carry professional indemnity insurance (West Yorkshire HA 1995). However, Complementary practitioners have been cautioned against adoption of the conventional medical model of statutory regulation (Stone 1996). It is argued they should continue developing their own standards of training, accreditation, voluntary self-regulation and thus professionalism, and avoid the philosophical and financial cost of an 'inappropriate statutory straitjacket'.

Efficacy: source and nature of the evidence

To our knowledge there has been no scientific evaluation of whole diagnostic and therapeutic systems such as those embodied in traditional Chinese medicine (TCM), macrobiotic medicine, naturopathy, or homeopathy. We have attempted to introduce and evaluate some studies applicable to the use of Complementary medicine for women's health. In many cases we draw on studies which were not designed to investigate Complementary medicine *per se*, but which are nonetheless relevant. Some of the more accessible evidence is concerned with nutritional aspects of Complementary approaches. It should be noted that although dietary manipulation is central to macrobiotic therapy, it is one of several elements dictated by, for instance, TCM or naturopathy.

The layout of this review mirrors this volume's chapters. The single, problem-based approach to some degree runs counter to many Alternative systems which emphasize that the significance of a symptom such as dysmenorrhoea, or a disease such as breast cancer, may be apparent only when taken in the context of the whole person.

In pursuit of objectivity, this review draws whenever possible on the randomized control trial (RCT). However, much is recognized and written about the limitations of the RCT. Additional investigative approaches such as epidemiology, observational and case-control studies, the $n=1$ trial, and experimental work are all needed to try and tease out the active, and the most potent, ingredients of holistic health care. A survey, carried out first in GP trainees and then in dually-qualified Complementary and medical practitioners, has investigated what evidence they considered important before accepting that an Alternative technique might benefit their patients. A controversial finding was that, for the majority, the most important factor was personal experience of method use with patients, outweighing the importance of case-control or clinical trial evidence. This may indicate how strongly practitioners are influenced by their own, not necessarily representative experience. Equally, it may show that practitioners modify the message they receive from scientific trials, which are seldom free from design or analytical flaws, according to their own experience. It also emerged that the practitioners' views concerning the nature of valid evidence were determined in part by age group and by their affiliation to either hospital, university, or primary care.

Sources of information on Complementary medicine

Bibliographic

Clinical and experimental research relevant to Complementary medicine is widely scattered in a number of databases worldwide. Several of the major biomedical bibliographic databases now contain significant numbers of citations on Alternative medicine; both Medline and Embase (the European nearest equivalent to Medline) contain in the region of 50 000 to 60 000 references each, although with considerable overlap. Coverage in Medline has increased in recent years due to the policy of indexing the entire contents of journals, as opposed to the earlier policy of indexing only those articles that fitted pre-approved categories. Accessibility will be further enhanced by the establishment of a Cochrane Field of Complementary and Alternative Medicine since Medline have agreed to include all RCTs identified by hand searches performed by the Cochrane initiative, irrespective of journal of origin. However, references can still be difficult to retrieve as MeSH (Medical Subject Heading) terms are based on disease categories and conventional medical terminology. Recently, some progress has been made to incorporate Alternative medicine terms, and full text searching of the citations and abstracts affords yet more flexibility. In Medline, the catch-all term (when 'exploded') is 'Alternative medicine', not 'Complementary medicine'.

There are three relatively recent peer review journals specific to Complementary medicine, two of which were reviewed in the *Journal of the American Medical Association* (Simpson and Bick 1996) and one of which has been adopted for indexing by Medline.

The Cochrane Pregnancy and Childbirth Database includes some evaluations of Complementary therapies. One anticipates expansion of this resource as suitable studies are identified or performed.

A comprehensive list of UK organizations involved in specific forms of Complementary medicine, and charitable organizations promoting research in this area, is provided in a useful *Handbook of Complementary medicine* (Fulder 1996).

Internet

Further electronic resources are openly and publicly available on the Internet. The most reliable are academic, non-commercial sites which increasingly act as a necessary adjunct to library facilities for academics and professionals. One site of particular interest for women's health issues is the Centers for Disease Control, USA, Women's Health Page: (http:www.cdc.gov.diseases/women/html). Some specific health sites have large subsets of information relating to women's conditions, for instance: the Aeiveos Home Page on Aging (*sic*), put out as an academically-oriented public information resource by a biotechnology research and education company: (http:www.aeiveos.com/). An overview of all information resources relevant to women's health and details of how to access them is available on the Internet through the Rosenthal Centre Directory of Databases. The url (unique resource location) is: (http:cpmcnet.columbia.edu/ dept/rosenthal). Sites and 'urls' for all Internet sites change frequently but there is usually a trail of information left for the user to locate the new site.

The exponential growth of electronic information media coincides with both the development of health consumerism and the growing interest in Complementary medicine. On the Internet, new health care consumers are actively seeking and swapping information. Electronic access to full text articles, reviews, advice sheets, discussion groups, and increasing numbers of medical journals has enabled consumers as well as professionals to research the latest medical information, resulting in increasing patient sophistication. This new medium has proved particularly appropriate for those who seek to take control of their own health care decisions in partnership with professionals. The 'downside' of all this is that GPs may be asked by patients about theories and products about which they know little. The GP must be aware that resources on the Web are heterogeneous and variable in quality, and that there is little to limit the making of extravagant claims and dissemination of promotional material. Guidelines on how to evaluate and selectively utilize promotional material are available, however, from the Rosenthal Directory, and the three peer-reviewed journals of Complementary medicine referred to earlier (p. 611).

Breast disease

Breast cancer – causation and prevention

Influence of diet

Epidemiological studies show large differences between countries in the incidence of breast cancer. Race, lifestyle, and diet have all been implicated. Japan is reported to have the lowest risk of hormone-dependent cancers, and the importance of diet is suggested by the observation that following transition from a Japanese to a Western diet, the risk of breast cancer increases (Kolonel 1988; Adlercreutz *et al.* 1991; Lee *et al.* 1991) The diet recommended in macrobiotic medicine is very close to the traditional Japanese diet and as with the traditional Chinese diet, and vegetarian or semi-vegetarian diets, carries with it a low risk of hormone-dependent cancers. These dietary groups are characterized by a lower prevalence of obesity and saturated fat intake, the former and possibly the latter being risk factors for breast cancer. A further factor which may afford protection to those in the low-risk groups is the intake of naturally-occurring oestradiol (E2)-like compounds of plant origin. These diphenolic phytoestrogens, which include the lignans and isoflavonoids, are converted by intestinal bacteria to biologically active compounds. Their effects in humans are those of a weak oestrogen with, in addition, proven antioxidant and anti-proliferative activity (Knight and Eden 1996). The highest intakes of these compounds are found in countries or regions with a low cancer incidence.

Lignans are found in wholegrain cereals, seeds, nuts, vegetables, legumes, and fruits. Isoflavonoids are less widely distributed but occur in high concentrations in soybean products, chick peas, and possibly other legumes. The consumption of soy products in some Japanese populations reaches 200 mg/day. Total isoflavone intake in Asia ranges between 25–45 mg/day, compared with an intake of less than 5 mg/day in Western countries (Knight and Eden 1996). Soy products contain differing amounts of phytoestrogens; tofu, for example, contains 10 times more phytoestrogens than soy drinks. Fermentation decreases the content but increases the bioavailability and excretion of isoflavones in soy (Hutchins *et al.* 1995a). In the macrobiotic medical system, great importance is attributed to a diet consisting of grains (50%), vegetables (20%), legumes (10%), fish, fruit, or nuts (10%), and seasoning with fermented soy products such as miso, tempeh, or tamari (Kushi 1978).

Isoflavonoids and lignans have been shown to influence intracellular enzymes, protein synthesis, growth factor action, malignant cell proliferation, differentiation, and angiogenesis (Knight and Eden 1996). There is increasing interest in their possible role as natural cancer protective compounds. They also influence sex hormone metabolism and biological activity. Fibre intake and phyto-oestrogen metabolite excretion show a positive correlation with the concentration of plasma sex hormone-binding globulin and a negative correlation with plasma percentage of free oestradiol and free testosterone (Adlercreutz *et al.* 1987). In addition, being weak oestrogens, it has been hypothesized that phyto-oestrogen metabolites may have anti-oestrogen effects through competitive binding to oestrogen receptors. It is suggested that such a mechanism would attenuate the adverse consequences of obesity and might partly explain the low cancer incidence in Hispanic women (Horn 1995). A contrasting hypothesis is that dietary oestrogen intake might promote the growth of breast cancer cells, and antagonize the action of tamoxifen (Welshons *et al.* 1987). A study of Chinese women in Singapore found that soy product intake seemed to protect pre-menopausal women, but not post-menopausal women, from breast cancer (Lee *et al.* 1991).

There is considerable evidence that plasma levels and excretion of phyto-oestrogen metabolites are determined by dietary manipulation of the sort integral to many forms of Complementary medicine. It can be shown under controlled dietary conditions that urinary lignan and isoflavonoid excretion change in response to alterations in vegetable, fruit, and legume intake (Hutchins *et al.* 1995b). Following soybean consumption, some isoflavonoids are secreted in amounts equivalent to classical oestrogens. When a total of 53 subjects adhering to macrobiotic or lactovegetarian diets were compared with those having an omnivorous diet, the excretion of phyto-oestrogen metabolites was eightfold higher in the macrobiotics, and twice as high in the lactovegetarians. The lowest levels of excretion were found in a group of post-menopausal breast cancer patients (Adlercreutz *et al.* 1986).

Vitamins and co-factors

A prospective study of 89 494 nurses found a high intake of dietary Vitamin A to be associated with a 16% reduction in risk of breast cancer (Hunter *et al.* 1993). No association was found between dietary vitamin C and E intake and risk of breast disease. Vitamin A supplements ($\geq$10 000 iu/day) appear to decrease the risk of breast cancer only in those with a low dietary intake (<6 630 iu/day), in whom they reduced the incidence by a half. Vitamin C and E supplements, even at high dose and for long periods, appeared to have no effect on the incidence of breast cancer. Any conclusions concerning the possible beneficial effect of vitamin A must, in women of childbearing age, be tempered by evidence concerning the teratogenic potential of high doses (see Fertility, below). However, daily vitamin A intakes of <10 000 iu/day seem to carry no significant teratogenic risk, and carotenoids, which are vitamin A precursors, are not teratogenic (Smithells 1996).

The effect of beta-carotene, the naturally occurring form of Vitamin A in vegetables, has been examined not in relation to breast but to cervical cancer. In a case control study utilising 191 pairs of women in Italy, women with the lowest intake of dietary beta-carotene had a six-fold higher risk of developing invasive cervical cancer. (LaVecchia, Franceschi *et al.* 1984) Beta-carotene itself might only be a marker for other cancer-protective carotenoids as two lung cancer prophylaxis trials have shown no benefit, and even a possible risk associated with β-carotene supplements.

Life events

The holistic view common to all Complementary medicine holds that state of mind is linked with, and can be causally related to, disease. Some support for the holistic view comes from a well-designed, case-control study of 119 women under investigation for breast disease (Chen *et al.* 1995). Using pre-defined qualitative and quantitative definitions, details of 'life events and difficulties' experienced in the preceding 5 years were collected by researchers blinded to the results of breast biopsy. Severe life-events were associated with a threefold increase in risk of breast cancer, and a 12-fold increase when adjustments were made for age, menopausal status, and other potential confounding factors.

Exercise

A case-control study matched 545 women with breast cancer who had been diagnosed before age 40 with similar women without breast cancer (Bernstein *et al.* 1994). Women who had averaged 3.8 hours or more a week in physical exercise since puberty had a risk of breast cancer only 42% of that of inactive women.

Breast cancer – palliation and prognosis

Post-mastectomy pain and lymphoedema

A very small, randomized controlled study suggests that topical capsaicin is helpful in neurogenic post-mastectomy pain syndrome (Watson and Evan 1992). Five of 13 patients receiving the capsaicin cream reported good to excellent results compared with only one of 10 patients in the placebo group.

Secondary lymphoedema can be improved by massage. The efficacy of manual massage has been compared with that of pneumatic devices. In one study of 60 patients with post-mastectomy arm oedema, 12 manual lymphatic massage treatments over the course of a month resulted in a significant reduction in oedema lasting at least 3 months (Zanolla *et al.* 1984). A pneumatic device with constant pressure used for 6 hours a day was also effective, while a pneumatic device with variable pressure was ineffective. Patients might find a massage three times a week preferable to the wearing of a device for 6 hours a day, although both appear effective.

Mood and pain in metastatic breast cancer

Few in the medical profession would disagree with any approach that improved mood and reduced pain in patients with breast cancer. Studies exist which suggest that the use of hypnotherapy or relaxation and imagery as an adjunct to routine oncological care is associated with an improvement in general condition and tolerance to chemotherapy (Spiegel and Bloom 1983; Bridge *et al.* 1988).

614

One study of 54 women with metastatic breast cancer compared the effect of group therapy with or without self-hypnosis training on mental suffering and pain sensation (Spiegel and Bloom 1983). Improvement was obtained in both treatment groups with the maximum effect seen in the group also learning self-hypnosis.

In another study, 154 breast cancer patients receiving therapy were randomized to three groups: one group received training in progressive muscle relaxation and deep breathing; another group added pleasant imagery to relaxation and deep breathing; whilst controls were encouraged to simply talk about themselves (Bridge *et al.* 1988). Before the trial began, women in all the groups scored similarly on validated measures of mood, depression, and anxiety. After 6 weeks, mood in the control group had deteriorated whilst mood in the intervention groups had improved, women in the relaxation and imagery group benefiting the most.

Many other supportive approaches might achieve the same laudable improvement in psychological parameters. A separate issue is whether this form of psychological therapy has any effect on disease outcome in terms of survival.

Survival in metastatic breast cancer

It is claimed by some practitioners of Complementary medicine and their patients that emotions and mental attitudes can influence disease prognosis. One group has examined the effect of altering patients' emotional state without attempting to change their expectations of survival and without employing any 'cancer-conquering' imagery (Spiegel *et al.* 1989). Psychologists used a programme of weekly support groups and self-hypnosis for pain, a programme which had earlier been shown to reduce anxiety, depression, and pain in women with metastatic breast cancer (Spiegel and Bloom 1983). The emphasis lay in encouraging patients to discuss the impact of cancer on their lives, express their feelings, develop strategies for coping with the mental and physical distress, and counter the tendency to social isolation. In a prospective, randomized study of women with metastatic breast cancer receiving routine oncological care, the 1-year psychological support programme appeared to double the length of survival. Fifty patients participated in the psychosocial intervention group while 36 acted as controls. Mean survival in the intervention group was 36.6 (SD 37.6) months compared with 18.9 (SD 10.8) months in the control group, a significant difference (p<0.0001). It was concluded by the authors that the study bears out observational studies describing the apparent impact of social isolation versus support on disease outcome. Studies they quote report improved outcome in communities with good supportive networks, and in married women as compared with unmarried women. In their own study the psychosocial intervention group showed a survival advantage despite this group's higher percentage of unmarried women (Spiegel, Bloom *et al.* 1989).

Further studies, including some randomized controlled trials, suggest that hypnotherapy alone improves symptom control in, and outcome from, other types of cancer (Fulder 1996). It is difficult to separate the efficacy of hypnotherapy from relaxation and imagery or even concentrated psychological support, but the message emerges that these related 'mind–body' approaches help patients greatly.

It is suspected that the neuroendocrine and immune systems may be a major link between the psyche and course of cancer, with some experimental evidence. Thus, in 13 patients with stage 1 breast cancer, a combination of relaxation, guided imagery, and biofeedback had a measurable effect on the immune system, including an increase in natural killer cells and lymphocytes (Gruber *et al.* 1993).

A multi-modality approach is that taken by the Bristol Cancer Help Centre (BCHC), which employs dietary manipulation, psychological techniques, and many forms of Complementary medicine. A controversial case control study published in 1990 suggested that patients attending the BCHC had poorer survival than selected controls (Bagenal *et al.* 1990). The study design and methods of analysis attracted much criticism and the consensus view is that the study was inconclusive.

Mastalgia

Evening primrose oil (EPO), high in the essential fatty acids linoleic and gamma-linoleic acid, is helpful for mastalgia. A retrospective study of 414 patients with either cyclical or non-cyclical mastalgia found EPO at 3 g/day (contains 240 g gamma-linoleic acid) to be as effective as bromocriptine, although less effective than danazol. The response rate for EPO was 58% in cyclical mastalgia and 38% in non-cyclical mastalgia. EPO was given initially for 6 months, and patients were counselled that it might take 4 months for it to exert an effect. EPO had fewer side-effects than either drug (Gately *et al.* 1992).

Contraception

Natural family planning

The theory and applications of natural family planning are now well researched and validated (Chapter 6). Sympto-thermal methods in menstruating women and the lactational amenorrhoea technique in the post-partum period provide a contraceptive option for the fully-trained and highly-motivated. These approaches enable some women to avoid exogenous forms of contraception, or can be combined with use of barrier contraceptives. This approach may be facilitated by the newly released Persona™ device which identifies fertile days by assay of urinary luteinizing hormone and estrone-3-glucuronide, a metabolite of oestradiol.

Natural family planning is not 'owned' by any Complementary medical discipline as such, but it often appeals to women who espouse a 'natural' ideology, and who are therefore reluctant to take hormones. The option should also be remembered when advising women with medical contraindications to hormonal contraception.

Subfertility and early pregnancy loss

Many patients and practitioners share a suspicion that psychological stress compromises fertility. In couples struggling to conceive, any form of therapy, whether Complementary or conventional, may have an anxiolytic effect. The opposite is also true, as many anxiety-filled IVF or GIFT patients will attest. There is a need to identify the impact of Complementary therapies on fertility, the degree to which any apparent effect is related to psychological support, and whether there are other modes of action.

Stress, anxiety, and fertility

One study has demonstrated an association between physiological and endocrine markers of stress and concurrent infertility (Harrison *et al.* 1986). Since a fertility problem undoubtedly causes anxiety, this study does not prove the hypothesis that stress may cause or exacerbate subfertility. The influence of behavioural therapy on conception rates has been examined in an uncontrolled study of couples with unexplained infertility (Domar *et al.* 1990a). The study population was 54 women with a mean age of 34 years (range 25–42 years) and mean duration of infertility of 3.3 years. Following a mind–body programme held in a hospital department, 34% fell pregnant within 6 months. This compares with a conception rate of 18% in a separate longitudinal study of a comparable patient population (Domar *et al.* 1990b). A controlled study is clearly required.

There is considerable data concerning the impact of orthodox social and psychological support in a different population; those women who had reached the first or second trimester of pregnancy, but in whom the fetus was judged to be at risk of having low birth weight. Studies in a total of 8000 women have been the subject of a recent systematic analysis, showing that in high-risk pregnancies social support interventions had no effect on medical outcome (Hodnett 1995).

Acupuncture

A comparison between auricular acupuncture and hormonal treatment has been carried out in 90 women with infertility associated with oligomenorrhoea or luteal insufficiency (Gerhard and Postneek 1992). The pregnancy rate of 22/45 achieved in the acupuncture group was similar to the rate of 20/45 in the hormone-treated group. Despite matching of age, duration of infertility, Body Mass Index, previous pregnancies, menstrual cycle, and tubal patency there was an imbalance between the two groups. Women in the acupuncture group had an excess of features such as adnexitis or reduced post-coital tests usually associated with a poorer outcome. Side-effects were reported only in the hormone group. The prevalence of endometriosis was higher in the women in whom neither modality of treatment proved effective compared with successfully-treated women. The lack of an untreated control group in this study limits the conclusions that can be drawn.

Herbalism

In an uncontrolled study of 60 women with uncomplicated luteal phase insufficiency treated with traditional Chinese herbs, the pregnancy rate was 56% (Lian 1991). In a separate case report, use of the herbal medicine, *Vitex agnus castus* was associated with symptoms suggestive of mild ovarian hyperstimulation syndrome (Cahill *et al.* 1994).

Caffeine intake

Many forms of Complementary medicine counsel against instant coffee or cola beverages as part of a general principle of avoiding processed foods. Most disciplines will allow, at least in some patients, a low intake of fresh coffee or tea, depending on the individual patient's health problems. No specific claims are made regarding the impact of caffeine intake on fertility. Indeed, more interest in this question has been shown by orthodox medical investigators. There are several studies concerning the effect of caffeine consumption on fertility or fecundity (time to conception). Their results are mixed but there is some support for a recommendation that women moderate their caffeine consumption.

Two studies which took account of caffeine from all sources suggested caffeine has a dose-dependent adverse effect on fecundity. For reference, 100 mg/day caffeine is equivalent to one cup of coffee (and several varieties of tea) or one litre of cola. In the earliest study, a caffeine intake of more than 100 mg/day appeared to halve the chances of conception per cycle (Wilcox *et al.* 1988). The second study found an intake ranging between one cup of coffee per week to two cups per day had no effect on time to conceive (Joesoef *et al.* 1990). In a third study, the chances of conception per cycle were reduced by 10% with an intake of under 300 mg/day, and by 27% with an intake of over 300 mg/day. This study suggested a dose-dependent effect with the odds ratio for delay of conception for 1 year or more being 1.39 (CI 0.9–2.1) for caffeine intakes of 1–150 mg/day; 1.88 (CI 1.13–3.11) for 151–300 mg/day; and 2.24 (CI 1.06–4.73) for over 300 mg/day (Hatch and Bracken 1993). A more recent study suggested a threshold of 300 mg/day above which an adverse effect was seen (OR 1.77, CI 1.33–2.37) (Stanton and Gray 1995). This and another (Alderete *et al.* 1995) study found the effect confined to non-smokers, smoking *per se* having a significant effect on conception rate which may have been overriding. Confusingly, another study found the effect confined to smokers (Olsen 1991). Further inconsistencies in the evidence exist, including a prospective study which found moderate levels of caffeine intake (400–700 mg/day) to be associated with higher fecundability than lower levels (OR 2.1, CI 1.2–3.7), and only those with an intake of over 700 mg/day to have reduced fecundability (OR 0.6, CI 0.3–0.97) (Florack *et al.* 1994) This study found moderate smoking (1–10 cigarettes per day) to be associated with a higher level of fecundability than non-smoking, and found that whilst alcohol had no effect on a woman's fecundability, for her partner more than 10 drinks per week had a beneficial effect compared with less than five drinks per week. (OR 1.6, 1–2.4).

There is also some work concerning caffeine intake and fetal well-being.

In pregnancy, coffee has a dose-dependent inverse effect on birth-weight, but only when intake levels are high (>seven cups per day) (Nehlig and Debry 1994). Moderate intake having no effect, it would seem reasonable for pregnant mothers to limit their intake to two to three cups per day. In this context it is interesting that many pregnant women lose the inclination to drink coffee, at least during the first trimester. Post-partum, caffeine stimulates breast-milk production. However, it also enters breast-milk, although measured quantities vary in different studies.

Folic acid intake and homocysteine

A diet including regular green vegetable and fresh fruit consumption is central to many Complementary philosophies. This advice is likely to be of particular importance to women hoping for a healthy pregnancy, since maternal folic acid administration is now known to reduce the incidence of neural tube defects (NTDs) in low and high-risk pregnancies (MRC Vitamin Study Group 1991). Women planning a pregnancy are advised to consume more folate-rich foods, preferably raw, in addition to taking folic acid supplements.

The precise mechanism by which folic acid exerts its protective effect is unclear. However, it has become clear that both folic acid and vitamin B^{12} are necessary for the metabolism of homocysteine. Homocysteine levels are higher in women who have given birth to infants with NTDs than in control women with healthy offspring (Steegers *et al.* 1994). Increased levels are normalized by administration of folic acid or Vitamin B^{12}. Hyperhomocysteinaemia was also found in 21% of 102 women who had suffered at least two spontaneous early miscarriages (Wouters *et al.* 1993).

Vitamin A

Shortly before and during early pregnancy, a total intake from all sources of Vitamin A >15 000 iu/day is associated with a significant increase in birth defects (Smithells 1996). Few women can achieve an intake of 10 000 iu/day from food alone, but in order to maintain the safety margin women are advised to avoid liver products or fish-liver oils. The source of Vitamin A is also important; vegetables contain carotene which appears to be safe, whilst animal sources contain retinol, the form known to be potentially teratogenic. The current recommendation for women wishing to take vitamin supplements prior to and during pregnancy is to avoid doses of >5000 iu/day. If a multivitamin contains retinol rather than carotene, it is particularly important to adhere to this recommendation.

Fertility awareness

The well-validated concepts underlying natural family planning can also be used to improve fertility awareness, as discussed elsewhere (Chapter 6). It provides a 'natural' approach, which is valued by couples, at least in the early stages of a fertility problem.

Premenstrual syndrome

The severity of premenstrual syndrome (PMS) and ability to cope with it varies with patients' psychosocial situation. Any approach to management which includes reassurance and empathy is often successful. In 5–10% of patients, symptoms are severe enough to disrupt activities, work, or relationships, and further measures may be required. Many GPs institute a trial of hormonal suppression of ovulation, or progesterone supplementation during the luteal phase. Outcomes are variable and many women seek alternatives, usually vitamin B[6] or evening primrose oil. The evidence concerning their efficacy is mixed but sufficient for many GPs to now recommend their use, first-line in the orthodox management of PMS (Chapter 9).

Evening primrose oil (EPO)

There is good evidence that EPO relieves cyclical mastalgia (see Breast disease, above). For the relief of other PMS symptoms, 3 g/day EPO was found in four small studies to be more effective than placebo (O'Brien 1993; Lewith 1996). It appeared that EPO was more effective for irritability and depression than for other PMS symptoms. As is often the case in this field, the studies were too small to have sufficient power to prove efficacy. A deficiency of omega-6 fatty acids, of which EPO is a source, may cause abnormal sensitivity to prolactin, a putative cause of PMS (Lewith 1996).

Other dietary interventions

Other dietary interventions include supplementation with vitamins B[6], A, or E or minerals such as magnesium or calcium. A recent review of clinical studies is available (Lewith 1996). Two large placebo-controlled studies into the effect of vitamin B[6] (50–200 mg daily) found a response in 80% of recipients. In these studies the incidence of placebo-responders was also exceptionally high at 70%. Three smaller double-blind crossover studies showing greater benefit in patients receiving vitamin B[6] provide slightly more persuasive evidence. These and further studies into Vitamins A or E raise the possibility of differential effects on the various types of PMS, but none are conclusive. In one small, double-blind, placebo-controlled trial, oral magnesium supplements (360 mg/day, day 15 to onset of menstruation) were found to relieve premenstrual mood changes as well as menstrual migraine (see below) (Facchinetti et al. 1991). Vitamin B[6] supplementation at 100 mg twice daily is reported to normalize low erythrocyte magnesium levels in women with PMS (Lewith 1996). One reason why Vitamin B[6], magnesium, and calcium might be important is that they are all involved in neurotransmitter metabolism.

It has been observed that women with PMS have a significantly higher intake of refined carbohydrates than non-sufferers or patients with mild PMS (Abraham 1982; et al. 1982). Refined sugar has been reported to increase the excretion of magnesium (Seelig 1971). There is a view, unsupported by any evidence, that PMS is in some way caused by hypoglycaemia, and can be combated by the consumption of regular carbohydrates. On the other hand, that there is some evidence that diet or dieting has a measurable effect on serotonin and perhaps other neurotransmitter levels, a field ripe for further exploration (see Chapter 18).

Natural progesterone

On the presumption that PMS is often due to progesterone deficiency and relative oestrogen excess, natural progesterone derived from Mexican wild yam root (Dioscorea sp) has been administered as a transdermal cream (Progest Cream™) in the latter third of the cycle (Lee 1996). Without any supporting data, the product is claimed to be effective and free from side-effects. Members of the genus Dioscorea contains a sterol precursor, diosgenin, said to be converted *in vivo* to human progesterone. A contrast is drawn with synthetic progestogens which are chemically dissimilar to human progesterone, having been modified to promote oral absorption, delay metabolism, and to provide prolonged duration of action (and to be patentable). Requests by women to their GPs, and electronic correspondence on the Internet reflects the growth of consumer interest in natural progesterone. Progest Cream™ is in increasing use in the USA and UK, available by mail order from Ireland, or on prescription, on a named patient basis, as an unlicensed medicine from a few GPs. Independent studies are needed.

Herbal medicine

Vitex agnus castus, or Chaste tree, is a herb used to treat PMS and menstrual disorders. It increases LH and inhibits FSH production, resulting in a lower oestrogen to progesterone ratio. An uncontrolled survey of *Vitex*-use in 1542 women with PMS reported complete relief of symptoms in over 90% of cases (Lewith 1996). Side-effects were noted in 1–2% of recipients.

Manipulative medicine

Osteopaths and chiropractors claim some success in treating PMS and menstrual disorders by means of spinal manipulation. At present, there are no clinical trials supporting these claims.

Reflexology

In a randomized controlled study of premenstrual symptoms treated with ear, hand, and foot reflexology, 35 women with PMS were assigned to weekly reflexology lasting 30 minutes for 8 weeks, or placebo reflexology (Oleson and Flocco 1993). Somatic and psychological indicators of PMS, recorded daily by patients for 2 months prior to, during, and after the treatment showed a significant decrease in the reflexology group.

Relaxation and imagery

A 5-month study of 46 women examined the effect on physical, emotional, and social indicators of three interventions (Goodale *et al.* 1990). The women were randomly assigned to a group learning to elicit the relaxation response, a reading group, or a group simply charting their symptoms. Improvements were noted in all three groups with the greatest effect seen in the relaxation group. Regular elicitation of the relaxation response seems to be an effective treatment for physical and psychological symptoms, and was most effective for women with severe symptoms in whom a 58% improvement was noted. Another 6-month study in 30 women with regular menstrual cycles employed a 3-month run-in period, and then 3 months of listening to an audio tape with progressive muscle relaxation exercise, followed by guided imagery and a suggestive message focusing on lengthening the menstrual cycle and delaying the onset of menstrual bleeding (Groer and Ohnesorge 1993). Only 15 women completed the study, but in these PMS symptoms were reduced and cycle length was significantly increased.

Homeopathy

Classical homeopathy is often used for the many psychological and physical symptom complexes attributed to PMS, but no studies were found in our on-line literature search.

Menstrual problems

Dysmenorrhoea

Acupuncture

Acupuncture appears effective for menstrual cramps. In a 1 year, randomized, controlled study of 43 women, subjects received either real acupuncture (at fixed, classical acupuncture points with no individual variation), sham acupuncture, extra consultations, or no intervention (Helms 1987). Ten of 11 in the true acupuncture group improved (defined by halving of the monthly pain score). Four of 11 in the sham acupuncture group improved, as did two of 11 in the group receiving extra consultations, and one out of the 10 who received no intervention. During the 9 months after treatment, there was a 41% drop in analgesic usage for those receiving true acupuncture, whilst in the other groups analgesic usage increased or stayed the same.

Manipulative medicine

A small dysmenorrhoea trial compared chiropractic manipulation in eight women with three controls (Thomason *et al.* 1979). Seven of the eight women treated twice-weekly with manipulation experienced decreased pain and disability, compared with none of the controls. A trial conducted in 40 women with dysmenorrhoea compared chiropractic with intensive sham manipulation applied to 'incorrect' sites. Women in the two groups reported equal reductions in perceived menstrual stress, and equivalent reductions in plasma levels of prostaglandin F2a were observed (Kokjohn *et al.* 1992). This study suggests improvement with manual techniques but does not enable comparison with placebo.

Migraines related to the menstrual cycle

Population studies find the prevalence of migraines to be 17% in women, compared with 6% in men, with a concentration of attacks between menarche and the menopause, suggesting a hormonal influence (MacGregor 1996a). This section is concerned not with non-migrainous headaches which occur as part of PMS, or migraine caused or exacerbated by the oral contraceptive pill, but with two other distinct conditions: menstrual migraine and menstrually-related migraine (MacGregor 1996a).

Menstrual migraine

A small proportion of female migraine sufferers have true menstrual migraine attacks, occurring regularly in the 2 days before and 3 days after the onset of menses, and at no other time (MacGregor 1996b). A pilot study carried out in migraine clinic attendees, using these strict criteria, found a prevalence of menstrual migraine of 7.2% (MacGregor *et al*. 1990c). This condition has been linked with declining oestrogen levels and managed with some success by percutaneous or transdermal oestradiol supplementation, although such products are not yet licensed for this indication (MacGregor 1996 *a* and *b*). Most women with menstrual migraine are 35–45 years of age (MacGregor 1996a) and therefore subject to the slow physiological decline in oestrogen levels occurring at this time. Given the proven oestrogenic action of soy and some other vegetable products (see above), one wonders whether diet has a role to play here. Another mechanism implicated in menstrual migraine is the secretion of prostaglandins from the myometrium into the systemic circulation during the luteal phase, with maximum entry during the first 48 hours of menstruation. There are double-blind, placebo-controlled studies showing that prostaglandin inhibitors effectively prevent menstrual migraine in some women and may be particularly useful if patients also experience dysmenorrhoea (MacGregor 1996a). This finding suggests that dietary manipulations able to influence prostaglandins might possibly help, but there seems to be little investigation in this area.

Magnesium supplements

Women with menstrual migraine may be helped by oral magnesium supplements. A double-blind, placebo-controlled study of 20 women found a significant reduction of days with headaches (as well as other premenstrual complaints) in women taking magnesium at a dose of 360 mg/day; started on day 15 and continued until the next menses. The effect lasted for some months beyond the time of supplementation. Intracellular magnesium levels were significantly lower in these migraine sufferers than in controls (Facchinetti *et al*. 1991). These findings, together with other studies concerning intra and extracellular magnesium levels in migraine patients, suggest that a lower migraine threshold may be related to magnesium deficiency.

Menstrually-related migraine

Thirty-five per cent of migraine clinic attendees have menstrually-related migraine (also known as premenstrual migraine), which is thus more common than menstrual migraine (MacGregor *et al.* 1990c). The attack rate is increased in the luteal phase, with relief at the onset of menstruation (MacGregor 1996a). Although attacks can occur throughout the cycle, and may be triggered by well-known factors such as chocolate, soft cheeses, etc., the threshold for triggering seems to be lower in the luteal phase.

Dietary restrictions

Approximately 25% of migraine sufferers believe that their attacks can be provoked by foodstuffs. Dietary changes can reduce the frequency of all types of migraine other than true menstrual migraine. An uncontrolled trial of 60 migraine patients given an elimination diet reported a dramatic improvement in symptoms: 85% became headache-free when 13 common foods were avoided (Grant 1979). The foodstuffs most commonly responsible were wheat, oranges, eggs, tea, coffee, chocolate, milk, beef, corn, cane sugar, yeast, mushrooms and peas. Chocolate, caffeine, red wine, and mature cheese are well-known triggers, but not other foods implicated in this study.

Biofeedback

There are extensive data on the effectiveness of biofeedback for most types of migraine (Blanchard and Andrasik 1987). Using biofeedback, the patient learns how to increase hand temperature by dilating blood vessels in the hands, thus affecting blood flow to the head which reduces the pain.

Herbal medicine

There are clinical trials supporting the use of feverfew (*Tanacetum parthenium*) for migraine. In a randomized study of 17 patients whose normal practice was to eat feverfew leaves daily to prevent migraine, subjects randomized to placebo had a significant increase in the frequency and severity of migraines, while those in the feverfew group experienced no change (Johnson, 1985). This small study reveals only the effect of withdrawing feverfew from regular users.

In a larger, crossover trial, 76 migraine patients were given either one capsule of dried feverfew (equivalent to two medium-sized leaves) or placebo daily for 4 months, before crossover for a further 4 months (Murphy *et al.* 1988). In the 59 patients completing the trial, migraine attacks diminished during the months on feverfew. Patients with common migraine showed a 24% reduction in attack rate, and patients with classical migraine a 32% reduction. The severity of remaining attacks was reduced although the duration of individual attacks remained the same.

Some migraine sufferers grow feverfew and eat a few leaves every day. In a small percentage of users, feverfew may cause mouth ulcers, swelling of the mouth, lips, or tongue, and loss of taste (Awang 1989). The herb is available in capsule form which may reduce, but does not eliminate, these local adverse effects. Of note, in the crossover trial described above, more oral symptoms were reported by patients whilst taking placebo than whilst taking feverfew (Murphy *et al.* 1988).

Homeopathy

Homeopathy may also help migraine. In a double-blind, placebo-controlled study of 60 migraine sufferers, individualized homeopathic prescriptions were given once every 2 weeks for 8 weeks (Brigo and Sepelloni 1991). In the placebo group, the attack rate dropped from 9.9 to 7.9 attacks per month after 2 months (the effect remained at follow-up 2 months after the study ended). In the treated group, the attack rate dropped from 10 to 3 per month by the end of the study, and at 2-month follow-up the rate was 1.8 per month. The intensity of attacks also decreased significantly in the treated group.

Chiropractic

A randomized, controlled trial of 83 migraine sufferers, compared a group receiving chiropractic manipulation with a group receiving cervical manipulation by a conventional practitioner, and a group taught head and shoulder exercises. All groups improved in the frequency, duration, or induced-disability of migraine attacks. Although the severity of migraine was reduced more (by 40%) in those receiving chiropractic, compared with a 34% reduction in the exercise group, the difference was not statistically significant (Parker *et al.* 1978).

Menopause

Menopausal symptoms

Influence of diet

There are large international variations in the incidence of menopausal symptoms. Lowest rates occur in Asian countries. The incidence of hot flushes, for instance, is 70–80% in Europe, 57% in Malaysia, 18% in China, and 14% in Singapore (Knight and Eden 1996). There is a similar international variation in the incidence of osteoporosis and hip fractures, the lowest being in Asian women. Race, body habitus, culture, lifestyle, and diet may all have a contributory influence. As with breast cancer, the low incidence of menopausal symptoms in Asian countries correlates with high dietary consumption of soy products. Oestrogenization of vaginal epithelium in response to 6-week dietary supplementation with soy flour and linseed has been demonstrated in a pilot study of 25 post-menopausal women (Wilcox *et al.* 1990). The post-menopausal increase in cystitis and vaginal infection has been attributed to the increase in vaginal pH and consequent colonization with pathogenic bacteria (Cardozo 1996). Oral oestrogen lowers vaginal pH and topical oestriol reduces the incidence of urinary tract infections. Dietary phytoestrogens might therefore reduce the incidence of cystitis and vaginitis in post-menopausal women.

Natural progesterone cream

Natural progesterone cream applied transdermally is claimed by its chief proponent, John Lee, MD, to increase osteoblast activity and cause a measurable increase in bone mineral density as assessed by dual photon densitometry (Lee

1996). The claim is said to be supported by a study which has been multiply published, but in inadequate detail. The study was an unselected case series of 100 post-menopausal women, aged 38–83 years. Little objective evidence of osteoporosis is presented beyond the statement that 'the majority had already experienced height loss, some as much as five inches'. Bone densitometry in 63 of the women was reported to show an average increase in density of 15.4% over a 3-year period. In addition to treatment with natural progesterone cream, an unspecified number of women were taking oestrogen. Women were also advised to stop smoking, exercise three times weekly for 30 minutes, and take supplements of calcium, vitamins C and D, and beta carotene, all potential confounders (Fugh-Berman and Kronenberg 1996).

Those criticisms apart, there is some support for Lee's claims that natural progesterone is important in the maintenance of bone density. It is also apparent that not all synthetic progestogens share this property. There are indeed progesterone receptors on bone and, *in vitro* at least, natural progesterone stimulates osteoblasts. In a study of 66 pre-menopausal women, those with short luteal phases had decreased spinal bone density and loss of up to 2–4% of bone a year (Prior, *et al.* 1990). Amenorrhoeic athletes given 10 mg medroxyprogesterone acetate (Provera) for 10 days a month show significant increases in trabecular bone (Prior *et al.* 1994). Lactation reduces bone density temporarily, and progestogen-only contraception seems to reduce post-partum bone loss (Caird *et al.* 1994).

Oral natural progesterone capsules or skin cream (Progest Cream™) are also used, particularly in the US, for treatment of hot flushes and for vaginal dryness without, as yet, formal evidence of effectiveness. It remains to be established whether oral and topical natural progesterone supplements have a beneficial effect on menopausal symptoms and bone density, their side-effect profile, and if benefits are confirmed, the effective dose of oral progesterone and transdermal preparations.

Manipulative medicine

One placebo-controlled trial suggested a form of osteopathy was helpful for menopausal symptoms (Lewith 1996).

Biofeedback

Women have been successfully trained to control their hot flushes using the techniques of biofeedback (Freedman and Woodward 1992). The impact on hot flushes is confirmed by skin conductance measurements. This control may be of value in women unwilling or unable to receive HRT, or who are receiving HRT but nonetheless experience occasional hot flushes.

Cardiovascular and cerebrovascular disease

Diet and dietary supplements

Several observational studies suggest that vegetarianism is associated with an average reduction in mortality of 30%, but a recent report found the daily consumption of fresh fruit and raw salad rather than vegetarianism *per se* to be protective (Key *et al.* 1996). In this 25 year cohort study of 10 671 health conscious men and women, daily fresh fruit and raw salad consumption was associated with a 21–32% reduction in overall mortality, cardiovascular and cerebrovascular disease compared with less frequent consumption. The study controlled for smoking but not for physical exercise or socio-economic status. However, the method of subject recruitment may have minimized variation in those two potential confounders.

The lipid-lowering and potential cardioprotective properties of soy are being explored (Knight and Eden 1996). A meta-analysis of 38 controlled trials found that consumption of soy protein significantly reduced total cholesterol, low density lipoprotein, and triglycerides without decreasing high-density lipoprotein (Anderson *et al.* 1995). Substitution of soy protein for meat lowered cholesterol even when total fat and calorie intake remain the same. A crossover study in rhesus monkeys suggests that the beneficial constituents in soy protein are the alcohol-extractable components including the isoflavonic phytoestrogens (Anthony *et al.* 1996). Inclusion of phytoestrogen-intact soy protein in an atherogenic diet had a favourable effect on plasma lipid and lipoprotein concentrations unlike soy subjected to removal of alcohol-extractable components. The phytoestrogens had no measurable adverse effects on the reproductive systems of either males or females.

Other studies have suggested a possible cardioprotective role for specific nutrients such as vitamin C, beta-carotene, and vitamin E. This work is relevant to women who choose to take supplements rather than, or in addition to, dietary change. One of the largest effects was observed in the Nurse's Health Trial, a prospective study involving 87 245 women (Stampfer *et al.* 1993) Women taking specific vitamin E supplements containing 100 iu or more for at least two years had a 41% reduction in ischaemic heart disease. Although 100 iu is a modest amount for supplementation, it is difficult to obtain this quantity in food. In other cases, supplements may lack the benefits of the original food source. For instance, a recent randomized clinical trial found the consumption of 900 mg of a single brand of 'odour-controlled' dried garlic powder tablets to have no lipid-lowering effect in patients with hyperlipidaemia. In contrast, meta-analyses of studies employing a range of garlic preparations including garlic tablets, garlic oil and raw garlic have concluded the opposite. Since there is a marked variation in anti-platelet activity between whole garlic and commercial garlic extracts, the manufacturing process may affect other biological properties, perhaps accounting for some of the conflicting reports (Myers and Smith 1996). Although garlic also has confirmed hypotensive, fibrinolytic, and anti-oxidant properties, no study to date has had sufficient power to examine effects on cardiovascular disease endpoints.

Alzheimer's disease

An observational study of 1124 elderly women suggests post-menopausal oestrogen use delays the onset and decreases the risk of Alzheimer's disease (AD) (Tang *et al.* 1996). If the suggestion is borne out by randomized controlled studies then the influence of dietary phytoestrogens will be of interest. In this context, cross-cultural comparisons of AD prevalence may be illuminating if based on accurate diagnostic criteria.

Vaginal discharge and sexually-transmitted diseases

AIDS

Available surveys suggest that usage of Complementary medicine is even higher amongst AIDS patients than the general population. Of 287 patients questioned (67 women), 31% used Complementary therapies (Bates *et al.* 1996). Other, smaller studies suggest higher usage. Nowhere is health consumerism better illustrated than in AIDS. The AIDS community has been highly vocal in demanding not just more from the research effort, but more information about Alternative treatments. In the US, Buyers' Clubs have been set up to help PWAs (persons with AIDS) obtain treatments which may be banned or difficult to obtain, such as marijuana for appetite stimulation and control of nausea. They have swapped information on nutritional manipulation and mega-vitamin and mineral supplementation to combat wasting syndrome. The reaction of the medical profession to these recommendations is often negative, with emphasis placed on the potential ill-effects of dietary supplements when taken in excess or in combination with some prescribed drugs. Within the AIDS community information is available concerning experimentation with herbs, natural hormones, and fungi believed to act as immune enhancers. There is also interest in a psychotropic drug called ibogaine, derived from the West African iboga plant and credited with the property of interrupting narcotic addiction when administered only once or twice a year, in contrast with the need for daily methadone administration. Massage, reflexology, and meditation are considered generally beneficial. AIDS activists claim, with some justification, that many of the recent improvements in life span and quality of life have been due more to community efforts than to biomedical research, facilitated by the rapid communication and feedback made possible by the Internet. One such source of information exchange used extensively is the Critical Path AIDS Project (http:www.critpath.org/critpath.htm).

Candidiasis

This condition is sometimes diagnosed by patients attending Complementary practitioners and is ascribed to diets high in carbohydrates, refined sugar, or yeast. It does not necessarily correspond to the vaginal, oral, or visceral forms of *Candida* infection recognized by conventional medical science. No trials of the effect of dietary intervention on *Candida* infection have been conducted. Only two strands of evidence support a dietary approach; the first, the known predisposition of diabetics to *Candida* infection; the second, preliminary evidence that a proportion of women with recurrent, severe mucocutaneous *Candida* infection have undiagnosed coeliac disease, and following serological identification (using endomysial antibody), benefit from elimination of wheat and other gluten sources from the diet (Dr G. Bird, personal communication).

Urinary tract infection (UDT)

Cranberry juice

Women suffering recurrent UTIs are in particular need of effective preventive measures and many women seek an alternative to antibiotics. High-risk groups include diaphragm-users, sexually active and elderly women. Cranberry juice is a folk remedy once widely used for both symptomatic relief and prevention. The first randomized, double-blind, placebo-controlled trial was carried out in 153 elderly women with a mean age of 78 years (Avorn et al. 1994). In a 6-month study, women were randomized to either 300 ml/day of a commercially-available cranberry juice cocktail, or a placebo juice matched for taste, appearance, and vitamin C content. Those drinking cranberry juice showed a statistically significant halving of the number of urine specimens containing bacteriuria ($\geq 10^5$ cfu/ml) with pyuria. There was also a modest reduction in the frequency with which symptomatic UTI was diagnosed and antibiotics prescribed. Cranberry juice was more effective in treating than preventing bacteriuria and pyuria.

Possible mechanisms of action include urinary acidification, but consistent acidification may require consumption of up to 2000 ml/day. One study demonstrating the acidifying effect of cranberry juice on urine also showed that anticipated problems with increased number of bowel movements, weight gain, and increased voiding frequency, did not occur (Kinney and Blount 1979). Recent interest has shifted to inhibition of bacterial adherence to bladder wall or gut mucosa with, in the latter case, a postulated reduction in gut bacterial load (Avorn et al. 1994). Two compounds in cranberry juice inhibit adherence (Zafriri et al. 1989): fructose, present in most fruit juices; and a non-dialyzable polymeric compound isolated from cranberry and blueberry juice (both belonging to Vaccinia genus) but not from orange, grapefruit, pineapple, guava, or mango juice (Ofek et al. 1991). When a total of 77 clinical isolates of Escherichia coli were tested, cranberry juice inhibited adherence to uroepithelial cells by at least 75% in over 60% of clinical isolates (Sobota 1984). Fifteen of 22 subjects showed significant anti-adherence activity in the urine 1–3 hours after drinking 15 oz (430 ml) of cranberry cocktail. Together, these studies imply the need for intake of perhaps six cups of juice a day (one cup is 400–600 ml). Cranberry juice tablets are now commercially available but have not yet been evaluated in clinical trials.

There are many reports of herbal medicines used for the treatment of UTI, and in some cases active ingredients with potent anti-microbial properties have been isolated. The paucity of data concerning safety constrains further discussion in this general overview.

Live yoghurt

In post-menopausal women, the rise in vaginal pH promotes an alteration in the normal vaginal flora with decreased lactobacilli and increased colonization with pathogenic faecal flora. This contributes to the increase in incidence of urinary tract infections, especially in the sexually active (Cardozo 1996). Whether oral lactobacilli supplements or topical treatment with live yoghurt have any beneficial effect in this group of women has not been formally investigated.

Urinary incontinence

Pelvic floor exercises and biofeedback

For stress incontinence, pelvic floor exercises are now generally used as first-line treatment before surgery is considered, with significant improvements reported in 42–52% of patients (Klarskov *et al.* 1986; Elia and Bergman 1993) (Chapter 16). In a uncontrolled study of 48 women, the combination of pelvic floor exercises with biofeedback was found to improve 62% of patients (McIntosh *et al.* 1993). Several small studies find biofeedback alone to be effective in the treatment of stress incontinence, with reported reductions in urinary loss of 80–90%. In a controlled study of 135 women, urinary losses were reduced by 54% in the pelvic floor exercise group and by 61% in the biofeedback group, whilst increased by 9% in the control group (Burns *et al.* 1993). Complete cure was reported by 16% in the pelvic exercise group, 23% in the biofeedback group, and 3% in the control group.

Smoking cessation

Acupuncture

Auricular acupuncture is one of the most widely-used techniques for smoking cessation, and available studies suggest it is as effective as nicotine supplements or behaviour therapy. Cessation rates of 20–40% are reported for all these modalities. However, acupuncture, like other methods, suffers from a gradual decrease of therapeutic effect over time and a high relapse rate. Trials lacking follow-up are therefore of limited clinical significance. One-year success rates of only 8–10% have been reported for all three modalities in a comparative study of acupuncture, nicotine supplements, and placebo (Clavel-Chapelon *et al.* 1992). Hypnosis is commonly used to aid smoking cessation but there is no evidence that it is superior to other approaches.

Relaxation imagery

The high relapse rates and the fact that smokers identify stress as a major contributory factor highlight the need for smokers to develop additional long-term coping strategies and substitute behaviours. A randomized, controlled trial carried out in 76 subjects who had completed a local smoking cessation programme compared the effect of a further 3 months of instruction in relaxation imagery in the experimental group with regular meetings in the control group. The practice of relaxation imagery was associated with a reduction in perceived stress and prolongation of smoking abstinence (Wynd 1992).

Emotional problems

Anxiety

The anxiolytic effects of massage, aromatherapy, reflexology, meditation, relaxation, and imagery are widely assumed, and supporting evidence can be found (Fulder 1996). Virtually every other Complementary approach has also been used in this context. Further research in the area of massage and aromatherapy is likely to be spearheaded by midwives and the nursing profession who have already studied its applications in childbirth, in cancer patients, and in the intensive care unit (Fulder 1996).

Depression

Since up to 83% of patients report an increase in general well-being following consultation with a Complementary therapist (Francis 1995), an improvement in mild depression might be anticipated, but awaits confirmation. In the case of herbalism there is one example of proven efficacy. A recent systematic review found extracts of St John's wort (*Hypericum perforatum*) to be more effective than placebo for treating mild to moderate depressive disorders (Linde *et al.* 1996). No equivalent studies are available for severe depression. Comparison of *Hypericum* alone with low doses of amitriptyline, imipramine, or maprotiline found no statistical difference in efficacy, and a lower incidence of side-effects with *Hypericum*. Extensive use of the herb in Germany has not resulted in published reports of toxicity. Like synthetic antidepressants, Hypericum extracts need 2–4 weeks to take effect.

Conclusion

To quote a view expressed in *Stedman's medical dictionary*: 'the real value of homeopathy was to demonstrate the healing powers of nature, and the therapeutic virtue of placebos'. Arguably all medicine, Complementary or conventional, should, whenever possible, harness both these forces. Studies which suggest an effect exceeding that of placebo are appearing in many fields of Complementary medicine, and future advances need to incorporate the best from all approaches to health and disease.

References and further reading

Abraham, G. (1982). Nutritional factors in the aetiology of the premenstrual syndrome. *Journal of Reproductive Medicine*, **28**, 446–64.

Adlercreutz, H., Fotsis, T., *et al.* (1986). Determination of urinary lignans and phytoestrogen metabolites, potential antiestrogens and anticarcinogens in urine of women on various habitual diets. *J Steroid Biochem*, **25**(5B): 791–7.

Adlercreutz, H., Hockerstedt, K., *et al.* (1987). Effect of dietary components, including lignans and phytoestrogens, on enterohepatic circulation and liver metabolism of estrogens and on sex hormone binding globulin (SHBG). *J Steroid Biochem*, **27**(4–6), 1135–44.

Adlercreutz, H., Honjo, H., *et al.* (1991). Urinary excretion of lignans and isoflavonoid phytoestrogens in Japanese men and women consuming a traditional Japanese diet. *American Journal of Clinical Nutrition*, **54**(6), 1093–100.

Alderete, E., Eskenazi, B., *et al.* (1995). Effect of cigarette smoking and coffee drinking on time to conception. *Epidemiology*, **6**(4), 403–8.

Anderson, J., Eskenazi, B., *et al.* (1995). Meta-analysis of the effect of soy protein intake on serum lipids. *New England Journal of Medicine*, **333**, 276–82.

Anthony, M. S., Clarkson, T. B., *et al.* (1996). Soybean isoflavones improve cardio-vascular risk factors without affecting the reproductive system of peripubertal rhesus monkeys. *Journal of Nutrition*, **126**(1), 43–50.

Avorn, J., Monane, M. *et al.* (1994). Reduction of bacteruria and pyuria after ingestion of cranberry juice. *Journal of the American Medical Association*, **271**(10), 751–4.

Awang, D. (1989). Herbal medicine: feverfew. *Canadian Pharm Journal*, **122**, 266–70.

Bagenal, F.S., Easton, D. F., *et al.* (1990). Survival of patients with breast cancer attending Bristol Cancer Help Centre. [See comments.] *Lancet*, **336**(8715): 606–10.

Bates, B., Kissinger, P., *et al.* (1996). Complementary therapy use amongst HIV infected patients. *AIDS Patient Care and STDs*, February, 32–36.

Bernstein, L., Henderson, B., *et al.* (1994). Physical exercise and reduced risk of breast cancer in young women. *Journal of the National Cancer Institute*, **86**(18), 1403–8.

Blanchard, E. and Andrasik, F. (ed.). (1987). Biofeedback treatment of patients with vascular headache. In *Biofeedback: studies in clinical efficacy*. Plenum, New York.

Bodeker, G. (1994). *Traditional health knowledge and public policy*. UNESCO.

Bridge, L. R., Benson, P., *et al.* (1988). Relaxation and imagery in the treatment of breast cancer. *British Medical Journal*, **297**(6657), 1169–72.

Brigo, B. and Sepelloni, G. (1991). Homeopathic treatment of migraines: a randomised, double-blind, controlled study of sixty cases. *Berlin Journal on Research in Homeopathy*, **1**(2): 98–105.

Burns, P., Pranikof, K., *et al.* (1993). A comparison of the effectiveness of biofeedback and pelvic muscle exercise treatment of stress incontinence in older community-dwelling women. *Journal of Gerontology*, **48**(4), M167–M174.

Cahill, D. J., Fox, R., *et al.* (1994). Multiple follicular development associated with herbal medicine. *Human Reproduction*, **9**(8), 1469–70.

Caird, L., Reid-Thomas, V., *et al.* (1994). Oral progestogen-only contraception may protect against loss of bone mass in breast-feeding women. *Clin Endo*, **41**, 739–45.

Cardozo, L. (1996). Postmenopausal cystitis. *British Medical Journal*, **313**, 129.

Chen, C., David, A., *et al.* (1995). Adverse life-events and breast cancer: case control study. *British Medical Journal*, **311,** 1527–30.

Clavel-Chapelon, F., Paoletti, C., *et al.* (1992). A randomised 2× 2 factorial design to evaluate different smoking cessation methods. *Rev Epidemiol Sante Publique*, **40**(3), 187–90.

Committee on Safety of Medicines/Medicines Control Agency. *Current problems in pharmaco-vigilance*, 22: 10.

De Smet, P. (1995). Should herbal medicine-like products be licensed as medicines? *British Medical Journal*, **310,** 1023–4.

Dickinson, D. (1996). The growth of Complementary therapy. A consumer-led boom. In *Complementary medicine: an objective appraisal* (ed. E. Ernst Butterworth). Heinemann, Oxford.

Domar, A., Seibel, M., *et al.* (1990b). Letter to the editor. *Fertility and Sterility*, **54,**(6), 1183–4.

Domar, A. D., Siebel, M., *et al.* (1990a). The mind/body program for infertility: a new behavioral treatment approach for women with infertility [see comments]. *Fertility and Sterility*, **53**(2), 246–9.

Eisenberg, D. (1993). Unconventional medicine in the United States: prevalence, costs and patterns of use. *New England Journal of Medicine*, **328**(4), 246–83.

Elia, G. and Bergman, A. (1993). Pelvic muscle exercises: when do they work? *Obstetrics and Gynaecology*, **81**(2), 283–6.

Ellis, J., Mulligan, I. *et al.* (1995). In-patient general medicine is evidence based. *Lancet*, **346,** 407–10.

Facchinetti, F., Scanes, G., *et al.* (1991). Magnesium prophylaxis of menstrual migraine: effects on intracellular magnesium. *Headache*, **31**(5), 298–301.

Florack, E., Zielhuis, G., *et al.* (1994). Cigarette smoking, alcohol consumption, and caffeine intake and fecundability. *Prev Med*, **23**(2), 175–80.

Francis, J. (1995). *Report on Consumers' Association members' usage of and satisfaction with Alternative Medicine Practitioners.*

Freedman, R. R. and Woodward, S. (1992). Behavioral treatment of menopausal hot flushes: evaluation by ambulatory monitoring. *American Journal of Obstetrics and Gynecology*, **167**(2), 436–9.

Fugh-Berman, A. and Kronenberg, F. (1996). Natural hormones. In *Herbalism and Medicine*, College of Physicians and Surgeons, Columbia University.

Fulder, S. (1996). *The handbook of Complementary medicine.* Oxford University Press, Oxford.

Fulder, S. and Munro, R. (1985). Complementary medicine in the United Kingdom: patients, practitioners and consultations. *Lancet*, **2,** 542–5.

Furnham, A. and Vincent, C. (1995). The health beliefs and behaviours of three groups of Complementary medicine and a general practice group of patients. *Journal of Alternative and Complementary Medicine*, **1**(4), 347–59.

Gately, C., Miers, M., *et al.* (1992). Drug treatments for mastalgia: 17 years of experience in the Cardiff mastalgia clinic. *Journal of the Royal Society of Medicine*, **85**, 12–15.

Gerhard, I. and Postneek, F. (1992). Auricular acupuncture in the treatment of female infertility. *Gynecology and Endocrinology*, **6**(3), 171–81.

Gill, P., Dowell, A., *et al.* (1996). Evidence-based general practice: a retrospective study of interventions in one training practice. *British Medical Journal*, **312**, 819–21.

GMC (1995). Delegating care to non-medical staff and students. *Duties of a doctor. Guidance from the General Medical Council.* GMC, London.

Goei, G., *et al.* (1982). Dietary patterns of patients with premenstrual tension. *Journal of Applied Nutrition*, **34**(1), 4–11.

Goodale, I. L., Domar, A. D. *et al.* (1990). Alleviation of premenstrual syndrome symptoms with the relaxation response. *Obstetrics and Gynecology*, **75**(4), 649–55.

Grant, E. C. (1979). Food allergies and migraine. *Lancet*, **1**(8123), 966–9, Correction in (8126), 1154.

Groer, M. and Ohnesorge, C. (1993). Menstrual-cycle lengthening and reduction in premenstrual distress through guided imagery. *Journal of Holistic Nursing*, **11**(3), 286–94.

Gruber, B. L., Hersh, S. P., *et al.* (1993). Immunological responses of breast cancer patients to behavioral interventions. *Biofeedback Self Regul*, **18**(1), 1–22.

Harrison, R. F., O'Moore, R. R. *et al.* (1986). Stress and fertility: some modalities of investigation and treatment in couples with unexplained infertility in Dublin. *International Journal of Fertility*, **31**(2), 153–9.

Hatch, E. and Bracken, M. (1993). Association of delayed conception with caffeine consumption. *American Journal of Epidemiology*, **138**(12), 1082–92.

Helms, J. M. (1987). Acupuncture for the management of primary dysmenorrhea. *Obstetrics and Gynecology*, **69**(1), 51–6.

Hodnett, E. (1995). *Support from care-givers during at-risk pregnancy.* Pregnancy and Childbirth Module (1995, issue 2) Cochrane Database of Systematic Reviews. The Cochrane Collaboration.

Horn, R. P. (1995). Phyto-oestrogens, body composition, and breast cancer. *Cancer Causes Control*, **6**(6), 567–73.

Hunter, D., Manson, J. *et al.* (1993). A prospective study of the intake of vitamins C, E and A and the risk of breast cancer. *New England Journal of Medicine*, **329**, 234–40.

Hutchins, A. M., Lampe, J. W., *et al.* (1995b). Vegetables, fruits, and legumes: effect on urinary isoflavonoid phytoestrogen and lignan excretion. *J Am Diet Asso*, **95**(7), 769–74.

Hutchins, A. M., Slavin, J. L. *et al.* (1995a). Urinary isoflavonoid phytoestrogen and lignan excretion after consumption of fermented and unfermented soy products. *J Am Diet Assoc* **95**(5): 545–51.

Joesoef, M. R., Beral, V. *et al.* (1990). Are caffeinated beverages risk factors for delayed conception? [See comments.] *Lancet*, **335** (8682), 136–7.

Johnson, E., Kadam, N. *et al.* (1985). Efficacy of feverfew as prophylactic treatment of migraine. *British Medical Journal*, **291**, 569–573.

Key, T., Thorogood, M. *et al.* (1996). Dietary habits and mortality in 11 000 vegetarians and health conscious people: results of 17 year follow up. *British Medical Journal*, **313**, 775–9.

Kinney, A. B. and Blount, M. (1979). Effect of cranberry juice on urinary pH. *Nurs Res*, **28**(5), 287–90.

Klarskov, P., Belving, D. *et al.* (1986). Pelvic floor exercises versus surgery for female stress incontinence. *Urologia Internationalis*, **41**, 129–32.

Knight, D. and Eden J. (1996). A review of the clinical effects of phytoestrogens. *Obstetrics and Gynaecology*, **87**, 897–904.

Kokjohn, K., Schmid, D. *et al.* (1992). The effect of spinal manipulation on pain and prostaglandin levels in women with primary dysmenorrhoea. *Journal of Manipulative and Physiological Therapeutics*, **15**, 279–85.

Kolonel, L. (1988). Variability in diet and its relation to risk in ethnic and migrant groups. *Basic Life Sciences*, **43**, 129–35.

Kushi, M. (1978). *Natural healing through macrobiotics.* Japan Publications Inc., Tokyo.

La Vecchia, C., Franceschi, S. *et al.* (1984). Dietary vitamin A and the risk of invasive cervical cancer. *International Journal of Cancer*, **34**, 319–22.

Lee, H., Gourley, L., *et al.* (1991). Dietary effects on breast cancer in Singapore. *Lancet*, **337**, 1197–200.

Lee, J. (1996). *Natural progesterone. The multiple roles of a remarkable hormone.* Jon Carpenter, Chipping Norton.

Lewith, G. (1996). Premenstrual syndrome and the menopause. In *Complementary medicine. An integrated approach.* (eds. G. Lewith, J. Kenyon, P. Lewis.) Oxford University Press, Oxford.

Lian, F. (1991). TCM treatment of luteal phase defect-an analysis of 60 cases. *Journal of Traditional Chinese Medicine*, **11**(2), 115–20.

Linde, K., Ramirez, G. *et al.* (1996). St John's wort for depression – an overview and meta-analysis of randomised clinical trials. *British Medical Journal*, **313**, 253–8.

MacGregor, E. (1996b). 'Menstrual' migraine: towards a definition. *Cephalalgia*, **16**, 11–21.

MacGregor, E. (1996a). Menstruation, sex hormones and migraine. *Clinics of North America*, WB Saunders.

MacGregor, E., Chia, H., *et al.* (1990c). Migraine and menstruation: a pilot study. *Cephalalgia,* **10,** 305–10.

MacLennan, A., Wilson, D., *et al.* (1996). Prevalence and cost of Alternative medicine in Australia. *Lancet,* **347,** 569–72.

McIntosh, L., Frahm, J., *et al.* (1993). Pelvic floor rehabilitation in the treatment of incontinence. *Journal Of Reproductive Medicine,* **38**(9): 662–5.

Mintel (1995). Sales of Alternative medicine increase. *British Medical Journal,* **310,** 1624.

MRC Vitamin Study Group (1991). Prevention of neural tube defects: results of the Medical Research Council Study Group. *Lancet,* **238,** 131–7.

Murphy, J., Heptinsall, S., *et al.* (1988). Randomised, double-blind, controlled trial of feverfew in migraine prevention. *Lancet,* **ii,** 189–92.

Murray, J. and Sheperd, S. (1993). Alternative or additional medicine? An exploratory study in general practice. *Social Sciences and Medicine,* **37**(8), 983–8.

Myers, S. and Smith, A. (1997). Cardioprotection and garlic. *Lancet,* **349,** 131–2.

Nehlig, A. and Debry, G. (1994). Effects of coffee and caffeine on fertility, reproduction, lactation, and development. Review of human and animal data. *Journal of Gynecol Obstet Biol Reprod Paris,* **23**(3), 241–56.

O'Brien, P. (1993). Helping women with premenstrual syndrome. *British Medical Journal,* **307,** 1471–5.

Ofek, I., J. Goldhar, *et al.* (1991). Anti-*Escherichia* adhesin activity of cranberry and blueberry juices. *New England Journal of Medicine,* **324,** 1599.

Oleson, T. and Flocco, W. (1993). Randomized controlled study of premenstrual symptoms treated with ear, hand, and foot reflexology. *Obstetrics and Gynecology,* **82**(6), 906–11.

Olsen, J. (1991). Cigarette smoking, tea and coffee drinking, and sebfecundity. *American Journal of Epidemiology,* **133**(7), 734–9.

Parker, G. B., Tupling, H., *et al.* (1978). A controlled trial of cervical manipulation of migraine. *Australian and New Zealand Journal of Medicine,* **8**(6), 589–93.

Prior, J., Vigna, Y., *et al.* (1994). Cyclic medroxyprogesterone treatment increases bone density: a controlled trial in active women with menstrual cycle disturbances. *American Journal of Medicine,* **96,** 521–30.

Prior, J., Vigna, Y., *et al.* (1990). Spinal bone loss and ovulatory disturbances. *New England Journal of Medicine,* **323,** 1221–7.

Royal College of General Practitioners (1986). *Morbidity statistics from general practice – third national study.* HMSO, London.

Seelig, N. (ed). (1971). *Human requirements of magnesium: factors that increase needs.* Springer Verlag, Paris.

Simpson, R. and Bick, D. (1996). Alternative therapies. *Journal of the American Medical Association,* **275**(13), 1034–5.

Smith, I. (1996). More than pin money. *Health Service Journal*, **Jan,** 24–5.

Smithells, D. (1996). Vitamins in early pregnancy. *British Medical Journal*, **313**, 128–9.

Sobota, A. E. (1984). Inhibition of bacterial adherence by cranberry juice: potential use for the treatment of urinary tract infections. *Journal of Urology*, **131**(5), 1013–6.

Spiegel, D. and Bloom, J. (1983). Group therapy and self-hypnosis reduce metastatic breast carcinoma pain. *Psychosomatic Medicine*, **45**(4), 333–9.

Spiegel, D., Bloom, J. *et al.* (1989). Effect of psychosocial treatment on survival of patients with metastaic breast cancer. *Lancet*, **2**, 888–91.

Stampfer, M., Hennekens, C. *et al.* (1993). Vitamin E consumption and the risk of coronary disease in women. *New England Journal of Medicine*, **328**, 1444–9.

Stanton, C. and Gray, R. (1995). Effects of caffeine consumption on delayed conception. *American Journal of Epidemiology*, **142**(12), 1322–9.

Steegers, T.R., Boers, G.H., *et al.* (1994). Maternal hyperhomocysteinemia: a risk factor for neural-tube defects? *Metabolism*, **43**(12), 1475–80.

Stone, J. (1996a). Complements slip. *The Health Service Journal*, **106** (5487), 26–7.

Stone, J. (1996b). Regulating Complementary medicine. *British Medical Journal*, **312**, 1492–3.

Tang, M. *et al.* (1996). Effect of oestrogen during menopause use on risk and age at onset of Alzheimer's disease. *Lancet*, **348**, 429–32.

Thomas, K., Carr, J., *et al.* (1991). Use of non-orthodox and conventional health care in Great Britain. *British Medical Journal*, **26**, 207–10.

Thomas, K., Fall, M., *et al.* (1995). National survey of access to Complementary health care via general practitioners. Sheffield Centre for Health and Related Research, Sheffield University.

Thomason, P., Fisher B., *et al.* (1979). Effectiveness of spinal manipulative therapy in treatment of primary dysmenorrhoea: a pilot study. *Journal of Manipulative and Physiological Therapeutics*, **2**(3), 140–5.

Vincent, C. and Furnham A. (1996). Why do patients turn to Complementary medicine? An empirical study. *British Journal of Clinical Psychology*, **35**, 37–48.

Watson, C. and Evan, R. (1992). The post-mastectomy pain syndrome and topical capsaicin: a randomized trial. *Pain*, **51**, 372–9.

Welshons, W. V., Murphy, C. S. *et al.* (1987). Stimulation of breast cancer cells *in vitro* by the environmental estrogen enterolactone and the phytoestrogen equol. *Breast Cancer Res Treat*, **10**(2), 169–75.

West Yorkshire Health Authority (1995). *Guidelines for the employment of Complementary therapists in the NHS*.

Wilcox, A., Weinberg, C., *et al.* (1988). Caffeinated beverages and decreased fertility. *Lancet*, **ii**, 1453–6.

Wilcox, G., Wahlqvist, M., *et al.* (1990). Oestrogenic effects of plant foods in post-menopausal women. *British Medical Journal,* **301**, 905–6.

Wouters, M. G., Boers, G. H., *et al.* (1993). Hyperhomocysteinemia: a risk factor in women with unexplained recurrent early pregnancy loss. *Fertility and Sterility* **60**(5), 820–5.

Wynd, C. A. (1992). Relaxation imagery used for stress reduction in the prevention of smoking relapse. *Journal of Advanced Nursing,* **17**(3), 294–302.

Zafriri, D., Ofek, I., *et al.* (1989). Inhibitory activity of cranberry juice on adherence of type 1 and type P fimbriated *Escherichia coli* to eucaryotic cells. *Antimicrob Agents Chemother* **33**(1): 92–8.

Zanolla, R., Monzeglio, C. *et al.* (1984). Evaluation of the results of three different methods of postmastectomy lymphedema treatment. *Journal of Surgical Oncology,* **26**(3), 210–3.

Index